ADVANCES IN DIETARY LIPIDS
AND HUMAN HEALTH
———

ADVANCES IN DIETARY LIPIDS AND HUMAN HEALTH

Edited by

DUO LI

Institute of Nutrition and Health, Qingdao University, Qingdao, Shandong, China
Department of Food Science and Nutrition, Zhejiang University, Hangzhou, Zhejiang, China
Department of Nutrition, Dietetics and Food, Monash University, Melbourne, VIC, Australia

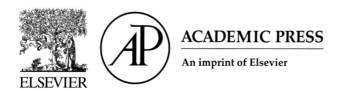

Academic Press is an imprint of Elsevier
125 London Wall, London EC2Y 5AS, United Kingdom
525 B Street, Suite 1650, San Diego, CA 92101, United States
50 Hampshire Street, 5th Floor, Cambridge, MA 02139, United States
The Boulevard, Langford Lane, Kidlington, Oxford OX5 1GB, United Kingdom

Copyright © 2022 Elsevier Inc. All rights reserved.

No part of this publication may be reproduced or transmitted in any form or by any means, electronic or mechanical, including photocopying, recording, or any information storage and retrieval system, without permission in writing from the publisher. Details on how to seek permission, further information about the Publisher's permissions policies and our arrangements with organizations such as the Copyright Clearance Center and the Copyright Licensing Agency, can be found at our website: www.elsevier.com/permissions.

This book and the individual contributions contained in it are protected under copyright by the Publisher (other than as may be noted herein).

Notices

Knowledge and best practice in this field are constantly changing. As new research and experience broaden our understanding, changes in research methods, professional practices, or medical treatment may become necessary.

Practitioners and researchers must always rely on their own experience and knowledge in evaluating and using any information, methods, compounds, or experiments described herein. In using such information or methods they should be mindful of their own safety and the safety of others, including parties for whom they have a professional responsibility.

To the fullest extent of the law, neither the Publisher nor the authors, contributors, or editors, assume any liability for any injury and/or damage to persons or property as a matter of products liability, negligence or otherwise, or from any use or operation of any methods, products, instructions, or ideas contained in the material herein.

ISBN 978-0-12-823914-8

For information on all Academic Press publications
visit our website at https://www.elsevier.com/books-and-journals

Publisher: Nikki Levy
Acquisitions Editor: Megan Ball
Editorial Project Manager: Kathrine Esten
Production Project Manager: Sruthi Satheesh
Cover Designer: Victoria Pearson

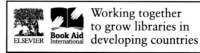

Typeset by STRAIVE, India

Contents

Contributors ix

1. Overview of dietary lipids and human health

DUO LI

1.1 Introduction 1
1.2 Dietary lipids 1
1.3 Dietary total fat intake and human health 3
1.4 Dietary saturated fat intake and human health 5
1.5 Dietary monounsaturated fat intake and human health 6
1.6 Dietary polyunsaturated fat intake and human health 6
1.7 Conclusion 10
References 11

2. Fatty acids and telomeres in humans

MICHAEL FENECH, PERMAL DEO, AND VARINDERPAL DHILLON

2.1 Introduction 13
2.2 Dietary fatty acids and telomeres 14
2.3 Cross-sectional and prospective studies 14
2.4 Randomized controlled trials 18
2.5 Discussion 19
2.6 Conclusion 22
References 22

3. The role of lipids in the brain

AMAL D. PREMARATHNA, ANURA P. JAYASOORIYA, AND ANDREW J. SINCLAIR

3.1 Introduction 27
3.2 Properties of brain fatty acids 32
3.3 Where are brain lipids synthesized? In the brain or imported from blood? 35
3.4 Effects of exogenous/dietary agents on brain lipids 36
3.5 Conclusions 40
References 40

4. Lipids and mental health

DANIEL TZU-LI CHEN, JOCELYN CHIA-YU CHEN, JANE PEI-CHEN CHANG, AND KUAN-PIN SU

4.1 Introduction 51
4.2 Metabolism of lipids in the brain 51
4.3 Lipids and inflammation and oxidative stress 53
4.4 Lipids, microbiota, and immune system 53
4.5 Lipids and nervous system 55
4.6 Can omega-3 fatty acids be used as treatment? How to use them? 56
4.7 Conclusion 65
References 66

5. Diet in different fat content and cardiometabolic health

YI WAN

5.1 Introduction 75
5.2 Diet with different fat-to-carbohydrate ratios and cardiometabolic health 76
5.3 What we previously conducted 78
5.4 Conclusions 80
References 80

6. Dietary lipids and malignant tumor of the digestive system

CANXIA HE AND XIAOHONG ZHANG

6.1 Dietary lipids and gastric cancer 83
6.2 Dietary lipids and liver carcinoma 87
6.3 N-3 PUFAs and colon cancer 91
6.4 Conclusion 101
References 101

7. Dietary lipids and breast cancer

JIAOMEI LI

7.1 Introduction 111
7.2 Epidemiological evidence regarding dietary lipids intake and breast cancer 112
7.3 Effects of n-3 PUFA on breast cancer development 114
7.4 Conclusions 121
References 121

8. Marine lipids and diabetes

YUNYI TIAN AND JU-SHENG ZHENG

8.1 Introduction 125
8.2 Marine n-3 PUFAs and T2D prevention 126
8.3 Marine n-3 PUFAs and T2D management 128
8.4 Marine n-3 PUFAs and gestational diabetes 131
8.5 Conclusion 131
References 131

9. Lipids and nonalcoholic fatty liver disease

XIAO-FEI GUO AND WEN-JUN MA

9.1 Introduction 135
9.2 Fatty acids and NAFLD 136
9.3 Factors affecting NAFLD on biomarkers of NAFLD 141
9.4 Dose–response relationship between n-3 PUFA intake and biomarkers 141
9.5 The underlying mechanisms why n-3 PUFAs protect against NAFLD 142
References 143

10. Dietary lipids and pulmonary diseases

ZUQUAN ZOU

10.1 Pulmonary diseases 147
10.2 Dietary lipids and clinically manifest asthma 148
10.3 Dietary lipids and pneumonia 149
10.4 Dietary lipids and chronic obstructive pulmonary disease 153
10.5 Dietary lipids and pulmonary fibrosis 154
10.6 Dietary lipids and lung cancer 155
10.7 How do dietary lipids influence pulmonary diseases? 156

10.8 Conclusion 160
References 160

11. Dietary lipids and hypertension

XIANG HU AND BO YANG

11.1 Introduction 165
11.2 General background on the relationship between lipids and hypertension 166
11.3 Meta-analytic evidence based on dietary intervention studies 169
11.4 Evidence based on the relevant epidemiological studies 175
11.5 Biological mechanisms for the antihypertensive effects of dietary n-3 lipids 181
11.6 Conclusion 185
References 185

12. Postprandial lipemia and the relationship to health

CATHERINE E. HUGGINS, ANTHONY P. JAMES, MAXINE P. BONHAM, KATYA M. CLARK, AND SARAH D. LEE

12.1 Introduction 193
12.2 Generation of an atherogenic postprandial phenotype 194
12.3 Mechanisms linking postprandial lipids to atherogenesis 196
12.4 Modulators of postprandial lipemia 198
12.5 Meal timing a novel mediator of postprandial triglycerides 203
12.6 Nonmodifiable factors: Evidence of ethnic/genetic influences on postprandial lipemia 204
12.7 Assessment of postprandial lipemia is important for CVD risk screening 204
12.8 Conclusion 205
References 205

13. The metabolites derived from lipids and their effects on human health

LI-LI XIU, LING-SHEN HUNG, LING WANG, JIAN-YING HUANG, AND XIANG-YANG WANG

13.1 Introduction 211
13.2 The gut microbiota and lipid metabolism 214

13.3 Effects of lipid metabolites on CVDs 216
13.4 Metabolites derived from lipids that correlate with cancer incidence 217
13.5 Metabolites derived from lipids that correlated with neurodegenerative disease 219
13.6 Conclusions 220
References 220

14. Marine n-3 polyunsaturated fatty acids and inflammatory diseases

YUANQING FU

14.1 Marine n-3 polyunsaturated fatty acids and inflammatory processes 225
14.2 Marine n-3 polyunsaturated fatty acids and inflammatory diseases 228
14.3 What are the gaps in evidence that need attention? 237
References 237

15. Lipids and birth defects

KELEI LI AND YAN SHI

15.1 Introduction 243
15.2 Evidence relating lipids to birth defects risk in human studies 244
15.3 Evidence relating lipids to birth defects in animal studies 245
15.4 The possible mechanism for the relationship between lipids and birth defects 245
15.5 Conclusion 247
References 247

16. Conjugated linolenic acids and their bioactivities

GAOFENG YUAN

16.1 Introduction 251
16.2 Natural sources and utilization of CLNA 251
16.3 The metabolism of CLNA 252
16.4 CLNA and carcinogenesis 253
16.5 CLNA and lipid metabolism 255
16.6 Effect of conjugated linolenic acid on obesity 258
16.7 Effect of conjugated linolenic acid on type 2 diabetes mellitus 260

16.8 Effect of conjugated linolenic acid on inflammatory bowel diseases 261
16.9 Antioxidant activity of CLNA 264
16.10 Conclusion 265
References 265

17. N-3 polyunsaturated fatty acid and homocysteine metabolism

TAO HUANG AND ZHENHUANG ZHUANG

17.1 Introduction 273
17.2 Epidemiological evidence regarding n-3 PUFAs, genetics, and homocysteine levels 274
17.3 Effects of n-3 PUFAs on homocysteine: Evidence from animal studies and cell culture 277
17.4 Experimental epidemiological evidence regarding the effects of n-3 PUFAs on homocysteine metabolism 279
17.5 Mechanisms by which n-3 PUFAs reduce homocysteine levels and future research 280
17.6 Conclusion 281
References 282

18. Effect of 1,3-diacylglycerol on cardiometabolic risk

TONGCHENG XU AND MIN JIA

18.1 Introduction 285
18.2 The 1,3-diacylglycerol 285
18.3 Effects of 1,3-diacylglycerol on cardiometabolic risk 287
18.4 Metabolism of 1,3-diacylglycerol 289
18.5 Supplementation of 1,3-diacylglycerol 290
18.6 Conclusion 291
References 291

19. Palmitoleic acid in health and disease

JUN TANG

19.1 Introduction 293
19.2 Is palmitoleic acid a novel lipid hormone? 294
19.3 Effects of palmitoleic acid on metabolic diseases 295
19.4 What are the gaps in evidence that need attention? 297
References 301

20. Ximenynic acid and its bioactivities

FANG CAI, DHANUSHKA HETTIARACHCHI, XIAOJIE HU, ANISH SINGH, YANDI LIU, AND BRUCE SUNDERLAND

20.1 Introduction 303
20.2 Bioactivities, functions, and applications of ximenynic acid 304
20.3 Safety of ximenynic acid 311
20.4 Physical characteristics and natural distribution 312
20.5 Preparation methods of natural ximenynic acid 314
20.6 Synthesis of ximenynic acid 319
20.7 Conclusion and future studies of ximenynic acid 321
References 323

21. Application of phytosterols in management of plasma cholesterol

WEN-SEN HE AND ZHEN-YU CHEN

21.1 Introduction 329
21.2 Structure diversity and sources of dietary phytosterols 329
21.3 Cholesterol-lowering effects 333
21.4 Cholesterol-lowering mechanisms 341
21.5 Commercial applications and regulated policy 345
21.6 Conclusive remarks and future perspectives 346
References 347

22. Lipids in breast milk and formulas

JIN SUN, CE QI, AND RENQIANG YU

22.1 Introduction 353
22.2 Composition of breast milk lipids 354
22.3 Composition of formulas in lipids 359
22.4 Breast milk and formula lipid nutrition 363
22.5 Conclusion 365
References 366

Index 369

Contributors

Maxine P. Bonham Department of Nutrition, Dietetics and Food, School of Clinical Sciences at Monash Health, Faculty of Medicine Nursing and Health Sciences, Monash University, Clayton, VIC, Australia

Fang Cai School of Life Sciences, Guizhou Normal University, Guiyang, China

Jane Pei-Chen Chang Department of Psychiatry and Mind-Body Interface Laboratory (MBI-Lab), China Medical University Hospital, Taichung, Taiwan; Department of Psychological Medicine, Institute of Psychiatry, Psychology and Neuroscience, King's College London, London, United Kingdom; School of Medicine, College of Medicine, China Medical University, Taichung, Taiwan

Daniel Tzu-Li Chen Division of Neuroscience, Graduate Institute of Biomedical Sciences, China Medical University; Department of Psychiatry and Mind-Body Interface Laboratory (MBI-Lab), China Medical University Hospital; School of Chinese Medicine, College of Chinese Medicine, China Medical University, Taichung, Taiwan

Jocelyn Chia-Yu Chen Department of Psychiatry and Mind-Body Interface Laboratory (MBI-Lab), China Medical University Hospital; School of Chinese Medicine, College of Chinese Medicine, China Medical University, Taichung, Taiwan

Zhen-Yu Chen School of Life Sciences, The Chinese University of Hong Kong, Shatin, New Territories, China

Katya M. Clark Nutrition & Dietetics, Curtin School of Population Health, Curtin University, Bentley, WA, Australia

Permal Deo Clinical and Health Sciences, University of South Australia, Adelaide, SA, Australia

Varinderpal Dhillon Clinical and Health Sciences, University of South Australia, Adelaide, SA, Australia

Michael Fenech Clinical and Health Sciences, University of South Australia, Adelaide, SA, Australia

Yuanqing Fu Laboratory of Precision Nutrition and Computational Medicine, School of Life Sciences, Westlake University, Hangzhou, China

Xiao-fei Guo Institute of Nutrition & Health; School of Public Health, Qingdao University, Qingdao, China

Canxia He School of Medicine, Ningbo University, Ningbo, China

Wen-Sen He School of Food and Biological Engineering, Jiangsu University, Zhenjiang, Jiangsu, China

Dhanushka Hettiarachchi School of Pharmacy, Curtin Health Innovation Research Institute, Curtin University, Perth, WA, Australia

Xiang Hu Department of Endocrine and Metabolic Diseases, The First Affiliated Hospital of Wenzhou Medical University; Institute of Lipids Medicine & School of Public Health and Management, Wenzhou Medical University, Wenzhou, China

Xiaojie Hu College of Life Science, Linyi University, Linyi, China

Jian-Ying Huang Department of Food Science and Technology, School of Food Science and Biotechnology, Zhejiang Gongshang University, Hangzhou, China

Tao Huang Department of Epidemiology and Biostatistics, School of Public Health, Peking University; Key Laboratory of Molecular Cardiovascular Sciences, Peking University, Ministry of Education; Center for Intelligent Public Health, Institute for Artificial Intelligence, Peking University, Beijing, China

Catherine E. Huggins Department of Nutrition, Dietetics and Food, School of Clinical Sciences at Monash Health, Faculty of Medicine Nursing and Health Sciences, Monash University, Clayton, VIC, Australia

Ling-Shen Hung Department of Food Science, College of Chemistry and Food Science, Yulin Normal University, Yulin, Guangxi, China

Anthony P. James Nutrition & Dietetics, Curtin School of Population Health, Curtin University, Bentley, WA, Australia

Anura P. Jayasooriya Department of Basic Veterinary Sciences, Faculty of Veterinary Medicine and Animal Science, University of Peradeniya, Peradeniya, Sri Lanka

Min Jia Grain & Oil Engineering Lab, Institute of Agro-food Science and Technology, Shangdong Academy of Agricultural Sciences, Jinan, China

Sarah D. Lee Department of Nutrition, Dietetics and Food, School of Clinical Sciences at Monash Health, Faculty of Medicine Nursing and Health Sciences, Monash University, Clayton, VIC, Australia

Duo Li Institute of Nutrition and Health, Qingdao University, Qingdao, Shandong; Department of Food Science and Nutrition, Zhejiang University, Hangzhou, Zhejiang, China; Department of Nutrition, Dietetics and Food, Monash University, Melbourne, VIC, Australia

Jiaomei Li Department of Nutrition and Food Hygiene, Zhejiang Chinese Medical University, Hangzhou, China

Kelei Li Institute of Nutrition and Health; Department of Nutrition and Food Hygiene, School of Public Health, Qingdao University, Qingdao, China

Yandi Liu School of Pharmacy, Curtin Health Innovation Research Institute, Curtin University, Perth, WA, Australia

Wen-Jun Ma Institute of Nutrition & Health; School of Public Health, Qingdao University, Qingdao, China

Amal D. Premarathna School of Natural Sciences and Health, Tallinn University, Tallinn, Estonia

Ce Qi Institute of Nutrition and Health, Qingdao University, Qingdao, China

Yan Shi Institute of Nutrition and Health; Department of Nutrition and Food Hygiene, School of Public Health, Qingdao University, Qingdao, China

Andrew J. Sinclair Department of Nutrition, Dietetics and Food, Monash University, Melbourne; Faculty of Health, Deakin University, Geelong, Australia

Anish Singh Institute of Nutrition & Health, Qingdao University, Qingdao, China

Kuan-Pin Su Division of Neuroscience, Graduate Institute of Biomedical Sciences, China Medical University; Department of Psychiatry and Mind-Body Interface Laboratory (MBI-Lab), China Medical University Hospital, Taichung, Taiwan; Department of Psychological Medicine, Institute of Psychiatry, Psychology and Neuroscience, King's College London, London, United Kingdom; School of Medicine, College of Medicine, China Medical University, Taichung; Depression Center, An-Nan Hospital, China Medical University, Tainan, Taiwan

Jin Sun Institute of Nutrition and Health, Qingdao University, Qingdao, China

Bruce Sunderland School of Pharmacy, Curtin Health Innovation Research Institute, Curtin University, Perth, WA, Australia

Jun Tang Laboratory of Precision Nutrition and Computational Medicine, School of Life Sciences, Westlake University, Hangzhou, China

Yunyi Tian School of Life Sciences, Westlake University, Hangzhou, China

Yi Wan Department of Food Science and Nutrition, Zhejiang University, Hangzhou, China

Ling Wang Department of Food Micrology, College of Food Science and Technology, Huazhong Agricultural University, Wuhan, Hubei, China

Xiang-Yang Wang Department of Food Science and Technology, School of Food Science and Biotechnology, Zhejiang Gongshang University, Hangzhou, China

Li-Li Xiu Department of Food Science and Technology, School of Food Science and Biotechnology, Zhejiang Gongshang University, Hangzhou, China

Tongcheng Xu Grain & Oil Engineering Lab, Institute of Agro-food Science and Technology, Shandong Academy of Agricultural Sciences, Jinan, China

Bo Yang Institute of Lipids Medicine & School of Public Health and Management, Wenzhou Medical University, Wenzhou, China

Renqiang Yu Department of Neonatology, The Affiliated Wuxi Maternity and Child Health Care Hospital of Nanjing Medical University, Wuxi, China

Gaofeng Yuan Department of Food Science, College of Food and Medicine, Zhejiang Ocean University, Zhoushan, China

Xiaohong Zhang School of Medicine, Ningbo University, Ningbo, China

Ju-Sheng Zheng School of Life Sciences, Westlake University, Hangzhou, China

Zhenhuang Zhuang Department of Epidemiology and Biostatistics, School of Public Health, Peking University, Beijing, China

Zuquan Zou Beilun District Center for Disease Control and Prevention, Ningbo, Zhejiang, China

CHAPTER 1

Overview of dietary lipids and human health

Duo Li

Institute of Nutrition and Health, Qingdao University, Qingdao, Shandong, China
Department of Food Science and Nutrition, Zhejiang University, Hangzhou, Zhejiang, China
Department of Nutrition, Dietetics and Food, Monash University, Melbourne, VIC, Australia

1.1 Introduction

In the past four decades, there has been extensive research on dietary lipids and non-communicable diseases and their risk factors. This chapter systematically reviewed the effects of dietary fat intake on human health based on the results of meta-analysis of recent randomized controlled trials or cohort studies. Meta-analysis combines the similar results of individual studies, enabling us to make full use of all information, and improves the accuracy and power of intervention/treatment effect evaluation (Moher, Liberati, Tetzlaff, & Altman, 2009). Uncommon dietary lipids, lipids in food with a very low content, such as trans-fatty acids, conjugated linoleic acids, furan fatty acids, and monoacylglycerols, and manufactory-produced structured lipids are not included in the chapter and the book.

1.2 Dietary lipids

Dietary lipids are important substances found in food. They play a major role in taste, texture, color, and flavor. In the human body, they maintain the integrity and function of cells and serve as energy storage. Dietary lipids are insoluble in water and soluble in many organic solvents. This property of nonpolarity and hydrophobicity is largely controlled by fatty acids. Most dietary lipids are molecules that contain or are derived from fatty acids. The lipid information required by the food database for calculating energy content and comparison between foods includes content and composition of total fat, fatty acids (including saturates, cis- and trans-monounsaturates, n-6 and n-3 polyunsaturates), and sterols. Fat-soluble vitamins will not be discussed in this book, even though these vitamins can be classified as lipids.

Dietary lipids can be divided into two categories: the nonpolar lipids (such as triacylglycerol and cholesteryl esters) and the polar lipids (amphiphilic, because they contain both hydrophobic and hydrophilic domains in the same molecule, such as phospholipids). More than 95% of dietary lipids are acylglycerols, and triacylglycerol (TG) is most predominant one, in which the three hydroxyl groups of glycerol are esterified with one fatty acid. They contain fatty acids with different chain lengths and saturation levels. Vegetable oils, such as soybean and sunflower oil, are mainly composed of TG with unsaturated fatty acids, so they are liquid at room temperature. TG contains only saturated fatty acids, such as tristearin, the main component of beef fat, which is a white greasy solid at room temperature. Monoacylglycerols, diacyglycerols, and free fatty acids are present only in relatively minor amounts and occur largely as metabolic intermediates in the biosynthesis and degradation of glycerol-containing lipids.

All animal foods, including seafood, contain different amounts of cholesterol, because all animal cells make cholesterol. The main dietary sources of cholesterol include yolk and whole egg, red meat, offal, seafood, and dairy products. Human breast milk also contains generous cholesterol. Cholesterol is synthesized by plant cells only as an intermediate (precursor) of other compounds, such as phytosterols. Therefore, there is little or no cholesterol in plant food. Vegetable oil is a main source of dietary phytosterols. The most common dietary phytosterols are β-sitosterol, campesterol, stigmasterol, and stigmastanol. Phospholipids are divided into two main classes: glycerophospholipids and phosphosphingolipids, depending on whether they contain a glycerol or a sphingosine backbone. The main dietary glycerophospholipids are phosphatidylethanolamine (cephalin, PE), phosphatidylcholine (lecithin, PC), phosphatidylserine (PS), and phosphatidylinositol (PI). The main phosphosphingolipids are ceramides and sphingomyelins. Major sources of dietary phospholipids are soya, rapeseed, sunflower, eggs, milk, seafood, eggs, etc. (Fig. 1.1).

Plant/vegetable seed oil and animal fat are the most predominant dietary fat for human beings. Fatty acids are the functional group of most dietary lipids. Natural dietary fatty acids can be classified as saturated, monounsaturated fatty acids (MUFA), and polyunsaturated fatty acids (PUFA). Animal fats are a major source of saturated fatty acids, as well as coconut oil and certain tropical plant oil such as palm oil. Oleic acid (C18:1) is the most abundant monounsaturated fatty acid in the diet, and olive oil is probably the most well-known source of C18:1.

PUFA has four families, that is, n-7, n-9, n-6, and n-3, derived from the four parent fatty acids, palmitoleic acid (C16:1n-7), oleic acid (C18:1n-9), linoleic acid (C18:2n-6, LA), and a-linolenic acid (C18:3n-3, ALA). C18:2n-6 and C18:3n-3 are essential fatty acids for humans. C18:2n-6 is the predominant PUFA in the global food chain, which is commonly found in plant/vegetable seed oils. C18:3n-3 is less abundant than C18:2n-6, and is the predominant n-3 PUFA found in plant food and commonly found in some plant/vegetable oils such as flaxseed, perilla, chia seed, canola, soybean, and walnut oils. C18:3n-3 and C18:2n-6 can be converted in vivo to C20 and C22 long chain (LC) PUFA in humans (Li, 2015). Eicosapentaenoic acid (C20:5n-3, EPA) is a predominant LC n-3 PUFA in most fish and fish/marine oils, docosahexaenoic acid (C22:6n-3, DHA) is most abundant LC n-3 PUFA in tuna and tuna oil (Sinclair, Oon, Lim, Li, & Mann, 1998), while docosapentaenoic acid (C22:5n-3, DPA) is a major LC n-3 PUFA in certain seafood such as abalone (Su, Antonas, & Li, 2004), lean meat, and meat products (Li, Ng, Mann, & Sinclair, 1998). Stearidonic acid (18:4n-3, SDA) is found in Ribes berries and Boraginaceae families (Li & Hu, 2011) (Fig. 1.2).

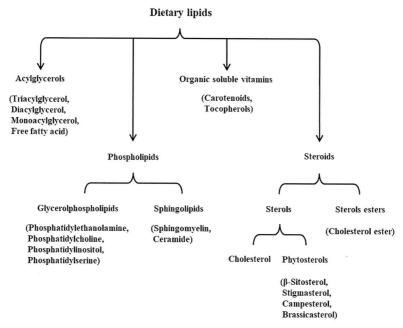

FIG. 1.1 Classification of main dietary lipid. *No permission required.*

1.3 Dietary total fat intake and human health

FAO/WHO recommended that the dietary intake of total fat should not exceed 30% of total energy for the general population, and 35% for heavy physical personnel (FAO, 2010). Compared with conventional or guideline-recommended dietary fat intake, increasing total fat intake can significantly increase body weight, body mass index (BMI), waist circumference, serum total cholesterol (TC), and low density lipoprotein cholesterol (LDL-C) under the condition of equal calories.

In a systematic review and meta-analysis, which included 32 RCTs, 31 studies in healthy adults, and 1 in children, involving approximately 54,000 participants with an intervention period of 6 months to >8 years, excluding the studies with only subject BMI >25 kg/m², all included studies were from developed countries (21 from North America, 9 from Europe, and 1 from New Zealand), and there is no study from developing or transitional countries. With the isocaloric diets, the study found that reducing the dietary proportion of fat (30% energy) resulted in a slight but significant decrease in body weight, body mass index, and waist circumference compared with habitual dietary fat intake. This effect has been found in both adults and children. The effect did not change over time. Compared with habitual or modified fat diets, the low-fat diet could reduce serum concentrations of total cholesterol (TC) and low-density lipoprotein cholesterol (LDL-C), but had no significant effect on high-density lipoprotein cholesterol (HDL-C) and TG. There is no evidence that a low-fat diet is harmful to human health (Hooper et al., 2015).

A six-month randomized controlled feeding trial in two centers, three arms, from China, found consistent results with the above meta-analysis,

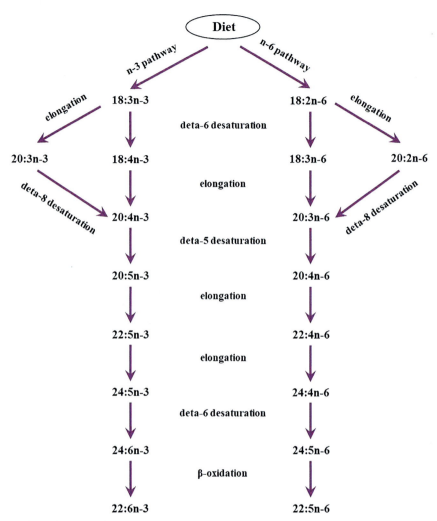

FIG. 1.2 Metabolism of essential fatty acids in vivo. *No permission required.*

in which, 307 healthy young adults, aged 18–35 years and with body mass index less than 28, were randomly assigned to the three isocaloric diets: the lower fat diet (carbohydrate 66%, fat 20% energy), the moderate fat diet (carbohydrate 56%, fat 30% energy), and the higher fat diet (carbohydrate 46%, fat 40% energy) with same protein (14% energy). The body weight, BMI, and waist circumference of the subjects in the low-fat and high-carbohydrate diet intervention group were significantly lower than those in the other two groups. Serum concentrations of TC, LDL-C, non-HDL-C, HDL-C, and plasma pro-inflammatory factors such as leukotriene B_4, thromboxane B_2, prostaglandin E_2, and high-sensitivity C-reactive protein were significantly lower in the low-fat and high-carbohydrate diet intervention group than those in the other two groups (Wan et al., 2019; Wan et al., 2017). Based on the results, the authors interpreted that the possible benefits of a high-fat diet in European and North American populations are not applicable to other ethnic groups, at least not to Chinese people.

There are several randomized controlled trials (RCTs) conducted by European and American researchers on patients with obesity or metabolic diseases using ketogenic and Atkins diets compared with traditional diets or diets recommended by dietary guidelines. They found that short-term, high-fat, and low-carbohydrate diets caused weight loss and serum TG reduction in obese or metabolic disease subjects (Gardner et al., 2007; Moreno, Crujeiras, Bellido, Sajoux, & Casanueva, 2016). Based on these findings, some people suggest that the restriction of carbohydrates, rather than the reduction of fat, should be recommended as the most appropriate nutritional method to control obesity and reduce the risk of cardiovascular and metabolic diseases. However, the genes encoding fat, carbohydrate, and metabolism-related enzymes in patients with obesity or metabolic diseases are different from those in healthy people, and the response of these volunteers to fat and carbohydrate is also different from that in healthy people, which may be ignored.

1.4 Dietary saturated fat intake and human health

Animal fat, butter, palm oil, and coconut oil have been considered as saturated fat. FAO/WHO recommends that the dietary intake of saturated fat should not exceed 10% of total energy. Replacement of MUFA and PUFA with isocaloric SFA significantly increased serum TC and LDL-C, resulting in a significantly increased risk of CVD events.

In a systematic review and meta-analysis of dietary saturated fat intake and cardiovascular disease included 15 RCTs with approximately 59,000 participants. Results from 11 long-term trials ($\geq$2 years) with 53,3000 subjects showed that reducing dietary intake of saturated fat acid (SFA) significantly reduced the risk of combined cardiovascular events by 21%. The meta-regression showed that a greater reduction in dietary intake of SFA led to a tremendous reduction in serum TC, resulting in a greater reduction in the risk of cardiovascular disease (CVD) events. Substituting the dietary energy in SFA with PUFA or carbohydrate seems to be a useful strategy, while the effect of replacing SFA with MUFA is unclear. The reduction in cardiovascular events due to reduced dietary intake of saturated fat was not affected by study duration, gender, or baseline level of cardiovascular risk. Reducing dietary intake of SFA can benefit people who are currently healthy, who have an increased risk of heart disease or stroke (e.g., people with high blood pressure, high serum TC, and LDL-C or diabetes), and who already have heart disease or stroke (Hooper et al., 2020). Another systematic review and meta-analysis of RCTs found when the dietary intake of SFA was reduced and replaced with PUFA, serum glucose, glycosylated hemoglobin A1c (HbA1c), C-peptide and homeostasis model assessment for insulin resistance (HOMA-IR) were significantly decreased (Imamura et al., 2016).

Palm oil is one of the most used saturated fats globally. It is composed of approximately 50% palmitic acid, 40% oleic acid, and 10% linoleic acid. A meta-analysis of RCTs found that palm oil significantly increased serum TC, LDL-C, and HDL-C, but not TG compared with MUFA and PUFA such as olive oil and safflower/sunflower oil (Hisham, Aziz, Huin, Haur, & Jamil, 2020).

Compared with C18:0, MUFAs and PUFAs enrich diets, apart from TC, LDL-C, and HDL-C, palm oil also significantly increased apolipoprotein B and apolipoprotein A-I. However, when compared with myristic/lauric acid-enriched diet, palm oil showed a significantly lower serum concentrations of TC, HDL-C, and apolipoprotein A-I (Fattore, Bosetti, Brighenti, Agostoni, & Fattore, 2014).

A WHO publication entitled "Effects of saturated fatty acids on serum lipids and lipoproteins: a systematic review and regression analysis" summarized that the mixture of SFA was replaced by cis-PUFA (mainly linoleic acid and α-linolenic acid) or cis-MUFA (mainly oleic acid), which was more beneficial on serum lipids and lipoproteins profile than replacing SFA with a mixture of carbohydrates. Especially for TC, LDL-C, and TG, PUFAs have the best effect. Compared with the mixture of carbohydrates, increasing dietary intake of individual C12:0, C14:0, or C16:0 increased serum concentrations of TC, LDL-C, and HDL-C, and decreased TG, while increasing C18:0 intake did not seem to have a significant effect on these serum concentrations of lipids and lipoproteins as compared with carbohydrate. Compared with carbohydrate, C12:0 decreased the ratios of TC:HDL-C and LDL-C:HDL-C (Mensink, 2016).

1.5 Dietary monounsaturated fat intake and human health

There is no recommended acceptable macronutrient distribution range for MUFA. On the premise that the total fat does not exceed 30% of the total energy, subtracting SFA and PUFA is the intake of MUFA for the general population. Isocalorically substituting SFA and carbohydrate with MUFA has a beneficial effect on metabolic risk factors in healthy adult subjects and type 2 diabetic patients.

In a systematic review and meta-analysis of RCTs, the metabolic effects of high-MUFA and high-carbohydrate diets were compared in 24 studies with 1460 participants, and high-MUFA and high-PUFA diets in 4 studies with 44 participants. Comparing a high-MUFA diet with a high-carbohydrate diet, there was significant reduction in fasting plasma glucose, TAG, body weight, and systolic blood pressure, and significant increases in HDL-C. Comparison of high-MUFA diet with high-PUFA diets showed significantly lower fasting plasma glucose (Qian, Korat, Malik, & Hu, 2016).

In another systematic review and meta-analysis of randomized controlled feeding trials, it included 102 trials, 239 diet arms, and 4220 adults. The dose-response effect of isocaloric substitution, adjusted dietary intakes of protein, trans-fat, and dietary fiber showed that HbA1c, 2-h postchallenge insulin, and HOMA-IR were significantly lowered when dietary carbohydrate was replaced by MUFA (Imamura et al., 2016).

1.6 Dietary polyunsaturated fat intake and human health

The recommended acceptable macronutrient distribution range for PUFA is 6%–11% of total energy. Isocaloric replacement of SFA with PUFA has a beneficial effect on reduction of the risk of cardiovascular and metabolic diseases. The effect of n-3 PUFA on NCDs has been extensively studied during the past three decades. Increasing dietary intake of n-3 PUFA can reduce the risk of cardiovascular disease, type 2 diabetes, breast cancer, acute respiratory distress syndrome, nonalcoholic fatty liver disease (NAFLD), and chronic kidney disease, reduce serum concentration of triacylglycerol and blood pressure, and improve cognitive and depression symptoms.

1.6.1 Dietary polyunsaturated fat intake and cardiovascular diseases and risk factors

N-3 PUFAs have beneficial effects on cardioprotection, and reducing cardiovascular mortality, CHD mortality, and events. In the most extensive systematic review and meta-analysis of n-3 PUFA for the primary and secondar prevention of cardiovascular disease, which included 86 RCTs and 162,796 participants, study length was between 12 and 88 months. Most trials used LC n-3 PUFA capsules, some adapted LC n-3 PUFA or C18:3n-3-rich or enriched foods or dietary advice compared with placebo control or habitual diet. Dosage ranged from 0.5 g to >5 g daily (19 RCTs gave at least 3 g LC n-3 PUFA a day). Results indicated that increased LC n-3 PUFA reduced cardiovascular mortality (RR = 0.92, 95% CI: 0.86–0.99), coronary heart disease mortality (RR = 0.90, 95% CI: 0.81–1.00), coronary heart disease events (RR = 0.91, 95% CI: 0.85–0.97), and serum triacylglycerol by ~15% in a dose-dependent manner. Increased dietary intake of ALA reduced risk of arrhythmia (RR = 0.73, 95% CI: 0.55–0.97) and lightly reduced risk of CVD events (RR = 0.91, 95% CI: 0.79–1.04) (Abdelhamid et al., 2020).

In a systematic review without a meta-analysis, the authors concluded that EPA and DHA significantly reduced serum triglycerides in five of the six randomized controlled trials compared with placebo. The reduction ranged from 12% to 26% compared with baseline. There is evidence that DHA may be more effective in reducing serum triglycerides than EPA (Innes & Calder, 2018).

The existing evidence provided by RCT shows that supplementation of LC n-3 PUFA can reduce systolic blood pressure, and diastolic blood pressure can be reduced when the supplement dose is greater than 2 g. In a meta-analysis of 70 RCTs, supplementation of EPA + DHA reduced both systolic (−1.52 mmHg; 95% CI = −2.25 to −0.79) and diastolic blood pressure (−0.99 mmHg; 95% CI = −1.54 to −0.44) compared with placebo. The strongest effect of EPA + DHA supplementation was observed in untreated hypertensive subjects with reduction of systolic blood pressure 4.51 mmHg (95% CI = −6.12 to −2.8) and diastolic blood pressure 3.05 mmHg (95% CI = −4.35 to −1.74), although both systolic blood pressure (−1.25 mmHg, 95% CI = −2.05 to −0.46) and diastolic blood pressure (−0.62 mmHg, 95% CI = −1.22 to −0.02) also decreased in normotensive subjects (Miller, Van Elswyk, & Alexander, 2014).

1.6.2 Dietary polyunsaturated fat intake and diabetes mellitus

Increased dietary intake of total PUFA and decreased ratio of n-6/n-3 PUFA have beneficial effects on reducing risk of diabetes. Replacing carbohydrate with PUFA significantly lowered HbA1c (−0.11%; −0.17, −0.05) and fasting insulin (−1.6 pmol/L; −2.8, −0.4). Replacing SFA with PUFA significantly lowered glucose, HbA1c, C-peptide, and HOMA. Based on gold-standard acute insulin response in 10 trials, PUFA significantly improved insulin secretion capacity (+0.5 pmol/L/min; 0.2, 0.8) whether replacing SFA, carbohydrate, or even MUFA (Imamura et al., 2016).

A meta-analysis of dietary PUFA intake and type 2 diabetes included 11 RCTs and a total of 458 participants (229 in each treatment and control group, respectively). Low-ratio n-6/n-3 PUFA supplementation can decrease the plasma insulin level (WMD: −3.010 mIU L^{-1}; 95% CI: −5.371 to −0.648 mIU L^{-1}) and insulin resistance index (WMD: −0.460; 95% CI: −0.908 to −0.012) (Li et al., 2019).

1.6.3 Dietary polyunsaturated fat intake and cancers

Dietary intake of total PUFA and individual PUFA may have different effects on different types of cancer. Pooled RCTs showed that neither dietary intake of total PUFA, n-3, nor n-6 PUFA was associated with cancer incidence. However, pooled prospective cohort studies suggested that increased dietary intake of LC n-3 PUFA is significantly associated with decreased risk of breast cancer.

In a systematic review, it included 47 RCTs with 108,194 participants. Increasing dietary intake of total PUFA may slightly increase, or no effect on the risk of cancer diagnosis (RR = 1.19, 95% CI 0.99–1.42) and cancer death (RR = 1.10, 95% CI: 0.48–2.49). LC n-3 PUFA has little or no effect on cancer diagnosis (RR = 1.02, 95% CI: 0.98–1.07), cancer death (RR = 0.97, 95% CI: 0.90–1.06), or breast cancer diagnosis (RR = 1.03, 95% CI: 0.89–1.20). Increasing ALA has little or no effect on cancer death (RR = 1.05, 95% CI: 0.74–1.49). Increasing dietary intake of LC n-3 PUFA (RR = 1.10, 95% CI: 0.97–1.24) and ALA (RR = 1.30, 95% CI: 0.72–2.32) may slightly increase risk of prostate cancer, or no significant effect (Hanson et al., 2020).

In another meta-analysis of n-3 PUFA and breast cancer, it included 26 publications with 883,585 participants and 20,905 cases of breast cancer from 21 independent prospective cohort studies. LC n-3 PUFA was significantly negatively associated with breast cancer risk (RR = 0.86, 95% CI: 0.78–0.94) in 17 publications from 16 independent cohort studies involving 527,392 participants and 16,178 breast cancer cases. Dose-response analysis showed a 5% reduction of breast cancer risk with 0.1 g/day (RR = 0.95, 95% CI: 0.90–1.00) or 0.1% energy/day (RR = 0.95, 0.90–1.00) increment of dietary intake of LC n-3 PUFA. Total n-3 PUFA intake was significantly negatively associated with risk of breast cancer (RR = 0.77, 95% CI: 0.60–0.99) only in studies without adjustment for BMI. For individual LC n-3 PUFA, the significant inverse association with risk of breast cancer was observed only in studies with shorter follow-up, RR = 0.82 (95% CI: 0.70–0.96) for C20:5n-3, and 0.74 (0.62–0.89) for C22:6n-3 (Zheng, Hu, Zhao, Yang, & Li, 2013).

1.6.4 Dietary polyunsaturated fat intake and respiratory diseases

The n-3 PUFAs have beneficial effects on respiratory diseases. Early use of n-3 PUFA in patients with acute respiratory disease can significantly reduce mortality.

In a systematic review, a meta-analysis evaluated the impact of n-3 PUFA on severe acute respiratory distress syndrome in 12 RCTs including 1280 patients. Results showed that *Horowitz index* was significantly increased with administration of n-3 PUFAs in early stage (WMD = 49.33, 95% CI: 20.88–77.78, $P = 0.0007$, $I^2 = 69\%$), measured by PaO_2-to-FiO_2 ratio (ratio of partial pressure of oxygen in blood (mmHg) and the fraction of oxygen in the inhaled air), lasts until the 7th to 8th day (WMD = 27.87; 95% CI: 0.75–54.99; $P = .04$; $I^2 = 57\%$). Continuous enteral infusion of n-3 PUFA significantly reduced mortality ($P = .02$). However, the analysis limited to enteral administration with or without bolus injection all improved early ratio of PaO_2 to FiO_2 ($P = .001$), and mechanical ventilation duration ($P = .03$) (Langlois, D'Aragon, Hardy, & Manzanares, 2019).

1.6.5 Dietary polyunsaturated fat intake and cognition

Higher intake of LC n-3 PUFA will increase cognitive function and improve symptoms of children and adolescents with Attention Deficit Hyperactivity Disorder (ADHD). The effect of n-3 PUFA on cognitive function depends on the specific study subjects and dosage. Increased tissue levels of LC n-3 PUFA are positively correlated with cognitive function.

The meta-analysis included 38 RCTs and 41 comparisons involving 49,757 participants. The results showed that LC n-3 PUFA had no or little effect on new neurocognitive impairment (RR = 0.98, 95% CI: 0.87–1.10), new cognitive impairment (RR = 0.99, 95% CI: 0.92–1.06), or overall cognition, which was assessed by mini mental state examination (MD 0.10, 95% CI: 0.03–0.16) (Brainard et al., 2020).

However, in a meta-analysis of the effects of LC n-3 PUFA on cognition in subjects aged 4–25 years, 33 studies were included, of which

21 were for developing subjects and 12 were for dysfunctional subjects. The results showed that in the study of children in typical developmental stages, daily supplementation of DHA+EPA ≥450 mg can significantly improve cognitive function. When the n-3 index (DHA+EPA red blood cell fatty acid composition) is greater than 6%, it has a positive impact on cognitive indicators (van der Wurff, Meyer, & de Groot, 2020).

N-3 PUFA improves symptoms of children and adolescents with Attention Deficit Hyperactivity Disorder (ADHD). In meta-analysis of 7 RCTs involving 534 young people with ADHD, the supplementation of n-3 PUFAs improved the clinical symptom score of ADHD ($g = 0.38$, $P < .0001$); in three RCTs involving 214 young people with ADHD, n-3 PUFA supplementation improved the cognitive indicators related to attention ($g = 1.09$, $P < .0001$). In addition, children and adolescents with ADHD had lower tissue levels of DHA (7 studies, $n = 412$, $g = -0.76$, $P = .0002$), EPA (7 studies, $n = 468$, $g = -0.38$, $P = .0008$), and a total of n-3 PUFAs (6 studies, $n = 396$, $g = -0.58$, $P = .0001$) (Chang, Su, Mondelli, & Pariante, 2018).

1.6.6 Dietary polyunsaturated fat intake and depression

LC n-3 PUFA has some beneficial effects on the risk of depressive or anxiety symptoms. The systematic review and meta-analysis of RCTs evaluated the effect of PUFA on prevention of depression and anxiety symptoms, which included 31 studies of LC n-3 PUFA ($n = 41,470$), one study of a-linolenic acid ($n = 4837$), and one of total PUFA ($n = 4997$). The results showed that LC n-3 PUFA may have little or no effect on the risk of depressive symptoms (HR = 1.01, 95% CI: 0.92–1.10, median dose 0.95 g/d, duration 12 months) or anxiety symptoms (SMD = 0.15, 95% CI: 0.05–0.26, median dose 1.1 g/d, duration 6 months) (Deane et al., 2021).

However, other studies have found that n-3 PUFA has a beneficial effect on depression. The meta-analysis included 18 RCTs with 4052 participants, and found that n-3 PUFA had a significant small effect on perinatal depressive symptoms compared with placebo (SMD = -0.236, 95% CI: -0.463 to -0.009; $P = .042$) (Mocking et al., 2020).

It seems that EPA has the effect of suppressing depression, while DHA does not. The meta-analysis of 26 RCTs including 2160 participants showed that n-3 PUFA was generally beneficial to depressive symptoms (SMD = -0.28, $P = .004$). Pure EPA (=100% EPA) and EPA main preparation (≥60% EPA) had effects on SMD = -0.50 ($P = .003$) and SMD = -1.03 ($P = .03$), respectively, while pure DHA and main DHA formula had no such benefit compared with placebo (Liao et al., 2019). Another meta-analysis of 8 RCTs involving 638 participants showed that n-3 PUFA has a significant effect on perinatal depression. The ratio of EPA/DHA ≥1.5 has a significant effect in mild-to-moderate maternal and postpartum depression (Zhang et al., 2020).

In another RCT network meta-analysis, 910 patients with major depression in 10 trials were treated with three adjuvant strategies: high-dose n-3 PUFA, low-dose n-3 PUFA, and placebo. The results showed that n-3 PUFA was superior to placebo (SMD: 1.243 ± 0.596; 95% CI: 0.060–2.414), and high-dose n-3 PUFA was more effective than low-dose n-3 PUFA, both of which were higher (SMD: 0.908 ± − 3.131; 95% CI: 0.262–1.581) and lower dose (SMD: 0.601 ± 0.286; 95% CI: 0.034–1.18) than placebo (Luo et al., 2020).

1.6.7 Dietary polyunsaturated fat intake and nonalcoholic fatty liver disease

The n-3 PUFAs have a beneficial effect on the risk of NAFLD. In a meta-analysis of fatty acid and NAFLD, 11 RCTs were included. The n-3 PUFA supplementation significantly reduced the serum concentrations of ALT, ASL, TAG with weighted mean differences (WMDs) of −7.53 U/L; 95% CI: −9.98, −5.08 U/L), −7.10 U/L, 95% CI: −11.67, −2.52 U/L, and −36.16 mg/dL, 95% CI: −49.15, −23.18 mg/dL, respectively. The liver fat content marginally reduced (−5.11%, 95% CI: −10.24, 0.02%, $P = .051$), but not fasting serum glucose. Dose-response analysis showed that 1 g per day increment of EPA + DHA was associated with 3.14 U/L reduction in ALT (95% CI: −5.25, −1.02 U/L), 2.43 U/L in AST (95% CI: −3.90, −0.90 U/L), 2.74% in liver fat (95% CI: −4.32, −1.16%), and 9.97 mg/dL in TAG (95% CI: −14.47, −5.48 mg/dL), respectively (Guo, Yang, Tang, & Li, 2018).

In another meta-analysis of n-3 PUFA supplementation and nonalcoholic fatty liver disease, it included 22 RCTs with 1366 participants. Supplementation of n-3 PUFAs significantly reduced liver fat compared with placebo (RR = 1.52; 95% CI: 1.09–2.13). Supplementation of n-3 PUFA also significantly reduced BMI with pooled mean difference and 95% CI were −0.46: −0.84, −0.08; and concentrations of serum/plasma TAG -28.57: −40.81, −16.33; TC -7.82: −14.86, −0.79 and HDL-C 3.55: 1.38–5.73, respectively (Lee, Fu, Yang, & Chi, 2020).

1.6.8 Dietary polyunsaturated fat intake and chronic kidney disease

The dietary intake of n-3 PUFA has a beneficial effect on the risk of chronic kidney disease. In a meta-analysis of 60 RCTs (4129 participants) of the effects of n-3 PUFA intake on cardiovascular death in patients with chronic kidney disease, all of the supplementation with a median follow-up of 6 months. Results suggested that n-3 PUFA supplementation reduced cardiovascular death for patients on hemodialysis (39 events; RR = 0.45, 95% CI: 0.23–0.89), and prevented end-stage kidney disease (29 events; RR = 0.30, 95% CI: 0.09–0.98) in patients with chronic kidney disease not receiving renal replacement therapy (Saglimbene et al., 2020).

1.6.9 Dietary polyunsaturated fat intake and inflammation

Inflammation is associated with many diseases. N-3 PUFA can be in vivo metabolized in the human body into special potent antiinflammatory lipid mediators, namely resolvins, protectins, and maresins. Increased dietary intake of n-3 PUFA or n-3/n-6 ratio will reduce serum inflammatory factors such as tumor necrosis factor-α (TNF-α) and interleukin 6 (IL-6). In a meta-analysis which included 68 RCTs with a total of 4601 subjects, marine-derived LC n-3 PUFAs supplementation showed a lowering effect on TNF-a, IL-6, and CRP in three groups of subjects (subjects with chronic nonautoimmune disease, subjects with chronic autoimmune disease and healthy subjects). However, all results are with significant heterogeneity, $I^2 \geq 70\%$ (Li et al., 2014).

In another meta-analysis which included 31 RCTs, the results indicated that lower dietary intake of n-6/n-3 PUFA ratio significantly decreased the serum concentrations of TNF-α (SMD = −0.270; 95% CI: −0.433, −0.106; $P = .001$) and IL-6 (SMD = −0.153; 95% CI: −0.260, −0.045; $P = .005$) (Wei, Meng, Li, Wang, & Chen, 2021).

1.7 Conclusion

Dietary fat provides energy and essential fatty acids, participates in all physiological functions, and is closely related to human development and health. In order to prevent noncommunicable diseases, the total dietary fat intake of the general population should not exceed 30% of the total energy, and unsaturated fats should be used to substitute saturated fats, increasing dietary intake of food rich in n-3 PUFA, such as fish and other seafood, walnuts, flax, chia and perilla seeds, and their oils.

References

Abdelhamid, A. S., Brown, T. J., Brainard, J. S., Biswas, P., Thorpe, G. C., Moore, H. J., et al. (2020). Omega-3 fatty acids for the primary and secondary prevention of cardiovascular disease. *Cochrane Database of Systematic Reviews*, 2020(3). https://doi.org/10.1002/14651858.CD003177.pub5.

Brainard, J. S., Jimoh, O. F., Deane, K. H. O., Biswas, P., Donaldson, D., Maas, K., et al. (2020). Omega-3, omega-6, and polyunsaturated fat for cognition: Systematic review and meta-analysis of randomized trials. *Journal of the American Medical Directors Association*, 21(10), 1439–1450.e21. https://doi.org/10.1016/j.jamda.2020.02.022.

Chang, J. P. C., Su, K. P., Mondelli, V., & Pariante, C. M. (2018). Omega-3 polyunsaturated fatty acids in youths with attention deficit hyperactivity disorder: A systematic review and meta-analysis of clinical trials and biological studies. *Neuropsychopharmacology*, 43(3), 534–545. https://doi.org/10.1038/npp.2017.160.

Deane, K. H. O., Jimoh, O. F., Biswas, P., O'Brien, A., Hanson, S., Abdelhamid, A. S., et al. (2021). Omega-3 and polyunsaturated fat for prevention of depression and anxiety symptoms: Systematic review and meta-analysis of randomised trials. *British Journal of Psychiatry*, 218(3), 135–142. https://doi.org/10.1192/bjp.2019.234.

FAO. (2010). *Fats and fatty acids in human nutrition: Report of an expert consultation*. Vol. 97. Food and Agriculture Organization of the United Nations.

Fattore, E., Bosetti, C., Brighenti, F., Agostoni, C., & Fattore, G. (2014). Palm oil and blood lipid-related markers of cardiovascular disease: A systematic review and meta-analysis of dietary intervention trials. *American Journal of Clinical Nutrition*, 99(6), 1331–1350. https://doi.org/10.3945/ajcn.113.081190.

Gardner, C. D., Kiazand, A., Alhassan, S., Kim, S., Stafford, R. S., Balise, R. R., et al. (2007). Comparison of the Atkins, Zone, Ornish, and LEARN diets for change in weight and related risk factors among overweight premenopausal women: The A to Z weight loss study: A randomized trial. *Journal of the American Medical Association*, 297(9), 969–977. https://doi.org/10.1001/jama.297.9.969.

Guo, X. F., Yang, B., Tang, J., & Li, D. (2018). Fatty acid and non-alcoholic fatty liver disease: Meta-analyses of case-control and randomized controlled trials. *Clinical Nutrition*, 37(1), 113–122. https://doi.org/10.1016/j.clnu.2017.01.003.

Hanson, S., Thorpe, G., Winstanley, L., Abdelhamid, A. S., Hooper, L., Abdelhamid, A., et al. (2020). Omega-3, omega-6 and total dietary polyunsaturated fat on cancer incidence: Systematic review and meta-analysis of randomised trials. *British Journal of Cancer*, 122(8), 1260–1270. https://doi.org/10.1038/s41416-020-0761-6.

Hisham, M. D. B., Aziz, Z., Huin, W. K., Haur, C., & Jamil, A. H. A. (2020). The effects of palm oil on serum lipid profiles: A systematic review and meta-analysis. *Asia Pacific Journal of Clinical Nutrition*, 29(3), 523–536. https://doi.org/10.6133/apjcn.202009_29(3).0011.

Hooper, L., Abdelhamid, A., Bunn, D., Brown, T., Summerbell, C. D., & Skeaff, C. M. (2015). Effects of total fat intake on body weight. *Cochrane Database of Systematic Reviews*, 2015(8). https://doi.org/10.1002/14651858.CD011834.

Hooper, L., Martin, N., Jimoh, O. F., Kirk, C., Foster, E., & Abdelhamid, A. S. (2020). Reduction in saturated fat intake for cardiovascular disease. *Cochrane Database of Systematic Reviews*, 2020(8). https://doi.org/10.1002/14651858.CD011737.pub3.

Imamura, F., Micha, R., Wu, J. H. Y., de Oliveira Otto, M. C., Otite, F. O., Abioye, A. I., et al. (2016). Effects of saturated fat, polyunsaturated fat, monounsaturated fat, and carbohydrate on glucose-insulin homeostasis: A systematic review and meta-analysis of randomised controlled feeding trials. *PLoS Medicine*, 13(7). https://doi.org/10.1371/journal.pmed.1002087.

Innes, J. K., & Calder, P. C. (2018). The differential effects of eicosapentaenoic acid and docosahexaenoic acid on cardiometabolic risk factors: A systematic review. *International Journal of Molecular Sciences*, 19(2). https://doi.org/10.3390/ijms19020532.

Langlois, P. L., D'Aragon, F., Hardy, G., & Manzanares, W. (2019). Omega-3 polyunsaturated fatty acids in critically ill patients with acute respiratory distress syndrome: A systematic review and meta-analysis. *Nutrition*, 61, 84–92. https://doi.org/10.1016/j.nut.2018.10.026.

Lee, C. H., Fu, Y., Yang, S. J., & Chi, C. C. (2020). Effects of Omega-3 polyunsaturated fatty acid supplementation on non-alcoholic fatty liver: A systematic review and meta-analysis. *Nutrients*, 12(9), 1–20. https://doi.org/10.3390/nu12092769.

Li, D. (2015). Omega-3 polyunsaturated fatty acids and non-communicable diseases: Meta-analysis based systematic review. *Asia Pacific Journal of Clinical Nutrition*, 24(1), 10–15. https://doi.org/10.6133/apjcn.2015.24.1.21.

Li, D., & Hu, X. (2011). Fatty acid content of commonly available nuts and seeds. In *Nuts and seeds in health and disease prevention* (pp. 35–42). Elsevier Inc. https://doi.org/10.1016/B978-0-12-375688-6.10004-0.

Li, K., Huang, T., Zheng, J., Wu, K., Li, D., & Schunck, W.-H. (2014). Effect of marine-derived n-3 polyunsaturated fatty acids on C-reactive protein, interleukin 6 and tumor necrosis factor α: A meta-analysis. *PLoS One*, 9(2). https://doi.org/10.1371/journal.pone.0088103, e88103.

Li, D., Ng, A., Mann, N. J., & Sinclair, A. J. (1998). Contribution of meat fat to dietary arachidonic acid. *Lipids*, 33(4), 437–440. https://doi.org/10.1007/s11745-998-0225-7.

Li, N., Yue, H., Jia, M., Liu, W., Qiu, B., Hou, H., et al. (2019). Effect of low-ratio n-6/n-3 PUFA on blood glucose:

A meta-analysis. *Food and Function, 10*(8), 4557–4565. https://doi.org/10.1039/c9fo00323a.

Liao, Y., Xie, B., Zhang, H., He, Q., Guo, L., Subramaniapillai, M., et al. (2019). Efficacy of omega-3 PUFAs in depression: A meta-analysis. *Translational Psychiatry, 9*(1). https://doi.org/10.1038/s41398-019-0515-5.

Luo, X. D., Feng, J. S., Yang, Z., Huang, Q. T., Lin, J. D., Yang, B., et al. (2020). High-dose omega-3 polyunsaturated fatty acid supplementation might be more superior than low-dose for major depressive disorder in early therapy period: A network meta-analysis. *BMC Psychiatry, 20*(1). https://doi.org/10.1186/s12888-020-02656-3.

Mensink, R. P. (2016). *Effects of saturated fatty acids on serum lipids and lipoproteins: A systematic review and regression analysis*. Geneva: World Health Organization.

Miller, P. E., Van Elswyk, M., & Alexander, D. D. (2014). Long-chain Omega-3 fatty acids eicosapentaenoic acid and docosahexaenoic acid and blood pressure: A meta-analysis of randomized controlled trials. *American Journal of Hypertension, 27*(7), 885–896. https://doi.org/10.1093/ajh/hpu024.

Mocking, R. J. T., Steijn, K., Roos, C., Assies, J., Bergink, V., Ruhé, H. G., et al. (2020). Omega-3 fatty acid supplementation for perinatal depression: A meta-analysis. *The Journal of Clinical Psychiatry, 81*(5). https://doi.org/10.4088/JCP.19r13106.

Moher, D., Liberati, A., Tetzlaff, J., & Altman, D. G. (2009). Preferred reporting items for systematic reviews and meta-analyses: The PRISMA statement. *PLoS Medicine, 6*(7). https://doi.org/10.1371/journal.pmed.1000097, e1000097.

Moreno, B., Crujeiras, A. B., Bellido, D., Sajoux, I., & Casanueva, F. F. (2016). Obesity treatment by very low-calorie-ketogenic diet at two years: Reduction in visceral fat and on the burden of disease. *Endocrine, 54*(3), 681–690. https://doi.org/10.1007/s12020-016-1050-2.

Qian, F., Korat, A. A., Malik, V., & Hu, F. B. (2016). Metabolic effects of monounsaturated fatty acid-enriched diets compared with carbohydrate or polyunsaturated fatty acid-enriched diets in patients with type 2 diabetes: A systematic review and meta-analysis of randomized controlled trials. *Diabetes Care, 39*(8), 1448–1457. https://doi.org/10.2337/dc16-0513.

Saglimbene, V. M., Wong, G., van Zwieten, A., Palmer, S. C., Ruospo, M., Natale, P., et al. (2020). Effects of omega-3 polyunsaturated fatty acid intake in patients with chronic kidney disease: Systematic review and meta-analysis of randomized controlled trials. *Clinical Nutrition, 39*(2), 358–368. https://doi.org/10.1016/j.clnu.2019.02.041.

Sinclair, A., Oon, K., Lim, L., Li, D., & Mann, N. (1998). The omega-3 fatty acid content of canned, smoked and fresh fish in Australia. *Australian Journal of Nutrition and Dietetics, 55*, 116–120.

Su, X. Q., Antonas, K. N., & Li, D. (2004). Comparison of n-3 polyunsaturated fatty acid contents of wild and cultured Australian abalone. *International Journal of Food Sciences and Nutrition, 55*(2), 149–154. https://doi.org/10.1080/09637480410001666469.

van der Wurff, I. S. M., Meyer, B. J., & de Groot, R. H. M. (2020). Effect of omega-3 long chain polyunsaturated fatty acids (N-3 LCPUFA) supplementation on cognition in children and adolescents: A systematic literature review with a focus on n-3 LCPUFA blood values and dose of DHA and EPA. *Nutrients, 12*(10), 1–28. https://doi.org/10.3390/nu12103115.

Wan, Y., Wang, F., Yuan, J., Li, J., Jiang, D., Zhang, J., et al. (2017). Effects of macronutrient distribution on weight and related cardiometabolic profile in healthy non-obese Chinese: A 6-month, randomized controlled-feeding trial. *eBioMedicine, 22*, 200–207. https://doi.org/10.1016/j.ebiom.2017.06.017.

Wan, Y., Wang, F., Yuan, J., Li, J., Jiang, D., Zhang, J., et al. (2019). Effects of dietary fat on gut microbiota and faecal metabolites, and their relationship with cardiometabolic risk factors: A 6-month randomised controlled-feeding trial. *Gut, 68*(8), 1417–1429. https://doi.org/10.1136/gutjnl-2018-317609.

Wei, Y., Meng, Y., Li, N., Wang, Q., & Chen, L. (2021). The effects of low-ratio n-6/n-3 PUFA on biomarkers of inflammation: A systematic review and meta-analysis. *Food and Function, 12*(1), 30–40. https://doi.org/10.1039/d0fo01976c.

Zhang, M. M., Zou, Y., Li, S. M., Wang, L., Sun, Y. H., Shi, L., et al. (2020). The efficacy and safety of omega-3 fatty acids on depressive symptoms in perinatal women: A meta-analysis of randomized placebo-controlled trials. *Translational Psychiatry, 10*(1). https://doi.org/10.1038/s41398-020-00886-3.

Zheng, J. S., Hu, X. J., Zhao, Y. M., Yang, J., & Li, D. (2013). Intake of fish and marine n-3 polyunsaturated fatty acids and risk of breast cancer: Meta-analysis of data from 21 independent prospective cohort studies. *British Medical Journal, 347*(7917). https://doi.org/10.1136/bmj.f3706 (Online).

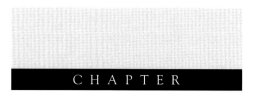

CHAPTER 2

Fatty acids and telomeres in humans

Michael Fenech, Permal Deo, and Varinderpal Dhillon
Clinical and Health Sciences, University of South Australia, Adelaide, SA, Australia

2.1 Introduction

Telomeres located at the ends of chromosomes are highly conserved, long hexamer (TTAGGG) repeat DNA sequences that are essential for chromosomal stability because they protect ends of the chromosome from fusion and degradation (Blackburn, Epel, & Lin, 2015). Telomerase, an intra-nuclear enzyme, is important for telomere formation, maintenance, and restoration (Blackburn, 2005, 2010). Without telomere maintenance and replication, telomeric DNA would be lost every time a cell divides. Attrition of telomeres and/or DNA breaks in the telomere results in cellular senescence, characterized by alterations in gene expression that promote a pro-inflammatory state (Allsopp & Harley, 1995; Coppé, Desprez, Krtolica, & Campisi, 2010).

Telomere length decreases over time due to the telomere end-replication problem and may serve as a biomarker of the aging process (Blasco, 2005; Raynaud, Sabatier, Philipot, Olaussen, & Soria, 2008; Shay, 2018). Telomere length maintenance is largely influenced by genetic, epigenetic, and various environmental and endogenous factors, such as oxidative stress, which may further influence telomere integrity (Blasco, 2007; Fouquerel et al., 2019; Opresko, Fan, Danzy, Wilson, & Bohr, 2005).

Telomere attrition has also been associated with physical inactivity, smoking, psychological stress, body composition (BMI), and lower socioeconomic status (Needham et al., 2013; Shalev et al., 2013; Valdes et al., 2005). Genome-wide association studies have shown that genetic variation within the gene coding for telomerase RNA component (TERC) affects telomere length in humans (Codd et al., 2010; Shen et al., 2011). The exact mechanisms determining telomere attrition remain incompletely understood. However, dietary factors involved as cofactors in DNA replication and repair and in response to oxidative stress may play an important role in influencing the rate of telomere shortening (Dhillon, Bull, & Fenech, 2016). Evidence is emerging that diet is an important variable affecting the rate of telomere attrition, with the most robust evidence so far indicating a protective role for the Mediterranean diet and dietary patterns with a low inflammatory index (Canudas et al., 2020; García-Calzón et al., 2015; Shivappa, Wirth, Hurley, & Hébert, 2017).

This chapter is a narrative review of the current evidence relating to the association of telomere length with dietary or supplemental fatty acid intake or fatty acid status in humans. Evidence from observational cross-sectional and prospective studies and randomized controlled trials has been evaluated.

2.2 Dietary fatty acids and telomeres

Omega-3 fatty acids improve cardiovascular health by lowering cholesterol and triglycerides in the blood and preventing cardiac arrhythmias and, furthermore, contribute to healthy aging by attenuating excessive inflammation via their central role in the synthesis of pro-resolving protectin, maresin, and resolvin mediators (Innes & Calder, 2020; Serhan, 2014). Because dietary fatty acids can influence the risk of cardiometabolic diseases and inflammation, both of which are consistently associated with increased telomere attrition (Haycock et al., 2014; Zhang et al., 2016), it is plausible that telomere length may also be associated with dietary fatty acid intake. Furthermore, unsaturated fatty acids are prone to oxidation to form reactive lipid hydroperoxides (malondialdehyde, epoxyaldehydes, 2-alkenals, and 4-oxo-2-alkenals) that form DNA adducts such as the deoxyguanine (dG) adducts M1dG, $1,N^2$-propano-dG, $1,N^2$-etheno (ε)-dG, 7-(2-oxo-alkyl)-εdG, respectively (Kawai & Nuka, 2018). Formation of DNA adducts on the telomere sequence may lead to DNA replication stress which can result in inefficient telomere replication and/or DNA strand breaks in the telomere, leading to acentric chromosome fragment formation and loss of the fragment together with its associated telomere. Another plausible indirect mechanism is the formation of lipid-derived advanced glycation end-products that may adduct on the telomere and/or promote inflammation and oxidative stress via the RAGE and NF$\kappa\beta$ axis (Fishman, Sonmez, Basman, Singh, & Poretsky, 2018; Fu et al., 1996; Refsgaard, Tsai, & Stadtman, 2000; Slatter, Avery, & Bailey, 2004; Slatter, Bolton, & Bailey, 2000; Vistoli et al., 2013). Fig. 2.1 illustrates plausible mechanisms by which fatty acids may influence loss of telomere integrity and promote cellular aging.

2.3 Cross-sectional and prospective studies

Thirteen observational studies have been reported, 12 are cross-sectional studies, and one is a prospective study. Total fat and saturated fatty acids were found to be inversely associated with telomere length in men (Tiainen et al., 2012). In another study, monounsaturated fatty acids were found to be significantly inversely associated with telomere length (Kark, Goldberger, Kimura, Sinnreich, & Aviv, 2012). In yet another study, dietary intake of linoleic acid was found to be inversely associated with telomere length (Cassidy et al., 2010). However, the study by Song and associates showed that intake of short-to-medium-chain saturated fatty acids is inversely associated with telomere length, but no significant association was found with long-chain saturated fatty acids or PUFAs or MUFAs (Song et al., 2013).

In 287 participants (55% males, 6–18 years), who were randomly selected from the GENOI study, dietary intake of polyunsaturated fatty acids was significantly and inversely associated with telomere length; however, no association with dietary intake of total fats, saturated fatty acids, and monounsaturated fatty acids was reported with telomere length (García-Calzón et al., 2015). In the Seychelles Child Development Study, prenatal PUFA status was not associated with telomere length of the mother or child; however, a higher prenatal n-6:n-3 PUFA ratio was significantly associated with longer telomere length in the mothers ($\beta = 0.001$, $P = .048$) (Yeates et al., 2017). It has also been reported that telomere length decreased with increased trans-fatty acids, most significantly with increased palmitelaidic acid and linolelaidic acid (Mazidi, Banach, & Kengne, 2018). Another study, in elderly subjects with recent myocardial infarction, reported a weak but significant positive correlation between linoleic acid and telomere length. However, other

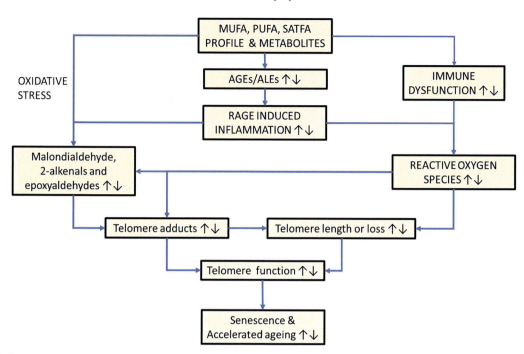

FIG. 2.1 Plausible mechanisms by which fatty acids may influence loss of telomere integrity and promote cellular aging. *No permission required.*

long-chain fatty acids and the n-3/n-6 ratio were not associated with telomere length (Kalstad et al., 2019). In a cross-sectional study, involving a total of 1,246 subjects aged 25–74 years, elaidic acid and n-3 PUFA were negatively associated with telomere length and n-6 PUFA was positively associated (Zhao et al., 2020). Recently, it has been reported that the majority of saturated and monounsaturated fatty acids measured in red blood cells (RBCs) were negatively associated with telomere length in leukocytes whereas polyunsaturated fatty acids (more specifically arachidonic acid) were positively associated with telomere length (V. S. Dhillon, Deo, Chua, Thomas, & Fenech, 2021). In contrast, an increased concentration of arachidonic acid in RBCs was reported to be significantly associated with decreased telomere length in Mediterranean elders (Freitas-Simoes et al., 2019). In a study of obese and nonobese children, it was reported that leukocyte telomere length was positively associated with concentrations of total saturated fatty acids and DHA in RBCs ($P<.05$), and negatively with the AA/DHA ratio ($P<.05$) (Liu, Liu, Shi, Fan, & Qi, 2021).

There is only one prospective study that investigated the association of fatty acids with telomere length. In this study, the Heart and Soul study, increased intake of omega-3 fatty acids (EPA, DHA), over a 6-year period, was associated with a significantly reduced rate of telomere shortening (Farzaneh-Far et al., 2010). Further details of the above studies are provided in Table 2.1. Fig. 2.2 provides a condensed landscape of these various studies showing the great diversity of statistically significant outcomes involving different fatty acid classes and specific fatty acids. The weight of evidence from this sparse observational data tends to suggest an association between shorter telomeres, and increased saturated fatty acids, monounsaturated fatty acids, and trans-fatty acids.

TABLE 2.1 Observational cross-sectional and prospective studies on association of fatty acids with telomere length.

References	Study design	Population	Tissue/method	Results
Cassidy et al. (2010)	Cross-sectional substudy from a prospective cohort study	2284 female participants from Nurses' Health Study from US aged 30–55 years	PBL/qPCR	Linoleic acid intake was inversely associated with telomere length after multivariate adjustments ($P=.001$; P for trend $=0.05$)
Tiainen et al. (2012)	Cross-sectional	1942 males and females aged 57–70 years from the Helsinki Birth Cohort Study (Finland)	PBL/qPCR	Total fat and SFA were inversely associated with leukocyte telomere length in men adjusting for age and energy intake ($b=-0.001$; $P=.04$)
Kark et al. (2012)	Cross-sectional substudy from a longitudinal observational study	405 men and 204 women; mean age at baseline (30.1 years) and follow-up (43.2 years) from Jerusalem LRC Prevalence Study (Israel)	Buffy coat/Southern blot	MUFA was significantly inversely associated with LTL in men only ($b=-0.104$; $P=.042$) after adjusting for covariates
Song et al. (2013)	Cross-sectional substudy from a longitudinal observational study	4029 healthy postmenopausal women aged 58+ years from WHI Observational study cohort (California, US)	PBL/qPCR	Intake of short-to-medium-chain fatty acids (SMSFAs; aliphatic tails of ≤12 carbons) was inversely associated with telomere length. No significant associations were found with long-chain saturated fatty acids, monounsaturated fatty acids, and polyunsaturated fatty acids
García-Calzón, Moleres, et al. (2015) and García-Calzón, Zalba, et al. (2015)	Cross-sectional study	207 participants aged between 6 and 18 years randomly selected from GENOI cohort (Spain)	Buffy coat/qPCR	Dietary intake of PUFA is significantly inversely associated with telomere length. However, no association of dietary intake of total fats, SFA, and MUFA with telomere length
Yeates et al. (2017)	Observational study	229 expectant mother in 28-week gestation (Seychelles)	PBL/qPCR	n3 and n6 PUFAs are inversely but not significantly associated with telomere length. However, higher n6:n3 ratio is significantly associated with longer telomere length
Mazidi et al. (2018)	Observational study	5446 participants with average age of 47.1 years from National Health and Nutrition Examination Survey (NHANES) aged	PBL/qPCR	Concentration of trans-fatty acids such as palmitelaidic acid and linolelaidic acid decreased with increasing length of telomeres ($P=.05$) after adjustments for factors such as age, gender, ethnicity, BMI, and smoking

Study	Design	Population	Sample/Method	Findings
Freitas-Simoes et al. (2019)	Cross-sectional substudy from a randomized controlled trial	344 subjects with mean age of 68.8 years from Walnut and Healthy Aging trial (Spain)	PBMC/FISH	An increasing proportion of arachidonic acid in RBCs is significantly ($P=.02$) associated with shorter telomeres in Mediterranean elders
Kalstad et al. (2019)	Cross-sectional substudy of data from omega-3 fatty acids in elderly patients with myocardial infarction (OMEMI) trial	299 patients aged between 70 and 82 years (Norway)	PBL/qPCR	There was a weak but significant correlation between linoleic acid and telomere length ($r=0.139$; $P=.017$). However, other long-chain fatty acids and n-6/n-3 ratio is not associated with telomere length
Zhao et al. (2020)	Cross-sectional	1246 participants aged between 25 and 74 years (China)	PBL/qPCR	Elaidic acid (C18:1) and n-3 PUFA were negatively associated with relative telomere length after adjustments for age, gender, race, smoking, and exercise
Dhillon et al. (2021)	Cross-sectional study	174 healthy elderly participants with mean age of 53.71 years, from South Australian (Australia)	PBL/qPCR	Majority of saturated fatty acids and monounsaturated fatty acids were negatively associated with telomere length whereas polyunsaturated fatty acids were positively associated with telomere length. Multiple regression analysis revealed that arachidonic acid is significantly, independently, positively correlated with telomere length ($b=0.262$; $P=0.000$).
Liu et al. (2021)	Cross-sectional Study	Forty-six preschool children with obesity aged 3–4 years were included in the study, with equal numbers of age- and gender-matched children with normal weight as control	PBMC/qPCR	Correlative analysis showed that leukocyte telomere length had a positive association with total saturated fatty acids ($r=0.49$, $P<.05$) and DHA ($r=0.44$, $P<.05$), and a negative association with the AA/DHA ratio ($r=-0.36$, $P<.05$)
Farzaneh-Far et al. (2010)	Prospective cohort	608 outpatients in California (US) with stable coronary artery disease—Heart and Soul Study. Study duration: 6 years	PBL/qPCR	Log omega-3 fatty acids were associated with a decrease in telomere shortening (OR: 0.68; 95% CI: 0.47–0.98)

	LONGER TELOMERE	SHORTER TELOMERE
SATFA	Liu et al [51]	Tianen et al [40] Song et al [43] Dhillon et al [49]
MUFA	NONE REPORTED	Kark et al [41] Dhillon et al [49]
PUFA	Dhillon et al [49]	Garcia-Calzon et al [44]
n6PUFA	NONE REPORTED	Zhao et al [48]
n6:n3 PUFA ratio	Yeates et al [45]	Dhillon et al [49]
TRANSFA	NONE REPORTED	Mazidi et al [46] Zhao et al [48]
ω-3PUFA	Liu et al [51] Faranzeh-Far et al [52]	Zhao et al [48]
Linoleic acid	Kalstad et al [47]	Cassidy et al [42]
Arachidonic acid	Dhillon et al [49]	Freitag-Simoes et al [50]
AA:DHA ratio	NONE REPORTED	Liu et al [51]

FIG. 2.2 Significant associations of fatty acids with telomere length—Observational studies. *No permission required.*

2.4 Randomized controlled trials

Only six randomized controlled trials (RCTs) have been reported, all of them involving supplementation with n-3 fatty acids. Four of these RCTs investigated effects on telomere length as a primary or secondary outcome measure, and the remaining two studied the effect on telomerase activity. An increase of 21 and 50 bp in telomere length was reported among individuals who respectively received low and high doses of n-3 fatty acids compared to the placebo group who reported a loss of 43 bp in telomere length (Kiecolt-Glaser et al., 2013). An intervention trial involving long-chain n-3 fatty acids supplementation among people with mild cognitive impairment did not show any association with telomere attrition (O'Callaghan et al., 2014); however, increased erythrocyte DHA levels were associated with reduced telomere attrition ($r = -0.67$; $P = .02$) in the group treated with DHA. An RCT on chronic kidney disease patients reported no effect of n-3 fatty acids or CoQ on neutrophil or PBMC telomere length; however, neutrophil telomere length corrected for neutrophil count was increased after n-3 fatty acids supplementation ($P = .015$) (Barden et al., 2016). In another study, maternal n-3 LC PUFA supplementation did not influence offspring telomere length at birth or at 12y (See et al., 2016).

Two RCTs explored the effects of n-3 fatty acid supplementation on telomerase activity. The first study in diabetic patients showed that supplementation with DHA resulted in a significant decrease in telomere length (Toupchian et al., 2018). In the second RCT study, performed in schizophrenia patients, telomerase activity in peripheral blood mononuclear cells (PBMCs) increased significantly in the group receiving the EPA + DHA supplement relative to the placebo group (Pawełczyk et al., 2018). Telomere length was not measured in these two studies. Further details regarding these RCTs are provided in Table 2.2.

2.5 Discussion

Results from various cross-sectional, observational, prospective, and randomized trials described above did not provide robust evidence that dietary intake of specific fatty acid groups, or specific fatty acids, is substantially protective against or aggravates telomere shortening. Furthermore, there was great heterogeneity between studies with regards to (i) health status, (ii) age-range, (iii) duration of RCT interventions, and (iv) cells used to measure telomere length, all of which are important factors that can affect telomere length (Aviv, 2004; Sanders & Newman, 2013). For example, although the majority of reported observational studies involved healthy subjects, the RCTs

TABLE 2.2 Randomized controlled trials on the effects of ω-3 fatty acid supplementation on telomere length or telomerase activity.

References	Study design	Cohort and treatment	Tissue/method	Results
Kiecolt-Glaser et al. (2013)	Double-blind randomized controlled trial of 4 months' duration	106 healthy sedentary overweight men and women, aged 40–85 years randomized to one of these treatments: (1) 2.5 g/day n-3 PUFAs, (2) 1.25 g/day n-3 PUFAs, or (3) placebo capsules that mirrored the proportions of fatty acids in the typical American diet	PBL/qPCR	Telomere length had an increase of 21 bp for the low-dose n-3 PUFA group and an increase of 50 bp in the high-dose n-3 PUFA group compared to a decrease of 43 bp for placebo; differences between groups were not significant. Telomere length increased with decreasing n-6:n-3 ratios, $P=.02$
O'Callaghan et al. (2014)	Randomized controlled trial, pilot study of 6 months' duration	33 elderly participants aged >65 years with mild cognitive impairment from Adelaide (Australia) randomized to receive one of these treatments: (1) a supplement rich in the long-chain ω-3 PUFA eicosapentaenoic acid (EPA; 1.67 g EPA + 0.16 g docosahexaenoic acid DHA/d; $n=12$) or (2) DHA supplement (1.55 g DHA + 0.40 g EPA/d; $n=12$), or (3) ω-6 PUFA supplement linoleic acid (LA; 2.2 g/d; $n=9$) for 6 months	Whole blood/qPCR	The intervention trial with long-chain ω-3 fatty acids did not show an increase in telomere length, and there was a trend toward telomere shortening during the intervention period. Increased erythrocyte DHA levels were associated with reduced telomere attrition ($r=-0.67$; $P=.02$) in the DHA group
Barden et al. (2016)	Randomized, double-blind	87 chronic kidney disease patients were randomized	Telomere length was measured in neutrophils	There was no effect of n-3 fatty acids or CoQ on

Continued

TABLE 2.2 Randomized controlled trials on the effects of ω-3 fatty acid supplementation on telomere length or telomerase activity—cont'd

References	Study design	Cohort and treatment	Tissue/method	Results
	controlled trial. Duration 8 weeks	to: (i) n-3 fatty acids (4 g); (ii) CoQ (200 mg); (iii) both supplements; or (iv) control (4 g olive oil), daily for 8 weeks	and peripheral blood mononuclear cells (PBMCs) at baseline and 8 weeks, with and without correction for cell counts	neutrophil or PBMC telomere length. However, telomere length corrected for neutrophil count was increased after n-3 fatty acids ($P = .015$)
See et al. (2016)	Randomized controlled trial, from 20-week gestation until delivery	Double-blind, placebo-controlled, parallel group study involving 98 pregnant atopic women who were randomized to 4 g/day of n-3 LCPUFA or control (olive oil)	Offspring cord blood at birth and peripheral blood at 12 years. PBL/qPCR	Maternal n-3 LCPUFA supplementation did not influence offspring telomere length at birth or at 12y
Toupchian et al. (2018)	Randomized, double-blind placebo-controlled trial. Duration 8 weeks	Diabetic patients aged 30–70 years were randomly assigned to receive either (i) 2.4 g of DHA-enriched fish oil or (ii) a placebo	Telomerase activity measured in PBMC using TRAP assay	Telomerase activity decreased ($P < .001$) during the intervention in the DHA treatment group
Pawełczyk et al. (2018)	Randomized placebo-controlled trial, duration 26 weeks	66 first episode schizophrenia patients aged 16–35 years who were randomized to either (i) 2.2 g/day of n-3 PUFA (i.e., 1320 mg eicosapentaenoic and 880 mg docosahexaenoic acid) or (ii) olive oil placebo	Telomerase levels of PBMC were assessed at weeks 8 and 26 of the intervention	A significantly greater increase in PBMC telomerase levels in the intervention group compared to placebo was observed ($P < .001$). Changes in telomerase levels significantly and inversely correlated with improvement in depressive symptoms and severity of the illness

which provide more robust evidence of causality were performed in largely disparate health/life-stage groups (obese, pregnant, coronary artery disease, mild cognitive impairment, chronic kidney disease, diabetes, and schizophrenia), and none of them have yet been replicated. The duration of RCTs ranged from 8 to 26 weeks without justification for the RCT duration chosen, which arguably should be based on the kinetics of the rate of change in telomere in length in the cell type chosen and the turnover of the cells within the body, which can range from 5.4 days for neutrophils to at least 450 days in human memory CD8 T cells (Akondy et al., 2017; Pillay et al., 2010). None of the observational studies adequately corrected for important variables that may affect telomere length such as homocysteine status, oxidative stress, and inflammation measured as C-reactive protein (van der Spek et al., 2019; Zhang et al.,

2016). In general, although age-related telomere shortening is evident in most studies, it has also been shown that telomeres can either elongate or shorten in-vivo depending on a wide range of micronutrients and their intake as well as caloric intake (Crous-Bou, Molinuevo, & Sala-Vila, 2019; Paul et al., 2009; Welendorf et al., 2019).

Furthermore, telomere length varies between leucocyte subsets, making it possible that observed changes in telomere length may be confounded by changes in leucocyte subset counts which may be affected by nutrient intake and disease status (Afari & Bhat, 2016; Can & Can, 2019; Kaya et al., 2019). Although all studies that we reviewed used blood cells to measure telomere length, they either used combined DNA from all types of leukocytes in the blood, or they used DNA from isolated lymphocytes or isolated neutrophils which differ significantly in telomere length (Robertson et al., 2000; Rufer et al., 1999). These variations in the cell type studied and the natural cyclical variation in telomere length in leukocytes create additional confounding and heterogeneity in the data which hinders the possibility of meta-analytical analysis of results from the various reported studies (Svenson et al., 2011).

There is, therefore, an urgent need to set some guidelines for the design of observational and RCT studies that aim to investigate the effect of fatty acids and other nutrients on telomere length. We make the following suggestions:

- Preferably use purified cell populations (e.g., isolated lymphocytes and/or isolated neutrophils; ideally also measure telomere length in epithelial tissue such as buccal cells).
- Measure major known confounding factors affecting telomere length (e.g., age, gender, obesity, homocysteine, C-reactive protein, folate, genetics, etc.) (Crous-Bou et al., 2019; McNally, Luncsford, & Armanios, 2019; Nelson & Codd, 2020; Paul et al., 2009; van der Spek et al., 2019; Welendorf et al., 2019; Zhang et al., 2016).
- Background diet, depending on its Mediterranean and inflammatory index score, can significantly affect telomere length (Canudas et al., 2020; García-Calzón, Zalba, et al., 2015; Sofi, Macchi, Abbate, Gensini, & Casini, 2013); it is therefore essential that participants with similar Mediterranean diet and inflammatory index scores are recruited so that the outcomes of the trial are properly framed within the context of the dietary group to which they appertain.
- Ideally, measure changes in telomere length using well-established techniques that measure not only average telomere length across the whole genome but also telomere length of specific chromosome arms (Lai, Wright, & Shay, 2018); measurement of telomere loss is also desirable because of its evident strong diagnostic value (M'kacher et al., 2020). Measurement of DNA adducts and DNA strand breaks in the telomere sequence may also shed light on the mechanisms by which fatty acids may improve or aggravate telomere integrity (Chung, Chen, & Nath, 1996; Fouquerel et al., 2019).
- Measure telomerase activity in the cell types investigated for telomere length.
- Intervention duration of 6 months or greater depending on the turnover rate and telomere length dynamics of the cell types investigated.

RCTs with fatty acids can potentially change the n-3:n-6 ratio, which in turn can alter the levels of inflammatory biomarkers such as TNF-a, IL-6, and IL-8. Therefore, it is important to include all these biomarkers in any future study which can explain the actual mechanism involving the telomere attrition rate. Also, it is important to include the complete profile of fatty acids in red blood cells (or preferably the target cells used to measure telomere length) at the beginning and end of the study as well.

2.6 Conclusion

The current evidence available regarding the effect of fatty acids on telomere length is still inadequate to provide reliable dietary or supplementation recommendations. We provide suggestions on improvements in observational and RCT study designs for the field to move forward in the hope that heterogeneity of future studies will be diminished and the mechanistic links between dietary intake of fatty acids and telomere integrity can be better revealed.

References

Afari, M. E., & Bhat, T. (2016). Neutrophil to lymphocyte ratio (NLR) and cardiovascular diseases: An update. *Expert Review of Cardiovascular Therapy*, 14(5), 573–577. https://doi.org/10.1586/14779072.2016.1154788.

Akondy, R. S., Fitch, M., Edupuganti, S., Yang, S., Kissick, H. T., Li, K. W., et al. (2017). Origin and differentiation of human memory CD8 T cells after vaccination. *Nature*, 552(7685), 362–367. https://doi.org/10.1038/nature24633.

Allsopp, R. C., & Harley, C. B. (1995). Evidence for a critical telomere length in senescent human fibroblasts. *Experimental Cell Research*, 219(1), 130–136. https://doi.org/10.1006/excr.1995.1213.

Aviv, A. (2004). Telomeres and human aging: Facts and fibs. *Science of Aging Knowledge Environment (SAGE KE)*, 2004(51), pe43. https://doi.org/10.1126/sageke.2004.51.pe43.

Barden, A., O'Callaghan, N., Burke, V., Mas, E., Beilin, L. J., Fenech, M., et al. (2016). N-3 fatty acid supplementation and leukocyte telomere length in patients with chronic kidney disease. *Nutrients*, 8(3). https://doi.org/10.3390/nu8030175.

Blackburn, E. H. (2005). Telomeres and telomerase: Their mechanisms of action and the effects of altering their functions. *FEBS Letters*, 579(4), 859–862. https://doi.org/10.1016/j.febslet.2004.11.036.

Blackburn, E. H. (2010). Telomeres and telomerase: The means to the end (Nobel lecture). *Angewandte Chemie, International Edition*, 49(41), 7405–7421. https://doi.org/10.1002/anie.201002387.

Blackburn, E. H., Epel, E. S., & Lin, J. (2015). Human telomere biology: A contributory and interactive factor in aging, disease risks, and protection. *Science*, 350(6265), 1193–1198. https://doi.org/10.1126/science.aab3389.

Blasco, M. A. (2005). Telomeres and human disease: Ageing, cancer and beyond. *Nature Reviews Genetics*, 6(8), 611–622. https://doi.org/10.1038/nrg1656.

Blasco, M. A. (2007). The epigenetic regulation of mammalian telomeres. *Nature Reviews Genetics*, 8(4), 299–309. https://doi.org/10.1038/nrg2047.

Can, E., & Can, C. (2019). The value of neutrophil-to-lymphocyte ratio (NLR) and platelet-to-lymphocyte ratio (PLR) parameters in analysis with fetal malnutrition neonates. *Journal of Perinatal Medicine*, 47(7), 775–779. https://doi.org/10.1515/jpm-2019-0016.

Canudas, S., Becerra-Tomás, N., Hernández-Alonso, P., Galié, S., Leung, C., Crous-Bou, M., et al. (2020). Mediterranean diet and telomere length: A systematic review and meta-analysis. *Advances in Nutrition*, 11(6), 1544–1554. https://doi.org/10.1093/advances/nmaa079.

Cassidy, A., De Vivo, I., Liu, Y., Han, J., Prescott, J., Hunter, D. J., et al. (2010). Associations between diet, lifestyle factors, and telomere length in women. *American Journal of Clinical Nutrition*, 91(5), 1273–1280. https://doi.org/10.3945/ajcn.2009.28947.

Chung, F. L., Chen, H. J. C., & Nath, R. G. (1996). Lipid peroxidation as a potential endogenous source for the formation of exocyclic DNA adducts. *Carcinogenesis*, 17(10), 2105–2111. https://doi.org/10.1093/carcin/17.10.2105.

Codd, V., Mangino, M., Van Der Harst, P., Braund, P. S., Kaiser, M., Beveridge, A. J., et al. (2010). Common variants near TERC are associated with mean telomere length. *Nature Genetics*, 42(3), 197–199. https://doi.org/10.1038/ng.532.

Coppé, J. P., Desprez, P. Y., Krtolica, A., & Campisi, J. (2010). The senescence-associated secretory phenotype: The dark side of tumor suppression. *Annual Review of Pathology: Mechanisms of Disease*, 5, 99–118. https://doi.org/10.1146/annurev-pathol-121808-102144.

Crous-Bou, M., Molinuevo, J. L., & Sala-Vila, A. (2019). Plant-rich dietary patterns, plant foods and nutrients, and telomere length. *Advances in Nutrition*, 10, S296–S303. https://doi.org/10.1093/advances/nmz026.

Dhillon, V., Bull, C., & Fenech, M. (2016). Telomeres, aging, and nutrition. In *Molecular basis of nutrition and aging: A volume in the molecular nutrition series* (pp. 129–140). Elsevier Inc. https://doi.org/10.1016/B978-0-12-801816-3.00010-8.

Dhillon, V. S., Deo, P., Chua, A., Thomas, P., & Fenech, M. (2021). Telomere length in healthy adults is positively associated with polyunsaturated fatty acids, including arachidonic acid, and negatively with saturated fatty acids. *The Journals of Gerontology. Series A, Biological Sciences and Medical Sciences*, 76(1), 3–6. https://doi.org/10.1093/GERONA/GLAA213.

Farzaneh-Far, R., Lin, J., Epel, E. S., Harris, W. S., Blackburn, E. H., & Whooley, M. A. (2010). Association of marine omega-3 fatty acid levels with telomeric aging in patients with coronary heart disease. *JAMA: The Journal of the American Medical Association*, 303(3), 250–257. https://doi.org/10.1001/jama.2009.2008.

Fishman, S. L., Sonmez, H., Basman, C., Singh, V., & Poretsky, L. (2018). The role of advanced glycation end-products in the development of coronary artery disease in patients with and without diabetes mellitus: A review. *Molecular Medicine*, 24(1). https://doi.org/10.1186/s10020-018-0060-3.

Fouquerel, E., Barnes, R. P., Uttam, S., Watkins, S. C., Bruchez, M. P., & Opresko, P. L. (2019). Targeted and persistent 8-oxoguanine base damage at telomeres promotes telomere loss and crisis. *Molecular Cell*, 75(1), 117–130.e6. https://doi.org/10.1016/j.molcel.2019.04.024.

Freitas-Simoes, T. M., Cofán, M., Blasco, M. A., Soberón, N., Foronda, M., Corella, D., et al. (2019). The red blood cell proportion of arachidonic acid relates to shorter leukocyte telomeres in Mediterranean elders: A secondary analysis of a randomized controlled trial. *Clinical Nutrition*, 38(2), 958–961. https://doi.org/10.1016/j.clnu.2018.02.011.

Fu, M. X., Requena, J. R., Jenkins, A. J., Lyons, T. J., Baynes, J. W., & Thorpe, S. R. (1996). The advanced glycation end product, N∈-(carboxymethyl)lysine, is a product of both lipid peroxidation and glycoxidation reactions. *Journal of Biological Chemistry*, 271(17), 9982–9986. https://doi.org/10.1074/jbc.271.17.9982.

García-Calzón, S., Moleres, A., Martínez-González, M. A., Martínez, J. A., Zalba, G., Marti, A., et al. (2015). Dietary total antioxidant capacity is associated with leukocyte telomere length in a children and adolescent population. *Clinical Nutrition*, 34(4), 694–699. https://doi.org/10.1016/j.clnu.2014.07.015.

García-Calzón, S., Zalba, G., Ruiz-Canela, M., Shivappa, N., Hébert, J. R., Martínez, J. A., et al. (2015). Dietary inflammatory index and telomere length in subjects with a high cardiovascular disease risk from the PREDIMED-NAVARRA study: Cross-sectional and longitudinal analyses over 5 y. *American Journal of Clinical Nutrition*, 102(4), 897–904. https://doi.org/10.3945/ajcn.115.116863.

Haycock, P. C., Heydon, E. E., Kaptoge, S., Butterworth, A. S., Thompson, A., & Willeit, P. (2014). Leucocyte telomere length and risk of cardiovascular disease: Systematic review and meta-analysis. *BMJ (Online)*, 349. https://doi.org/10.1136/bmj.g4227.

Innes, J. K., & Calder, P. C. (2020). Marine omega-3 (N-3) fatty acids for cardiovascular health: An update for 2020. *International Journal of Molecular Sciences*, 21(4). https://doi.org/10.3390/ijms21041362.

Kalstad, A. A., Tveit, S., Myhre, P. L., Laake, K., Opstad, T. B., Tveit, A., et al. (2019). Leukocyte telomere length and serum polyunsaturated fatty acids, dietary habits, cardiovascular risk factors and features of myocardial infarction in elderly patients. *BMC Geriatrics*, 19(1). https://doi.org/10.1186/s12877-019-1383-9.

Kark, J. D., Goldberger, N., Kimura, M., Sinnreich, R., & Aviv, A. (2012). Energy intake and leukocyte telomere length in young adults. *American Journal of Clinical Nutrition*, 95(2), 479–487. https://doi.org/10.3945/ajcn.111.024521.

Kawai, Y., & Nuka, E. (2018). Abundance of DNA adducts of 4oxo2alkenals, lipid peroxidation derived highly reactive genotoxins. *Journal of Clinical Biochemistry and Nutrition*, 62(1), 3–10. https://doi.org/10.3164/jcbn.17-90.

Kaya, T., Açıkgöz, S. B., Yıldırım, M., Nalbant, A., Altaş, A. E., & Cinemre, H. (2019). Association between neutrophil-to-lymphocyte ratio and nutritional status in geriatric patients. *Journal of Clinical Laboratory Analysis*, 33(1). https://doi.org/10.1002/jcla.22636.

Kiecolt-Glaser, J. K., Epel, E. S., Belury, M. A., Andridge, R., Lin, J., Glaser, R., et al. (2013). Omega-3 fatty acids, oxidative stress, and leukocyte telomere length: A randomized controlled trial. *Brain, Behavior, and Immunity*, 28, 16–24. https://doi.org/10.1016/j.bbi.2012.09.004.

Lai, T. P., Wright, W. E., & Shay, J. W. (2018). Comparison of telomere length measurement methods. *Philosophical Transactions of the Royal Society, B: Biological Sciences*, 373(1741). https://doi.org/10.1098/rstb.2016.0451.

Liu, X., Liu, X., Shi, Q., Fan, X., & Qi, K. (2021). Association of telomere length and telomerase methylation with n-3 fatty acids in preschool children with obesity. *BMC Pediatrics*, 21(1). https://doi.org/10.1186/s12887-020-02487-x.

M'kacher, R., Colicchio, B., Borie, C., Junker, S., Marquet, V., Heidingsfelder, L., et al. (2020). Telomere and centromere staining followed by m-fish improves diagnosis of chromosomal instability and its clinical utility. *Genes*, 11(5). https://doi.org/10.3390/genes11050475.

Mazidi, M., Banach, M., & Kengne, A. P. (2018). Association between plasma trans fatty acids concentrations and leucocyte telomere length in US adults. *European Journal of Clinical Nutrition*, 72(4), 581–586. https://doi.org/10.1038/s41430-017-0065-y.

McNally, E. J., Luncsford, P. J., & Armanios, M. (2019). Long telomeres and cancer risk: The price of cellular immortality. *Journal of Clinical Investigation*, 129(9), 3474–3481. https://doi.org/10.1172/JCI120851.

Needham, B. L., Adler, N., Gregorich, S., Rehkopf, D., Lin, J., Blackburn, E. H., et al. (2013). Socioeconomic status, health behavior, and leukocyte telomere length in the National Health and Nutrition Examination Survey, 1999–2002. *Social Science & Medicine*, 1–8. https://doi.org/10.1016/j.socscimed.2013.02.023.

Nelson, C. P., & Codd, V. (2020). Genetic determinants of telomere length and cancer risk. *Current Opinion in Genetics and Development*, 60, 63–68. https://doi.org/10.1016/j.gde.2020.02.007.

O'Callaghan, N., Parletta, N., Milte, C. M., Benassi-Evans, B., Fenech, M., & Howe, P. R. C. (2014). Telomere shortening in elderly individuals with mild cognitive impairment may be attenuated with ω-3 fatty acid supplementation:

A randomized controlled pilot study. *Nutrition*, *30*(4), 489–491. https://doi.org/10.1016/j.nut.2013.09.013.

Opresko, P. L., Fan, J., Danzy, S., Wilson, D. M., & Bohr, V. A. (2005). Oxidative damage in telomeric DNA disrupts recognition by TRF1 and TRF2. *Nucleic Acids Research*, *33*(4), 1230–1239. https://doi.org/10.1093/nar/gki273.

Paul, L., Cattaneo, M., D'Angelo, A., Sampietro, F., Fermo, I., Razzari, C., et al. (2009). Telomere length in peripheral blood mononuclear cells is associated with folate status in men. *Journal of Nutrition*, *139*(7), 1273–1278. https://doi.org/10.3945/jn.109.104984.

Pawełczyk, T., Grancow-Grabka, M., Trafalska, E., Szemraj, J., Żurner, N., & Pawełczyk, A. (2018). Telomerase level increase is related to n-3 polyunsaturated fatty acid efficacy in first episode schizophrenia: Secondary outcome analysis of the OFFER randomized clinical trial. *Progress in Neuro-Psychopharmacology and Biological Psychiatry*, *83*, 142–148. https://doi.org/10.1016/j.pnpbp.2017.12.008.

Pillay, J., Den Braber, I., Vrisekoop, N., Kwast, L. M., De Boer, R. J., Borghans, J. A. M., et al. (2010). In vivo labeling with 2H2O reveals a human neutrophil lifespan of 5.4 days. *Blood*, *116*(4), 625–627. https://doi.org/10.1182/blood-2010-01-259028.

Raynaud, C. M., Sabatier, L., Philipot, O., Olaussen, K. A., & Soria, J. C. (2008). Telomere length, telomeric proteins and genomic instability during the multistep carcinogenic process. *Critical Reviews in Oncology/Hematology*, *66*(2), 99–117. https://doi.org/10.1016/j.critrevonc.2007.11.006.

Refsgaard, H. H. F., Tsai, L., & Stadtman, E. R. (2000). Modifications of proteins by polyunsaturated fatty acid peroxidation products. *Proceedings of the National Academy of Sciences of the United States of America*, *97*(2), 611–616. https://doi.org/10.1073/pnas.97.2.611.

Robertson, J. D., Gale, R. E., Wynn, R. F., Dougal, M., Linch, D. C., Testa, N. G., et al. (2000). Dynamics of telomere shortening in neutrophils and T lymphocytes during ageing and the relationship to skewed X chromosome inactivation patterns. *British Journal of Haematology*, *109*(2), 272–279. https://doi.org/10.1046/j.1365-2141.2000.01970.x.

Rufer, N., Brümmendorf, T. H., Kolvraa, S., Bischoff, C., Christensen, K., Wadsworth, L., et al. (1999). Telomere fluorescence measurements in granulocytes and T lymphocyte subsets point to a high turnover of hematopoietic stem cells and memory T cells in early childhood. *Journal of Experimental Medicine*, *190*(2), 157–167. https://doi.org/10.1084/jem.190.2.157.

Sanders, J. L., & Newman, A. B. (2013). Telomere length in epidemiology: A biomarker of aging, age-related disease, both, or neither? *Epidemiologic Reviews*, *35*(1), 112–131. https://doi.org/10.1093/epirev/mxs008.

See, V. H. L., Mas, E., Burrows, S., O'Callaghan, N. J., Fenech, M., Prescott, S. L., et al. (2016). Prenatal omega-3 fatty acid supplementation does not affect offspring telomere length and F2-isoprostanes at 12 years: A double blind, randomized controlled trial. *Prostaglandins, Leukotrienes, and Essential Fatty Acids*, *112*, 50–55. https://doi.org/10.1016/j.plefa.2016.08.006.

Serhan, C. N. (2014). Pro-resolving lipid mediators are leads for resolution physiology. *Nature*, *510*(7503), 92–101. https://doi.org/10.1038/nature13479.

Shalev, I., Entringer, S., Wadhwa, P. D., Wolkowitz, O. M., Puterman, E., Lin, J., et al. (2013). Stress and telomere biology: A lifespan perspective. *Psychoneuroendocrinology*, *38*(9), 1835–1842. https://doi.org/10.1016/j.psyneuen.2013.03.010.

Shay, J. W. (2018). Telomeres and aging. *Current Opinion in Cell Biology*, *52*, 1–7. https://doi.org/10.1016/j.ceb.2017.12.001.

Shen, Q., Zhang, Z., Yu, L., Cao, L., Zhou, D., Kan, M., et al. (2011). Common variants near TERC are associated with leukocyte telomere length in the Chinese Han population. *European Journal of Human Genetics*, *19*(6), 721–723. https://doi.org/10.1038/ejhg.2011.4.

Shivappa, N., Wirth, M. D., Hurley, T. G., & Hébert, J. R. (2017). Association between the dietary inflammatory index (DII) and telomere length and C-reactive protein from the National Health and Nutrition Examination Survey-1999-2002. *Molecular Nutrition & Food Research*, *61*(4), 1600630. https://doi.org/10.1002/mnfr.201600630.

Slatter, D. A., Avery, N. C., & Bailey, A. J. (2004). Identification of a new cross-link and unique histidine adduct from bovine serum albumin incubated with malondialdehyde. *Journal of Biological Chemistry*, *279*(1), 61–69. https://doi.org/10.1074/jbc.M310608200.

Slatter, D. A., Bolton, C. H., & Bailey, A. J. (2000). The importance of lipid-derived malondialdehyde in diabetes mellitus. *Diabetologia*, *43*(5), 550–557. https://doi.org/10.1007/s001250051342.

Sofi, F., Macchi, C., Abbate, R., Gensini, G. F., & Casini, A. (2013). Mediterranean diet and health status: An updated meta-analysis and a proposal for a literature-based adherence score. *Public Health Nutrition*, *17*(12), 2769–2782. https://doi.org/10.1017/S1368980013003169.

Song, Y., You, N. C. Y., Song, Y., Kang, M. K., Hou, L., Wallace, R., et al. (2013). Intake of small-to-medium-chain saturated fatty acids is associated with peripheral leukocyte telomere length in postmenopausal women1-3. *Journal of Nutrition*, *143*(6), 907–914. https://doi.org/10.3945/jn.113.175422.

Svenson, U., Nordfjäll, K., Baird, D., Roger, L., Osterman, P., Hellenius, M.-L., et al. (2011). Blood cell telomere length is a dynamic feature. *PLoS ONE*, *6*(6). https://doi.org/10.1371/journal.pone.0021485, e21485.

Tiainen, A. M., Männistö, S., Blomstedt, P. A., Moltchanova, E., Perälä, M. M., Kaartinen, N. E., et al. (2012). Leukocyte telomere length and its relation to food and nutrient intake in an elderly population. *European Journal of Clinical Nutrition*, 66(12), 1290–1294. https://doi.org/10.1038/ejcn.2012.143.

Toupchian, O., Sotoudeh, G., Mansoori, A., Abdollahi, S., Ali Keshavarz, S., Djalali, M., et al. (2018). DHA-enriched fish oil upregulates cyclin-dependent kinase inhibitor 2A (P16 INK) expression and downregulates telomerase activity without modulating effects of PPARγ Pro12Ala polymorphism in type 2 diabetic patients: A randomized, double-blind, placebo-controlled clinical trial. *Clinical Nutrition*, 37(1), 91–98. https://doi.org/10.1016/j.clnu.2016.12.007.

Valdes, A. M., Andrew, T., Gardner, J. P., Kimura, M., Oelsner, E., Cherkas, L. F., et al. (2005). Obesity, cigarette smoking, and telomere length in women. *Lancet*, 366(9486), 662–664. https://doi.org/10.1016/S0140-6736(05)66630-5.

van der Spek, A., Broer, L., Draisma, H. H. M., Pool, R., Albrecht, E., Beekman, M., et al. (2019). Metabolomics reveals a link between homocysteine and lipid metabolism and leukocyte telomere length: the ENGAGE consortium. *Scientific Reports*, 9(1). https://doi.org/10.1038/s41598-019-47282-6.

Vistoli, G., De Maddis, D., Cipak, A., Zarkovic, N., Carini, M., & Aldini, G. (2013). Advanced glycoxidation and lipoxidation end products (AGEs and ALEs): An overview of their mechanisms of formation. *Free Radical Research*, 47(1), 3–27. https://doi.org/10.3109/10715762.2013.815348.

Welendorf, C., Nicoletti, C. F., Pinhel, M. A. D. S., Noronha, N. Y., de Paula, B. M. F., & Nonino, C. B. (2019). Obesity, weight loss, and its influence on telomere length: New insights for personalized nutrition. *Nutrition*, 66, 115–121. https://doi.org/10.1016/j.nut.2019.05.002.

Yeates, A. J., Thurston, S. W., Li, H., Mulhern, M. S., McSorley, E. M., Watson, G. E., et al. (2017). PUFA status and methylmercury exposure are not associated with leukocyte telomere length in mothers or their children in the seychelles child development study. *Journal of Nutrition*, 147(11), 2018–2024. https://doi.org/10.3945/jn.117.253021.

Zhang, J., Rane, G., Dai, X., Shanmugam, M. K., Arfuso, F., Samy, R. P., et al. (2016). Ageing and the telomere connection: An intimate relationship with inflammation. *Ageing Research Reviews*, 25, 55–69. https://doi.org/10.1016/j.arr.2015.11.006.

Zhao, Y., Wang, B., Wang, G., Huang, L., Yin, T., Li, X., et al. (2020). Functional interaction between plasma phospholipid fatty acids and insulin resistance in leukocyte telomere length maintenance. *Lipids in Health and Disease*, 19(1). https://doi.org/10.1186/s12944-020-1194-1.

CHAPTER 3

The role of lipids in the brain

Amal D. Premarathna[a], Anura P. Jayasooriya[b], and Andrew J. Sinclair[c,d]

[a]School of Natural Sciences and Health, Tallinn University, Tallinn, Estonia [b]Department of Basic Veterinary Sciences, Faculty of Veterinary Medicine and Animal Science, University of Peradeniya, Peradeniya, Sri Lanka [c]Department of Nutrition, Dietetics and Food, Monash University, Melbourne, Australia [d]Faculty of Health, Deakin University, Geelong, Australia

3.1 Introduction

3.1.1 Diversity of lipids in the brain

The brain is the most important organ of the human body and is extremely rich in many types of lipids, and with a large diversity of chemical mediators. It has more than 80 billion neurons which interconnect/communicate through electrical signaling and movement of neurotransmitters across synapses (Borroni, Vallés, & Barrantes, 2016; Sinclair, 2019). Critical functions of the brain include analytical capacity, initiation, processing, coordination, interpretation, perception, and emotional behavior of the subject (Fischer & Rose, 1994; Parr & Hopkins, 2000; Schnitzler & Gross, 2005; Watson & Breedlove, 2012).

Lipids represent 50%–60% of the dry weight in the brain, and there is an uneven distribution of lipids throughout the brain regions and cells contributing to dynamic nanodomains (Cermenati et al., 2015; Fujimoto & Parmryd, 2017). The lipids are distributed in gray matter 36%–40% lipid, white matter 49%–66% lipid, and myelin 78%–81% lipid (Aggarwal, Yurlova, & Simons, 2011; O'Brien & Sampson, 1965). All neuronal cell membranes and those in myelin contain cholesterol. The central nervous system consists of 2% of the body mass and yet contains 25% of the cholesterol in the whole body (Vance, Hayashi, & Karten, 2005).

Lipids play a fundamental role in critical structural development of the brain (Bullmore & Sporns, 2009) and regulation of crucial physiological processes of neuronal differentiation, cell proliferation, apoptosis, tissue repair, synaptogenesis, and neurotransmitter dynamics (Kim, Huang, & Spector, 2014; Postila & Róg, 2020; Sinclair, 2019). Generally, lipids contain a huge number of chemically different molecules arising from fatty acid arrangements with various backbone structures ranging from glycerolipids to sphingolipids (Cermenati et al., 2015). It has been estimated that there are more than 11,000 different molecular species of lipids in the human brain

(Li et al., 2017) which are essential for structural and functional activities of neuronal cells. The lipid categories found in the brain include fatty acyls, endocannabinoids, glycerolipids, glycerophospholipids, sphingolipids, sterols, prenol lipids, saccharolipids, and polyketides (Adibhatla & Hatcher, 2007). Among these, some unique lipid types in neuronal membranes deserve mention including phosphatidylserine (PS) rich in docosahexaenoic acid (DHA) (Kim et al., 2014), sphingomyelin rich in hydroxy-fatty acids (Schuette, Pierstorff, Huettler, & Sandhoff, 2001), glycerophospholipids (or phosphoglycerides) rich in DHA and arachidonic acid (AA) (O'Brien & Sampson, 1965), cerebrosides (Cha & Yeung, 2007), sulfatides and gangliosides (Wang, McVeagh, Petocz, & Brand-Miller, 2003). These various lipid types all contribute to the many aspects of brain function and development (Bullmore & Sporns, 2009).

Oligodendrocytes and myelin are extremely rich in sphingolipids: galactosylceramide (GalCer), sphingomyelin, and its sulfated derivate, sulfatide (Buccinnà et al., 2009). Gangliosides are abundant components of the neuronal membranes with up to 10%–12% of the lipid content of the neuronal membrane (Palmano, Rowan, Guillermo, Guan, & McJarrow, 2015). They have been proposed to influence neuronal function including neural tube formation, differentiation, myelin stability, neuronal development, synaptogenesis, and brain maturation (Cant, Del Favero, Sonnino, & Prinetti, 2011; Olsen & Færgeman, 2017; Palmano et al., 2015).

More than 45 years ago, it was reported that brains of more than 32 different mammals were highly enriched in DHA (Crawford, Casperd, & Sinclair, 1976; Sinclair, 1975b) with PS and phosphatidylethanolamine (PE) being the principal repositories for DHA in the brain (Cao, Xue, Xu, & Liu, 2005; Harauma, Salem, & Moriguchi, 2010). It has been shown that PE, PS, and phosphatidylinositol (PI) are frequently confined to the inner leaflet of membranes, while phosphatidylcholine (PC), glycolipids, and sphingomyelin are mainly in the outer membrane leaflet (Ikeda, Kihara, & Igarashi, 2006). In general terms, DHA is predominantly found in the gray matter of the brain where DHA-rich phospholipids have a unique role in the functioning of integral proteins in cell membranes, which in turn allows the optimal function of G-coupled membrane proteins such as receptors, voltage-gated ion channels, and enzymes of which there are many thousands on each of more than 80 billion neural cells. One of the downstream events related to DHA is that optimal neurotransmission could be due in part to brain energy metabolism (facilitation of glucose entry into the brain), which is significantly influenced by neural omega-3 status (Sinclair, 2019). Substantial increases of DHA and AA in the brain occur during the fetal and early postnatal periods, depending on the animal species (Farquharson et al., 1992; Martinez, 1992).

Phosphatidylserine is a unique lipid in the brain where it modulates synaptic receptors and supports neuronal survival and neurite growth (Kim et al., 2014). PS in neural tissue is rich in 18:0-DHA (up to 45%–65% of total PS). Activation of signaling proteins which support neuronal survival, neurite growth, and synaptogenesis, such as Akt, Raf-12, and protein kinase C, requires interactions of these proteins with PS (Kim et al., 2014). Additionally, neural membranes include several other classes of glycerophospholipids, including ethanolamine- and choline-plasmalogens, known as ether lipids. These ether lipids are found in both neuronal and myelin membranes. Recently, the role of plasmalogens in Alzheimer's disease has been reviewed (Su, Wang, & Sinclair, 2019). Brain lipids can influence the function of proteins (enzymes and receptors) in the cell membranes and can thereby regulate synaptic function of neurons (Müller et al., 2015). Additionally, endocannabinoids, sphingolipids, and lysophospholipids have been shown to be involved in cellular signaling and regulation of numerous ion pumps, channels, and transporters (Farooqui, Horrocks, & Farooqui, 2000; Fišar, 2009; Hussain et al., 2019).

Brain membrane lipids can provide necessary channel functions for membrane ion channels and also serve as precursors for various secondary lipid mediators such as 1,2-diacylglycerol (DAG), ceramide, lysophospholipids, and phosphatidic acid (Adibhatla & Hatcher, 2007), and specialized lipid mediators derived from brain polyunsaturated fatty acids (PUFA) such as lipoxins, neuroprotectins, resolvins, and maresins (Chiang & Serhan, 2020; Dyall, 2015).

In myelin, sphingomyelin and galactosphingolipids are important lipids (Grassi et al., 2016; Zöller et al., 2008), the content of which increases during myelin development (Marcus et al., 2006). Brain sphingomyelin contains long-chain saturated, monounsaturated, and hydroxy fatty acids which have important roles in the biological function of myelin and membranes in neurons and oligodendrocytes (Cremesti, Goni, & Kolesnick, 2002). Galactosylceramides and sulfatides in myelin represent around 20% (Poitelon, Kopec, & Belin, 2020). Galactosylceramides in myelin have high content of very long chain saturated and monounsaturated fatty acids. In most tissues, sphingolipids are relatively minor cell membrane lipids in contrast to the brain (Goñi & Alonso, 2006). Sphingolipids typically affect the structural differentiation in cellular membranes, regulate the function of several membrane-associated proteins (Piccinini et al., 2010), and support other important intra- and/or extracellular lipid mediators (Farooqui, 2009). Another feature of brain lipids is the concentration of cerebrosides and their unique fatty acid profile (monounsaturated hydroxy fatty acids); these lipids are especially marked in the cerebrum (Svennerholm & Ställberg-Stenhagen, 1968). Lipid mediators, such as ceramide, can be liberated from cerebrosides by ceramidase and sphingoglycolipids (Farooqui, 2009).

There is a crucial role for inositol phospholipids in brain membranes, including involvement in cell signaling (Giusto, Salvador, Castagnet, Pasquaré, & Ilincheta de Boschero, 2002). This occurs through the hydrolysis of phosphatidylinositol 4,5-bisphosphate by an enzyme of phospholipase C, releasing DAG (Cockcroft, 2009; Ivanova, Milne, Forrester, & Brown, 2004).

The gangliosides in the brain are primarily a group of sialic acid glycosphingolipids found in the plasma membrane of cells and are a significant component of the nervous system (nerve cells, muscle, gland cells, nervous tissues, etc.) (Robert, Tsai, & Ariga, 2012). It has been proposed that these have multiple roles in cell differentiation and proliferation, involved in apoptosis, neurogenesis and neural repair, calcium homeostasis, membrane receptors, and ion channels and the immune system (Robert et al., 2012). The above information shows that lipids in the brain, as found in the neuronal cell membranes and in myelin, are complex and have highly dynamic roles. For a comprehensive and contemporary discourse on measurement of lipids in the brain, readers are referred to Dawson (2015) which discusses a wide range of analytical techniques for measuring brain lipids.

3.1.2 Contrast lipid content and fatty acids in the brain to other tissues

The brain contains the second highest amount of lipids in the body (50%–60% of dry weight) next to the adipose tissue (Veloso et al., 2011); in adipose, 60%–85% of the weight is lipid, with 90%–99% being triglycerides, together with small amounts of free fatty acids, diglycerides, cholesterol, phospholipids, cholesterol esters, and monoglycerides (Langin, 2011). The fatty acid composition of adipose tissue reflects the dietary fatty acid intake in both humans and animals (Hodson, Skeaff, & Fielding, 2008); however, this is not true for the brain

(Crawford et al., 1976). In particular, it was found that the fatty acid composition of the liver and muscle varied significantly between many different mammalian species, presumably reflecting diet differences. However, the fatty acid composition of the brain was very similar between species, being characterized by high levels of AA and DHA and low levels of linoleic and linolenic acids (Crawford et al., 1976).

3.1.3 Lipids in different brain anatomical regions and cell types

The brain is comprised of many different regions, including the cerebrum or telencephalon, corpus callosum, thalamus, hypothalamus, hippocampus, cerebellum, basal ganglia, medulla oblongata, and the spinal cord, which all have specialized functions (Evans & Miller, 1993).

With the growing evidence for the critical role of lipids in brain function (Korade & Kenworthy, 2008), there are now a number of publications on the brain's lipidome composition (Bozek et al., 2015; Li et al., 2017; Rappley et al., 2009), lipidome differences between the brain and the other tissues (Bozek et al., 2015), and the lipid concentration differences among brain regions (Carrié, Clément, De Javel, Francès, & Bourre, 2000; Fraser, Tayler, & Love, 2010). Recently, Li et al. (2017) compared the lipidomic profiles in the human, chimpanzee, and macaque prefrontal cortex regions. They reported that 7589 lipid peaks showed significant changes across the life span in all three species, with more than 60% of these taking place in the first 20 y of life. They claimed to be able to predict the age of the individuals based on specific lipid markers, which in particular included polyprenols. Of all the lipid markers, polyprenols, including dolichol showed the greatest change between infants and adults. It was of interest that there were significant numbers of lipids that were found to distinguish between humans ($n = 54$ lipid peaks) and the other two species. The rate of change in the lipidome composition in human infants was approximately six times greater than in adults (aged between 20 and 60 years), with about 15% of the change in the first years being attributed to myelin-related lipids. Furthermore, there were 1824 lipids which showed concentration differences between humans and chimpanzees, and 3324 lipids which differed in concentration between humans and macaques. The first 10 years of human age was the period when these species differences were most evident. Zhang, Appelkvist, Kristensson, and Dallner (1996) studied changes in rat brain lipids (cerebral cortex, striatum, hippocampus, cerebellum, and brain stem) during development and aging. They reported substantial increases in total phospholipid, cholesterol, ubiquinone, dolichol, and vitamin E from birth to 60 days, followed by a stabilization or gradual increase in levels of some of these lipids until the age of 25 months. Most dramatically, dolichol increased in all brain regions and up to 100-fold from birth until 25 months. In contrast, ubiquinone increased significantly from birth and then stabilized after 50 days.

PUFA play a major role in the functioning of the brain during different life stages (Bazinet & Layé, 2014). Diau et al. (2005) conducted a systematic evaluation of the DHA and AA proportions in 26 regions of the brain of 40-week-old baboons. The highest concentrations of DHA and AA were in gray matter such as basal ganglia. The % DHA (of total FA) ranged from 15.8 (globus pallidus) to 4.5 (optic nerve), while the % AA (of total FA) ranged from 13.7 (amygdala) to 6.8 (optic tract). In rats, the level of PUFA (DHA, etc.) was found to be slightly higher in the frontal cortex than in the striatum, which could make the frontal cortex more sensitive to n-3 PUFA deficiency (Favrelière, Barrier, Durand, Chalon, & Tallineau, 1998). A recent study of the molecular species in different glycerophospholipids in the retina and six brain regions in C57Bl6 mice at 3 different ages showed that DHA-containing species decreased with age, and that all brain regions except the hippocampus showed an increased content of ethanolamine plasmalogens with age. Furthermore, the retina, but not the brain, contained high proportions of di-PUFA species with PS having as much as 30% (di-DHA). Very long chain PUFAs (>C24) were found in the retina (PC fraction), but not in the brain (Hopiavuori et al., 2017).

While it is true that the brain has many different cell types including neurons, astrocytes, glial cells, oligodendrocytes, ependymal cells, microglia, satellite cells, and Schwann cells, there have been few systematic studies aimed at determining similarities and differences in the lipid classes between different cells within the brain. Overall, brain cells are rich in lipids, with isolated rat neurons having 24% lipid on dry weight basis and astrocytes 39% (Norton & Poduslo, 1973); furthermore, cholesterol, dolichol, and ubiquinone were present in all regions of the brain (Runquist, Parmryd, Thelin, Chojnacki, & Dallner, 1995; Söderberg, Edlund, Kristensson, & Dallner, 1990; Zhang et al., 1996). Most of the cholesterol (70%–80%) in the brain is found in myelin, but cholesterol is also present in neurons and astrocytes (Vance et al., 2005). Myelin and glial cells (oligodendrocytes, etc.) are enriched in galactolipids and in sphingomyelin (Jackman, Ishii, & Bansal, 2009). However, astrocytes are characterized by a lower sphingolipid content and by the presence of a simpler glycolipid profile (Norton & Poduslo, 1973). It has been reported that cholesterol and ganglioside levels were decreased in the cell membranes of aged neurons (Ledesma, Martin, & Dotti, 2012). It is likely that new information on the lipid content and lipid molecular species will be revealed as research progresses by characterizing the lipids in thin slices of brain sections.

3.1.4 Mapping lipids in the brain using mass spectrometry techniques

The mammalian brain lipidome includes more than 10,000 individual species of lipid molecules which originate from the sphingolipids, phospholipids, glycolipids, and neutral lipids (Sparvero et al., 2012). The identification of lipid molecular species relies on the efficient extraction of lipids prior to their analysis by mass spectrometry (MS) and/or HPLC-MS (Cajka & Fiehn, 2014), which can provide precise data on the abundance of the different molecular species (Fauland et al., 2011). The complexity and vast number of lipid molecules can be determined by mass spectrometry technique on slices, enabling lipidomic analysis in different areas of the brain (Chan et al., 2009; Dawson, 2015; Li et al., 2017; Sparvero et al., 2012). In brain tissue, lipids detectable by using thin slices can be seen by quantitative autoradiography using 14C-AA or 14C-DHA (Basselin, Ramadan, & Rapoport, 2012). These and other techniques have been used to map and identify multiple lipids from brain tissue slices (Chen, Hui, Sturm, & Li, 2009). Recently, matrix-assisted laser desorption/ionization (MALDI) imaging mass spectrometry (IMS) has permitted scanning tissue slices to determine the distribution of lipids and metabolites in tissues (Akiko, Mayumi, & Makoto, 2012; Sparvero et al., 2012; Woods & Jackson, 2006). This technique consists of obtaining slices of $\sim$10–20 µm of a tissue, covering them with an appropriate MALDI matrix, and the resulting images represent separately spatial distribution and relative abundance of that particular lipid ion, which can be correlated with histological features (Norris & Caprioli, 2013). Using MALDI-TOF imaging mass spectrometry of the human frontal cortex, some lipids, such as PC 32:0 and PC 30:0, were present at a higher abundance in gray matter, while others such as phosphatidylglycerol (PG) 36:1, PC 36:0, PE 34:1, PE 40:4, and SM 42:2 were more abundant in white matter. In addition, this study provided detailed analysis of the distribution of many lipid species present in the human hippocampus in both gray and white matter (Veloso et al., 2011). MALDI-IMS has revealed the distribution of sulfatide molecular species in the human brain; these can contain both hydroxy- and nonhydroxy fatty acids, and they reported that the hydroxylated sulfatide species predominated in gray matter (Yuki et al., 2011). This technique has been used to study cerebrosides, which are highly abundant in myelin membranes (Stoffel & Bosio, 1997). Sparvero et al. (2012) showed a significant increase in the signal in the rat brain (partly from PS 18:0–22:6) using MALDI-MSI after 3 days of i.p. injections of DHA. It is also possible to map lipids in the brain using mass-spectral 3D imaging where it has been revealed that PC and sphingomyelin species were localized according to specific patterns in crustacean brain, suggesting structure function roles for different lipid species (Chen et al., 2009).

3.2 Properties of brain fatty acids

3.2.1 Saturated fatty acids and unsaturated fatty acids affect the brain and health

The general outcome of the many research studies reveals that saturated fats are less beneficial for health than unsaturated fatty acids (Lovejoy et al., 2002). Natural foods have variable lipid profiles - saturated fatty acids are found in high proportions in meat and dairy products (Scollan et al., 2006), and unsaturated fatty acids are more common in vegetables and fruits (Agudo & Pera, 1999). However, saturated and unsaturated fatty acids modulate brain function and metabolism by mechanisms that have not been fully elucidated (Bazinet & Layé, 2014). Some studies have suggested that saturated fatty acids might lead to reductions in cognitive abilities (Gomez-Pinilla, 2011; Wu, Ying, & Gomez-Pinilla, 2004); however, the exact mechanisms to account for these effects have not been revealed (Uauy, Hoffman, Peirano, Birch, & Birch, 2001).

3.2.2 The n-3 polyunsaturated fatty acids (PUFAs) and n-6 PUFA in the brain

The omega-6 polyunsaturated fatty acids (n-6 PUFAs) and omega-3 polyunsaturated fatty acids (n-3 PUFAs) account for 25%–30% of total brain fatty acids, and they are reported to be required for optimal performance of biochemical and physiological brain function and integrity (Chang, Ke, & Chen, 2009; Sinclair, 2019). In mammals, the 18-carbon short-chain n-6 and n-3 PUFAs cannot be synthesized de novo by humans or animals, and they must be obtained from food to supply the needs of the brain through the plasma (Neuringer & Connor, 1986). Dietary PUFAs such as α-linolenic acid (ALA; 18:3 n-3) and linoleic acid (LA; 18:2 n-6) are converted into long-chain PUFAs, DHA, and AA, respectively, in the liver prior to transport to the brain (Rapoport & Igarashi, 2009). The brain has low concentrations of ALA, LA, and eicosapentaenoic acid (EPA, C20:5 n-3) compared with high concentrations of AA, docosatetraenoic acid 22:4n-6, and DHA (Chen & Bazinet, 2015; Sinclair, 1975b).

3.2.3 Docosahexaenoic acid has multiple functions in the brain

The role of DHA in the brain and retina was recently reviewed by Sinclair (Sinclair, 2019). It is interesting that in DHA deficiency studies (resulting from dietary depletion of ALA), the animals showed reduced levels of DHA in cell membranes which is nearly quantitatively replaced by a 22-carbon omega-6 PUFA, docosapentaenoic acid (C22:5n-6) (Galli, Trzeciak, & Paoletti, 1971; Mohrhauer & Holman, 1963). This replacement PUFA (22:5n-6) has similar, but less potent, biophysical, and physiological properties to DHA. It has been suggested that omega-6 docosapentaenoic acid might be a buffer to prevent the damaging effects of DHA depletion on brain and visual function (Sinclair, 2019). The results from animal and cellular studies indicate that reduced DHA levels in brain phospholipids (and replacement by omega-6 docosapentaenoic acid) affect the flexibility/compression of the membrane lipids, which has a fundamental influence on the optimal function of integral membrane proteins (receptors, voltage-gated ion channels, and enzymes) (Seebungkert & Lynch, 2002). This impacts various second messenger systems, and from that alters neurotransmitter concentrations due to "weakened" signals from the initiating receptors. Since there are more than 80 billion neurons and many times more synaptic connections between neurons, a very small loss of "efficiency" in signal due to altered properties of membrane proteins is likely to result in meaningful changes in brain and visual function. One of the downstream effects that could also contribute to an impairment of neurotransmission might be due to suboptimal brain energy metabolism (glucose entry into the brain), which is significantly reduced in omega-3 deficiency (Da Silva et al., 2002). In terms of global effects of significantly reduced brain DHA levels resulting from dietary deficiency of n-3 fatty acids, significant changes have been observed in learning, coping with stress, behavior, responses to visual function, auditory function, and olfactory function (Sinclair, 2019).

3.2.4 Docosapentaenoic acid (n-3 DPA; 22:5n-3) and the brain

From the very early gas chromatography studies on the brain, n-3 DPA was reported in human gray and white matter glycerophospholipids (O'Brien & Sampson, 1965; Svennerholm, 1968), and brain gray matter of a wide variety of ruminant and nonruminant species from Africa (Crawford et al., 1976). The level of n-3 DPA in the brain is typically 1%–2% of total fatty acids and is more abundant than EPA. It is now clear that blood and tissue levels of n-3 DPA give no indication of its broad biological role. Specialized lipid mediators (SPMs) such as resolvins, maresins, and protectins of the n-3 DPA type are involved in resolution of inflammation and regulating immune function. The true functionality of this enigmatic n-3 fatty acid remains obscure until more is known about the properties of the unique n-3 DPA-derived SPMs (Ghasemi Fard, Cameron-Smith, & Sinclair, 2021). Two studies reveal that n-3 DPA plays a role in aging and epilepsy. Kelly et al. (2011) examined whether n-3 DPA could modulate the age-related increases in microglial activation and the associated increase in oxidative changes and therefore impact on synaptic function in aged rats. Both n-3 DPA and EPA downregulated microglial activation and decreased the activation of sphingomyelinase and caspase 3, and consequently attenuated the age-related decrease in spatial learning and long-term potentiation. DPA levels increased in cortical tissue of young and aged rats with both n-3 DPA and EPA. The authors concluded these data demonstrated a neuroprotective effect for n-3 DPA similar to that of EPA, perhaps through antioxidative effects. In terms of epilepsy, Frigerio et al. (2018) reported that intracerebroventricular injection of protectin PD1-n-3 DPA reduced the epilepsy severity (3-fold reduction of seizure time) in a mouse model. This was accompanied by significant improvements in body weight and recovery from a cognitive deficit, relative to placebo.

3.2.5 Arachidonic acid has multiple functions in the brain

AA is the second most abundant PUFA in the brain (Youdim, Martin, & Joseph, 2000), and it cannot be synthesized de novo. AA is found in the flesh of lean red meat and human milk, chicken, and egg yolk (Komprda, Zelenka, Fajmonova, Fialova, & Kladroba, 2005; Li, Ng, Mann, & Sinclair, 1998). The role of AA in the brain has been less extensively studied than that of DHA (Brenna & Diau, 2007; Schmitz & Ecker, 2008). In the case of DHA, it is possible to create a dietary deficiency of omega-3 fatty acids which leads to reductions in tissue and brain DHA levels. While it is possible to create a dietary omega-6 deficiency by restricting linoleic acid in the diet where this leads to loss of AA in tissues, this paradigm has rarely been studied (Belza, Anderson, Ryan, & Cunnane, 1999). During the last trimester of pregnancy, AA starts to rapidly accumulate in the infant's brain and continues to accumulate in the early years of life (until 2 years) (Innis et al., 2002; Martinez, 1992). AA is also a precursor for adrenic acid (22:4n-6) which might be necessary for myelin (structure and/or function) during the early postnatal period in infants (Wijendran et al., 2002).

While the effect of omega-3 PUFA deficiency on neural function has been extensively characterized in rodents and primates (Sinclair, 2019), there has been far less research on the role of AA in the brain, mainly because it is difficult to deplete brain AA levels through dietary deficiency studies. An example of the effect of simultaneous reductions of brain AA and DHA levels resulting from the use of delta-6 KO mice showed that the delta-6 KO mice had a significantly reduced performance in behavioral function tests. These mice were fed supplements of DHA, AA, and a combination of both, and the best performing groups were those fed DHA alone and DHA plus AA (Harauma et al., 2017). These data support the importance of balanced levels of AA and DHA in the brain. AA and DHA imbalances are known to occur with the use of high doses of fish oil which can reduce tissue and brain AA levels and also with omega-3 PUFA deficiency, which can elevate neural omega-6 PUFA and reduce DHA levels.

Clearly, brain AA is important structurally and also as a precursor of a wide range of oxygenated PUFA derivatives known as eicosanoids (prostaglandins, thromboxanes, lipoxins, leukotrienes, hydroxyeicosatetraenoic, and epoxyeicosatetraenoic acids) which are locally acting hormone-like compounds (Chiang & Serhan, 2020) and which play critical roles in many aspects of neural function including a role in sleep (PGD_2) (Onoe et al., 1988) and short- and long-term memory and spatial learning (in rats) (Chang et al., 2009; Schaeffer & Gattaz, 2005). Readers are referred to a publication which reviews the impacts on brain physiology and metabolism in genetically altered mice in whom various AA metabolizing enzymes have been deleted (Bosetti, Weerasinghe, Rosenberger, & Rapoport, 2003). There has been a sustained interest in lipoxin modulation of the proinflammatory responses in neural tissue with recent research suggesting analogs of lipoxin A4 might be even more potent in terms of inhibiting synthesis of pro-inflammatory cytokines, which increase the anti-inflammatory cytokines (Tułowiecka, Kotlęga, Bohatyrewicz, & Szczuko, 2021). Additional and critical neural functions of AA are the endocannabinoids (2-arachidonoyl-glycerol and anandamide), which are lipid messengers involved in fine-tuning of synaptic function (Duffy, Hayes, Fiore, & Moalem-Taylor, 2021); in addition, sn-1-stearoyl-2-arachidonoyl-glycerol, derived from phosphoinositides, is an important signal transduction molecule in the brain (Rusciano et al., 2021). On the other side of the ledger, neuroinflammation plays an important role in several neurodegenerative disorders and "hypermetabolism" of AA has been implicated. This remains a controversial area (Gorica & Calderone, 2021), though the following examples suggest there are indications of exaggerated metabolism of neural AA by COX-2 to PGE_2 in mood disorders (Basselin, Villacreses, Lee, Bell, & Rapoport, 2007; Bazinet, Rao, Chang, Rapoport, & Lee, 2006; Bosetti et al., 2003), and also in omega-3 deficiency (Begg, Sinclair, & Weisinger, 2012). However, it is clear that more systematic studies of AA in the brain might help to understand how this fatty acid contributes to brain development and function in human health.

3.3 Where are brain lipids synthesized? In the brain or imported from blood?

3.3.1 Brain lipids synthesized and uptake from blood into brain

Neurons and glial cells cannot perform the desaturation of shorter chain fatty acids, such as ALA, which is necessary for the synthesis of DHA (Zhang et al., 2011). However, astrocytes have been shown to synthesize DHA, but this was limited and apparently held up at the steps in the conversion of DPA to DHA (Innis & Dyer, 2002). Therefore, for DHA to be incorporated into the brain, it must originate from dietary sources (such as marine foods) or be synthesized in the liver from ALA (Rapoport, Rao, & Igarashi, 2007; Spector, 2001). There is still debate about which lipoproteins are the preferred carriers of DHA in the plasma to the brain: FFA bound to albumin, lysophospholipids containing DHA (1-lyso-2-DHA-phosphatidylcholine), or phospholipids found in plasma lipoproteins (Bazinet, Bernoud-Hubac, & Lagarde, 2019; Hachem et al., 2016; Sugasini, Thomas, Yalagala, Tai, & Subbaiah, 2017). In other words, DHA may be obtained directly from the diet or synthesized in the liver and then transported to the brain to maintain the cerebral DHA levels (Rapoport & Igarashi, 2009). It is of great interest that a transporter expressed on the blood brain barrier has been shown to be an important carrier of 1-lyso-2-DHA-phosphatidylcholine into the brain (Nguyen et al., 2014); the same authors described three families with defects in this transporter and those individuals with the mutation showed severe microcephaly and intellectual disability (Alakbarzade et al., 2015; Guemez-Gamboa et al., 2015).

There are some in *vitro* studies which show that some brain cells can synthesize DHA from n-3 PUFA precursors, primarily in astrocytes, and that these cells supply some of the newly formed DHA to the neurons and blood-brain barrier endothelium (Moore, 2001; SanGiovanni & Chew, 2005). It is also possible that endothelial cells in the brain may play a role in the synthesis of PUFA and in the specific delivery of DHA to the brain (Chen & Subbaiah, 2007; Qi, Hall, & Deckelbaum, 2002). There are no studies which have considered the relative uptake of PUFA from the blood into the brain compared with endogenous synthesis in some brain cells, although most believe the supply is mainly from blood lipids. Brain cholesterol levels are strictly controlled and brain cholesterol is almost exclusively derived from in situ synthesis as there is no evidence for the transfer of cholesterol from blood plasma to the brain (Chattopadhyay & Paila, 2007). While neurons can only synthesize a little cholesterol themselves, it has been proposed that they mostly rely on cholesterol-containing lipoproteins secreted by astrocytes (Pfrieger, 2003).

3.3.2 Fatty acid transport and metabolism of 14C-labeled polyunsaturated fatty acids in the developing brain

In-vivo experiments in suckling rat pups investigated the incorporation of radioactivity from orally administered LA, ALA, AA, and DHA into brain lipids (Sinclair, 1975a). It was revealed that AA and DHA were rapidly incorporated intact into the brain lipids, in contrast to LA and ALA which were significantly degraded with much of the 14C-label being found in saturated and monounsaturated fatty acids in the brain. This suggests extensive beta-oxidation of these 18-carbon fatty acids to acetate (acetyl-CoA) followed by synthesis of saturated and monounsaturated fatty acids. Later studies by Rapoport and Bazinet using labeled fatty acids via intracerebroventricular infusion confirmed that LA and EPA were rapidly beta-oxidized in the brain compared with DHA which was mainly incorporated into brain phospholipids (Chen & Bazinet, 2015). Data showed as brain growth increased so did myelination, and this was associated with increases in the major saturated and monounsaturated fatty acids in brain lipids (Deoni et al., 2011; Edmond, Higa, Korsak, Bergner, & Lee, 1998; Sinclair & Crawford, 1972); these fatty acids are almost exclusively produced locally by de novo biosynthesis (Cunnane et al., 2003; Menard, Goodman, Corso, Brenna, & Cunnane, 1998). It appears that sphingomyelin and cerebrosides are synthesized by two distinctive metabolic pathways. However, the systems for their fatty acid chain elongation must either be the same or similar to account for the similarities in their fatty acid compositions (Dhopeshwarkar & Mead, 1973). It would appear that the brain can make ceramide endogenously by biosynthetic pathways, as well as by hydrolysis of cerebroside and sphingomyelin (Kopaczyk & Radin, 1965; Lipsky & Pagano, 1983).

In essential fatty acid deficiency, there are losses of LA and AA in tissues including the brain; it is known that in these circumstances, that a novel unsaturated fatty acid is synthesized from oleic acid which yields a 20-carbon acid with the structure all-cis-5, 8, 11, eicosatrienoic acid in place of AA (Mohrhauer & Holman, 1963). This fatty acid is not normally present in tissues, and its accumulation provides a biochemical diagnosis of the occurrence and extent of essential fatty acid deficiency (Bourre, 2004). Since it is generally regarded that PUFAs cannot be synthesized de novo in brain tissue, it is assumed that the 5, 8, 11, eicosatrienoic acid is synthesized in the liver and transported to the brain via plasma lipids (Galli et al., 1971; Rapoport & Igarashi, 2009).

3.4 Effects of exogenous/dietary agents on brain lipids

3.4.1 Ethanol

Ethanol can cause significant brain damage (Tapert, Caldwell, & Burke, 2004), through effects on structural elements resulting in the malfunction of the brain (De La Monte & Kril, 2014). Heavy alcohol consumption can also lead to hepatic cirrhosis and result in nutritional deficiency that could lead to severe brain damage and dysfunction (Harper, 2009). Effects of ethanol consumption include altering the metabolism of certain brain fatty acids and evidence of lipid peroxidation (Kogure, Watson, Busto, & Abe, 1982). Chronic ethanol exposure in animal experiments has been shown to reduce levels of docosahexanoic acid (DHA; 22:6n-3) in the brain and increase levels of omega-6 docosapentaenoic acid (DPAn-6) (Pawlosky & Salem, 1995; Weiser, Wynalda, Salem, & Butt, 2015). These changes have been proposed to alter nervous system function (Pawlosky, Bacher, & Salem, 2001). The main omega-6 fatty acid in the brain, AA, was not changed in these animal studies. It has been shown that additional DHA did not reduce the impact of ethanol on brain inflammation and neurodegeneration in rats (Olsson, Shoaf, & Salem, 1998).

Brain mitochondrial membranes contain large amounts of lipids which play an essential role in the cellular activity in the brain (Federico et al., 2012). Moreover, high concentrations of ethanol (ethanol toxicity) have been proposed to interrupt mitochondrial ATP production, induce changes in fatty acid metabolism, and alterations of mtDNA (Begriche, Massart, Robin, Borgne-Sanchez, & Fromenty, 2011; Hoek, Cahill, & Pastorino, 2002). Ethanol can inhibit enzymes and interfere with the acute fluidizing effect of the plasma membranes of brain synaptosomes and erythrocytes (Crews, Majchrowicz, & Meeks, 1983; Sun & Sun, 1985). These data suggest that ethanol intake

3.4.2 Cholesterol and saturated fat-enriched diets

High intakes of cholesterol and/or saturated fats may have negative effects on normal brain functioning. Diets rich in saturated fats have been shown to decrease levels of brain-derived neurotrophic factor (BDNF), neuroplasticity, and cognitive performance (Molteni, Barnard, Ying, Roberts, & Gómez-Pinilla, 2002), increase inflammation in the hypothalamus (Valdearcos et al., 2014), and aggravate the outcome of traumatic brain injury (Wu, Molteni, Ying, & Gomez-Pinilla, 2003). However, the mechanisms by which saturated fats affect BDNF expression are basically unknown (Gomez-Pinilla, 2008). Furthermore, saturated fat consumption is associated with an increased risk for chronic "metabolic inflammation," marked by macrophage accumulation (Lichtenstein et al., 2010). Saturated fatty acids also influence the control of food intake, thermogenesis, and intermediary metabolism (Khan & Vanden Heuvel, 2003). Recent studies emphasize that changes in plasma lipids induced by chronic consumption of saturated fatty acids were associated with parallel changes in cerebral lipid homeostasis (Giles et al., 2016). Some evidence indicates that a high fat diet rich in saturated fats can lead to obesity with a resultant increase in lipid peroxidation (Beltowski, Wojcicka, Gorny, & Marciniak, 2000), which can result in adverse effects on neuronal function and cognition (Granholm et al., 2008; Wu et al., 2004). Additionally, the long-term consumption of a saturated fat-enriched diet results in changes in the brain lipidome (Giles et al., 2016) and learning ability (Yu et al., 2010).

Cholesterol imbalance in the brain has been associated with a range of neurodegenerative disorders including vascular dementia, Alzheimer's disease, and Huntington's disease (Puglielli, Tanzi, & Kovacs, 2003; Valenza & Cattaneo, 2006). Furthermore, blood vessel damage deprives brain cells of oxygen and nutrients, leading to error messages in the recycling of sterols and altering the expression of apolipoprotein E in the brain, which can result in harmful effects on neuronal cells (Ikonen, 2006). However, the biological mechanisms for the consequences of a diet rich in cholesterol and/or saturated fatty acids in the expression or suppression of brain markers are not well understood (Granholm et al., 2008).

3.4.3 Reactive oxygen species (ROS) and lipid peroxidation

Reactive oxygen species (ROS) cause oxidative damage to lipids and other substances such as nucleic acids, proteins, and carbohydrates (Blokhina, Virolainen, & Fagerstedt, 2003; Mariani, Polidori, Cherubini, & Mecocci, 2005). In the brain, oxidative stress leads to lipid peroxidation since the membranes are rich in PUFA (Yang et al., 2019). The brain processes consume large amounts of oxygen for energy production and have lower antioxidant defenses compared to other organs (Halliwell, 1996). ROS are produced during regular cellular metabolic functions, including superoxide anion radicals and hydrogen peroxide (Bergamini, Gambetti, Dondi, & Cervellati, 2004). ROS are involved in oxidative phosphorylation in several ways, such as the mitochondrial respiratory chain, xanthine oxidase, monoamine oxidase, and NAD(P)H oxidases (Nickel, Kohlhaas, & Maack, 2014; Siraki, Pourahmad, Chan, Khan, & O'Brien, 2002).

Lipid peroxidation can increase levels of reactive α, β-unsaturated aldehydes (malondialdehyde, 4-hydroxynonenal, and acrolein) (Catalá, 2009; Negre-Salvayre, Coatrieux, Ingueneau, & Salvayre, 2008). These groups have highly specific reactivity by covalently binding to protein thiol groups and altering their function (Furuhata, Nakamura, Osawa, & Uchida, 2002). Increased production of ROS reduces the antioxidant defenses, and there is evidence that oxidation damages brain cells and leads to failure in physiological function (Rose et al., 2012; Wu, Kosten, & Zhang, 2013). It has been reported that oxidative changes in the brain are associated with diseases such as Parkinson's disease, Alzheimer's disease, Huntington's disease, and amyotrophic lateral sclerosis (Mariani et al., 2005; Perry, Cash, & Smith, 2002). In these conditions, the lipid peroxidation in the brain membrane might change the brain's chemical composition and create toxic messengers, such as 4-hydroxynonenal (Gaschler & Stockwell, 2017). Interpretation of data from lipid peroxidation on brain lipids from in vivo and in vitro studies is extremely complicated, and clear molecular mechanisms of action in brain disorders are still to be discovered.

3.4.4 Effects of traumatic brain injury

Traumatic brain injury (TBI) is a major problem worldwide, and it results in major long-term consequences (James et al., 2019). The causes of TBI are various and include traffic accidents, falls, assaults, sporting injuries, and military combat. In the last decade, researchers have turned their attention to lipid biomarkers of TBI using a variety of lipidomic techniques, as reviewed recently by Nessel and Michael-Titus (2020). These researchers concluded that it is still very early days in this research and the hope is that a suite of lipid biomarkers reflecting different cell types in the brain could become useful in improved patient stratification in TBI. An example of the complexity of these studies is revealed by the findings from a mass spectrometry imaging study in a TBI model in rats where there were increases in DHA and lyso-phosphatidylethanolamine (22:6) in the injury area in the acute stage which subsequently decreased (Guo et al., 2017). However, there were opposing results for the levels of phosphatidylethanolamine (PE-P-18:0/22:6), (PE-18:0/22:6), and phosphatidylserine (18:0/22:6) which decreased and then increased in the chronic phase.

3.4.5 Effects of plasticizers and microparticulate plastics on brain function

Di-2-ethylhexyl phthalate (DEHP), dibutyl phthalate (DBP), and butyl-benzyl-phthalate (BBP) are extensively used as plasticizers in many products (Castle, Mercer, Startin, & Gilbert, 1988; Kawakami, Isama, & Matsuoka, 2011). Some phthalates are of great concern due to their putative adverse effects on humans and ubiquitous presence in the environment (Latini, Scoditti, Verrotti, De Felice, & Massaro, 2008). DEHP, as an example of the most widely used, is a peroxisome proliferator, which can activate the peroxisome proliferator-activated receptor (PPAR) (Lee et al., 1995) and induce a broad spectrum of responses such as cell proliferation, effects on apoptosis, and alterations in the metabolism of fatty acids (Corton, Anderson, & Stauber, 2000; Hurst & Waxman, 2003). The issue is broader than just DEHP since there are many different types of phthalates which have similar effects on metabolic function (Frederiksen, Skakkebæk, & Andersson, 2007). Some of these compounds are suspected of being endocrine disruptors and capable of affecting the reproduction of humans and animals (Casals-Casas & Desvergne, 2011; Kabir, Rahman, & Rahman, 2015). It has been reported that DEHP exposure is associated with altered fetal brain lipid composition, which may be an indicator of altered fetal neurodevelopment (Xu, Agrawal, Cook, & Knipp, 2007). Other research has reported decreased fatty acid uptake and transport of AA and DHA from maternal to fetal tissues, including the fetal brain, in an in vivo model after exposure to DEHP (Xu, Agrawal, Cook, & Knipp, 2008). It has been shown that DEHP is found in food products such as meat and lipid-rich foods, including fats and dairy products (Serrano, Braun, Trasande, Dills, & Sathyanarayana,

2014). DBP and diethyl phthalate (DEP) are widely used phthalates in medicinal products (Hill, Shaw, & Wu, 2001; Thomas, Thomas, & Gangolli, 1984). DEHP exposure might lead to metabolic disturbances, such as effects on the lipidome in the fetal brain, and this might have subsequent effects on brain function (Rowdhwal & Chen, 2018).

Thyroid hormones (THs) have a direct effect on metabolic activity in the body, including influencing enzyme activities related to the formation of myelin lipids (Walravens & Chase, 1969); it has been suggested that these hormones might determine the level of brain lipids in the developing brain. It is possible that DEHP can disturb the thyroid system and reduce the TH levels (triiodothyronine, thyroxine, and thyrotropin-releasing hormone) (Ye et al., 2017). Furthermore, endocrine-disrupting chemicals can produce complex effects on TH signaling in the brain (Miller, Crofton, Rice, & Zoeller, 2009). Based on a number of studies, some plasticizers might have effects on several metabolic processes and biological activities in the intact organism (Waring & Harris, 2005).

Microparticulate plastic is an ever-increasing issue in the marine environment with concerns being expressed about the impact of these on human health, including brain function (Banerjee & Shelver, 2021; Miller, Hamann, & Kroon, 2020; Prüst, Meijer, & Westerink, 2020; Sana, Dogiparthi, Gangadhar, Chakravorty, & Abhishek, 2020). While it is too early to discuss whether microparticulate plastics impact brain lipids in mammals, two studies have reported effects on brain damage and learning ability in fish (Chen et al., 2020; Mattsson et al., 2017). Additional studies are warranted to investigate the metabolic mechanism(s) of these phthalates on brain lipid profiles and microparticulates as these relate to neural function and development.

A recent report has highlighted that there is a significant direct release of microplastics from polypropylene feeding bottles during the preparation of infant formulas (Li et al., 2020). This study looked at microplastics following WHO guidelines for the preparation of infant formulas and found the microplastic levels to be 3- to 5-orders of magnitude greater than acceptable levels. This, together with the microparticulate plastic which contaminates the food supply through the water and the marine environment, gives cause for concern and further monitoring and action is required.

3.4.6 Methyl mercury (MeHg) on brain lipids

Methyl mercury (MeHg) is widely prevalent in the 21st century due to anthropogenic activities and acid rain (Wong, Duzgoren-Aydin, Aydin, & Wong, 2006). Human industrial works have led to scattering and bio-accumulation of MeHg in the ecosystem, particularly in the aquatic food cycle (Jackson, 1997). MeHg is regarded as a stable compound in the body (Syversen, 1974), distributed in all tissues including the brain, and it has been implicated as a mutagen, a neurotoxicant, and a teratogen in biologic organisms (Carroquino, Posada, & Landrigan, 2012). MeHg is associated with a variety of deleterious effects on health such as the blood/brain barrier (Aschner & Aschner, 1990), effect on receptor cells of sensory nerves (Castoldi, Coccini, Ceccatelli, & Manzo, 2001), cerebral palsy, mental retardation (Holmes, James, & Levy, 2009), connection with brain macromolecules, and various other effects on the central nervous system (Carocci, Rovito, Sinicropi, & Genchi, 2014). However, while MeHg is present in low amounts in the brain, its distribution is fairly uniform throughout the central nervous system (Choi, 1991; Hansen, Reske-Nielsen, Thorlacius-Ussing, Rungby, & Danscher, 1989). Mercury can induce changes in lipid profile/fatty acid, cholesterol production (Bano & Hasan, 1989), and in brain lipid peroxidation and cellular damage (El-Demerdash, 2001).

The particular sensitivity of the brain as a result of MeHg toxicity could be due to increased levels of lipid peroxidation compared with other organs (Yin et al., 2007). Lipid peroxidation has been detected in the brain as a result of MeHg poisoning, and it may be the initial neurotoxic effect in mammals (Yee & Choi, 1996). Hg^{2+} may be involved in mitochondrial electron transport processes by stimulating the lipid peroxidative stress and formation of free radicals (Roos, Seeger, Puntel, & Vargas Barbosa, 2012). Lipid oxidation of membrane lipids can affect the function of cellular/organelle membrane integrity, which may result in structural damage in cells, cell death, regional brain pathology injury, and disturbed sensory behavior (Girotti, 1998; Silva & Coutinho, 1972). Additionally, the results of several studies revealed that MeHg toxic effects can alter enzymes containing active sulfhydryl groups (Magour, 1986), such as with Na+/K+- ATPase, which has a major role in neuronal function (Sinclair, 2019).

3.5 Conclusions

It has been known for more than 136 years that the brain is rich in lipids (Thudichum, 1884). Recent developments in highly sensitive methods for analysis of complex lipid species have enabled significant progress in understanding of the localization of more than 10,000 lipid molecular species. The field is wide open for scientists from different disciplines to work together in unraveling the roles of these important biological molecules in the most complex organ in the body.

References

Adibhatla, R. M., & Hatcher, J. F. (2007). Role of lipids in brain injury and diseases. *Future Lipidology*, 2(4), 403–422. https://doi.org/10.2217/17460875.2.4.403.

Aggarwal, S., Yurlova, L., & Simons, M. (2011). Central nervous system myelin: Structure, synthesis and assembly. *Trends in Cell Biology*, 21(10), 585–593. https://doi.org/10.1016/j.tcb.2011.06.004.

Agudo, A., & Pera, G. (1999). Vegetable and fruit consumption associated with anthropometric, dietary and lifestyle factors in Spain. *Public Health Nutrition*, 2(3), 263–271. https://doi.org/10.1017/s136898009900035x.

Akiko, K., Mayumi, K., & Makoto, S. (2012). Matrix-assisted laser desorption/ionization (MALDI) imaging mass spectrometry (IMS): A challenge for reliable quantitative analyses. *MASS Spectrometry*, A0004. https://doi.org/10.5702/massspectrometry.a0004.

Alakbarzade, V., Hameed, A., Quek, D. Q. Y., Chioza, B. A., Baple, E. L., Cazenave-Gassiot, A., et al. (2015). A partially inactivating mutation in the sodium-dependent lysophosphatidylcholine transporter MFSD2A causes a non-lethal microcephaly syndrome. *Nature Genetics*, 47(7), 814–817. https://doi.org/10.1038/ng.3313.

Aschner, M., & Aschner, J. L. (1990). Mercury neurotoxicity: Mechanisms of blood-brain barrier transport. *Neuroscience and Biobehavioral Reviews*, 14(2), 169–176. https://doi.org/10.1016/S0149-7634(05)80217-9.

Banerjee, A., & Shelver, W. L. (2021). Micro- and nanoplastic induced cellular toxicity in mammals: A review. *Science of the Total Environment*, 755. https://doi.org/10.1016/j.scitotenv.2020.142518.

Bano, Y., & Hasan, M. (1989). Mercury induced time-dependent alterations in lipid profiles and lipid peroxidation in different body organs of cat-fish heteropneustes fossilis. *Journal of Environmental Science and Health, Part B*, 24(2), 145–166. https://doi.org/10.1080/03601238909372641.

Basselin, M., Ramadan, E., & Rapoport, S. I. (2012). Imaging brain signal transduction and metabolism via arachidonic and docosahexaenoic acid in animals and humans. *Brain Research Bulletin*, 87(2–3), 154–171. https://doi.org/10.1016/j.brainresbull.2011.12.001.

Basselin, M., Villacreses, N. E., Lee, H. J., Bell, J. M., & Rapoport, S. I. (2007). Chronic lithium administration attenuates up-regulated brain arachidonic acid metabolism in a rat model of neuroinflammation. *Journal of Neurochemistry*, 102(3), 761–772. https://doi.org/10.1111/j.1471-4159.2007.04593.x.

Bazinet, R. P., Bernoud-Hubac, N., & Lagarde, M. (2019). How the plasma lysophospholipid and unesterified fatty acid pools supply the brain with docosahexaenoic acid. *Prostaglandins Leukotrienes and Essential Fatty Acids*, 142, 1–3. https://doi.org/10.1016/j.plefa.2018.12.003.

Bazinet, R. P., & Layé, S. (2014). Polyunsaturated fatty acids and their metabolites in brain function and disease. *Nature Reviews Neuroscience*, 15(12), 771–785. https://doi.org/10.1038/nrn3820.

Bazinet, R. P., Rao, J. S., Chang, L., Rapoport, S. I., & Lee, H. J. (2006). Chronic carbamazepine decreases the incorporation rate and turnover of arachidonic acid but not docosahexaenoic acid in brain phospholipids of the unanesthetized rat: Relevance to bipolar disorder.

Biological Psychiatry, 59(5), 401–407. https://doi.org/10.1016/j.biopsych.2005.07.024.

Begg, D. P., Sinclair, A. J., & Weisinger, R. S. (2012). Thirst deficits in aged rats are reversed by dietary omega-3 fatty acid supplementation. *Neurobiology of Aging*, 33(10), 2422–2430. https://doi.org/10.1016/j.neurobiolaging.2011.12.001.

Begriche, K., Massart, J., Robin, M. A., Borgne-Sanchez, A., & Fromenty, B. (2011). Drug-induced toxicity on mitochondria and lipid metabolism: Mechanistic diversity and deleterious consequences for the liver. *Journal of Hepatology*, 54(4), 773–794. https://doi.org/10.1016/j.jhep.2010.11.006.

Beltowski, J., Wojcicka, G., Gorny, D., & Marciniak, A. (2000). The effect of dietary-induced obesity on lipid peroxidation, antioxidant enzymes and total plasma antioxidant capacity. *Journal of physiology and pharmacology*, 51.

Belza, K., Anderson, M., Ryan, M., & Cunnane, S. (1999). Carbon recycling from linoleate during severe dietary linoleate deficiency. *Lipids*, 34, S129–S130. https://doi.org/10.1007/BF02562260.

Bergamini, C. M., Gambetti, S., Dondi, A., & Cervellati, C. (2004). Oxygen, reactive oxygen species and tissue damage. *Current Pharmaceutical Design*, 10(14), 1611–1626. https://doi.org/10.2174/1381612043384664.

Blokhina, O., Virolainen, E., & Fagerstedt, K. V. (2003). Antioxidants, oxidative damage and oxygen deprivation stress: A review. *Annals of Botany*, 91, 179–194. https://doi.org/10.1093/aob/mcf118.

Borroni, M. V., Vallés, A. S., & Barrantes, F. J. (2016). The lipid habitats of neurotransmitter receptors in brain. *Biochimica et Biophysica Acta - Biomembranes*, 1858(11), 2662–2670. https://doi.org/10.1016/j.bbamem.2016.07.005.

Bosetti, F., Weerasinghe, G. R., Rosenberger, T. A., & Rapoport, S. I. (2003). Valproic acid down-regulates the conversion of arachidonic acid to eicosanoids via cyclooxygenase-1 and -2 in rat brain. *Journal of Neurochemistry*, 85(3), 690–696. https://doi.org/10.1046/j.1471-4159.2003.01701.x.

Bourre, J. M. (2004). Roles of unsaturated fatty acids (especially omega-3 fatty acids) in the brain at various ages and during ageing. *Journal of Nutrition, Health and Aging*, 8(3), 163–174.

Bozek, K., Wei, Y., Yan, Z., Liu, X., Xiong, J., Sugimoto, M., et al. (2015). Organization and evolution of brain Lipidome revealed by large-scale analysis of human, chimpanzee, macaque, and mouse tissues. *Neuron*, 85(4), 695–702. https://doi.org/10.1016/j.neuron.2015.01.003.

Brenna, J. T., & Diau, G. Y. (2007). The influence of dietary docosahexaenoic acid and arachidonic acid on central nervous system polyunsaturated fatty acid composition. *Prostaglandins Leukotrienes and Essential Fatty Acids*, 77(5–6), 247–250. https://doi.org/10.1016/j.plefa.2007.10.016.

Buccinnà, B., Piccinini, M., Prinetti, A., Scandroglio, F., Prioni, S., Valsecchi, M., et al. (2009). Alterations of myelin-specific proteins and sphingolipids characterize the brains of acid sphingomyelinase-deficient mice, an animal model of Niemann-pick disease type A. *Journal of Neurochemistry*, 109(1), 105–115. https://doi.org/10.1111/j.1471-4159.2009.05947.x.

Bullmore, E., & Sporns, O. (2009). Complex brain networks: Graph theoretical analysis of structural and functional systems. *Nature Reviews Neuroscience*, 10(3), 186–198. https://doi.org/10.1038/nrn2575.

Cajka, T., & Fiehn, O. (2014). Comprehensive analysis of lipids in biological systems by liquid chromatography-mass spectrometry. *TrAC - Trends in Analytical Chemistry*, 61, 192–206. https://doi.org/10.1016/j.trac.2014.04.017.

Cant, L., Del Favero, E., Sonnino, S., & Prinetti, A. (2011). Gangliosides and the multiscale modulation of membrane structure. *Chemistry and Physics of Lipids*, 164(8), 796–810. https://doi.org/10.1016/j.chemphyslip.2011.09.005.

Cao, D., Xue, R., Xu, J., & Liu, Z. (2005). Effects of docosahexaenoic acid on the survival and neurite outgrowth of rat cortical neurons in primary cultures. *Journal of Nutritional Biochemistry*, 16(9), 538–546. https://doi.org/10.1016/j.jnutbio.2005.02.002.

Carocci, A., Rovito, N., Sinicropi, M. S., & Genchi, G. (2014). Mercury toxicity and neurodegenerative effects. *Reviews of Environmental Contamination and Toxicology*, 229, 1–18. https://doi.org/10.1007/978-3-319-03777-6_1.

Carrié, I., Clément, M., De Javel, D., Francès, H., & Bourre, J. M. (2000). Specific phospholipid fatty acid composition of brain regions in mice: Effects of n-3 polyunsaturated fatty acid deficiency and phospholipid supplementation. *Journal of Lipid Research*, 41(3), 465–472.

Carroquino, M., Posada, M., & Landrigan, P. (2012). *Environmental toxicology: Children at risk* (pp. 239–291). Springer Science and Business Media LLC. https://doi.org/10.1007/978-1-4614-5764-0_11.

Casals-Casas, C., & Desvergne, B. (2011). Endocrine disruptors: From endocrine to metabolic disruption. *Annual Review of Physiology*, 73, 135–162. https://doi.org/10.1146/annurev-physiol-012110-142200.

Castle, L., Mercer, A. J., Startin, J. R., & Gilbert, J. (1988). Migration from plasticized films into foods 3. Migration of phthalate, sebacate, citrate and phosphate esters from films used for retail food packaging. *Food Additives and Contaminants*, 5(1), 9–20. https://doi.org/10.1080/02652038809373657.

Castoldi, A. F., Coccini, T., Ceccatelli, S., & Manzo, L. (2001). Neurotoxicity and molecular effects of methylmercury. *Brain Research Bulletin*, 55(2), 197–203. https://doi.org/10.1016/S0361-9230(01)00458-0.

Catalá, A. (2009). Lipid peroxidation of membrane phospholipids generates hydroxy-alkenals and oxidized phospholipids active in physiological and/or pathological conditions. *Chemistry and Physics of Lipids*, *157*(1), 1–11. https://doi.org/10.1016/j.chemphyslip.2008.09.004.

Cermenati, G., Mitro, N., Audano, M., Melcangi, R. C., Crestani, M., De Fabiani, E., et al. (2015). Lipids in the nervous system: From biochemistry and molecular biology to pathophysiology. *Biochimica et Biophysica Acta - Molecular and Cell Biology of Lipids*, *1851*(1), 51–60. https://doi.org/10.1016/j.bbalip.2014.08.011.

Cha, S., & Yeung, E. S. (2007). Colloidal graphite-assisted laser desorption/ionization mass spectrometry and MSn of small molecules. 1. Imaging of cerebrosides directly from rat brain tissue. *Analytical Chemistry*, *79*(6), 2373–2385. https://doi.org/10.1021/ac062251h.

Chan, K., Lanthier, P., Liu, X., Sandhu, J. K., Stanimirovic, D., & Li, J. (2009). MALDI mass spectrometry imaging of gangliosides in mouse brain using ionic liquid matrix. *Analytica Chimica Acta*, *639*(1–2), 57–61. https://doi.org/10.1016/j.aca.2009.02.051.

Chang, C. Y., Ke, D. S., & Chen, J. Y. (2009). Essential fatty acids and human brain. *Acta Neurologica Taiwanica*, *18*(4), 231–241.

Chattopadhyay, A., & Paila, Y. D. (2007). Lipid-protein interactions, regulation and dysfunction of brain cholesterol. *Biochemical and Biophysical Research Communications*, *354*(3), 627–633. https://doi.org/10.1016/j.bbrc.2007.01.032.

Chen, C. T., & Bazinet, R. P. (2015). β-Oxidation and rapid metabolism, but not uptake regulate brain eicosapentaenoic acid levels. *Prostaglandins Leukotrienes and Essential Fatty Acids*, *92*, 33–40. https://doi.org/10.1016/j.plefa.2014.05.007.

Chen, R., Hui, L., Sturm, R. M., & Li, L. (2009). Three dimensional mapping of neuropeptides and lipids in crustacean brain by mass spectral imaging. *Journal of the American Society for Mass Spectrometry*, *20*(6), 1068–1077. https://doi.org/10.1016/j.jasms.2009.01.017.

Chen, Q., Lackmann, C., Wang, W., Seiler, T., Hollert, H., & Shi, H. (2020). 2020 microplastics lead to hyperactive swimming behaviour in adult zebrafish. *Aquatic Toxicology*, *224*. https://doi.org/10.1016/j.aquatox.2020.105521. Epub.

Chen, S., & Subbaiah, P. V. (2007). Phospholipid and fatty acid specificity of endothelial lipase: Potential role of the enzyme in the delivery of docosahexaenoic acid (DHA) to tissues. *Biochimica et Biophysica Acta - Molecular and Cell Biology of Lipids*, *1771*(10), 1319–1328. https://doi.org/10.1016/j.bbalip.2007.08.001.

Chiang, N., & Serhan, C. N. (2020). Specialized pro-resolving mediator network: An update on production and actions. *Essays in biochemistry*. https://doi.org/10.1042/EBC20200018.

Choi, B. (1991). Effects of methylmercury on the developing brain. In *Advances in mercury toxicology* (pp. 315–337). Springer.

Cockcroft, S. (2009). Phosphatidic acid regulation of phosphatidylinositol 4-phosphate 5-kinases. *Biochimica et Biophysica Acta - Molecular and Cell Biology of Lipids*, *1791*(9), 905–912. https://doi.org/10.1016/j.bbalip.2009.03.007.

Corton, J. C., Anderson, S. P., & Stauber, A. (2000). Central role of peroxisome proliferator–activated receptors in the actions of peroxisome proliferators. *Annual Review of Pharmacology and Toxicology*, *40*(1), 491–518.

Crawford, M. A., Casperd, N. M., & Sinclair, A. J. (1976). The long chain metabolites of linoleic and linolenic acids in liver and brain in herbivores and carnivores. *Comparative Biochemistry and Physiology*, *54B*, 395–401.

Cremesti, A. E., Goni, F. M., & Kolesnick, R. (2002). Role of sphingomyelinase and ceramide in modulating rafts: Do biophysical properties determine biologic outcome? *FEBS Letters*, *531*(1), 47–53. https://doi.org/10.1016/S0014-5793(02)03489-0.

Crews, F. T., Majchrowicz, E., & Meeks, R. (1983). Changes in cortical synaptosomal plasma membrane fluidity and composition in ethanol-dependent rats. *Psychopharmacology*, *81*(3), 208–213. https://doi.org/10.1007/BF00427263.

Cunnane, S. C., Ryan, M. A., Nadeau, C. R., Bazinet, R. P., Musa-Veloso, K., & McCloy, U. (2003). Why is carbon from some polyunsaturates extensively recycled into lipid synthesis? *Lipids*, *38*(4), 477–484. https://doi.org/10.1007/s11745-003-1087-8.

Da Silva, A. X., Lavialle, F., Gendrot, G., Guesnet, P., Alessandri, J. M., & Lavialle, M. (2002). Glucose transport and utilization are altered in the brain of rats deficient in n-3 polyunsaturated fatty acids. *Journal of Neurochemistry*, *81*(6), 1328–1337. https://doi.org/10.1046/j.1471-4159.2002.00932.x.

Dawson, G. (2015). Measuring brain lipids. *Biochimica et Biophysica Acta - Molecular and Cell Biology of Lipids*, *1851*(8), 1026–1039. https://doi.org/10.1016/j.bbalip.2015.02.007.

De La Monte, S. M., & Kril, J. J. (2014). Human alcohol-related neuropathology. *Acta Neuropathologica*, *127*(1), 71–90. https://doi.org/10.1007/s00401-013-1233-3.

Deoni, S. C. L., Mercure, E., Blasi, A., Gasston, D., Thomson, A., Johnson, M., et al. (2011). Mapping infant brain myelination with magnetic resonance imaging. *Journal of Neuroscience*, *31*(2), 784–791. https://doi.org/10.1523/JNEUROSCI.2106-10.2011.

Dhopeshwarkar, G. A., & Mead, J. F. (1973). Uptake and transport of fatty acids into the brain and the role of the blood-brain barrier system. *Advances in Lipid Research*, *11*, 109–142. https://doi.org/10.1016/b978-0-12-024911-4.50010-6.

Diau, G. Y., Hsieh, A. T., Sarkadi-Nagy, E. A., Wijendran, V., Nathanielsz, P. W., & Brenna, J. T. (2005). The influence of long chain polyunsaturate supplementation on docosahexaenoic acid and arachidonic acid in baboon neonate central nervous system. *BMC Medicine*, *3*. https://doi.org/10.1186/1741-7015-3-11.

Duffy, S. S., Hayes, J. P., Fiore, N. T., & Moalem-Taylor, G. (2021). The cannabinoid system and microglia in health and disease. *Neuropharmacology*, *190*, 108555. https://doi.org/10.1016/j.neuropharm.2021.108555.

Dyall, S. C. (2015). Long-chain omega-3 fatty acids and the brain: A review of the independent and shared effects of EPA, DPA and DHA. *Frontiers in Aging Neuroscience*, *7*. https://doi.org/10.3389/fnagi.2015.00052.

Edmond, J., Higa, T. A., Korsak, R. A., Bergner, E. A., & Lee, W. N. P. (1998). Fatty acid transport and utilization for the developing brain. *Journal of Neurochemistry*, *70*(3), 1227–1234. https://doi.org/10.1046/j.1471-4159.1998.70031227.x.

El-Demerdash, F. (2001). Effects of selenium and mercury on the enzymatic activities and lipid peroxidation in brain, liver, and blood of rats. *Journal of Environmental Science and Health, Part B*, *36*(4), 489–499. https://doi.org/10.1081/PFC-100104191.

Evans, H. E., & Miller, M. E. (1993). *Miller's anatomy of the dog* (pp. 658–670). Philadelphia, PA: W.B. Saunders.

Farooqui, A. A. (2009). Lipid mediators in the neural cell nucleus: Their metabolism, signaling, and association with neurological disorders. *The Neuroscientist*, *15*(4), 392–407. https://doi.org/10.1177/1073858409337035.

Farooqui, A. A., Horrocks, L. A., & Farooqui, T. (2000). Glycerophospholipids in brain: Their metabolism, incorporation into membranes, functions, and involvement in neurological disorders. *Chemistry and Physics of Lipids*, *106*(1), 1–29. https://doi.org/10.1016/S0009-3084(00)00128-6.

Farquharson, J., Jamieson, E. C., Logan, R. W., Cockburn, F., Patrick, W. A., Fauland, et al. (1992). A comprehensive method for lipid profiling by liquid chromatography-ion cyclotron resonance mass spectrometry. *Journal of Lipid Research*, *340*(8823), 2314–2322. https://doi.org/10.1194/jlr.D016550.

Fauland, A., Köfeler, H., Trötzmüller, M., Knopf, A., Hartler, J., Eberl, A., et al. (2011). A comprehensive method for lipid profiling by liquid chromatography-ion cyclotron resonance mass spectrometry. *Journal of Lipid Research*, *52*(12), 2314–2322. https://doi.org/10.1194/jlr.D016550.

Favrelière, S., Barrier, L., Durand, G., Chalon, S., & Tallineau, C. (1998). Chronic dietary n-3 polyunsaturated fatty acids deficiency affects the fatty acid composition of plasmenylethanolamine and phosphatidylethanolamine differently in rat frontal cortex, striatum, and cerebellum. *Lipids*, *33*(4), 401–407. https://doi.org/10.1007/s11745-998-0221-y.

Federico, A., Cardaioli, E., Da Pozzo, P., Formichi, P., Gallus, G. N., & Radi, E. (2012). Mitochondria, oxidative stress and neurodegeneration. *Journal of the Neurological Sciences*, *322*(1–2), 254–262. https://doi.org/10.1016/j.jns.2012.05.030.

Fišar, Z. (2009). Phytocannabinoids and endocannabinoids. *Current Drug Abuse Reviews*, *2*(1), 51–75. https://doi.org/10.2174/1874473710902010051.

Fischer, K. W., & Rose, S. P. (1994). Dynamic development of coordination of components in brain and behavior: A framework for theory and research. In G. Dawson, & K. W. Fischer (Eds.), *Human behavior and the developing brain* (pp. 3–66). The Guilford Press.

Fraser, T., Tayler, H., & Love, S. (2010). Fatty acid composition of frontal, temporal and parietal neocortex in the normal human brain and in Alzheimer's disease. *Neurochemical Research*, *35*(3), 503–513. https://doi.org/10.1007/s11064-009-0087-5.

Frederiksen, H., Skakkebæk, N. E., & Andersson, A. M. (2007). Metabolism of phthalates in humans. *Molecular Nutrition and Food Research*, *51*(7), 899–911. https://doi.org/10.1002/mnfr.200600243.

Frigerio, F., Pasqualini, G., Craparotta, I., Marchini, S., Van Vliet, E. A., Foerch, P., et al. (2018). N-3 Docosapentaenoic acid-derived protectin D1 promotes resolution of neuroinflammation and arrests epileptogenesis. *Brain*, *141*(11), 3130–3143. https://doi.org/10.1093/brain/awy247.

Fujimoto, T., & Parmryd, I. (2017). Interleaflet coupling, pinning, and leaflet asymmetry-major players in plasma membrane nanodomain formation. *Frontiers in Cell and Developmental Biology*, *4*. https://doi.org/10.3389/fcell.2016.00155.

Furuhata, A., Nakamura, M., Osawa, T., & Uchida, K. (2002). Thiolation of protein-bound carcinogenic aldehyde. An electrophilic acrolein-lysine adduct that covalently binds to thiols. *Journal of Biological Chemistry*, *277*(31), 27919–27926. https://doi.org/10.1074/jbc.M202794200.

Galli, C., Trzeciak, H. I., & Paoletti, R. (1971). Effects of dietary fatty acids on the fatty acid composition of brain ethanolamine phosphoglyceride: Reciprocal replacement of n-6 and n-3 polyunsaturated fatty acids. *Biochimica et Biophysica Acta (BBA)/Lipids and Lipid Metabolism*, *248*(3), 449–454. https://doi.org/10.1016/0005-2760(71)90233-5.

Gaschler, M. M., & Stockwell, B. R. (2017). Lipid peroxidation in cell death. *Biochemical and Biophysical Research Communications*, *482*(3), 419–425. https://doi.org/10.1016/j.bbrc.2016.10.086.

Ghasemi Fard, S., Cameron-Smith, D., & Sinclair, A. J. (2021). N-3 Docosapentaenoic acid: The iceberg n-3 fatty acid. *Current Opinion in Clinical Nutrition and Metabolic Care*, *23*. https://doi.org/10.1097/MCO.0000000000000722.

Giles, C., Takechi, R., Mellett, N. A., Meikle, P. J., Dhaliwal, S., & Mamo, J. C. (2016). The effects of long-term saturated fat enriched diets on the brain lipidome. *PLoS One*, *11*(12). https://doi.org/10.1371/journal.pone.0166964.

Girotti, A. W. (1998). Lipid hydroperoxide generation, turnover, and effector action in biological systems. *Journal of Lipid Research*, *39*(8), 1529–1542.

Giusto, N. M., Salvador, G. A., Castagnet, P. I., Pasquaré, S. J., & Ilincheta de Boschero, M. G. (2002). Age-associated changes in central nervous system glycerolipid composition and metabolism. *Neurochemical Research, 27*(11), 1513–1523. https://doi.org/10.1023/A:1021604623208.

Gomez-Pinilla, F. (2008). Brain foods: The effects of nutrients on brain function. *Nature Reviews Neuroscience, 9*(7), 568–578. https://doi.org/10.1038/nrn2421.

Gomez-Pinilla, F. (2011). Collaborative effects of diet and exercise on cognitive enhancement. *Nutrition and Health, 20*(3–4), 165–170. https://doi.org/10.1177/026010601102000401.

Goñi, F. M., & Alonso, A. (2006). Biophysics of sphingolipids I. membrane properties of sphingosine, ceramides and other simple sphingolipids. *Biochimica et Biophysica Acta - Biomembranes, 1758*(12), 1902–1921. https://doi.org/10.1016/j.bbamem.2006.09.011.

Gorica, E., & Calderone, V. (2021). Arachidonic acid derivatives and neuroinflammation. *CNS & Neurological Disorders - Drug Targets, 20*. https://doi.org/10.2174/1871527320666210208130412.

Granholm, A. C., Bimonte-Nelson, H. A., Moore, A. B., Nelson, M. E., Freeman, L. R., & Sambamurti, K. (2008). Effects of a saturated fat and high cholesterol diet on memory and hippocampal morphology in the middle-aged rat. *Journal of Alzheimer's Disease, 14*(2), 133–145. https://doi.org/10.3233/JAD-2008-14202.

Grassi, S., Prioni, S., Cabitta, L., Aureli, M., Sonnino, S., & Prinetti, A. (2016). The role of 3-O-sulfogalactosylceramide, sulfatide, in the lateral organization of myelin membrane. *Neurochemical Research, 41*(1–2), 130–143. https://doi.org/10.1007/s11064-015-1747-2.

Guemez-Gamboa, A., Nguyen, L. N., Yang, H., Zaki, M. S., Kara, M., Ben-Omran, T., et al. (2015). Inactivating mutations in MFSD2A, required for omega-3 fatty acid transport in brain, cause a lethal microcephaly syndrome. *Nature Genetics, 47*(7), 809–813. https://doi.org/10.1038/ng.3311.

Guo, S., Zhou, D., Zhang, M., Li, T., Liu, Y., Xu, Y., et al. (2017). Monitoring changes of docosahexaenoic acid-containing lipids during the recovery process of traumatic brain injury in rat using mass spectrometry imaging. *Scientific Reports, 7*(1). https://doi.org/10.1038/s41598-017-05446-2.

Hachem, M., Géloën, A., Van, A. L., Foumaux, B., Fenart, L., Gosselet, F., et al. (2016). Efficient docosahexaenoic acid uptake by the brain from a structured phospholipid. *Molecular Neurobiology, 53*(5), 3205–3215. https://doi.org/10.1007/s12035-015-9228-9.

Halliwell, B. (1996). Antioxidants in human health and disease. *Annual Review of Nutrition, 16*, 33–50. https://doi.org/10.1146/annurev.nu.16.070196.000341.

Hansen, J. C., Reske-Nielsen, E., Thorlacius-Ussing, O., Rungby, J., & Danscher, G. (1989). Distribution of dietary mercury in a dog. Quantitation and localization of total mercury in organs and central nervous system. *Science of the Total Environment, 78*(C), 23–43. https://doi.org/10.1016/0048-9697(89)90020-X.

Harauma, A., Hatanaka, E., Yasuda, H., Nakamura, M. T., Salem, N., & Moriguchi, T. (2017). Effects of arachidonic acid, eicosapentaenoic acid and docosahexaenoic acid on brain development using artificial rearing of delta-6-desaturase knockout mice. *Prostaglandins Leukotrienes and Essential Fatty Acids, 127*, 32–39. https://doi.org/10.1016/j.plefa.2017.10.001.

Harauma, A., Salem, N., & Moriguchi, T. (2010). Repletion of n-3 fatty acid deficient dams with α-linolenic acid: Effects on fetal brain and liver fatty acid composition. *Lipids, 45*(8), 659–668. https://doi.org/10.1007/s11745-010-3443-y.

Harper, C. (2009). The neuropathology of alcohol-related brain damage. *Alcohol and Alcoholism, 44*(2), 136–140. https://doi.org/10.1093/alcalc/agn102.

Hill, S., Shaw, B., & Wu, A. (2001). The clinical effects of plasticizers, antioxidants, and other contaminants in medical polyvinylchloride tubing during respiratory and non-respiratory exposure. *Clinica Chimica Acta, 304*(1–2), 1–8. https://doi.org/10.1016/s0009-8981(00)00411-3.

Hodson, L., Skeaff, C. M., & Fielding, B. A. (2008). Fatty acid composition of adipose tissue and blood in humans and its use as a biomarker of dietary intake. *Progress in Lipid Research, 47*(5), 348–380. https://doi.org/10.1016/j.plipres.2008.03.003.

Hoek, J. B., Cahill, A., & Pastorino, J. G. (2002). Alcohol and mitochondria: A dysfunctional relationship. *Gastroenterology, 122*(7), 2049–2063. https://doi.org/10.1053/gast.2002.33613.

Holmes, P., James, K. A. F., & Levy, L. S. (2009). Is low-level environmental mercury exposure of concern to human health? *Science of the Total Environment, 408*(2), 171–182. https://doi.org/10.1016/j.scitotenv.2009.09.043.

Hopiavuori, B. R., Agbaga, M. P., Brush, R. S., Sullivan, M. T., Sonntag, W. E., & Anderson, R. E. (2017). Regional changes in CNS and retinal glycerophospholipid profiles with age: A molecular blueprint. *Journal of Lipid Research, 58*(4), 668–680. https://doi.org/10.1194/jlr.M070714.

Hurst, C. H., & Waxman, D. J. (2003). Activation of PPARα and PPARγ by environmental phthalate monoesters. *Toxicological Sciences, 74*(2), 297–308. https://doi.org/10.1093/toxsci/kfg145.

Hussain, G., Wang, J., Rasul, A., Anwar, H., Imran, A., Qasim, M., et al. (2019). Role of cholesterol and sphingolipids in brain development and neurological diseases. *Lipids in Health and Disease, 18*(1). https://doi.org/10.1186/s12944-019-0965-z.

Ikeda, M., Kihara, A., & Igarashi, Y. (2006). Lipid asymmetry of the eukaryotic plasma membrane: Functions and related enzymes. *Biological and Pharmaceutical Bulletin, 29*(8), 1542–1546. https://doi.org/10.1248/bpb.29.1542.

Ikonen, E. (2006). Mechanisms for cellular cholesterol transport: Defects and human disease. *Physiological Reviews*, 86(4), 1237–1261. https://doi.org/10.1152/physrev.00022.2005.

Innis, S. M., Adamkin, D. H., Hall, R. T., Kalhan, S. C., Lair, C., Lim, M., et al. (2002). Docosahexaenoic acid and arachidonic acid enhance growth with no adverse effects in preterm infants fed formula. *Journal of Pediatrics*, 140(5), 547–554. https://doi.org/10.1067/mpd.2002.123282.

Innis, S. M., & Dyer, R. A. (2002). Brain astrocyte synthesis of docosahexaenoic acid from n-3 fatty acids is limited at the elongation of docosapentaenoic acid. *Journal of Lipid Research*, 43(9), 1529–1536. https://doi.org/10.1194/jlr.M200120-JLR200.

Ivanova, P. T., Milne, S. B., Forrester, J. S., & Brown, H. A. (2004). LIPID arrays: New tools in the understanding of membrane dynamics and lipid signaling. *Molecular Interventions*, 4(2).

Jackman, N., Ishii, A., & Bansal, R. (2009). Oligodendrocyte development and myelin biogenesis: Parsing out the roles of glycosphingolipids. *Physiology*, 24(5), 290–297. https://doi.org/10.1152/physiol.00016.2009.

Jackson, T. A. (1997). Long-range atmospheric transport of mercury to ecosystems, and the importance of anthropogenic emissions - A critical review and evaluation of the published evidence. *Environmental Reviews*, 5(2), 99–120. https://doi.org/10.1139/a97-005.

James, S. L., Bannick, M. S., Montjoy-Venning, W. C., Lucchesi, L. R., Dandona, L., Dandona, R., et al. (2019). Global, regional, and national burden of traumatic brain injury and spinal cord injury, 1990-2016: A systematic analysis for the global burden of disease study 2016. *The Lancet Neurology*, 18(1), 56–87. https://doi.org/10.1016/S1474-4422(18)30415-0.

Kabir, E. R., Rahman, M. S., & Rahman, I. (2015). A review on endocrine disruptors and their possible impacts on human health. *Environmental Toxicology and Pharmacology*, 40(1), 241–258. https://doi.org/10.1016/j.etap.2015.06.009.

Kawakami, T., Isama, K., & Matsuoka, A. (2011). Analysis of phthalic acid diesters, monoester, and other plasticizers in polyvinyl chloride household products in Japan. *Journal of Environmental Science and Health, Part A*, 46(8), 855–864. https://doi.org/10.1080/10934529.2011.579870.

Kelly, L., Grehan, B., Chiesa, DOWNER, E., Sahyoun, G., & Lynch, M. A. (2011). The polyunsaturated fatty acids, EPA and DPA exert a protective effect in the hippocampus of the aged rat. *Neurobiology of Aging*, 32(12), 2318.

Khan, S. A., & Vanden Heuvel, J. P. (2003). Reviews: Current topics role of nuclear receptors in the regulation of gene expression by dietary fatty acids (review). *Journal of Nutritional Biochemistry*, 14(10), 554–567. https://doi.org/10.1016/S0955-2863(03)00098-6.

Kim, H. Y., Huang, B. X., & Spector, A. A. (2014). Phosphatidylserine in the brain: Metabolism and function. *Progress in Lipid Research*, 56(1), 1–18. https://doi.org/10.1016/j.plipres.2014.06.002.

Kogure, K., Watson, B. D., Busto, R., & Abe, K. (1982). Potentiation of lipid peroxides by ischemia in rat brain. *Neurochemical Research*, 7(4), 437–454. https://doi.org/10.1007/BF00965496.

Komprda, T., Zelenka, J., Fajmonova, E., Fialova, M., & Kladroba, D. (2005). Arachidonic acid and long-chain $n-3$ polyunsaturated fatty acid contents in meat of selected poultry and fish species in relation to dietary fat sources. *Journal of Agricultural and Food Chemistry*, 53(17), 6804–6812. https://doi.org/10.1021/jf0504162.

Kopaczyk, K., & Radin, N. (1965). In vivo conversions of cerebroside and ceramide in rat brain. *Journal of Lipid Research*, 6, 140–145.

Korade, Z., & Kenworthy, A. K. (2008). Lipid rafts, cholesterol, and the brain. *Neuropharmacology*, 55(8), 1265–1273. https://doi.org/10.1016/j.neuropharm.2008.02.019.

Langin, D. (2011). In and out: Adipose tissue lipid turnover in obesity and dyslipidemia. *Cell Metabolism*, 14(5), 569–570. https://doi.org/10.1016/j.cmet.2011.10.003.

Latini, G., Scoditti, E., Verrotti, A., De Felice, C., & Massaro, M. (2008). Peroxisome proliferator-activated receptors as mediators of phthalate-induced effects in the male and female reproductive tract: Epidemiological and experimental evidence. *PPAR Research*, 1–13. https://doi.org/10.1155/2008/359267.

Ledesma, M. D., Martin, M. G., & Dotti, C. G. (2012). Lipid changes in the aged brain: Effect on synaptic function and neuronal survival. *Progress in Lipid Research*, 51(1), 23–35. https://doi.org/10.1016/j.plipres.2011.11.004.

Lee, S. S. T., Pineau, T., Drago, J., Lee, E. J., Owens, J. W., Kroetz, D. L., et al. (1995). Targeted disruption of the α isoform of the peroxisome proliferator- activated receptor gene in mice results in abolishment of the pleiotropic effects of peroxisome proliferators. *Molecular and Cellular Biology*, 15(6), 3012–3022. https://doi.org/10.1128/MCB.15.6.3012.

Li, Q., Bozek, K., Xu, C., Guo, Y., Sun, J., Pääbo, S., et al. (2017). Changes in Lipidome composition during brain development in humans, chimpanzees, and macaque monkeys. *Molecular Biology and Evolution*, 34(5), 1155–1166. https://doi.org/10.1093/molbev/msx065.

Li, D., Ng, A., Mann, N., & Sinclair, A. (1998). Contribution of meat fat to dietary arachidonic acid. *Lipids*, 33(4), 437–440. https://doi.org/10.1007/s11745-998-0225-7.

Li, D., Shi, Y., Yang, L., Xiao, L., Kehoe, D., Gun'ko, Y., et al. (2020). Microplastic release from the degradation of polypropylene feeding bottles during infant formula preparation. *Nature Food*, 1, 746–754. https://doi.org/10.1038/s43016-020-00171-y.

Lichtenstein, L., Mattijssen, F., De Wit, N. J., Georgiadi, A., Hooiveld, G. J., Van Der Meer, R., et al. (2010). Angptl4 protects against severe proinflammatory effects of saturated fat by inhibiting fatty acid uptake into mesenteric lymph node macrophages. *Cell Metabolism*, *12*(6), 580–592. https://doi.org/10.1016/j.cmet.2010.11.002.

Lipsky, N., & Pagano, R. (1983). Sphingolipid metabolism in cultured fibroblasts: Microscopic and biochemical studies employing a fluorescent ceramide analogue. *Proceedings of the National Academy of Sciences*, *80*(9), 2608–2612. https://doi.org/10.1073/pnas.80.9.2608.

Lovejoy, J. C., Smith, S. R., Champagne, C. M., Most, M. M., Lefevre, M., DeLany, J. P., et al. (2002). Effects of diets enriched in saturated (Palmitic), monounsaturated (Oleic), or trans (Elaidic) fatty acids on insulin sensitivity and substrate oxidation in healthy adults. *Diabetes Care*, *25*(8), 1283–1288. https://doi.org/10.2337/diacare.25.8.1283.

Magour, S. (1986). Studies on the inhibition of brain synaptosomal Na+/K+-ATPase by mercury chloride and methyl mercury chloride. *Archives of Toxicology. Supplement [Archiv Für Toxikologi Supplement]*, *9*, 393–396. https://doi.org/10.1007/978-3-642-71248-7_77.

Marcus, J., Honigbaum, S., Shroff, S., Honke, K., Rosenbluth, J., & Dupree, J. L. (2006). Sulfatide is essential for the maintenance of CNS myelin and axon structure. *Glia*, *53*(4), 372–381. https://doi.org/10.1002/glia.20292.

Mariani, E., Polidori, M., Cherubini, A., & Mecocci, P. (2005). Oxidative stress in brain aging, neurodegenerative and vascular diseases: An overview. *Journal of Chromatography B*, *827*(1), 65–75. https://doi.org/10.1016/j.jchromb.2005.04.023.

Martinez, M. (1992). Tissue levels of polyunsaturated fatty acids during early human development. *The Journal of Pediatrics*, *120*(4), S129–S138. https://doi.org/10.1016/S0022-3476(05)81247-8.

Mattsson, K., Johnson, E. V., Malmendal, A., Linse, S., Hansson, L. A., & Cedervall, T. (2017). Brain damage and behavioural disorders in fish induced by plastic nanoparticles delivered through the food chain. *Scientific Reports*, *7*(1). https://doi.org/10.1038/s41598-017-10813-0.

Menard, C. R., Goodman, K. J., Corso, T. N., Brenna, J. T., & Cunnane, S. C. (1998). Recycling of carbon into lipids synthesized de novo is a quantitatively important pathway of α-[U-13C] linolenate utilization in the developing rat brain. *Journal of Neurochemistry*, *71*(5), 2151–2158. https://doi.org/10.1046/j.1471-4159.1998.71052151.x.

Miller, M. D., Crofton, K. M., Rice, D. C., & Zoeller, R. T. (2009). Thyroid-disrupting chemicals: Interpreting upstream biomarkers of adverse outcomes. *Environmental Health Perspectives*, *117*(7), 1033–1041. https://doi.org/10.1289/ehp.0800247.

Miller, M. E., Hamann, M., & Kroon, F. J. (2020). Bioaccumulation and biomagnification of microplastics in marine organisms: A review and meta-analysis of current data. *PLoS One*, *15*(10). https://doi.org/10.1371/journal.pone.0240792.

Mohrhauer, H., & Holman, R. T. (1963). Alteration of the fatty acid composition of brain lipids by varying levels of dietary essential fatty acjds. *Journal of Neurochemistry*, *10*(7), 523–530. https://doi.org/10.1111/j.1471-4159.1963.tb09855.x.

Molteni, R., Barnard, R. J., Ying, Z., Roberts, C. K., & Gómez-Pinilla, F. (2002). A high-fat, refined sugar diet reduces hippocampal brain-derived neurotrophic factor, neuronal plasticity, and learning. *Neuroscience*, *112*(4), 803–814. https://doi.org/10.1016/S0306-4522(02)00123-9.

Moore, S. A. (2001). Polyunsaturated fatty acid synthesis and release by brain-derived cells in vitro. *Journal of Molecular Neuroscience*, *16*(2–3), 195–200. https://doi.org/10.1385/JMN:16:2-3:195.

Müller, C. P., Reichel, M., Mühle, C., Rhein, C., Gulbins, E., & Kornhuber, J. (2015). Brain membrane lipids in major depression and anxiety disorders. *Biochimica et Biophysica Acta - Molecular and Cell Biology of Lipids*, *1851*(8), 1052–1065. https://doi.org/10.1016/j.bbalip.2014.12.014.

Negre-Salvayre, A., Coatrieux, C., Ingueneau, C., & Salvayre, R. (2008). Advanced lipid peroxidation end products in oxidative damage to proteins. Potential role in diseases and therapeutic prospects for the inhibitors. *British Journal of Pharmacology*, *153*(1), 6–20. https://doi.org/10.1038/sj.bjp.0707395.

Nessel, I., & Michael-Titus, A. T. (2020). Lipid profiling of brain tissue and blood after traumatic brain injury: A review of human and experimental studies. *Seminars in Cell and Developmental Biology*. https://doi.org/10.1016/j.semcdb.2020.08.004.

Neuringer, M., & Connor, W. (1986). N-3 fatty acids in the brain and retina: Evidence for their essentiality. *Nutrition Reviews*, *44*(9), 285–294. https://doi.org/10.1111/j.1753-4887.1986.tb07660.x.

Nguyen, L. N., Ma, D., Shui, G., Wong, P., Cazenave-Gassiot, A., Zhang, X., et al. (2014). Mfsd2a is a transporter for the essential omega-3 fatty acid docosahexaenoic acid. *Nature*, *509*(7501), 503–506. https://doi.org/10.1038/nature13241.

Nickel, A., Kohlhaas, M., & Maack, C. (2014). Mitochondrial reactive oxygen species production and elimination. *Journal of Molecular and Cellular Cardiology*, *73*, 26–33. https://doi.org/10.1016/j.yjmcc.2014.03.011.

Norris, J. L., & Caprioli, R. M. (2013). Analysis of tissue specimens by matrix-assisted laser desorption/ionization imaging mass spectrometry in biological and clinical research. *Chemical Reviews*, *113*(4), 2309–2342. https://doi.org/10.1021/cr3004295.

Norton, W. T., & Poduslo, S. E. (1973). Myelination in rat brain: Changes in myelin composition during brain maturation. *Journal of Neurochemistry*, *21*(4), 759–773. https://doi.org/10.1111/j.1471-4159.1973.tb07520.x.

O'Brien, J. S., & Sampson, E. L. (1965). Lipid composition of the normal human brain: Gray matter, white matter, and myelin. *Journal of Lipid Research*, *6*(4), 537–544.

Olsen, A. S. B., & Færgeman, N. J. (2017). Sphingolipids: Membrane microdomains in brain development, function and neurological diseases. *Open Biology*, 7(5). https://doi.org/10.1098/rsob.170069.

Olsson, N. U., Shoaf, S. E., & Salem, N. (1998). The effect of dietary polyunsaturated fatty acids and alcohol on neurotransmitter levels in rat brain. *Nutritional Neuroscience*, 1(2), 133–140. https://doi.org/10.1080/1028415X.1998.11747222.

Onoe, H., Ueno, R., Fujita, I., Nishino, H., Oomura, Y., & Hayaishi, O. (1988). Prostaglandin D2, a cerebral sleep-inducing substance in monkeys. *Proceedings of the National Academy of Sciences of the United States of America*, 85(11), 4082–4086. https://doi.org/10.1073/pnas.85.11.4082.

Palmano, K., Rowan, A., Guillermo, R., Guan, J., & McJarrow, P. (2015). The role of gangliosides in neurodevelopment. *Nutrients*, 7(5), 3891–3913. https://doi.org/10.3390/nu7053891.

Parr, L. A., & Hopkins, W. D. (2000). Brain temperature asymmetries and emotional perception in chimpanzees, pan troglodytes. *Physiology & Behavior*, 71(3–4), 363–371.

Pawlosky, R. J., Bacher, J., & Salem, N. (2001). Ethanol consumption alters electroretinograms and depletes neural tissues of docosahexaenoic acid in rhesus monkeys: Nutritional consequences of a low n-3 fatty acid diet. *Alcoholism: Clinical and Experimental Research*, 25(12), 1758–1765. https://doi.org/10.1111/j.1530-0277.2001.tb02187.x.

Pawlosky, R. J., & Salem, N. (1995). Ethanol exposure causes a decrease in docosahexaenoic acid and an increase in docosapentaenoic acid in feline brains and retinas. *American Journal of Clinical Nutrition*, 61(6), 1284–1289. https://doi.org/10.1093/ajcn/61.6.1284.

Perry, G., Cash, A. D., & Smith, M. A. (2002). Alzheimer disease and oxidative stress. *Journal of Biomedicine and Biotechnology*, 2002(3), 120–123. https://doi.org/10.1155/S1110724302203010.

Pfrieger, F. W. (2003). Outsourcing in the brain: Do neurons depend on cholesterol delivery by astrocytes? *BioEssays*, 25(1), 72–78. https://doi.org/10.1002/bies.10195.

Piccinini, M., Scandroglio, F., Prioni, S., Buccinnà, B., Loberto, N., Aureli, M., et al. (2010). Deregulated sphingolipid metabolism and membrane organization in neurodegenerative disorders. *Molecular Neurobiology*, 41(2–3), 314–340. Humana Press https://doi.org/10.1007/s12035-009-8096-6.

Poitelon, Y., Kopec, A. M., & Belin, S. (2020). Myelin fat facts: An overview of lipids and fatty acid metabolism. *Cell*, 9(4), 812. https://doi.org/10.3390/cells9040812.

Postila, P. A., & Róg, T. (2020). A perspective: Active role of lipids in neurotransmitter dynamics. *Molecular Neurobiology*, 57(2), 910–925. https://doi.org/10.1007/s12035-019-01775-7.

Prüst, M., Meijer, J., & Westerink, R. H. S. (2020). The plastic brain: Neurotoxicity of micro- and nanoplastics. *Particle and Fibre Toxicology*, 17(1). https://doi.org/10.1186/s12989-020-00358-y.

Puglielli, L., Tanzi, R. E., & Kovacs, D. M. (2003). Alzheimer's disease: The cholesterol connection. *Nature Neuroscience*, 6(4), 345–351. https://doi.org/10.1038/nn0403-345.

Qi, K., Hall, M., & Deckelbaum, R. J. (2002). Long-chain polyunsaturated fatty acid accretion in brain. *Current Opinion in Clinical Nutrition and Metabolic Care*, 5(2), 133–138. https://doi.org/10.1097/00075197-200203000-00003.

Rapoport, S. I., & Igarashi, M. (2009). Can the rat liver maintain normal brain DHA metabolism in the absence of dietary DHA? *Prostaglandins Leukotrienes and Essential Fatty Acids*, 81(2–3), 119–123. https://doi.org/10.1016/j.plefa.2009.05.021.

Rapoport, S. I., Rao, J. S., & Igarashi, M. (2007). Brain metabolism of nutritionally essential polyunsaturated fatty acids depends on both the diet and the liver. *Prostaglandins Leukotrienes and Essential Fatty Acids*, 77(5–6), 251–261. https://doi.org/10.1016/j.plefa.2007.10.023.

Rappley, I., Myers, D. S., Milne, S. B., Ivanova, P. T., Lavoie, M. J., Brown, H. A., et al. (2009). Lipidomic profiling in mouse brain reveals differences between ages and genders, with smaller changes associated with α-synuclein genotype. *Journal of Neurochemistry*, 111(1), 15–25. https://doi.org/10.1111/j.1471-4159.2009.06290.x.

Robert, K., Tsai, Y., & Ariga, T. (2012). Functional roles of gangliosides in neurodevelopment: An overview of recent advances. *Neurochemical Research*, 37(6), 1230–1244.

Roos, D., Seeger, R., Puntel, R., & Vargas Barbosa, N. (2012). Role of calcium and mitochondria in MeHg-mediated cytotoxicity. *Journal of Biomedicine and Biotechnology*, 2012. https://doi.org/10.1155/2012/248764.

Rose, S., Melnyk, S., Pavliv, O., Bai, S., Nick, T., Frye, R., et al. (2012). Evidence of oxidative damage and inflammation associated with low glutathione redox status in the autism brain. *Translational Psychiatry*, 2(7), e134. https://doi.org/10.1038/tp.2012.61.

Rowdhwal, S. S. S., & Chen, J. (2018). Toxic effects of Di-2-ethylhexyl phthalate: An overview. *BioMed Research international*, 2018. https://doi.org/10.1155/2018/1750368.

Runquist, M., Parmryd, I., Thelin, A., Chojnacki, T., & Dallner, G. (1995). Distribution of branch point prenyltransferases in regions of bovine brain. *Journal of Neurochemistry*, 65(5), 2299–2306. https://doi.org/10.1046/j.1471-4159.1995.65052299.x.

Rusciano, I., Marvi, M. V., Owusu Obeng, E., Mongiorgi, S., Ramazzotti, G., Follo, M. Y., et al. (2021). Location-dependent role of phospholipase C signaling in the brain: Physiology and pathology. *Advances in Biological Regulation*, 79. https://doi.org/10.1016/j.jbior.2020.100771.

Sana, S. S., Dogiparthi, L. K., Gangadhar, L., Chakravorty, A., & Abhishek, N. (2020). Effects of microplastics and nanoplastics on marine environment and human health. *Environmental Science and Pollution Research, 27*(36), 44743–44756. https://doi.org/10.1007/s11356-020-10573-x.

SanGiovanni, J. P., & Chew, E. Y. (2005). The role of omega-3 long-chain polyunsaturated fatty acids in health and disease of the retina. *Progress in Retinal and Eye Research, 24*(1), 87–138. https://doi.org/10.1016/j.preteyeres.2004.06.002.

Schaeffer, E. L., & Gattaz, W. F. (2005). Inhibition of calcium-independent phospholipase A2 activity in rat hippocampus impairs acquisition of short- and long-term memory. *Psychopharmacology, 181*(2), 392–400. https://doi.org/10.1007/s00213-005-2256-9.

Schmitz, G., & Ecker, J. (2008). The opposing effects of n-3 and n-6 fatty acids. *Progress in Lipid Research, 47*(2), 147–155. https://doi.org/10.1016/j.plipres.2007.12.004.

Schnitzler, A., & Gross, J. (2005). Normal and pathological oscillatory communication in the brain. *Nature Reviews Neuroscience, 6*(4), 285–296. https://doi.org/10.1038/nrn1650.

Schuette, C. G., Pierstorff, B., Huettler, S., & Sandhoff, K. (2001). Sphingolipid activator proteins: Proteins with complex functions in lipid degradation and skin biogenesis. *Glycobiology, 11*(6), 81R–90R.

Scollan, N., Hocquette, J. F., Nuernberg, K., Dannenberger, D., Richardson, I., & Moloney, A. (2006). Innovations in beef production systems that enhance the nutritional and health value of beef lipids and their relationship with meat quality. *Meat Science, 74*(1), 17–33. https://doi.org/10.1016/j.meatsci.2006.05.002.

Seebungkert, B., & Lynch, J. W. (2002). Effects of polyunsaturated fatty acids on voltage-gated K+ and Na+ channels in rat olfactory receptor neurons. *European Journal of Neuroscience, 16*(11), 2085–2094. https://doi.org/10.1046/j.1460-9568.2002.02288.x.

Serrano, S. E., Braun, J., Trasande, L., Dills, R., & Sathyanarayana, S. (2014). Phthalates and diet: A review of the food monitoring and epidemiology data. *Environmental Health: A Global Access Science Source, 13*(1). https://doi.org/10.1186/1476-069X-13-43.

Silva, J. P., & Coutinho, O. P. (1972). Free radicals in the regulation of damage and cell death- -basic mechanisms and prevention. *Drug Discoveries & Therapeutics, 4*(3).

Sinclair, A. J. (1975a). Incorporation of radioactive polyunsaturated fatty acids into liver and brain of developing rat. *Lipids, 10*(3), 175–184. https://doi.org/10.1007/BF02534156.

Sinclair, A. J. (1975b). Long-chain polyunsaturated fatty acids in the mammalian brain. *Proceedings of the Nutrition Society, 34*(3), 287–291. https://doi.org/10.1079/pns19750051.

Sinclair, A. J. (2019). Docosahexaenoic acid and the brain- what is its role? *Asia Pacific Journal of Clinical Nutrition, 28*(4).

Sinclair, A. J., & Crawford, M. A. (1972). The accumulation of arachidonate and docosahexaenoate in the developing rat brain. *Journal of Neurochemistry, 19*(7), 1753–1758. https://doi.org/10.1111/j.1471-4159.1972.tb06219.x.

Siraki, A. G., Pourahmad, J., Chan, T. S., Khan, S., & O'Brien, P. J. (2002). Endogenous and endobiotic induced reactive oxygen species formation by isolated hepatocytes. *Free Radical Biology and Medicine, 32*(1), 2–10. https://doi.org/10.1016/S0891-5849(01)00764-X.

Söderberg, M., Edlund, C., Kristensson, K., & Dallner, G. (1990). Lipid compositions of different regions of the human brain during aging. *Journal of Neurochemistry, 54*(2), 415–423. https://doi.org/10.1111/j.1471-4159.1990.tb01889.x.

Sparvero, L. J., Amoscato, A. A., Dixon, C. E., Long, J. B., Kochanek, P. M., Pitt, B. R., et al. (2012). Mapping of phospholipids by MALDI imaging (MALDI-MSI): Realities and expectations. *Chemistry and Physics of Lipids, 165*(5), 545–562. https://doi.org/10.1016/j.chemphyslip.2012.06.001.

Spector, A. A. (2001). Plasma free fatty acid and lipoproteins as sources of polyunsaturated fatty acid for the brain. *Journal of Molecular Neuroscience, 16*(2–3), 159–165. https://doi.org/10.1385/JMN:16:2-3:159.

Stoffel, W., & Bosio, A. (1997). Myelin glycolipids and their functions. *Current Opinion in Neurobiology, 7*(5), 654–661. https://doi.org/10.1016/S0959-4388(97)80085-2.

Su, X. Q., Wang, J., & Sinclair, A. J. (2019). Plasmalogens and Alzheimer's disease: A review. *Lipids in Health and Disease, 18*(1). https://doi.org/10.1186/s12944-019-1044-1.

Sugasini, D., Thomas, R., Yalagala, P. C. R., Tai, L. M., & Subbaiah, P. V. (2017). Dietary docosahexaenoic acid (DHA) as lysophosphatidylcholine, but not as free acid, enriches brain DHA and improves memory in adult mice. *Scientific Reports, 7*(1). https://doi.org/10.1038/s41598-017-11766-0.

Sun, G. Y., & Sun, A. Y. (1985). Ethanol and membrane lipids. *Alcoholism: Clinical and Experimental Research, 9*(2), 164–180. https://doi.org/10.1111/j.1530-0277.1985.tb05543.x.

Svennerholm, L. (1968). Distribution and fatty acid composition of phosphoglycerides in normal human brain. *Journal of Lipid Research, 9*(5), 570–579.

Svennerholm, L., & Ställberg-Stenhagen, S. (1968). Changes in the fatty acid composition of cerebrosides and sulfatides of human nervous tissue with age. *Journal of Lipid Research, 9*(2), 215–225.

Syversen, T. L. M. (1974). Biotransformation of hg-203 labelled methyl mercuric chloride in rat brain measured by specific determination of Hg2+. *Acta Pharmacologica et Toxicologica, 35*(4), 277–283. https://doi.org/10.1111/j.1600-0773.1974.tb00747.x.

Tapert, S. F., Caldwell, L., & Burke, C. (2004). Alcohol and the adolescent brain: Human studies. *Alcohol Research & Health, 28*(4).

Thomas, J. A., Thomas, M. J., & Gangolli, S. D. (1984). Biological effects of DI-(2-ethylhexyl) phthalate and other phthalic acid esters. *Critical Reviews in Toxicology, 13*(4), 283–317. https://doi.org/10.3109/10408448409023761.

Thudichum, J. (1884). A treatise on the chemical constitution of the brain: Based throughout upon original researches. *Glasgow Medical Journal, 22*(5), 363–364.

Tułowiecka, N., Kotlęga, D., Bohatyrewicz, A., & Szczuko, M. (2021). Could Lipoxins represent a new standard in ischemic stroke treatment? *International Journal of Molecular Sciences, 22*(8), 4207. https://doi.org/10.3390/ijms22084207.

Uauy, R., Hoffman, D. R., Peirano, P., Birch, D. G., & Birch, E. E. (2001). Essential fatty acids in visual and brain development. *Lipids, 36*(9), 885–895. https://doi.org/10.1007/s11745-001-0798-1.

Valdearcos, M., Robblee, M. M., Benjamin, D. I., Nomura, D. K., Xu, A. W., & Koliwad, S. K. (2014). Microglia dictate the impact of saturated fat consumption on hypothalamic inflammation and neuronal function. *Cell Reports, 9*(6), 2124–2138. https://doi.org/10.1016/j.celrep.2014.11.018.

Valenza, M., & Cattaneo, E. (2006). Cholesterol dysfunction in neurodegenerative diseases: Is Huntington's disease in the list? *Progress in Neurobiology, 80*(4), 165–176. https://doi.org/10.1016/j.pneurobio.2006.09.005.

Vance, J. E., Hayashi, H., & Karten, B. (2005). Cholesterol homeostasis in neurons and glial cells. *Seminars in Cell and Developmental Biology, 16*(2), 193–212. https://doi.org/10.1016/j.semcdb.2005.01.005.

Veloso, A., Fernández, R., Astigarraga, E., Barreda-Gómez, G., Manuel, I., Giralt, M. T., et al. (2011). Distribution of lipids in human brain. *Analytical and Bioanalytical Chemistry, 401*(1), 89–101. https://doi.org/10.1007/s00216-011-4882-x.

Walravens, P., & Chase, H. P. (1969). Influence of thyroid on formation of myelin lipids. *Journal of Neurochemistry, 16*(10), 1477–1484. https://doi.org/10.1111/j.1471-4159.1969.tb09900.x.

Wang, B., McVeagh, P., Petocz, P., & Brand-Miller, J. (2003). Brain ganglioside and glycoprotein sialic acid in breastfed compared with formula-fed infants. *American Journal of Clinical Nutrition, 78*(5), 1024–1029. https://doi.org/10.1093/ajcn/78.5.1024.

Waring, R. H., & Harris, R. M. (2005). Endocrine disrupters: A human risk. *Molecular and cellular endocrinology, 244*(1–2), 2–9. https://doi.org/10.1016/j.mce.2005.02.007.

Watson, N. V., & Breedlove, S. M. (2012). *The mind's machine: Foundations of brain and behavior*. Sinauer Associates.

Weiser, M. J., Wynalda, K., Salem, N., & Butt, C. M. (2015). Dietary DHA during development affects depression-like behaviors and biomarkers that emerge after puberty in adolescent rats. *Journal of Lipid Research, 56*(1), 151–166. https://doi.org/10.1194/jlr.M055558.

Wijendran, V., Huang, M. C., Diau, G. Y., Boehm, G., Nathanielsz, P. W., & Brenna, J. T. (2002). Efficacy of dietary arachidonic acid provided as triglyceride or phospholipid as substrates for brain arachidonic acid accretion in baboon neonates. *Pediatric Research, 51*(3), 265–272. https://doi.org/10.1203/00006450-200203000-00002.

Wong, C. S. C., Duzgoren-Aydin, N. S., Aydin, A., & Wong, M. H. (2006). Sources and trends of environmental mercury emissions in Asia. *Science of the Total Environment, 368*(2–3), 649–662. https://doi.org/10.1016/j.scitotenv.2005.11.024.

Woods, A., & Jackson, S. N. (2006). Direct probing using matrix-assisted laser desorption/ionization mass spectrometry. *The AAPS Journal, 8*, 391–395.

Wu, J. Q., Kosten, T. R., & Zhang, X. Y. (2013). Free radicals, antioxidant defense systems, and schizophrenia. *Progress in Neuro-Psychopharmacology and Biological Psychiatry, 46*, 200–206. https://doi.org/10.1016/j.pnpbp.2013.02.015.

Wu, A., Molteni, R., Ying, Z., & Gomez-Pinilla, F. (2003). A saturated-fat diet aggravates the outcome of traumatic brain injury on hippocampal plasticity and cognitive function by reducing brain-derived neurotrophic factor. *Neuroscience, 119*(2), 365–375. https://doi.org/10.1016/S0306-4522(03)00154-4.

Wu, A., Ying, Z., & Gomez-Pinilla, F. (2004). The interplay between oxidative stress and brain-derived neurotrophic factor modulates the outcome of a saturated fat diet on synaptic plasticity and cognition. *European Journal of Neuroscience, 19*(7), 1699–1707. https://doi.org/10.1111/j.1460-9568.2004.03246.x.

Xu, Y., Agrawal, S., Cook, T. J., & Knipp, G. T. (2007). Di-(2-ethylhexyl)-phthalate affects lipid profiling in fetal rat brain upon maternal exposure. *Archives of Toxicology, 81*(1), 57–62. https://doi.org/10.1007/s00204-006-0143-8.

Xu, Y., Agrawal, S., Cook, T. J., & Knipp, G. T. (2008). Maternal Di-(2-ethylhexyl)-phthalate exposure influences essential fatty acid homeostasis in rat placenta. *Placenta, 29*(11), 962–969. https://doi.org/10.1016/j.placenta.2008.08.011.

Yang, B., Fritsche, K. L., Beversdorf, D. Q., Gu, Z., Lee, J. C., Folk, W. R., et al. (2019). Yin-yang mechanisms regulating lipid peroxidation of docosahexaenoic acid and arachidonic acid in the central nervous system. *Frontiers in Neurology, 10*. https://doi.org/10.3389/fneur.2019.00642.

Ye, H., Ha, M., Yang, M., Yue, P., Xie, Z., & Liu, C. (2017). Di2-ethylhexyl phthalate disrupts thyroid hormone homeostasis through activating the Ras/Akt/TRHr pathway and inducing hepatic enzymes. *Scientific Reports, 7*. https://doi.org/10.1038/srep40153.

Yee, S., & Choi, B. H. (1996). Oxidative stress in neurotoxic effects of methylmercury poisoning. *Neurotoxicology, 17*(1), 17–26.

Yin, Z., Milatovic, D., Aschner, J. L., Syversen, T., Rocha, J. B. T., Souza, D. O., et al. (2007). Methylmercury induces oxidative injury, alterations in permeability and glutamine transport in cultured astrocytes. *Brain Research, 1131*(1), 1–10. https://doi.org/10.1016/j.brainres.2006.10.070.

Youdim, K. A., Martin, A., & Joseph, J. A. (2000). Essential fatty acids and the brain: Possible health implications. *International Journal of Developmental Neuroscience, 18*(4–5), 383–399. https://doi.org/10.1016/S0736-5748(00)00013-7.

Yu, H., Bi, Y., Ma, W., He, L., Yuan, L., Feng, J., et al. (2010). Long-term effects of high lipid and high energy diet on serum lipid, brain fatty acid composition, and memory and learning ability in mice. *International Journal of Developmental Neuroscience, 28*(3), 271–276. https://doi.org/10.1016/j.ijdevneu.2009.12.001.

Yuki, D., Sugiura, Y., Zaima, N., Akatsu, H., Hashizume, Y., Yamamoto, T., et al. (2011). Hydroxylated and non-hydroxylated sulfatide are distinctly distributed in the human cerebral cortex. *Neuroscience, 193*, 44–53. https://doi.org/10.1016/j.neuroscience.2011.07.045.

Zhang, Y., Appelkvist, E. L., Kristensson, K., & Dallner, G. (1996). The lipid compositions of different regions of rat brain during development and aging. *Neurobiology of Aging, 17*(6), 869–875. https://doi.org/10.1016/S0197-4580(96)00076-0.

Zhang, W., Li, P., Hu, X., Zhang, F., Chen, J., & Gao, Y. (2011). Omega-3 polyunsaturated fatty acids in the brain: Metabolism and neuroprotection. *Frontiers in Bioscience, 16*(7), 2653–2670. https://doi.org/10.2741/3878.

Zöller, I., Meixner, M., Hartmann, D., Büssow, H., Meyer, R., Gieselmann, V., et al. (2008). Absence of 2-hydroxylated sphingolipids is compatible with normal neural development but causes late-onset axon and myelin sheath degeneration. *Journal of Neuroscience, 28*(39), 9741–9754. https://doi.org/10.1523/JNEUROSCI.0458-08.2008.

CHAPTER 4

Lipids and mental health

Daniel Tzu-Li Chen[a,b,c], Jocelyn Chia-Yu Chen[b,c], Jane Pei-Chen Chang[b,d,e], and Kuan-Pin Su[a,b,d,e,f]

[a]Division of Neuroscience, Graduate Institute of Biomedical Sciences, China Medical University, Taichung, Taiwan [b]Department of Psychiatry and Mind-Body Interface Laboratory (MBI-Lab), China Medical University Hospital, Taichung, Taiwan [c]School of Chinese Medicine, College of Chinese Medicine, China Medical University, Taichung, Taiwan [d]Department of Psychological Medicine, Institute of Psychiatry, Psychology and Neuroscience, King's College London, London, United Kingdom [e]School of Medicine, College of Medicine, China Medical University, Taichung, Taiwan [f]Depression Center, An-Nan Hospital, China Medical University, Tainan, Taiwan

4.1 Introduction

Mental health is important at every stage of life. It typically refers to our emotional, psychological, and social well-being, and can affect our thinking, feelings, and behaviors. Many factors contribute to mental health problems, including (1) biological factors, such as genes or brain chemistry, (2) life experiences, such as trauma or abuse, and (3) family history of mental health problems (Dixon, 2019). Recently, emerging evidence shows that dietary patterns, especially the lipids, greatly influence our mental health. Approximately 70% of the fatty acid pool is made de novo, and 30% must be obtained through diet. The composition of lipids, including cholesterol and polyunsaturated fatty acids (PUFAs), can be affected by both cellular function and diet. Therefore, the importance of diet cannot be over-emphasized.

4.2 Metabolism of lipids in the brain

It is well known that the brain plays the most essential role in our mental health. In order to understand how dietary lipids influence us, we have to start from their metabolism in the brain. Lipids can provide essential fatty acids (EFAs), and we are going to focus on the two EFAs for humans: alpha-linolenic acid (ALA; an omega-3 fatty acid) and linoleic acid (LA; an omega-6 fatty acid).

Food contains different types of fatty acids, such as saturated fatty acids (SAFAs), monounsaturated fatty acids (MUFAs), and PUFAs. PUFAs, one of the most important dietary lipids, are considered to be inert structural components of the human brain, which form the cell membrane. Long-chain PUFAs (LC-PUFAs), including arachidonic acid (ARA), docosahexaenoic acid (DHA), and eicosapentaenoic acid (EPA), are largely esterified to the membrane of neurons and glial cells (astrocytes, microglia, and oligodendrocytes) in our central nervous system (CNS) (Chianese et al., 2018). The brain is enriched in ARA and DHA; the former represents 5–11% of total brain phospholipids, while the latter represents 13–22% (Joffre et al., 2016). Each of them is the main metabolites of omega-6 (n-6) and omega-3 (n-3) PUFAs intake on diet. ARA and DHA accumulate during brain development, and the accumulation period corresponds to neuronal maturation and gray matter expansion (Layé et al., 2018). Thus, the balance of ARA and DHA is quite important to keep the brain function in balance. However, the capacity of the brain to synthesize LC-PUFAs is limited; therefore, they have to be provided through the diet either as precursors, that is LA and ALA, which can be widely found in vegetable oils and grain products, or as preformed ARA and DHA, which can be widely found in meat products and fish. Animal models have shown that ARA and DHA in the brain can partially replace each other according to the dietary intake (Joffre et al., 2016). N-3 and n-6 PUFAs undergo different but similar pathways; ALA and LA can synthesize DHA and ARA through a series of elongation and desaturation steps regulated by genes (Fig. 4.1). The metabolism mainly takes place in both microsomes and peroxisomes of the liver. However, the brain also has the ability to synthesize LC-PUFAs, which may have an impact on our mental health.

Among lipids, n-3 PUFAs, mainly EPA and DHA, have recently been proposed as a potential prevention and intervention for some psychiatric

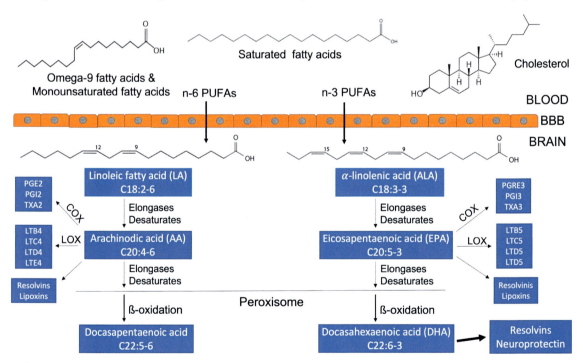

FIG. 4.1 Metabolic pathways of n-3 PUFAs and n-6 PUFAs in brain *No Permission Required* LA and ALA are converted to long-chain fatty acids through desaturation and elongation in the brain. DHA is synthesized in the peroxisome through the cycle of β-oxidation. AA and EPA synthesize prostanoids and leukotrienes, respectively, by the enzymes COX and LOX. AA, EPA, and DHA can also synthesize resolvins. These reactions primarily occur in the liver, but take place in the brain as well, once n-3 PUFAs and n-6 PUFAs pass through BBB.

disorders. The current literature suggests the following: (1) n-3 PUFAs help regulate our inflammation and reduce the oxidative stress in our brain; (2) n-3 PUFAs help balance the function of the gut microbiota; and (3) n-3 PUFAs help modulate and protect our nervous system. In fact, the impacts of n-3 PUFAs to our body are multi-aspect, that is, not only mental health, but cardiovascular diseases (Chang & Su, 2010), skeletal muscle health (Jeromson et al., 2015), and liver diseases (Spooner & Jump, 2019).

4.3 Lipids and inflammation and oxidative stress

The human brain operates at a very high metabolic rate and uses a substantial proportion of total energy and nutrient intake. The brain represents only 2% of the total body weight for human beings, but accounts for around 20% of our total oxygen consumption (Steiner, 2020). Oxidative stress (OS) is an inevitable result of life in an oxygen-rich environment (Farr & Kogoma, 1991). The influence of the OS is a width and diversity, and the consequences of a high OS level may range from cell damage to severe physiological diseases, such as gastrointestinal (GI) mucosal diseases (Bhattacharyya et al., 2014), vascular diseases (Sena et al., 2018), and neurodegenerative diseases (Uttara et al., 2009). With high oxygen consumption and lipid-rich content, the brain is highly susceptible to OS. OS, on the other hand, has been suggested to contribute to the development of several neuropsychiatric disorders, including anxiety and depressive disorders (Salim, 2017).

Meta-analysis has shown the OS increased in depression (Black et al., 2015). Clinical studies have also confirmed an increased level of several biomarkers of inflammation and OS, for example, interleukin (IL)-6, tumor necrosis factor (TNF)-α, 8-OH 2-deoxyguanosine, and F2-isoprostanes, in major depressive disorders (MDDs) (Lindqvist et al., 2017). A clinical trial observed increased compensatory antioxidant mechanisms in stable patients with schizophrenia at early stages (González-Blanco et al., 2018). This finding suggested that there might be a causal relationship between OS and negative symptoms. On the other hand, dietary lipids help to regulate inflammation. For example, PUFAs in the brain have been associated with reduction of neuroinflammation. Lipids can regulate inflammation via several mechanisms involving the cell membrane and intracellular receptors. For example, PUFAs control cell signaling by changing membrane fluidity and lipid rafts (Munro, 2003) and therefore affect genetic pathway related to inflammation such as nuclear factor κ B (NFκB) (Calder, 2011). Lipid rafts are plasma membrane microdomains enriched in cholesterol and sphingolipids that are involved in the lateral compartmentalization of molecules at the cell surface, and lipid rafts have been suggested to affect neurotransmission and neuroinflammation. Moreover, EPA and DHA have been shown to give rise to resolvins, a kind of anti-inflammatory substances which can resolve inflammation (Calder, 2010).

N-3 PUFAs (EPA) also have the ability to counteract the inflammatory actions of n-6 PUFAs (ARA). For example, ARA is released from cell membrane phospholipids and acts as a substrate for cyclooxygenase (COX) and lipoxygenase (LOX) to yield the eicosanoid family of pro-inflammatory mediators, such as prostaglandins (PGs), thromboxanes (TXs), and leukotrienes (LTs) (Calder, 2017). Meanwhile, EPA has been shown to inhibit ARA metabolism. ARA can therefore switch to lipoxins (LXs), which can limit the progress of the initial phase of the inflammation (Chianese et al., 2018).

4.4 Lipids, microbiota, and immune system

The gut microbiota has been suggested to play an important role in our mental health and has also been reported to regulate our immune system. Accumulating evidence has shown that the microbiota plays an essential role in the establishment of our immune system. Microbiota influences the development and functioning of multiple host systems, for instance, innate and adaptive immune responses (Matamoros, Gras-Leguen, Le Vacon, Potel, & de La Cochetiere, 2013) and the regulation of homeostasis (Olszak et al., 2012). These kinds of effects started from the colonization of the gut in the early stages of life, with a continuing, both pathologically and psychologically, influence throughout the life span. Numerous factors have been reported to influence the gut microbiota, including genetics, health status, birth mode, and the environment. However, diet and nutritional status have been widely reported as the most critical influential factor for the gut microbiota at every stage of life (Sandhu et al., 2017). Moreover, several studies further support the importance of diet by showing that healthy dietary patterns, including during pregnancy and early life stages (Jacka et al., 2013), can decrease the prevalence and risk of psychiatric disorders (Lai et al., 2014; Psaltopoulou et al., 2013). A recent clinical trial further supported the importance of a healthy diet by showing that a Mediterranean style diet supplemented with fish oil can improve depressive symptoms in adults and that healthy dietary changes help improve our mental health, including reduction of depression and anxiety symptoms (Parletta et al., 2019). On the other hand, several types of dietary pattern, including a western-style diet, which is defined as high intake of saturated fats (e.g., butter, palm and coconut oils, cheese, and red meat) and sucrose and low intake of fiber may increase the risk of depression through alteration of the microbiota and activation of the immune response (Li et al., 2017).

The connection between the gut and the brain, also known as the "gut-brain axis (GBA)," has recently been widely investigated. There are multiple pathways, including the neuroendocrine, immune, and nervous systems, to affect the cross talk between the gut and the brain. These pathways are dynamic and complex. Dysfunction of GBA may cause several pathological, including both psychological and physiological, consequences. For instance, it has been reported that the biopsychosocial patterns, such as response to stress and CNS activity, have been changed in patients with GI disorders (Drossman, 1998). Recent studies reported a clear link between microbiota changes and cognition, and GBA dysregulation has been associated with depression and anxiety disorders (Kim & Shin, 2018). Additionally, the use of probiotics, prebiotics, or dietary change has been shown to improve mood and reduce anxiety in both healthy people and patient groups (Butler, Mörkl, Sandhu, Cryan, & Dinan, 2019).

N-3 PUFAs may help balance the pathogenic and nonpathogenic gut microbiota across the life span. To be specific, dietary n-3 PUFAs supplements help prevent stress-induced neuropsychiatric disorders during adolescence, and this protection has been shown to be maintained through adulthood. Moreover, n-3 PUFAs have been shown to regulate behaviors, such as impaired social communication and depression-related behaviors, in animal models (Robertson et al., 2017). Additionally, short-chain fatty acids (SCFAs), produced when dietary fiber is fermented, are the main energy for cells in the gut. It has been shown that SCFAs can promote the metabolism of B cells (Kim, Qie, Park, & Kim, 2016), which provide humoral immunity by secreting antibodies. SCFAs can also improve the function and ratio of regulatory T (Treg) cells (Arpaia et al., 2013), and balance the differentiation between T helper 17 (Th17) cells and Treg cells (Berod et al., 2014). Th17 and Treg cells both play an essential role in regulating our immune system; the former can cause inflammation, while the latter can inhibit immune reaction. Emerging evidence has shown that, together with proper dietary lipids, such as n-3 PUFAs, may have a positive impact on our immune system and our mental health through the regulation of GBA.

4.5 Lipids and nervous system

Lipids have a direct impact on the brain by modifying neuronal processes. Long-term consumption of high-fat diets can also induce insulin resistance, obesity, and diabetes (Isken et al., 2010). Animal studies have further demonstrated the effects of short-term consumption of high-fat diets on the hypothalamus, where peptides and neurotransmitters interact closely. For example, increased levels of insulin, serotonin (5-HT), leptin, and their relative receptor proteins in the hypothalamus were observed in the high-fat-diet-fed rats (Banas et al., 2009). Moreover, the inflammatory signals in the hippocampus are also increased in the mice fed with short-term high-fat diets (Nakandakari et al., 2019). These results support the concept that high-fat diets cause a rapid alteration in specific mechanisms in the hypothalamus.

Fatty acids are the major components and the key to maintaining the function of cellular membranes. The intake of different ratios of n-6/n-3 PUFAs can influence the structure of the brain. It was found that the levels of PUFAs in the prefrontal cortex, hippocampus, and hypothalamus reflected the fatty acid composition of the diet (Horman et al., 2020). DHA comprises about 14% of total fatty acids in the body and is concentrated in neuronal membranes and synapses (Brunner et al., 2002). It has been demonstrated that one of the most important functions of DHA and cholesterol is to form lipid rafts (Du et al., 2016), which play an important role in modulating synaptic plasticity and neurite outgrowth. Without a doubt, the nervous system, especially the CNS, plays an essential role in our mental status, and for the CNS to function optimally, neurotransmitters are the key players. Several psychiatric disorders have been associated with the dysfunction of neurotransmitter signaling and the imbalance of the neurotransmitters. For instance, the deficiency of 5-HT has been associated with depression (López-Muñoz & Alamo, 2009). Previous studies have demonstrated that the chronic deficiency of dietary n-3 PUFAs could lead to an increase in 5-HT$_2$ and a decrease in dopamine 2 (D$_2$) receptor density in the frontal cortex (Chalon et al., 2001; Delion et al., 1994), which has been considered as a pathological risk for depression. As the dominant components of lipid rafts, DHA and EPA have been suggested to be able to regulate both dopaminergic and serotoninergic neurotransmission (Chang & Su, 2010).

Along with neurotransmission, the hypothalamic–pituitary–adrenal (HPA) axis is another complex neuroendocrine system controlling numerous systemic functions that may contribute to the development of psychiatric disorders. Stress has been shown as a risk factor for the development of psychiatric disorders, including depressive and anxiety disorders (Slavich & Irwin, 2014). On the other hand, the HPA axis and the autonomic nervous system (ANS) can interact with the CNS, being responsible to counteract stress and regulating the mood (Rotenberg & McGrath, 2016). In animal models, rats fed with n-3 PUFAs-deficient diets displayed HPA axis hyper-reactivity after being exposed to stress, and also had an increased level of plasmatic corticosterone (PC, a kind of stress-induced hormone). On the other hand, n-3 PUFAs supplementation has been shown to help reduce PC levels (Ferraz et al., 2011). Therefore, n-3 PUFAs may be able to reduce stress-induced phenomena via alteration of the HPA axis. HPA axis dysfunction, such as dysregulation of mineralocorticoid receptors (MRs) and glucocorticoid receptors (GRs), has also been associated with both bipolar disorder and MDD. For instance, the increased synthesis of glucocorticoid in response to stress-induced physiological changes was observed in both bipolar disorder and MDD (Ulrich-Lai et al., 2015). Additionally, the HPA axis has been suggested to activate the neuroendocrine system by invoking corticotrophin-releasing hormone (CRH) released from hypothalamic paraventricular nucleus (PVN) neurons (Herman et al., 2016), which modulates our reaction against stress. Thus, the well-functioning of the HPA axis can be seen as the key to protect our mental health.

Stress may also induce changes in the gut microbiota and affect neurotransmitters, such as Gamma-aminobutyric acid (GABA), linking to anxiety and depression (Zalar et al., 2018). GBA, on the other hand, has been reported to link with the HPA axis. Moreover, studies have shown that the gut microbiota can influence the organization of the HPA axis via activating the neural pathways and CNS signaling systems, which further influences the stress response (Foster & McVey Neufeld, 2013). Several studies suggest that various stressors can influence the intestinal integrity in both animal models and humans, while probiotic treatment has been shown to regulate the activity of the HPA axis and the response to stress (Du et al., 2020). Moreover, probiotic treatment helps attenuate HPA axis response to acute psychological stress in mice (Ait-Belgnaoui et al., 2012) and prevent abnormal brain activity related to chronic stress in mice (Ait-Belgnaoui et al., 2014). Intriguingly, observations on humans also confirm the link. For example, pregnant women with a history of childhood adversities have greater differential abundance of *Prevotella*, which is associated with inflammation, in their gut microbiota and were less likely to be cortisol responders (Hantsoo et al., 2019). Cortisol responders were defined as those who significantly respond to cortisol. The results indicated that the gut microbiota may influence the activity of the HPA axis through regulating inflammation. Another animal model further showed that mice with sufficient n-3 PUFAs diets displayed greater fecal *Bifidobacterium* and *Lactobacillus* abundance, which indicate lesser inflammation, and dampened HPA axis activity.

In summary, the dysfunction of the HPA axis, which can be influenced by our diet and stress, may be the key risk factor for several major psychiatric disorders, while the alteration of the gut microbiota, possibly via the administration of n-3 PUFAs, may help restore the functions of HPA axis and the GBA, and act as a potential intervention to prevent and treat neuropsychiatric disorders.

4.6 Can omega-3 fatty acids be used as treatment? How to use them?

Psychiatric disorders account for a large burden of disability worldwide, and the prevalence rates are still increasing (Whiteford et al., 2010). There have been numerous clinical studies examining n-3 PUFAs as potential interventions for prevention and treatment of psychiatric disorders. The following is a brief summary of current research evidence of n-3 PUFAs in depression, anxiety disorders, attention-deficit hyperactivity disorder (ADHD), dementia, and other common psychiatric disorders.

4.6.1 Depression

Major depressive disorder (MDD) is a common and serious mood disorder. For patients to be diagnosed with MDD, they have to have 5 out of the 9 diagnostic criteria of MDD of The Diagnostic and Statistical Manual of Mental Disorders 5th edition (DSM-5) (see Box 4.1), with at least one of the following symptoms: (1) persistent feelings of sadness and hopelessness, and/or (2) loss of interests almost all day, and with a duration for at least 2 weeks (American Psychiatric Association, 2013). MDD disturbs our daily lives by affecting our sleep quality (either insomnia or hypersomnia), appetite (either a decrease or an increase in appetite), energy level (usually feeling more fatigue), and concentration (usually a decrease in attention). According to WHO, MDD will be one of the 2 top causes of disability in humans globally by 2030 (World Health Organization, 2017).

> **BOX 4.1**
>
> ## DSM-5 Diagnostic Criteria for Major depressive disorder (MDD).
>
> The individual must be experiencing five or more symptoms during the same 2-week period, and at least one of the symptoms should be either (1) depressed mood or (2) loss of interest or pleasure.
>
> 1. Depressed mood most of the day, nearly every day.
> 2. Markedly diminished interest or pleasure in all, or almost all, activities most of the day, nearly every day.
> 3. Significant weight loss or weight gain when not dieting, or decrease or increase in appetite nearly every day.
> 4. A slowing down of thought and a reduction of physical movement (observable by others, not merely subjective feelings of restlessness or being slowed down).
> 5. Fatigue or loss of energy nearly every day.
> 6. Feelings of worthlessness or excessive or inappropriate guilt nearly every day.
> 7. Diminished ability to think or concentrate, or indecisiveness, nearly every day.
> 8. Recurrent thoughts of death, recurrent suicidal ideation without a specific plan, or a suicide attempt or a specific plan for committing suicide.
> 9. Insomnia or hypersomnia
>
> To receive a diagnosis of depression, these symptoms must cause the individual clinically significant distress or impairment in social, occupational, or other important areas of functioning. The symptoms must also not be a result of substance abuse or another medical condition.

Thus, prevention and treatment for MDD has been called to be top priority in several countries. Current pharmacotherapy of MDD is mainly based on the "monoamine hypothesis," which states that the deficiency of monoamine neurotransmitters, mainly serotonin, in the brain causes depression or depression-like behavior. Selective serotonin reuptake inhibitors (SSRIs) and serotonin-norepinephrine reuptake inhibitors (SNRIs) are currently used as first-line treatment to treat depression. However, less than 50% of the patients achieve full remission with this type of treatment (Berton & Nestler, 2006), suggesting that monoamine-based antidepressant theory is not at all satisfactory when it comes to treating depression.

Other depressive disorders include disruptive mood dysregulation disorder, persistent depressive disorder (dysthymia), premenstrual dysphoric disorder, substance/medication-induced depressive disorder, depressive disorder due to another medical condition, other specified depressive disorder, and unspecified depressive disorder (American Psychiatric Association, 2013). However, MDD is one of the most common subtypes of depressive disorders and affects more than one-tenth of the population. MDD affects more females than males and is one of the five leading causes of years lived with disability (YLDs) in 2016 (Theo et al., 2017).

It is noted that adult patients with depression have a lower n-3 PUFAs index, that is lower serum level of n-3 PUFAs in patients with MDD (Appleton et al., 2015). In a cross-national epidemiological study, Hibbeln et al. found an inverse correlation between prevalence rates of MDD and dietary n-3 PUFAs intake (Hibbeln,

1998). Intake of fish and long-chain n-3 PUFAs were proved to lower the odds of depression symptoms, with a U-shape relationship, which means moderate intake (around 0.5–1 g/day) can be beneficial to prevent depression (Sánchez-Villegas et al., 2018). Many clinical trials and studies have also examined the efficacy (Lespérance et al., 2011; Su et al., 2003, 2013; Su, 2015) and the tolerability (Chang, Tseng, et al., 2018) of n-3 PUFAs in depression, and abundant evidence supported n-3 PUFAs as a potential alternative treatment strategy in depressive disorders (Lin et al., 2010; Nemets et al., 2002; Peet & Horrobin, 2002). Several meta-analyses (Appleton et al., 2015; Bai et al., 2018; Grosso et al., 2014; Mocking et al., 2016) have also confirmed the efficacy of n-3 PUFAs in different age and clinical groups with MDD, including pregnant women with MDD (Su et al., 2008). Related biomarkers, including lower EPA and DHA level, and increased n-6/n-3 PUFAs ratio were also observed in patients with prenatal depression (Chang, Lin, et al., 2018). Accordingly, the expert consensus panel has also supported the use of n-3 PUFAs as MDD treatment for special clinical groups including pregnant women, children, and the elderly (Guu et al., 2019).

On the other hand, the preventive effect of n-3 PUFAs was still under debate. For instance, 1.8 g/day of n-3 PUFAs intake did not show positive effect on preventing maternal depression in a 16-week trial (Vaz et al., 2017). Another review summarized that EPA failed to prevent depression in those who did not meet the criteria for a clinical diagnosis of MDD but with depression symptoms (Hallahan et al., 2016). By contrast, a randomized controlled trial shows that EPA is effective in the prevention of MDD in patients with hepatitis C virus (HCV) receiving interferon (IFN)-α therapy (Su et al., 2014). An explanation for this discrepancy in the protective effect of MDD may be due to the differences in the EPA/DHA ratio and the severity of MDD. For instance, a meta-analysis showed that n-3 PUFAs showed efficacy in trials that used a strictly criteria for MDD and trials that used an n-3 PUFAs formula with a > 60% EPA. Thus, the efficacy of using n-3 PUFAs as intervention for MDD has been widely supported, especially in those with more severe MDD and a higher EPA/DHA ratio in the n-3 PUFAs supplementation; more studies are warranted in the future to support the prevention effect of n-3 PUFAs.

As for the mechanism for using n-3 PUFAs as treatment, several key pathways have been proposed. For instance, DHA deficiency is associated with dysfunctions of neuronal membrane stability and transmission of neurotransmitters (Su, 2009). EPA is important in regulating the immune function by reducing ARA level on cell membrane and prostaglandin E2 (PGE2) synthesis (Kuan-Pin, 2008). Therefore, n-3 PUFAs provide the great interface between mind and body through neuroimmune system.

4.6.1.1 How to use EPA/DHA in different stages of depression?

Patients willing to use n-3 PUFAs should only do so after professional diagnosis and medical test. In general, several reviews (Appleton et al., 2015) and meta-analyses (Mocking et al., 2016; Yang et al., 2015) suggest that n-3 PUFAs are better used as an adjunctive treatment than monotherapy in adult patients with MDD.

The following is the clinical guideline of n-3 PUFAs in the treatment of MDD proposed by International Society for Nutritional Psychiatric Research (ISNPR) (Guu et al., 2019):

- Acute Stage of MDD (Level 1): The recommended therapeutic dosages should aim for 1–2 g/day of total EPA from pure EPA or 1–2 g/day EPA from an EPA/DHA (>2:1) combination. The dose is recommended to be increased in 2 weeks for non- or partial responders, and titrated up to the maximum dose in 4–6 weeks if tolerable. For nonresponders, it is recommended to evaluate the quality of n–3 PUFAs supplementary products.

- Recurrent MDD and maintenance treatment (Level 2): Patients with MDD usually require maintenance treatment after the acute depressive episode. Although there is no enough evidence showing that n-3 PUFAs have efficacy of preventing recurrent MDD, n–3 PUFAs could be recommended as a potential prophylactic treatment for high-risk populations (alongside standard medical care) due to their tolerability profiles. Also, the duration of acute n–3 PUFAs treatment could be extended to include maintenance treatment to potentially prevent recurrence. Of course, further follow-up studies are certainly needed.

4.6.2 Anxiety disorders

According to DSM-5, anxiety disorders include disorders that share features of excessive fear and anxiety and related behavioral disturbances. Fear is the emotional response to real or perceived imminent threat, whereas anxiety is anticipation of future threat (American Psychiatric Association, 2013). Anxiety disorders can be subdivided into generalized anxiety disorder, panic disorder/agoraphobia, and social anxiety disorder. Anxiety is the most commonly experienced symptom; moreover, approximately one-third of the population are affected by an anxiety disorder during their lifetime (Bandelow, 2015). According to a German study in 2014, specific (isolated) phobias are the most common anxiety disorders (10.3% of 12-month prevalence) (Jacobi et al., 2014). Based on the investigation by WHO in 2015, the proportion of the global population with anxiety disorders is estimated to be 264 million (about 3.6%) and is more common among females than males (4.6% compared to 2.6% at the global level) (World Health Organization, 2017). Without a doubt, anxiety disorders can be seen as one of the most widely affected psychiatric disorders around the world. Current treatments include psychotherapy and pharmacotherapy (mostly antidepressants, such as SSRIs and SNRIs, and benzodiazepines). However, each of these approaches has limitations including adverse effects (GI disturbances, for instance, such as diarrhea or constipation) and unsatisfied efficacy.

Animal studies have supported that n-3 PUFAs-deficient diet may induce anxiety-like symptoms and abnormal social behavior in adult offspring (Lafourcade et al., 2011). In clinical observation, patients with anxiety disorders also have lower n-3 PUFAs and higher ratio of n-6 to n-3 PUFAs in both their blood and the brain (Green et al., 2006), which is similar to animal and clinical studies of n-3 PUFAs levels in MDD (Thesing et al., 2018). Therefore, anxiety and depressive disorders may share the similar mechanisms mediated by n-3 PUFAs (Larrieu & Layé, 2018). A review had highlighted the possible mechanisms of n-3 PUFAs on anxiety: (1) anti-inflammatory function, (2) regulation of neuroendocrine system, and (3) cortisol modulation (Polokowski et al., 2020). However, relatively few studies focus solely on anxiety disorders. Further basic studies are needed to confirm the link between n-3 PUFAs and anxiety disorders.

As for the clinical aspect, a meta-analysis has examined approximately 2000 participants and showed that the anxiolytic effect of n-3 PUFAs was more effective with a higher dosage, in this case at least 2000 mg/day (Su et al., 2018). Unlike MDD, it is not as common to use n-3 PUFAs as an intervention for anxiety disorders. Although some meta-analyses show that n-3 PUFAs supplementation has the effect in preventing anxiety symptoms in certain circumstances, such as substance abusers (Buydens-Branchey & Branchey, 2006), patients with acute myocardial infarction (Haberka et al., 2013), and in medical students (Kiecolt-Glaser et al., 2011), another meta-analysis of clinical randomized trials did not support the prevention effect of n-3 PUFAs in anxiety disorders (Deane et al., 2021). Therefore, we currently can only conclude that the effects of n-3 PUFAs as treatments in anxiety disorders may be dose-dependent and should be indicated for individuals with specific anxiety disorder diagnoses, while the exact dosage warrants future investigation.

4.6.3 Attention-deficit/hyperactivity disorder (ADHD)

Attention-deficit/hyperactivity disorder (ADHD) is a common neurodevelopmental disorder that features inattention, hyperactivity, and impulsivity. These symptoms often impair school, social, or work performance. Current treatments for ADHD include both behavioral therapy and pharmacotherapy. For pharmacotherapy, methylphenidate (MPH) is used as a first-line treatment along with atomoxetine (ATX) (Quintana et al., 2007). In terms of the mechanisms of these two medications, MPH inhibits the reuptake of dopamine and norepinephrine which increased dopaminergic and noradrenergic activity in the prefrontal cortex (Garnock-Jones & Keating, 2009), while ATX is the selective inhibitor of presynaptic norepinephrine reuptake in the prefrontal cortex. Although MPH has been shown good clinical efficacy in ADHD, there is still about 20–40% of ADHD patients do not benefit from the treatment (Pliszka et al., 2006). Hence, novel treatments such as cognitive, herbal, acupuncture, and dietary interventions may have a role as alternative treatments. Among the alternative treatments, n-3 PUFAs in ADHD patients have recently received great attention.

Children with ADHD have significantly lower concentrations of plasma n-3 PUFAs. Furthermore, lower red blood cells (RBCs) n-3 PUFAs and a higher n-6/n-3 ratio have been reported in ADHD. Lower n-3 PUFAs levels have been positively associated with the severity of ADHD symptoms in children (Colter et al., 2008). These findings were further supported by a recent meta-analysis showing that youth with ADHD have lower levels of DHA, EPA, n-3 PUFAs, and AA when compared with normal controls, which suggest that n-3 PUFAs supplementation may play a role in treating ADHD. The n-3 PUFAs dosage used in the ADHD clinical trials ranged widely, for example, supplementation may range from 2.7 to 640 mg for DHA and 80 to 650 mg for EPA. The meta-analysis further showed n-3 PUFAs improved inattention and total ADHD symptoms despite the supplementation dosage, while only supplementation with an EPA dosage of greater than 500 mg/day was shown to improve hyperactivity symptoms. Furthermore, high-dose EPA (1.2 g/day) improved focused attention and vigilance in patients with low endogenous EPA levels. Another study showed that the addition of PUFAs can help lower the dosage of MPH to achieve the same improvement (Derbyshire, 2017). A panel of experts reached the consensus that a total of at least 750 mg of combined DHA and EPA should be prescribed for children with ADHD who wish to receive n-3 PUFAs supplementation (Banaschewski et al., 2018). In terms of the duration of the treatment, a combination of DHA and EPA with a longer than 15-week duration showed the most efficacy (Agostoni et al., 2017). A recently published guideline of n-3 PUFAs in children with ADHD further suggested that a combination of EPA and DHA with a dose over 750 mg/day and a higher dose of EPA up to 1200 mg/day for those with inflammation or allergic diseases were suggested for a duration of 16–24 weeks (Chang & Su, 2020).

Concerning the mechanism, some studies have found inflammatory abnormalities in ADHD such as higher IL-6 (Chang et al., 2020) and IL-10 levels (Donfrancesco et al., 2016). On the other hand, another study shows that n-3 supplementation in ADHD children reduces IL-6 and C-reactive protein (CRP) levels (Hariri et al., 2012), which correlates to the theoretical model that PUFAs may affect ADHD symptoms via an anti-inflammatory action. A recent study also indicated that ADHD may be related to HPA axis dysregulation. Therefore, the stratification of ADHD children by n-3 PUFAs levels or immune biomarkers could be a promising personalized approach to optimize the effects of n-3 PUFAs supplementation.

4.6.4 Dementia

Dementia is defined as a neurocognitive disorder with the manifestation of meaningful decline compared with the previous level of cognitive performance (Fiest et al., 2016). Nowadays, the global annual period prevalence rate of dementia reached about 6.9% (Brodaty & Donkin, 2009). The high prevalence rate not only indicates the daily life quality impairment of the patient but also an increase in the burden of the family caregivers (Liara et al., 2014). Among the different types of dementia, Alzheimer's disease (AD) and vascular dementia are the two most common types (Casey et al., 2010). Currently, drugs that have been approved by the Food and Drug Administration (FDA) for treating AD include cholinesterase inhibitors and N-methyl-D-aspartate (NMDA) receptor antagonist. However, they are both supportive and palliative treatments with high costs (Casey et al., 2010). Therefore, novel dietary treatments such as vitamin E and n-3 PUFAs (DHA and EPA) consumption have been investigated as potential treatment options (Dysken et al., 2014).

Concerning AD, it is closely linked to changes in lipid metabolism. Among all the hallmarks of AD, amyloid-β (Aβ) deposition is the main pathological hallmark of AD (Grimm et al., 2017). It has been shown that EPA can enhance Aβ degradation mediated by increasing the gene expression of insulin-degrading enzyme (IDE). EPA can also affect the gene expression of many inflammation-related genes in immune cells such as microglial cells in the brain (Vors et al., 2017). Likewise, the effect of DHA on IDE results in increased Aβ degradation. Clinically, however, the findings have been controversial. For example, a meta-analysis showed that higher dietary intake of long-chain n-3 PUFAs is not significantly associated with a lower risk of AD. Moreover, a randomized trial indicated that supplementation with DHA did not slow the rate of cognitive and functional decline in patients with mild-to-moderate AD (Quinn et al., 2010). Nonetheless, a former study showed that n-3 PUFAs 1.8 g/day improved cognitive function in the mild cognitive impairment (MCI) group, a prodromal state that could precede the progress of AD.

In patients with vascular dementia, reduced blood flow to the brain may further affect cognitive abilities such as executive functioning (Venkat et al., 2015). Furthermore, the most common cause of the reduced blood flow is chronic inflammation resulting from atherosclerosis that induces cerebral infarction. On the other hand, n-3 PUFAs when compared to placebo have been shown to reduce circulating high sensitivity CRP in patients with vascular dementia (Bhatt et al., 2019). Thus, n-3 PUFAs may be able to reduce the risk for vascular dementia by lowering the risk for chronic inflammation with their anti-inflammatory and anti-thrombotic and anti-atherosclerotic process properties (Chang & Deckelbaum, 2013). When it comes to the supplementation dosage of n-3 PUFAs for primary and secondary prevention of vascular dementia, studies showed only with n-3 PUFAs administration ranging between 1.8 and 4 g/day can lead to a significant reduction in CV morbidity and mortality (Bhatt et al., 2019). Moreover, studies showed that supplementation with at least 1.2 g EPA and DHA in high risk of dementia population not only decrease the incidence of dementia but also ameliorate the working memory performance and processing speed (Bo, 2017; Boespflug et al., 2016; Hooper et al., 2017).

Briefly, although the promising benefit of n-3 PUFAs is mostly accepted for vascular dementia, there is little evidence regarding the beneficial effect of n-3 PUFAs supplementation in the cognitive decline of AD. However, n-3 PUFAs have shown some promising effects in MCI

(Rosa, 2018). Hence, n-3 PUFAs should be featured as the prevention strategy rather than the treatment strategy in dementia, and more clinical trials focusing on the prevention of dementia in high-risk groups with different dosages and durations of n-3 PUFAs are warranted.

4.6.5 Other disorders

4.6.5.1 Bipolar disorders (BDs)

According to DSM-5, BDs are defined as a group of brain disorders that cause extreme fluctuation in the mood, energy, and ability to function in an individual. BD include three different conditions—bipolar I, bipolar II, and cyclothymic disorder (see Box 4.2) (American Psychiatric Association, 2013). A cross-nation study found that lower n-3 dietary intake (i.e., fish) was associated with higher prevalence rates of BD (Noaghiul & Hibbeln, 2003). Lower level of n-3 PUFAs has also been shown in symptomatic BD and has shown correlations with clinical severities (Saunders et al., 2016). As for the treatments, growing evidence shows that n-3 PUFAs may be potential as the treatment of BD. Two clinical trials have confirmed the efficacy of n-3 PUFAs supplement for depressive symptom, but not manic symptoms, of BD (Frangou et al., 2006; Stoll et al., 1999). By contrast, manic and depressive symptoms of juvenile patients with pediatric BD were reduced by n-3 PUFAs intake (Clayton et al., 2009). On the other hand, a small clinical trial showed that the combined treatment of n-3 PUFAs and inositol reduced symptoms of mania and depression in prepubertal children with mild-to-moderate BD (Wozniak et al., 2015). Thus, the efficacy of n-3 PUFAs for depressive symptoms in BD is widely confirmed, while the efficacy for manic symptoms is still under debate. Therefore, n-3 PUFAs can be viewed as a potential add-on to the standard treatment for depressive episodes of BD.

4.6.5.2 Post-traumatic stress disorder (PTSD)

PTSD, now included in the category of trauma- and stressor-related disorders in DSM-5, may occur in people who have experienced or witnessed a traumatic event such as a natural disaster, a serious accident, a terrorist act, war/combat, or rape, or who have been threatened with death, sexual violence, or serious injury (American Psychiatric Association, 2013). Moreover, PTSD is strongly linked to suicide behavior. In a cross-sectional study, lower DHA was observed in PTSD patients compared to controls after correcting for diet (de Vries et al., 2016). Moreover, several reviews concluded that n-3 PUFAs supplement is an easy way to protect individuals against stress-related psychiatric disorders, including PTSD (Du et al., 2016). A clinical trial in Japan further found that post-trauma supplementation of n-3 PUFAs might be effective for the secondary prevention of psychophysiological symptoms of PTSD (Matsumura et al., 2017). On the other hand, another clinical trial by the same team reported that DHA supplementation was not superior to placebo for the secondary prevention of PTSD symptoms (Matsuoka et al., 2015). Thus, the efficacy of n-3 PUFAs in PTSD, with limited clinical trials, remains controversial.

BOX 4.2

Conditions of Bipolar disorders in DSM-5.

1. Bipolar I disorder: A manic-depressive disorder that can exist both with and without psychotic episodes
2. Bipolar II disorder: It consists of depressive and manic episodes which alternate and are typically less severe and do not inhibit function
3. Cyclothymic disorder: A cyclic disorder that causes brief episodes of hypomania and depression

4.6.5.3 Schizophrenia

Schizophrenia is defined as a severe, chronic mental disorder characterized by disturbances in thought, perception, and behavior. The lifetime prevalence of schizophrenia is approximately 0.3–0.7% (American Psychiatric Association, 2013) (see Box 4.3). In basic studies, a review concludes that the abnormal phospholipid metabolism may be involved in the pathogenesis of schizophrenia (Knöchel et al., 2015). Antipsychotic medications are the first-line treatments for schizophrenia. Growing evidence indicates that n-3 PUFAs have the potential of preventing or mitigating the symptom of schizophrenia. There have been several clinical trials but with mixed results. Accordingly, a meta-analysis revealed no beneficial effect of EPA augmentation in established schizophrenia (Fusar-Poli & Berger, 2012). Recently, most of the clinical studies are other diseases combined with schizophrenia, such as metabolic syndrome and inflammatory indices (Behdani et al., 2018; Xu et al., 2019), confirmed the efficacy of n-3 PUFAs. However, we cannot conclude the long-term or prevention effects of n-3 PUFAs on schizophrenia. Further and larger clinical trials are needed.

4.6.5.4 Autism spectrum disorder (ASD)

ASD is a severe disruption of the normal development process and is often diagnosed before the age of three. ASD is viewed as a spectrum or a continuum of disorders, with varying degrees of severity and levels of functioning. ASD included autistic disorder, childhood disintegrative disorder, pervasive developmental disorder-not otherwise specified (PDD-NOS), and Asperger syndrome (American Psychiatric Association, 1994). The pathology of ASD is complex. Besides genetic factors, nutrients are as important. A meta-analysis of 15 clinical trials concluded that those with ASD have lower index of n-3 PUFAs (Mazahery et al., 2019). Another meta-analysis also revealed the similar results (Cheng et al., 2019). Additionally, several reviews confirmed that n-3 PUFAs are associated with multiple mechanisms, including lipidomics (El-Ansary et al., 2020), neurodevelopment (Martins et al., 2020), and microbiota (Madore et al., 2016). However, results from clinical trials are mixed—some reported with positive or potential efficacy of n-3 PUFAs (Mazahery et al., 2017), while others did not (Fraguas et al., 2019; Sathe et al., 2017). Thus, the evidence for n-3 PUFAs as monotherapy for ASD warrants more studies in the future. On the other hand, a recently published guideline suggested that a combination of EPA+DHA of 1300–1500 mg/day for 16–24 weeks may be used as an add-on therapy to target specific symptoms, such as lethargy and hyperactivity, in children with ASD (Chang & Su, 2020).

4.6.5.5 Eating disorders (ED)

EDs are defined as a persistent disturbance of eating which will eventually lead to nutritional deficiency and impairment in psychosocial functioning (Satogami et al., 2019). DSM-5 classified ED into six types which included pica, rumination disorder, avoidant/restrictive food

---

BOX 4.3

Brief outline for schizophrenia in DSM-5.

1. Two or more of the following for at least one month (or longer period of time), and at least one of them must be a 1, 2, or 3:
   a. delusions
   b. hallucinations
   c. disorganized speech
   d. grossly disorganized or catatonic behavior
   e. negative symptoms, such as diminished emotional expression
2. Impairment in one of the major areas of functioning for a significant period of time since the onset of the disturbance: work, interpersonal relations, or self-care.

intake disorder, anorexia nervosa (AN), bulimia nervosa (BN), and binge-eating disorder (BED) (Christine et al., 2013). We will focus on AN, BN, and BED in this section. A recent study showed that the prevalence estimates of lifetime AN, BN, and BED were 0.8%, 0.28%, and 0.85%, respectively (Udo & Grilo, 2018). Hence, in addition to medication as well as cognitive-behavior therapy, n-3 PUFAs supplementation may offer an alternative treatment option for these three disorders. Patients with ED have been reported to have higher plasma levels of n-3 PUFAs and lower n-6 PUFAs as well as a lower n-6 PUFAs/n-3 PUFAs ratio (Satogami et al., 2019). A study carried out on children and adolescents with ED, where the participants received a daily total of 500mg n-3 PUFAs (300mg EPA and 200mg DHA) for 8 weeks, showed an increase in mean percent ideal body weight without obvious side effect (Woo et al., 2017). However, the data of clinical use of n-3 PUFAs in patients with ED are too scarce to draw any consistent conclusion (Bozzatello et al., 2019).

4.6.5.6 Addiction

Addiction is usually divided into two categories, which include substance addiction and nonsubstance addiction. To be more specific, nonsubstance addiction covers pathological gambling, food addiction, Internet addiction, and mobile phone addiction (Zou et al., 2017), while substance addiction indicates a pathological pattern of behaviors related to the use of the substance. Regardless of substance-related or nonsubstance-related, psychopathological mechanisms may all be attributed to the intense activation of the reward system that may result in the neglect of daily activities (Grant & Chamberlain, 2016). For many patients, addiction is a chronic or relapsing condition that lasts many years after diagnosis (Vaillant, 2003). Moreover, nearly 40–60% of patients treated for alcohol or other drug dependence return to regular use within 1 year following the treatment (Hubbard et al., 2003). Therefore, regarding the connection between dopaminergic neurotransmission and n-3 PUFAs, studies have been conducted to solve the recent predicament concerning the treatment for patients with addiction. Noteworthy, nicotine dependence is the most widely discussed addiction with the use of n-3 PUFAs as treatment. A study indicated that the peripheral n-3 PUFAs level is much lower in smokers than in nonsmokers (Scaglia et al., 2016). Furthermore, the patient showed a significant reduction in their levels of addiction with the daily supplement of 210.99mg EPA and 129.84mg of DHA for 4 months (Zaparoli et al., 2016). Thus, the use of PUFAs for patients with addiction, such as nicotine use, shows promising results.

4.6.6 Safety for using EPA/DHA as intervention in different genders and ages

Although n-3 PUFAs have been widely reported for their tolerability and relative less adverse effects when compared with standard treatment in neuropsychiatric disorders, there are still some potential adverse effects associated with n-3 PUFAs. The potential adverse effects of n-3 PUFAs include several categories. We list several common adverse effects confirmed based on a meta-analysis (Chang, Tseng, et al., 2018) and a guideline (Guu et al., 2019) in Table 4.1. Therefore, it is recommended

TABLE 4.1 Common adverse effects for n-3 PUFAs intervention.

Category	Common adverse effects
Gastrointestinal	Eructation, nausea, and dysgeusia
Dermatological	Skin eruption, itching, exanthema, and eczema
Biochemical	Higher level of LDL-C, fasting blood glucose, GPT, and BUN
Hematological	Lower level of hemoglobin, hematocrit, and anticoagulation problems

Abbreviations: *BUN*, blood urea nitrogen; *GPT*, glutamic-pyruvic transaminase; *LDL-C*, low-density lipoprotein cholesterol.

to monitor adverse effects systematically, including the gastrointestinal and dermatological conditions, and obtaining a comprehensive metabolic panel in patients receiving higher doses of n-3 PUFAs.

4.7 Conclusion

Lipids, especially n-3 PUFAs, play an essential role in both function and structure of brain, where in charge of our emotion and mental health. Moreover, n-3 PUFAs can regulate not merely brain function, but (1) inflammation and oxidative stress, (2) microbiota, (3) immune system, and (4) nervous system as well (Box 4.4). Chronic deficiency of n-3 PUFAs is one of the major risk factors for the development of psychiatric disorders. Therefore, n-3 PUFAs, especially EPA, intake should be an effective intervention and prevention for psychiatric disorders. We summarized the current evidence accordingly in Table 4.2.

BOX 4.4

Summary of how dietary lipids regulate our mental health.

1. N-3 PUFAs, especially EPA, can limit the progress of inflammation, which may inhibit the development of psychiatric disorders.
2. There is a bidirectal connection "gut-brain axis" between gut and brain, and n-3 PUFAs can help balance the pathogenic and nonpathogenic gut microbiota.
3. N-3 PUFAs and SCFAs can promote the metabolism of B cells and balance the immune system through regulating Th cells and Treg cells.
4. Lipids have direct impact on the brain by modifying neuronal processes.

   DHA and EPA regulate both dopaminergic and serotoninergic neurotransmission, which strongly link to psychiatric disorders.

   Stress or improper diet may induce the dysfunction of HPA axis, and n-3 PUFAs may help stabilize its activity.

TABLE 4.2 Brief summary for using n-3 PUFAs in psychiatry disorders.

Disorders	Level of evidence and recommendation	Explanation
Depression	Strong for intervention. Moderate for prevention	Strongly recommended to use in MDD, and the guideline is also provided. Recommended to use as intervention in depression or prevention depression-like behaviors, but the standard dosage was not provided yet
Anxiety	Strong for intervention. Moderate for prevention	Recommended to use high dosage in anxiety disorders, but no guideline provided. Positive efficacy results were reported only in certain circumstances as prevention
ADHD	Strong for intervention. Unclear for prevention	Recommended to use with the dosage over 750 mg for treating ADHD. Limited studies for prevention
Dementia	Unclear for intervention. Moderate for prevention	Strongly recommended to use as prevention in vascular dementia. Positive efficacy as intervention was reported in mild cognitive function impairment population

Continued

TABLE 4.2 Brief summary for using n-3 PUFAs in psychiatry disorders.—cont'd

Disorders	Level of evidence and recommendation	Explanation
Bipolar	Moderate for intervention. Unclear for prevention	The efficacy was recommended to use in depressive symptoms, while manic symptoms remain unclear. Not enough evidence supports for prevention
PTSD	Unclear for intervention. Unclear for prevention	Limited studies for both intervention and prevention n-3 PUFAs may be potential for treatment
Schizophrenia	Moderate for intervention. Unclear for prevention	Efficacy was only confirmed in schizophrenia combined with other diseases. n-3 PUFAs may be potential for treatment
Autism	Moderate for intervention. Unclear for prevention	Recommended to use as an add-on therapy, with guideline provided
Eating disorder	Moderate for intervention. Unclear for prevention	Limited studies for prevention. n-3 PUFAs may be potential for treatment with the duration of 8 weeks
Addiction	Moderate for intervention. Unclear for prevention	Limited studies for prevention. n-3 PUFAs may be potential for treatment with the duration of 4 months

Abbreviations: *ADHD*, attention deficit/hyperactivity disorder; *MDD*, major depressive disorder; *PTSD*, post-traumatic stress disorder.

References

Agostoni, C., Mazzocchi, A., Leone, L., Ciappolino, V., Delvecchio, G., Altamura, C. A., et al. (2017). The first model of keeping energy balance and optimal psycho affective development: Breastfed infants. *Journal of Affective Disorders*, 224, 10–15. https://doi.org/10.1016/j.jad.2017.01.001.

Ait-Belgnaoui, A., Colom, A., Braniste, V., Ramalho, L., Marrot, A., Cartier, C., et al. (2014). Probiotic gut effect prevents the chronic psychological stress-induced brain activity abnormality in mice. *Neurogastroenterology and Motility*, 26(4), 510–520. https://doi.org/10.1111/nmo.12295.

Ait-Belgnaoui, A., Durand, H., Cartier, C., Chaumaz, G., Eutamene, H., Ferrier, L., et al. (2012). Prevention of gut leakiness by a probiotic treatment leads to attenuated HPA response to an acute psychological stress in rats. *Psychoneuroendocrinology*, 37(11), 1885–1895. https://doi.org/10.1016/j.psyneuen.2012.03.024.

American Psychiatric Association. (1994). *Diagnostic and statistical manual of mental disorders: Fourth edition*. American Psychiatric Association.

American Psychiatric Association. (2013). *Diagnostic and statistical manual of mental disorders*. American Psychiatric Association.

Appleton, K. M., Sallis, H. M., Perry, R., Ness, A. R., & Churchill, R. (2015). Omega-3 fatty acids for depression in adults. *Cochrane Database of Systematic Reviews*, 2015(11). https://doi.org/10.1002/14651858.CD004692.pub4.

Arpaia, N., Campbell, C., Fan, X., Dikiy, S., van der Veeken, J., deRoos, P., et al. (2013). Metabolites produced by commensal bacteria promote peripheral regulatory T-cell generation. *Nature*, 504(7480), 451–455. https://doi.org/10.1038/nature12726.

Bai, Z. G., Bo, A., Wu, S. J., Gai, Q. Y., & Chi, I. (2018). Omega-3 polyunsaturated fatty acids and reduction of depressive symptoms in older adults: A systematic review and meta-analysis. *Journal of Affective Disorders*, 241, 241–248. https://doi.org/10.1016/j.jad.2018.07.057.

Banas, S. M., Rouch, C., Kassis, N., Markaki, E. M., & Gerozissis, K. (2009). A dietary fat excess alters metabolic and neuroendocrine responses before the onset of metabolic diseases. *Cellular and Molecular Neurobiology*, 29(2), 157–168. https://doi.org/10.1007/s10571-008-9307-9.

Banaschewski, T., Belsham, B., Bloch, M. H., Ferrin, M., Johnson, M., Kustow, J., et al. (2018). Supplementation with polyunsaturated fatty acids (PUFAs) in the management of attention deficit hyperactivity disorder (ADHD). *Nutrition and Health*, 24(4), 279–284. https://doi.org/10.1177/0260106018772170.

Bandelow, B. (2015). Epidemiology of anxiety disorders in the 21st century. *Dialogues in Clinical Neuroscience*, 327–335. https://doi.org/10.31887/dcns.2015.17.3/bbandelow.

Behdani, F., Roudbaraki, S. N., Saberi-Karimian, M., Tayefi, M., Hebrani, P., Akhavanrezayat, A., et al. (2018). Assessment of the efficacy of omega-3 fatty acids on metabolic and inflammatory parameters in patients with schizophrenia taking clozapine and sodium valproate. *Psychiatry Research*, *261*, 243–247. https://doi.org/10.1016/j.psychres.2017.12.028.

Berod, L., Friedrich, C., Nandan, A., Freitag, J., Hagemann, S., Harmrolfs, K., et al. (2014). De novo fatty acid synthesis controls the fate between regulatory T and T helper 17 cells. *Nature Medicine*, *20*(11), 1327–1333. https://doi.org/10.1038/nm.3704.

Berton, O., & Nestler, E. J. (2006). New approaches to antidepressant drug discovery: Beyond monoamines. *Nature Reviews Neuroscience*, *7*(2), 137–151. https://doi.org/10.1038/nrn1846.

Bhatt, D. L., Steg, P. G., Miller, M., Brinton, E. A., Jacobson, T. A., Ketchum, S. B., et al. (2019). Cardiovascular risk reduction with icosapent ethyl for hypertriglyceridemia. *New England Journal of Medicine*, *380*(1), 11–22. https://doi.org/10.1056/NEJMoa1812792.

Bhattacharyya, A., Chattopadhyay, R., Mitra, S., & Crowe, S. E. (2014). Oxidative stress: An essential factor in the pathogenesis of gastrointestinal mucosal diseases. *Physiological Reviews*, *94*(2), 329–354. https://doi.org/10.1152/physrev.00040.2012.

Black, C. N., Bot, M., Scheffer, P. G., Cuijpers, P., & Penninx, B. W. J. H. (2015). Is depression associated with increased oxidative stress? A systematic review and meta-analysis. *Psychoneuroendocrinology*, *51*, 164–175. https://doi.org/10.1016/j.psyneuen.2014.09.025.

Bo, Y. (2017). The n-3 polyunsaturated fatty acids supplementation improved the cognitive function in the Chinese elderly with mild cognitive impairment: A double-blind randomized controlled trial. *Nutrients*, *9*(1).

Boespflug, E. L., McNamara, R. K., Eliassen, J. C., Schidler, M. D., & Krikorian, R. (2016). Fish oil supplementation increases event-related posterior cingulate activation in older adults with subjective memory impairment. *The Journal of Nutrition, Health & Aging*, *20*(2), 161–169. https://doi.org/10.1007/s12603-015-0609-6.

Bozzatello, P., Rocca, P., Mantelli, E., & Bellino, S. (2019). Polyunsaturated fatty acids: What is their role in treatment of psychiatric disorders? *International Journal of Molecular Sciences*, *20*(21). https://doi.org/10.3390/ijms20215257.

Brodaty, H., & Donkin, M. (2009). Family caregivers of people with dementia. *Dialogues in Clinical Neuroscience*, *11*(2), 217–228.

Brunner, J., Parhofer, K. G., Schwandt, P., & Bronisch, T. (2002). Cholesterol, essential fatty acids, and suicide. *Pharmacopsychiatry*, *35*(1), 1–5. https://doi.org/10.1055/s-2002-19834.

Butler, M. I., Mörkl, S., Sandhu, K. V., Cryan, J. F., & Dinan, T. G. (2019). The gut microbiome and mental health: What should we tell our patients?: Le microbiote Intestinal et la Santé Mentale : que Devrions-Nous dire à nos Patients? *The Canadian Journal of Psychiatry*, *64*(11), 747–760. https://doi.org/10.1177/0706743719874168.

Buydens-Branchey, L., & Branchey, M. (2006). n-3 polyunsaturated fatty acids decrease anxiety feelings in a population of substance abusers. *Journal of Clinical Psychopharmacology*, *26*(6), 661–665. https://doi.org/10.1097/01.jcp.0000246214.49271.f1.

Calder, P. C. (2010). Omega-3 fatty acids and inflammatory processes. *Nutrients*, *2*(3), 355–374. https://doi.org/10.3390/nu2030355.

Calder, P. C. (2011). Fatty acids and inflammation: The cutting edge between food and pharma. *European Journal of Pharmacology*, *668*(1), S50–S58. https://doi.org/10.1016/j.ejphar.2011.05.085.

Calder, P. C. (2017). Omega-3 fatty acids and inflammatory processes: From molecules to man. *Biochemical Society Transactions*, *45*(5), 1105–1115. https://doi.org/10.1042/BST20160474.

Casey, D. A., Antimisiaris, D., & O'Brien, J. (2010). Drugs for Alzheimer's disease: Are they effective? *P & T*, *35*(4), 208–211. http://www.ptcommunity.com/ptJournal/fulltext/35/4/PTJ3504208.pdf.

Chalon, S., Vancassel, S., Zimmer, L., Guilloteau, D., & Durand, G. (2001). Polyunsaturated fatty acids and cerebral function: Focus on monoaminergic neurotransmission. *Lipids*, *36*(9), 937–944. https://doi.org/10.1007/s11745-001-0804-7.

Chang, C. L., & Deckelbaum, R. J. (2013). Omega-3 fatty acids: Mechanisms underlying "protective effects" in atherosclerosis. *Current Opinion in Lipidology*, *24*(4), 345–350. https://doi.org/10.1097/MOL.0b013e3283616364.

Chang, J. P. C., Lin, C. Y., Lin, P. Y., Shih, Y. H., Chiu, T. H., Ho, M., et al. (2018). Polyunsaturated fatty acids and inflammatory markers in major depressive episodes during pregnancy. *Progress in Neuro-Psychopharmacology and Biological Psychiatry*, *80*, 273–278. https://doi.org/10.1016/j.pnpbp.2017.05.008.

Chang, J. P. C., Mondelli, V., Satyanarayanan, S. K., Chiang, Y. J., Chen, H. T., Su, K. P., et al. (2020). Cortisol, inflammatory biomarkers and neurotrophins in children and adolescents with attention deficit hyperactivity disorder (ADHD) in Taiwan. *Brain, Behavior, and Immunity*, *88*, 105–113. https://doi.org/10.1016/j.bbi.2020.05.017.

Chang, J. P. C., & Su, K. P. (2010). The lipid raft hypothesis: The relation among omega-3 fatty acids, depression and cardiovascular diseases. Review. *Taiwanese Journal of Psychiatry*, *24*, 168–180.

Chang, J. P. C., & Su, K. P. (2020). Nutritional neuroscience as mainstream of psychiatry: The evidence-based treatment guidelines for using omega-3 fatty acids as a new treatment for psychiatric disorders in children and adolescents. *Clinical Psychopharmacology and Neuroscience*, *18*(4), 469–483. https://doi.org/10.9758/CPN.2020.18.4.469.

Chang, C. H., Tseng, P. T., Chen, N. Y., Lin, P. C., Lin, P. Y., Chang, J. P. C., et al. (2018). Safety and tolerability of prescription omega-3 fatty acids: A systematic review and meta-analysis of randomized controlled trials. *Prostaglandins, Leukotrienes, and Essential Fatty Acids, 129*, 1–12. https://doi.org/10.1016/j.plefa.2018.01.001.

Cheng, J., Eskenazi, B., Widjaja, F., Cordero, J. F., & Hendren, R. L. (2019). Improving autism perinatal risk factors: A systematic review. *Medical Hypotheses, 127*, 26–33. https://doi.org/10.1016/j.mehy.2019.03.012.

Chianese, R., Coccurello, R., Viggiano, A., Scafuro, M., Fiore, M., Coppola, G., et al. (2018). Impact of dietary fats on brain functions. *Current Neuropharmacology, 16*(7), 1059–1085. https://doi.org/10.2174/1570159X15666171017102547.

Christine, C., Timothy, W. B., & Evelyn, A. (2013). From DSM-IV to DSM-5. *Current Opinion in Psychiatry*, 532–536. https://doi.org/10.1097/YCO.0b013e328365a321.

Clayton, E. H., Hanstock, T. L., Hirneth, S. J., Kable, C. J., Garg, M. L., & Hazell, P. L. (2009). Reduced mania and depression in juvenile bipolar disorder associated with long-chain ω-3 polyunsaturated fatty acid supplementation. *European Journal of Clinical Nutrition, 63*(8), 1037–1040. https://doi.org/10.1038/ejcn.2008.81.

Colter, A. L., Cutler, C., & Meckling, K. A. (2008). Fatty acid status and behavioural symptoms of attention deficit hyperactivity disorder in adolescents: A case-control study. *Nutrition Journal, 7*(1). https://doi.org/10.1186/1475-2891-7-8.

de Vries, G. J., Mocking, R., Lok, A., Assies, J., Schene, A., & Olff, M. (2016). Fatty acid concentrations in patients with posttraumatic stress disorder compared to healthy controls. *Journal of Affective Disorders, 205*, 351–359. https://doi.org/10.1016/j.jad.2016.08.021.

Deane, K. H. O., Jimoh, O. F., Biswas, P., O'Brien, A., Hanson, S., Abdelhamid, A. S., et al. (2021). Omega-3 and polyunsaturated fat for prevention of depression and anxiety symptoms: Systematic review and meta-analysis of randomised trials. *The British Journal of Psychiatry, 218*(3), 135–142. https://doi.org/10.1192/bjp.2019.234.

Delion, S., Chalon, S., Herault, J., Guilloteau, D., Besnard, J. C., & Durand, G. (1994). Chronic dietary α-linolenic acid deficiency alters dopaminergic and serotoninergic neurotransmission in rats. *Journal of Nutrition, 124*(12), 2466–2476. https://doi.org/10.1093/jn/124.12.2466.

Derbyshire, E. (2017). Do omega-3/6 fatty acids have a therapeutic role in children and young people with ADHD? *Journal of Lipids, 2017*, 6285218. https://doi.org/10.1155/2017/6285218.

Dixon, M. (2019). *Restored by grace: A journey like no other*. Life-Rich Publishing.

Donfrancesco, R., Nativio, P., Borrelli, E., Giua, E., Andriola, E., Villa, M. P., et al. (2016). Serum cytokines in paediatric neuropsychiatric syndromes: Focus on attention deficit hyperactivity disorder. *Minerva Pediatrica, 73*(5), 398–404.

Drossman, D. A. (1998). Presidential address: Gastrointestinal illness and the biopsychosocial model. *Psychosomatic Medicine, 60*(3), 258–267. https://doi.org/10.1097/00006842-199805000-00007. PMID: 9625212.

Du, Y., Gao, X. R., Peng, L., & Ge, J. F. (2020). Crosstalk between the microbiota-gut-brain axis and depression. *Heliyon, 6*(6). https://doi.org/10.1016/j.heliyon.2020.e04097.

Du, J., Zhu, M., Bao, H., Li, B., Dong, Y., Xiao, C., et al. (2016). The role of nutrients in protecting mitochondrial function and neurotransmitter signaling: Implications for the treatment of depression, PTSD, and suicidal behaviors. *Critical Reviews in Food Science and Nutrition, 56*(15), 2560–2578. https://doi.org/10.1080/10408398.2013.876960.

Dysken, M. W., Sano, M., Asthana, S., Vertrees, J. E., Pallaki, M., Llorente, M., et al. (2014). Effect of vitamin E and memantine on functional decline in Alzheimer disease: The TEAM-AD VA cooperative randomized trial. *JAMA: The Journal of the American Medical Association, 311*(1), 33–44. https://doi.org/10.1001/jama.2013.282834.

El-Ansary, A., Chirumbolo, S., Bhat, R. S., Dadar, M., Ibrahim, E. M., & Bjørklund, G. (2020). The role of lipidomics in autism spectrum disorder. *Molecular Diagnosis & Therapy, 24*(1), 31–48. https://doi.org/10.1007/s40291-019-00430-0.

Farr, S. B., & Kogoma, T. (1991). Oxidative stress responses in Escherichia coli and Salmonella typhimurium. *Microbiological Reviews, 55*(4), 561–585. https://doi.org/10.1128/mmbr.55.4.561-585.1991.

Ferraz, A. C., Delattre, A. M., Almendra, R. G., Sonagli, M., Borges, C., Araujo, P., et al. (2011). Chronic ω-3 fatty acids supplementation promotes beneficial effects on anxiety, cognitive and depressive-like behaviors in rats subjected to a restraint stress protocol. *Behavioural Brain Research, 219*(1), 116–122. https://doi.org/10.1016/j.bbr.2010.12.028.

Fiest, K. M., Jetté, N., Roberts, J. I., Maxwell, C. J., Smith, E. E., Black, S. E., et al. (2016). The prevalence and incidence of dementia: A systematic review and meta-analysis. *Canadian Journal of Neurological Sciences, 43*(1), S3–S50. https://doi.org/10.1017/cjn.2016.18.

Foster, J. A., & McVey Neufeld, K. A. (2013). Gut-brain axis: How the microbiome influences anxiety and depression. *Trends in Neurosciences, 36*(5), 305–312. https://doi.org/10.1016/j.tins.2013.01.005.

Fraguas, D., Díaz-Caneja, C. M., Pina-Camacho, L., Moreno, C., Durán-Cutilla, M., Ayora, M., et al. (2019). Dietary interventions for autism spectrum disorder: A meta-analysis. *Pediatrics, 144*(5). https://doi.org/10.1542/peds.2018-3218.

Frangou, S., Lewis, M., & McCrone, P. (2006). Efficacy of ethyl-eicosapentaenoic acid in bipolar depression: Randomised double-blind placebo-controlled study. *British Journal of Psychiatry*, 188, 46–50. https://doi.org/10.1192/bjp.188.1.46.

Fusar-Poli, P., & Berger, G. (2012). Eicosapentaenoic acid interventions in schizophrenia: Meta-analysis of randomized, placebo-controlled studies. *Journal of Clinical Psychopharmacology*, 32(2), 179–185. https://doi.org/10.1097/JCP.0b013e318248b7bb.

Garnock-Jones, K. P., & Keating, G. M. (2009). Atomoxetine. *Pediatric Drugs*, 11(3), 203–226. https://doi.org/10.2165/00148581-200911030-00005.

González-Blanco, L., García-Portilla, M. P., García-Álvarez, L., de la Fuente-Tomás, L., Iglesias García, C., Sáiz, P. A., et al. (2018). Biomarcadores de estrés oxidativo y dimensiones clínicas en los 10 primeros años de esquizofrenia. *Revista de Psiquiatría y Salud Mental*, 11(3), 130–140. https://doi.org/10.1016/j.rpsm.2018.03.003.

Grant, J. E., & Chamberlain, S. R. (2016). Expanding the definition of addiction: DSM-5 vs. ICD-11. *CNS Spectrums*, 21(4), 300–303. https://doi.org/10.1017/S1092852916000183.

Green, P., Hermesh, H., Monselise, A., Marom, S., Presburger, G., & Weizman, A. (2006). Red cell membrane omega-3 fatty acids are decreased in nondepressed patients with social anxiety disorder. *European Neuropsychopharmacology*, 16(2), 107–113. https://doi.org/10.1016/j.euroneuro.2005.07.005.

Grimm, M. O. W., Michaelson, D. M., & Hartmann, T. (2017). Omega-3 fatty acids, lipids, and ApoE lipidation in Alzheimer's disease: A rationale for multi-nutrient dementia prevention. *Journal of Lipid Research*, 58(11), 2083–2101. https://doi.org/10.1194/jlr.R076331.

Grosso, G., Pajak, A., Marventano, S., Castellano, S., Galvano, F., Bucolo, C., et al. (2014). Role of omega-3 fatty acids in the treatment of depressive disorders: A comprehensive meta-analysis of randomized clinical trials. *PLoS One*, 9(5). https://doi.org/10.1371/journal.pone.0096905.

Guu, T. W., Mischoulon, D., Sarris, J., Hibbeln, J., McNamara, R. K., Hamazaki, K., et al. (2019). International society for nutritional psychiatry research practice guidelines for omega-3 fatty acids in the treatment of major depressive disorder. *Psychotherapy and Psychosomatics*, 88(5), 263–273. https://doi.org/10.1159/000502652.

Haberka, M., Mizia-Stec, K., Mizia, M., Gieszczyk, K., Chmiel, A., Sitnik-Warchulska, K., et al. (2013). Effects of n-3 polyunsaturated fatty acids on depressive symptoms, anxiety and emotional state in patients with acute myocardial infarction. *Pharmacological Reports*, 65(1), 59–68. https://doi.org/10.1016/S1734-1140(13)70964-2.

Hallahan, B., Ryan, T., Hibbeln, J. R., Murray, I. T., Glynn, S., Ramsden, C. E., et al. (2016). Efficacy of omega-3 highly unsaturated fatty acids in the treatment of depression. *British Journal of Psychiatry*, 209(3), 192–201. https://doi.org/10.1192/bjp.bp.114.160242.

Hantsoo, L., Jašarević, E., Criniti, S., McGeehan, B., Tanes, C., Sammel, M. D., et al. (2019). Childhood adversity impact on gut microbiota and inflammatory response to stress during pregnancy. *Brain, Behavior, and Immunity*, 75, 240–250. https://doi.org/10.1016/j.bbi.2018.11.005.

Hariri, M., Djazayery, A., Djalali, M., Saedisomeolia, A., Rahimi, A., & Abdolahian, E. (2012). Effect of n-3 supplementation on hyperactivity, oxidative stress and inflammatory mediators in children with attention-deficit-hyperactivity disorder. *Malaysian Journal of Nutrition*, 18(3), 329–335. http://nutriweb.org.my/publications/mjn0018_3/5%20Mitra%20_344ADHDChildren(edSP)(RV)_P329-335.pdf.

Herman, J. P., McKlveen, J. M., Ghosal, S., Kopp, B., Wulsin, A., Makinson, R., et al. (2016). Regulation of the hypothalamic-pituitary- adrenocortical stress response. *Comprehensive Physiology*, 6(2), 603–621. https://doi.org/10.1002/cphy.c150015.

Hibbeln, J. R. (1998). Fish consumption and major depression [9]. *Lancet*, 351(9110), 1213. https://doi.org/10.1016/S0140-6736(05)79168-6.

Hooper, C., de Souto Barreto, P., Coley, N., Cantet, C., Cesari, M., Andrieu, S., et al. (2017). Cognitive changes with omega-3 polyunsaturated fatty acids in non-demented older adults with low omega-3 index. *The Journal of Nutrition, Health & Aging*, 21(9), 988–993. https://doi.org/10.1007/s12603-017-0957-5.

Horman, T., Fernandes, M. F., Tache, M. C., Hucik, B., Mutch, D. M., & Leri, F. (2020). Dietary N-6/N-3 ratio influences brain fatty acid composition in adult rats. *Nutrients*, 12(6), 1–10. https://doi.org/10.3390/nu12061847.

Hubbard, R. L., Craddock, S. G., & Anderson, J. (2003). Overview of 5-year follow-up outcomes in the drug abuse treatment outcome studies (DATOS). *Journal of Substance Abuse Treatment*, 25(3), 125–134. https://doi.org/10.1016/S0740-5472(03)00130-2.

Isken, F., Klaus, S., Osterhoff, M., Pfeiffer, A. F. H., & Weickert, M. O. (2010). Effects of long-term soluble vs. insoluble dietary fiber intake on high-fat diet-induced obesity in C57BL/6J mice. *Journal of Nutritional Biochemistry*, 21(4), 278–284. https://doi.org/10.1016/j.jnutbio.2008.12.012.

Jacka, F. N., Ystrom, E., Brantsaeter, A. L., Karevold, E., Roth, C., Haugen, M., et al. (2013). Maternal and early postnatal nutrition and mental health of offspring by age 5 years: A prospective cohort study. *Journal of the American Academy of Child and Adolescent Psychiatry*, 52(10), 1038–1047. https://doi.org/10.1016/j.jaac.2013.07.002.

Jacobi, F., Höfler, M., Strehle, J., Mack, S., Gerschler, A., Scholl, L., et al. (2014). Psychische störungen in der allgemeinbevölkerung. Studie zur gesundheit erwachsener in Deutschland und ihr zusatzmodul psychische gesundheit (DEGS1-MH). *Nervenarzt, 85*(1), 77–87. https://doi.org/10.1007/s00115-013-3961-y.

Jeromson, S., Gallagher, I. J., Galloway, S. D. R., & Hamilton, D. L. (2015). Omega-3 fatty acids and skeletal muscle health. *Marine Drugs, 13*(11), 6977–7004. https://doi.org/10.3390/md13116977.

Joffre, C., Grégoire, S., De Smedt, V., Acar, N., Bretillon, L., Nadjar, A., et al. (2016). Modulation of brain PUFA content in different experimental models of mice. *Prostaglandins, Leukotrienes, and Essential Fatty Acids, 114*, 1–10. https://doi.org/10.1016/j.plefa.2016.09.003.

Kiecolt-Glaser, J. K., Belury, M. A., Andridge, R., Malarkey, W. B., & Glaser, R. (2011). Omega-3 supplementation lowers inflammation and anxiety in medical students: A randomized controlled trial. *Brain, Behavior, and Immunity, 25*(8), 1725–1734. https://doi.org/10.1016/j.bbi.2011.07.229.

Kim, M., Qie, Y., Park, J., & Kim, C. H. (2016). Gut microbial metabolites fuel host antibody responses. *Cell Host & Microbe, 20*(2), 202–214. https://doi.org/10.1016/j.chom.2016.07.001.

Kim, Y.-K., & Shin, C. (2018). The microbiota-gut-brain axis in neuropsychiatric disorders: Pathophysiological mechanisms and novel treatments. *Current Neuropharmacology, 16*(5), 559–573. https://doi.org/10.2174/1570159X15666170915141036.

Knöchel, C., Voss, M., Grüter, F., Alves, G. S., Matura, S., Sepanski, B., et al. (2015). Omega 3 fatty acids: Novel neurotherapeutic targets for cognitive dysfunction in mood disorders and schizophrenia? *Current Neuropharmacology, 13*(5), 663–680. https://doi.org/10.2174/1570159X13666150630173047.

Kuan-Pin, S. (2008). Mind-body interface: The role of N-3 fatty acids in psychoneuroimmunology, somatic presentation, and medical illness comorbidity of depression. *Asia Pacific Journal of Clinical Nutrition, 17*(S1), 151–157. https://doi.org/10.6133/apjcn.2008.17.s1.37.

Lafourcade, M., Larrieu, T., Mato, S., Duffaud, A., Sepers, M., Matias, I., et al. (2011). Nutritional omega-3 deficiency abolishes endocannabinoid-mediated neuronal functions. *Nature Neuroscience, 14*(3), 345–350. https://doi.org/10.1038/nn.2736.

Lai, J. S., Hiles, S., Bisquera, A., Hure, A. J., McEvoy, M., & Attia, J. (2014). A systematic review and meta-analysis of dietary patterns and depression in community-dwelling adults. *The American Journal of Clinical Nutrition, 99*(1), 181–197. https://doi.org/10.3945/ajcn.113.069880.

Larrieu, T., & Layé, S. (2018). Food for mood: Relevance of nutritional omega-3 fatty acids for depression and anxiety. *Frontiers in Physiology, 9*, 1047. https://doi.org/10.3389/fphys.2018.01047.

Layé, S., Nadjar, A., Joffre, C., & Bazinet, R. P. (2018). Anti-inflammatory effects of omega-3 fatty acids in the brain: Physiological mechanisms and relevance to pharmacology. *Pharmacological Reviews, 70*(1), 12–38. https://doi.org/10.1124/pr.117.014092.

Lespérance, F., Frasure-Smith, N., St-André, E., Turecki, G., Lespérance, P., & Wisniewski, S. R. (2011). The efficacy of omega-3 supplementation for major depression: A randomized controlled trial. *Journal of Clinical Psychiatry, 72*(8), 1054–1062. https://doi.org/10.4088/JCP.10m05966blu.

Li, Y., Lv, M.-R., Wei, Y.-J., Sun, L., Zhang, J.-X., Zhang, H.-G., et al. (2017). Dietary patterns and depression risk: A meta-analysis. *Psychiatry Research, 253*, 373–382. https://doi.org/10.1016/j.psychres.2017.04.020.

Liara, R., Idiane, R., & Matheus, R.-C. (2014). Global epidemiology of dementia: Alzheimer's and vascular types. *BioMed Research International*, 1–8. https://doi.org/10.1155/2014/908915.

Lin, P. Y., Huang, S. Y., & Su, K. P. (2010). A meta-analytic review of polyunsaturated fatty acid compositions in patients with depression. *Biological Psychiatry, 68*(2), 140–147. https://doi.org/10.1016/j.biopsych.2010.03.018.

Lindqvist, D., Dhabhar, F. S., James, S. J., Hough, C. M., Jain, F. A., Bersani, F. S., et al. (2017). Oxidative stress, inflammation and treatment response in major depression. *Psychoneuroendocrinology, 76*, 197–205. https://doi.org/10.1016/j.psyneuen.2016.11.031.

López-Muñoz, F., & Alamo, C. (2009). Monoaminergic neurotransmission: The history of the discovery of antidepressants from 1950s until today. *Current Pharmaceutical Design, 15*(14), 1563–1586. https://doi.org/10.2174/138161209788168001.

Madore, C., Leyrolle, Q., Lacabanne, C., Benmamar-Badel, A., Joffre, C., Nadjar, A., et al. (2016). Neuroinflammation in autism: Plausible role of maternal inflammation, dietary omega 3, and microbiota. *Neural Plasticity, 2016*. https://doi.org/10.1155/2016/3597209.

Martins, B. P., Bandarra, N. M., & Figueiredo-Braga, M. (2020). The role of marine omega-3 in human neurodevelopment, including autism spectrum disorders and attention-deficit/hyperactivity disorder–a review. *Critical Reviews in Food Science and Nutrition, 60*(9), 1431–1446. https://doi.org/10.1080/10408398.2019.1573800.

Matamoros, S., Gras-Leguen, C., Le Vacon, F., Potel, G., & de La Cochetiere, M.-F. (2013). Development of intestinal microbiota in infants and its impact on health. *Trends in Microbiology, 21*(4), 167–173. https://doi.org/10.1016/j.tim.2012.12.001.

Matsumura, K., Noguchi, H., Nishi, D., Hamazaki, K., Hamazaki, T., & Matsuoka, Y. J. (2017). Effects of omega-3 polyunsaturated fatty acids on psychophysiological symptoms of post-traumatic stress disorder in accident survivors: A randomized, double-blind, placebo-controlled trial. *Journal of Affective Disorders*, 224, 27–31. https://doi.org/10.1016/j.jad.2016.05.054.

Matsuoka, Y., Nishi, D., Hamazaki, K., Yonemoto, N., Matsumura, K., Noguchi, H., et al. (2015). Docosahexaenoic acid for selective prevention of posttraumatic stress disorder among severely injured patients: A randomized, placebo-controlled trial. *Journal of Clinical Psychiatry*, 76(8), e1015–e1022. https://doi.org/10.4088/JCP.14m09260.

Mazahery, H., Conlon, C. A., Beck, K. L., Mugridge, O., Kruger, M. C., Stonehouse, W., et al. (2019). A randomised controlled trial of vitamin D and omega-3 long chain polyunsaturated fatty acids in the treatment of irritability and hyperactivity among children with autism spectrum disorder. *Journal of Steroid Biochemistry and Molecular Biology*, 187, 9–16. https://doi.org/10.1016/j.jsbmb.2018.10.017.

Mazahery, H., Stonehouse, W., Delshad, M., Kruger, M. C., Conlon, C. A., Beck, K. L., et al. (2017). Relationship between long chain n-3 polyunsaturated fatty acids and autism spectrum disorder: Systematic review and meta-analysis of case-control and randomised controlled trials. *Nutrients*, 9(2). https://doi.org/10.3390/nu9020155.

Mocking, R. J. T., Harmsen, I., Assies, J., Koeter, M. W. J., Ruhé, H. G., & Schene, A. H. (2016). Meta-analysis and meta-regression of omega-3 polyunsaturated fatty acid supplementation for major depressive disorder. *Translational Psychiatry*, 6(3). https://doi.org/10.1038/tp.2016.29.

Munro, S. (2003). Lipid rafts: Elusive or illusive? *Cell*, 115(4), 377–388. https://doi.org/10.1016/S0092-8674(03)00882-1.

Nakandakari, S. C. B. R., Muñoz, V. R., Kuga, G. K., Gaspar, R. C., Sant'Ana, M. R., Pavan, I. C. B., et al. (2019). Short-term high-fat diet modulates several inflammatory, ER stress, and apoptosis markers in the hippocampus of young mice. *Brain, Behavior, and Immunity*, 79, 284–293. https://doi.org/10.1016/j.bbi.2019.02.016.

Nemets, B., Stahl, Z., & Belmaker, R. H. (2002). Addition of omega-3 fatty acid to maintenance medication treatment for recurrent unipolar depressive disorder. *American Journal of Psychiatry*, 159(3), 477–479. https://doi.org/10.1176/appi.ajp.159.3.477.

Noaghiul, S., & Hibbeln, J. R. (2003). Cross-national comparisons of seafood consumption and rates of bipolar disorders. *American Journal of Psychiatry*, 160(12), 2222–2227. https://doi.org/10.1176/appi.ajp.160.12.2222.

Olszak, T., An, D., Zeissig, S., Vera, M. P., Richter, J., Franke, A., et al. (2012). Microbial exposure during early life has persistent effects on natural killer T cell function. *Science*, 336(6080), 489–493. https://doi.org/10.1126/science.1219328.

Parletta, N., Zarnowiecki, D., Cho, J., Wilson, A., Bogomolova, S., Villani, A., et al. (2019). A Mediterranean-style dietary intervention supplemented with fish oil improves diet quality and mental health in people with depression: A randomized controlled trial (HELFIMED). *Nutritional Neuroscience*, 22(7), 474–487. https://doi.org/10.1080/1028415X.2017.1411320.

Peet, M., & Horrobin, D. F. (2002). A dose-ranging study of the effects of ethyl-eicosapentaenoate in patients with ongoing depression despite apparently adequate treatment with standard drugs. *Archives of General Psychiatry*, 59(10), 913–919. https://doi.org/10.1001/archpsyc.59.10.913.

Pliszka, S. R., Crismon, M. L., Hughes, C. W., Corners, C. K., Emslie, G. J., Jensen, P. S., et al. (2006). The Texas children's medication algorithm project: Revision of the algorithm for pharmacotherapy of attention-deficit/hyperactivity disorder. *Journal of the American Academy of Child and Adolescent Psychiatry*, 45(6), 642–657. https://doi.org/10.1097/01.chi.0000215326.51175.eb.

Polokowski, A. R., Shakil, H., Carmichael, C. L., & Reigada, L. C. (2020). Omega-3 fatty acids and anxiety: A systematic review of the possible mechanisms at play. *Nutritional Neuroscience*, 23(7), 494–504. https://doi.org/10.1080/1028415X.2018.1525092.

Psaltopoulou, T., Sergentanis, T. N., Panagiotakos, D. B., Sergentanis, I. N., Kosti, R., & Scarmeas, N. (2013). Mediterranean diet, stroke, cognitive impairment, and depression: A meta-analysis. *Annals of Neurology*, 74(4), 580–591. https://doi.org/10.1002/ana.23944.

Quinn, J. F., Raman, R., Thomas, R. G., Yurko-Mauro, K., Nelson, E. B., Van Dyck, C., et al. (2010). Docosahexaenoic acid supplementation and cognitive decline in Alzheimer disease: A randomized trial. *JAMA : The Journal of the American Medical Association*, 304(17), 1903–1911. https://doi.org/10.1001/jama.2010.1510.

Quintana, H., Cherlin, E. A., Duesenberg, D. A., Bangs, M. E., Ramsey, J. L., Feldman, P. D., et al. (2007). Transition from methylphenidate or amphetamine to atomoxetine in children and adolescents with attention-deficit/hyperactivity disorder-A preliminary tolerability and efficacy study. *Clinical Therapeutics*, 29(6), 1168–1177. https://doi.org/10.1016/j.clinthera.2007.06.017.

Robertson, R. C., Seira Oriach, C., Murphy, K., Moloney, G. M., Cryan, J. F., Dinan, T. G., et al. (2017). Omega-3 polyunsaturated fatty acids critically regulate behaviour and gut microbiota development in adolescence and adulthood. *Brain, Behavior, and Immunity*, 59, 21–37. https://doi.org/10.1016/j.bbi.2016.07.145.

Rosa, L. (2018). The gut-brain axis in Alzheimer's disease and omega-3. A critical overview of clinical trials. *Nutrients*, 10(9).

Rotenberg, S., & McGrath, J. J. (2016). Inter-relation between autonomic and HPA axis activity in children and adolescents. *Biological Psychology*, *117*, 16–25. https://doi.org/10.1016/j.biopsycho.2016.01.015.

Theo, V., Abajobir, A. A., Abate, K. H., Abbafati, C., Abbas, K. M., Abd-Allah, F., et al. (2017). Global, regional, and national incidence, prevalence, and years lived with disability for 328 diseases and injuries for 195 countries, 1990–2016: A systematic analysis for the Global Burden of Disease Study 2016. *The Lancet*, 1211–1259. https://doi.org/10.1016/s0140-6736(17)32154-2.

Salim, S. (2017). Oxidative stress and the central nervous system. *Journal of Pharmacology and Experimental Therapeutics*, *360*(1), 201–205. https://doi.org/10.1124/jpet.116.237503.

Sánchez-Villegas, A., Álvarez-Pérez, J., Toledo, E., Salas-Salvadó, J., Ortega-Azorín, C., Zomeño, M. D., et al. (2018). Seafood consumption, omega-3 fatty acids intake, and life-time prevalence of depression in the PREDIMED-plus trial. *Nutrients*, *10*(12). https://doi.org/10.3390/nu10122000.

Sandhu, K. V., Sherwin, E., Schellekens, H., Stanton, C., Dinan, T. G., & Cryan, J. F. (2017). Feeding the microbiota-gut-brain axis: Diet, microbiome, and neuropsychiatry. *Translational Research*, *179*, 223–244. https://doi.org/10.1016/j.trsl.2016.10.002.

Sathe, N., Andrews, J. C., McPheeters, M. L., & Warren, Z. E. (2017). Nutritional and dietary interventions for autism spectrum disorder: A systematic review. *Pediatrics*, *139*(6). https://doi.org/10.1542/peds.2017-0346.

Satogami, K., Tseng, P. T., Su, K. P., Takahashi, S., Ukai, S., Li, D. J., et al. (2019). Relationship between polyunsaturated fatty acid and eating disorders: Systematic review and meta-analysis. *Prostaglandins, Leukotrienes, and Essential Fatty Acids*, *142*, 11–19. https://doi.org/10.1016/j.plefa.2019.01.001.

Saunders, E. F. H., Ramsden, C. E., Sherazy, M. S., Gelenberg, A. J., Davis, J. M., & Rapoport, S. I. (2016). Omega-3 and omega-6 polyunsaturated fatty acids in bipolar disorder: A review of biomarker and treatment studies. *The Journal of Clinical Psychiatry*, *77*(10), e1301–e1308. https://doi.org/10.4088/JCP.15r09925.

Scaglia, N., Chatkin, J., Chapman, K. R., Ferreira, I., Wagner, M., Selby, P., et al. (2016). The relationship between omega-3 and smoking habit: A cross-sectional study. *Lipids in Health and Disease*, *15*(1). https://doi.org/10.1186/s12944-016-0220-9.

Sena, C. M., Leandro, A., Azul, L., Seiça, R., & Perry, G. (2018). Vascular oxidative stress: Impact and therapeutic approaches. *Frontiers in Physiology*, *9*. https://doi.org/10.3389/fphys.2018.01668.

Slavich, G. M., & Irwin, M. R. (2014). From stress to inflammation and major depressive disorder: A social signal transduction theory of depression. *Psychological Bulletin*, *140*(3), 774–815. https://doi.org/10.1037/a0035302.

Spooner, M. H., & Jump, D. B. (2019). Omega-3 fatty acids and nonalcoholic fatty liver disease in adults and children: Where do we stand? *Current Opinion in Clinical Nutrition and Metabolic Care*, *22*(2), 103–110. https://doi.org/10.1097/MCO.0000000000000539.

Steiner, P. (2020). Brain fuel utilization in the developing brain. *Annals of Nutrition and Metabolism*, *75*(1), 8–18. https://doi.org/10.1159/000508054.

Stoll, A. L., Severus, W. E., Freeman, M. P., Rueter, S., Zboyan, H. A., Diamond, E., et al. (1999). Omega 3 fatty acids in bipolar disorder: A preliminary double-blind, placebo-controlled trial. *Archives of General Psychiatry*, *56*(5), 407–412. https://doi.org/10.1001/archpsyc.56.5.407.

Su, K. P. (2009). Biological mechanism of antidepressant effect of omega-3 fatty acids: How does fish oil act as a "mind-body interface"? *Neurosignals*, *17*(2), 144–152. https://doi.org/10.1159/000198167.

Su, K. P. (2015). Personalized medicine with omega-3 fatty acids for depression in children and pregnant women and depression associated with inflammation. *Journal of Clinical Psychiatry*, *76*(11), e1476–e1477. https://doi.org/10.4088/JCP.15l10011.

Su, K. P., Huang, S. Y., Chiu, T. H., Huang, K. C., Huang, C. L., Chang, H. C., et al. (2008). Omega-3 fatty acids for major depressive disorder during pregnancy: Results from a randomized, double-blind, placebo-controlled trial. *Journal of Clinical Psychiatry*, *69*(4), 644–651. https://doi.org/10.4088/JCP.v69n0418.

Su, K. P., Huang, S. Y., Chiu, C. C., & Shen, W. W. (2003). Omega-3 fatty acids in major depressive disorder: A preliminary double-blind, placebo-controlled trial. *European Neuropsychopharmacology*, *13*(4), 267–271. https://doi.org/10.1016/S0924-977X(03)00032-4.

Su, K. P., Lai, H. C., Yang, H. T., Su, W. P., Peng, C. Y., Chang, J. P. C., et al. (2014). Omega-3 fatty acids in the prevention of interferon- Alpha-induced depression: Results from a randomized, controlled trial. *Biological Psychiatry*, *76*(7), 559–566. https://doi.org/10.1016/j.biopsych.2014.01.008.

Su, K. P., Tseng, P. T., Lin, P. Y., Okubo, R., Chen, T. Y., Chen, Y. W., et al. (2018). Association of use of omega-3 polyunsaturated fatty acids with changes in severity of anxiety symptoms: A systematic review and meta-analysis. *JAMA Network Open*, *1*(5). https://doi.org/10.1001/jamanetworkopen.2018.2327, e182327.

Su, K. P., Wang, S. M., & Pae, C. U. (2013). Omega-3 polyunsaturated fatty acids for major depressive disorder. *Expert Opinion on Investigational Drugs*, *22*(12), 1519–1534. https://doi.org/10.1517/13543784.2013.836487.

Thesing, C. S., Bot, M., Milaneschi, Y., Giltay, E. J., & Penninx, B. W. J. H. (2018). Omega-3 and omega-6 fatty acid levels in depressive and anxiety disorders.

Psychoneuroendocrinology, *87*, 53–62. https://doi.org/10.1016/j.psyneuen.2017.10.005.

Udo, T., & Grilo, C. M. (2018). Prevalence and correlates of DSM-5–defined eating disorders in a nationally representative sample of U.S. Adults. *Biological Psychiatry*, *84*(5), 345–354. https://doi.org/10.1016/j.biopsych.2018.03.014.

Ulrich-Lai, Y. M., Fulton, S., Wilson, M., Petrovich, G., & Rinaman, L. (2015). Stress exposure, food intake and emotional state. *Stress*, *18*(4), 381–399. https://doi.org/10.3109/10253890.2015.1062981.

Uttara, B., Singh, A. V., Zamboni, P., & Mahajan, R. T. (2009). Oxidative stress and neurodegenerative diseases: A review of upstream and downstream antioxidant therapeutic options. *Current Neuropharmacology*, *7*(1), 65–74. https://doi.org/10.2174/157015909787602823.

Vaillant, G. E. (2003). A 60-year follow-up of alcoholic men. *Addiction*, *98*(8), 1043–1051. https://doi.org/10.1046/j.1360-0443.2003.00422.x.

Vaz, J. D. S., Farias, D. R., Adegboye, A. R. A., Nardi, A. E., & Kac, G. (2017). Omega-3 supplementation from pregnancy to postpartum to prevent depressive symptoms: A randomized placebo-controlled trial. *BMC Pregnancy and Childbirth*, *17*(1). https://doi.org/10.1186/s12884-017-1365-x.

Venkat, P., Chopp, M., & Chen, J. (2015). Models and mechanisms of vascular dementia. *Experimental Neurology*, *272*, 97–108. https://doi.org/10.1016/j.expneurol.2015.05.006.

Vors, C., Allaire, J., Marin, J., Lépine, M. C., Charest, A., Tchernof, A., et al. (2017). Inflammatory gene expression in whole blood cells after EPA vs. DHA supplementation: Results from the ComparED study. *Atherosclerosis*, *257*, 116–122. https://doi.org/10.1016/j.atherosclerosis.2017.01.025.

Whiteford, H. A., Degenhardt, L., Rehm, J., Baxter, A. J., Ferrari, A. J., Erskine, H. E., et al. (2010). Global burden of disease attributable to mental and substance use disorders: Findings from the global burden of disease study. *Lancet*, *382*(9904), 61611–61616. https://doi.org/10.1016/s0140-6736.

Woo, J., Couturier, J., Pindiprolu, B., Picard, L., Maertens, C., Leclerc, A., et al. (2017). Acceptability and tolerability of omega-3 fatty acids as adjunctive treatment for children and adolescents with eating disorders. *Eating Disorders*, *25*(2), 114–121. https://doi.org/10.1080/10640266.2016.1260379.

World Health Organization. (2017). *Depression and other common mental disorders: Global health estimates*. World Health Organization. https://apps.who.int/iris/handle/10665/254610.

Wozniak, J., Faraone, S. V., Chan, J., Tarko, L., Hernandez, M., Davis, J., et al. (2015). A randomized clinical trial of high eicosapentaenoic acid omega-3 fatty acids and inositol as monotherapy and in combination in the treatment of pediatric bipolar spectrum disorders: A pilot study. *Journal of Clinical Psychiatry*, *76*(11), 1548–1555. https://doi.org/10.4088/JCP.14m09267.

Xu, F., Fan, W., Wang, W., Tang, W., Yang, F., Zhang, Y., et al. (2019). Effects of omega-3 fatty acids on metabolic syndrome in patients with schizophrenia: A 12-week randomized placebo-controlled trial. *Psychopharmacology*, *236*(4), 1273–1279. https://doi.org/10.1007/s00213-018-5136-9.

Yang, J. R., Han, D., Qiao, Z. X., Tian, X., Qi, D., & Qiu, X. H. (2015). Combined application of eicosapentaenoic acid and docosahexaenoic acid on depression in women: A meta-analysis of double-blind randomized controlled trials. *Neuropsychiatric Disease and Treatment*, *11*, 2055–2061. https://doi.org/10.2147/NDT.S86581.

Zalar, B., Haslberger, A., & Peterlin, B. (2018). The role of microbiota in depression—A brief review. *Psychiatria Danubina*, *30*(2), 136–141. https://doi.org/10.24869/spsih.2018.136.

Zaparoli, J. X., Sugawara, E. K., De Souza, A. A. L., Tufik, S., & Galduróz, J. C. F. (2016). Omega-3 levels and nicotine dependence: A cross-sectional study and clinical trial. *European Addiction Research*, *22*(3), 153–162. https://doi.org/10.1159/000439525.

Zou, Z., Wang, H., d'Oleire Uquillas, F., Wang, X., Ding, J., & Chen, H. (2017). Definition of substance and non-substance addiction. In *Vol. 1010. Advances in experimental medicine and biology* (pp. 21–41). New York LLC: Springer. https://doi.org/10.1007/978-981-10-5562-1_2.

CHAPTER 5

Diet in different fat content and cardiometabolic health

Yi Wan

Department of Food Science and Nutrition, Zhejiang University, Hangzhou, China

5.1 Introduction

5.1.1 Types of dietary fats and their food sources

Dietary fats and oil come from both animal and plant food sources. The fatty acid composition of dietary fat varies largely in different food sources. In general, dietary fats from animal sources tends to be relatively high in saturated fatty acids (SFAs), and fats of plant origin is high in unsaturated fatty acids like monounsaturated fatty acids (MUFAs) and polyunsaturated fatty acids (PUFAs).

In the US diet, the top dietary sources of SFAs, MUFAs, α-linolenic acid, and n-3 PUFAs were regular cheese, nuts and seeds, salad dressing and vegetable oils, and marine fish (Lichtenstein, 2019). However, in China, vegetable oil was the primary food source of dietary fats, contributing to more than 40% of total fat, more than 30% of SFAs, more than 40% of MUFAs, and around 60% of PUFAs (Shen et al., 2017). Meat and meat product intake is the secondary food sources for dietary fats in China (Shen et al., 2017). Food sources of dietary fats in China are different from those reported in the USA and other countries (Elmadfa & Kornsteiner, 2009; Harika, Eilander, Alssema, Osendarp, & Zock, 2013; Hulshof et al., 1999). The dietary habit results in large differences in dietary fatty acid profiles between China and other countries. A vast literature based on ecological studies, prospective cohorts, and randomized controlled trials investigating the relationship between dietary fats and intermediate cardiometabolic risk factors or diseases has documented that the types of dietary fats strongly influenced cardiometabolic health (Wang & Hu, 2017).

5.1.2 Trends in dietary fats intake

The parallel increases in dietary carbohydrate intake and incidences of overweight/obesity and cardiometabolic diseases have led to the suggestion that this dietary macronutrient change, especially a reduction in total fat intake (Austin, Ogden, & Hill, 2011), might be a risk factor for obesity and cardiometabolic health in the USA and many western countries (Livesey et al., 2019; Mozaffarian, Hao, Rimm, Willett, & Hu, 2011; Te, Mallard, & Mann, 2012). Findings from observational studies and randomized controlled trials have also suggested that diets with a moderate carbohydrate intake but relatively high unsaturated fat improved blood lipid profiles and lowered coronary heart disease risk among participants at high cardiometabolic risk (Halton et al., 2006; Jenkins et al., 2009). However, in China, overnutrition has considerably replaced malnutrition during a similar period (Du, Wang, Zhang, Zhai, & Popkin, 2014; Zhai et al., 2014). Overweight/obesity and cardiometabolic diseases prevail in China, whereas the prevalence is particularly low when compared with the USA and most Western countries during the same period (Adair, Gordon-Larsen, Du, Zhang, & Popkin, 2014). Intake of dietary fat doubled from 1982 to 2011 with a corresponding reduction in carbohydrate consumption (Zhai et al., 2014). Despite possible inherent or acquired biological differences between different populations or individuals, the differences in trends and food sources of dietary fats and carbohydrate in China and developed countries might also lead to a varied impact of diets with different fat-to-carbohydrate ratios on overweight/obesity incidence and cardiometabolic health.

5.2 Diet with different fat-to-carbohydrate ratios and cardiometabolic health

Underdeveloped or developing countries have a relatively lower prevalence of overweight/obesity, cardiometabolic diseases, and cancers than Westernized counties (Roth et al., 2020; Sung et al., 2021). When individuals move from countries with low overweight/obesity and cardiometabolic disease rates to malnutrition countries, their risks of developing overweight/obesity and cardiometabolic diseases are close to that of the new residents in the next one or two generations (Goel, McCarthy, Phillips, & Wee, 2004). This shift in chronic diseases rates has led to the suggestion that environmental exposure, particularly adopting a higher-fat Western diet, might be related to overweight/obesity and cardiometabolic risk. On the other hand, emerging evidence suggests that a diet with a high fat-to-carbohydrate ratio, particularly a ketogenic diet, might have therapeutic effects in a population with increased cardiometabolic risk (Kosinski & Jornayvaz, 2017).

The health effects of dietary fat on human health have been a longstanding research topic of interest (Ludwig, Willett, Volek, & Neuhouser, 2018). A low-fat diet might confer beneficial effects on controlling body weight. In the Women's Health Initiative Dietary Modification Trial, 1-year intervention of a low-fat diet ($\leq$20% of total energy) was associated with a moderate reduction in weight and body composition (Carty et al., 2011). Another randomized controlled trial found that weight loss was greater in a lower-fat (20% of total energy), higher-carbohydrate diet (65% of total energy) group than a lower-carbohydrate (45% of total energy), higher-fat diet (35% of total energy) group and a walnut-rich (18% of total energy), higher-fat (45% of total energy), lower-carbohydrate (35% of total energy) diet group after 1-year intervention among postmenopausal women (Rock et al., 2016). However, it should be noted that the design of the trial played an important role in the interpretation of the findings. A meta-analysis of randomized controlled trials comparing a low-fat diet with a higher-fat diet and reporting weight change outcomes for more than 1 year in adults, suggested that the intensity of the intervention is critical in the long-term effect of low-fat diets on body weight. Compared to dietary interventions of similar intensity, evidence from randomized controlled trials does not support low-fat diets over other dietary interventions in terms of long-term weight loss (Tobias et al., 2015). A low-fat diet might also have a favorable effect on reducing the risk of type 2 diabetes (T2D) through weight management, as obesity is clearly associated with T2D development (Kahn, Hull, & Utzschneider,

2006). In the Diabetes Prevention Program, the lifestyle intervention group led to at least 7% reductions in body weight achieved by following a low-calorie, low-fat diet and increasing physical activity, which was associated with a 58% lower risk of T2D. However, the effects of a low-fat diet cannot be entirely disentangled from weight management and other related factors (Knowler et al., 2002).

However, individuals with glucose intolerance, insulin resistance, or insulin hypersecretion are likely to have more weight loss after following a high-fat, low-carbohydrate diet intervention (Hjorth, Zohar, Hill, & Astrup, 2018; Ludwig & Ebbeling, 2018). Those with lower insulin concentrations and accelerated rates have a higher metabolic fuel availability for the brain, leading to greater satiety during the intervention period (Ludwig & Ebbeling, 2018). Short- and medium-term randomized controlled trials found that a diet with reduced carbohydrates tends to confer more favorable effects than a low-fat, high-carbohydrate diet on clinical markers associated with insulin resistance (Mansoor, Vinknes, Veierod, & Retterstol, 2016; Volek et al., 2009; Volek, Fernandez, Feinman, & Phinney, 2008). In an 8-week randomized controlled trial among T2D patients, liver fat content decreased more in a high-fat diet (42% of total energy, also high in MUFA) group than a low-fat (28% of total energy), high-fiber diet group among T2D patients (Bozzetto et al., 2012). Another trial comparing the effectiveness and safety of a weight-loss diet showed that moderately obese subjects in the low-carbohydrate diet (fat approximates 40% of total energy) group lost more weight and had more favorable effects on blood lipids and glycemic control than those in the low-fat diet (fat approximates 30% of total energy) group after a 2-year diet intervention (Shai et al., 2008). In patients with metabolic syndrome, those consuming a diet with carbohydrate restriction to ketogenic levels (50 g/day) lost more weight than those in the low-fat (24% of total energy), calorie-restricted diet group (Volek et al., 2009). The very-low-carbohydrate diet also improved blood lipids in T2D patients (Bhanpuri et al., 2018) and lowered inflammatory markers among obese subjects (Forsythe et al., 2008). A meta-analysis of five randomized controlled trials with at least 6 months of intervention showed that the low-carbohydrate diet appeared to be as effective as the low-fat diet in weight loss for a duration of up to 1 year (Nordmann et al., 2006). The low-carbohydrate diet was also associated with favorable changes in triglyceride and high-density lipoprotein (HDL) cholesterol values, but unfavorable changes in total cholesterol and low-density lipoprotein (LDL) cholesterol levels (Nordmann et al., 2006). Reduction in dietary carbohydrates might provide therapeutic benefits for the choice of treatment for obesity or T2D patients. However, the long-term safety of a very-high-fat, low-carbohydrate diet has not been fully assessed.

Different types of dietary fatty acids have divergent impacts on the risk of cardiovascular disease (CVD), and the effects are also influenced by the comparison or replacement of macronutrients (Wang & Hu, 2017). Generally, high-fat, low-carbohydrate diets are typically high in SFAs. Higher intake of saturated fat has been suggested to be associated with a higher risk of CVD and total mortality in the general population, although the effects of dietary SFAs vary due to the nature of the substituted macronutrients (Dehghan et al., 2017; Mensink, Zock, Kester, & Katan, 2003; Siri-Tarino, Sun, Hu, & Krauss, 2010). When substituted for overall carbohydrates, SFAs increase both LDL cholesterol and HDL cholesterol concentration but usually have no significant impact on the ratio of total to HDL cholesterol—a more important marker in estimating the risk of coronary artery disease (Mensink et al., 2003). It should be noted that the quality of carbohydrates influences the substituting effects of SFAs on lipid profile (Levitan et al., 2008). Findings from prospective cohort studies investigating the effect of replacing SFAs with PUFAs or carbohydrates with a low glycemic index, found significant benefits in CVD risk (Hu et al., 1997; Jakobsen et al., 2009; Li et al., 2015). Current evidence from randomized controlled trials regarding the effects of low-fat diets on CVD risk is limited. Most of the previous randomized controlled trials investigated the effect on CVD risk factors (Mansoor et al., 2016). In the Women's Health Initiative Dietary Modification Trial primarily investigating whether a low-fat diet that is high in fruit, vegetables, and grains could decrease the risk of breast and colorectal cancers, the low-fat diet did not significantly reduce the risk of coronary diseases, stroke, or CVD in postmenopausal women, but significantly lowered LDL cholesterol and metabolic syndrome scores (Howard et al., 2006). However, participants without prior CVD or baseline hypertension had a 30% reduced risk of CVD, whereas women with prior CVD or baseline hypertension appeared to be not sensitive to a change to a low-fat dietary pattern, suggesting that a low-fat diet might confer a greater effect on prevention than treatment (Howard et al., 2006; Ritenbaugh et al., 2003). Long-term randomized controlled trials primarily tracking CVD risk are needed in the future.

5.3 What we previously conducted

5.3.1 Effects of diets with different fat content on weight change and cardiometabolic risk factors

Given the different trends and food sources of dietary fats and carbohydrates between the Chinese population and those in North America and Europe, our group previously conducted a 6-month randomized, controlled-feeding trial to compare the effects of diets with different fat-to-carbohydrate ratios on weight control and related cardiometabolic profiles in Chinese young adults (Wan et al., 2017). We designed three isocaloric diets with various dietary fat-to-carbohydrate ratios. The targeted percentage of total energy derived from fat and carbohydrate was 20% and 66% in the lower-fat, higher-carbohydrate diet, 30% and 56% in the moderate-fat, moderate-carbohydrate diet, and 40% and 46% in the higher-fat, lower-carbohydrate diet, respectively. The target macronutrient distribution was achieved by replacing a proportion of energy derived from carbohydrate with fat (soybean oil, rich in n-6 PUFAs). All food and beverages were provided throughout the 6-month intervention. We found that among healthy young Chinese adults, the lower-fat, higher-carbohydrate diet is likely to be associated with a lower risk of excessive weight gain and a more favorable lipid profile than the higher-fat, lower-carbohydrate diet (Wan et al., 2017). Extensive use of soybean oil led the high-fat, low-carbohydrate diet in our trial to be a diet high in n-6 PUFAs (24% of total energy), which is much higher than the recommended range for PUFAs with 6–11% total energy (Burlingame, Nishida, Uauy, & Weisell, 2009). Therefore, the increased fat content in the higher-fat diet was mainly n-6 PUFAs in comparison with the lower-fat, higher-carbohydrate diet. Increased consumption of dietary n-6 PUFAs might trigger the inflammatory process via biosynthesis of proinflammatory arachidonic-acid-derived eicosanoids, including prostaglandins, thromboxane, and leukotrienes (Patterson, Wall, Fitzgerald, Ross, & Stanton, 2012). In our trial, we observed increased plasma level of thromboxane B_2, the fecal concentration of arachidonic acid, and the enriched predicted microbial lipopolysaccharide biosynthesis and arachidonic acid metabolism pathways after the higher-fat, lower-carbohydrate diet intervention, which was in line with previous studies suggesting that the n-6 PUFAs might involve in the intestinal dysbiosis and inflammation (Ghosh, Molcan, Decoffe, Dai, & Gibson, 2013; Kaliannan, Wang, Li, Kim, & Kang, 2015).

5.3.2 Effects of diets with different fat contents on gut microbiota and microbial metabolites

Gut microbiota composition and fecal metabolomic profiles were measured to assess whether the gut microbiota was affected by the dietary intervention and in turn influenced the host metabolism. The higher-fat, lower-carbohydrate diet conferred unfavorable effects on gut microbiota composition and microbial metabolites (Wan et al., 2019). At the phylum level, the higher-fat, lower-carbohydrate diet increased the relative abundance of the Bacteroidetes phylum, whereas the lower-fat, higher-carbohydrate diet decreased Firmicutes phylum abundance. At the genus level, the abundance of *Bacteroides* and *Alistipes* increased, and *Faecalibacterium* genus was decreased after 6 months of the higher-fat, lower-carbohydrate diet consumption. Meanwhile, fecal concentrations of palmitic acids, stearic acid, and arachidonic acid were increased, whereas the butyric acid decreased after following the higher-fat, lower-carbohydrate diet for 6 months (Wan et al., 2019).

Besides, the higher-fat, lower-carbohydrate diet was associated with increased levels of plasma proinflammatory factors such as high-sensitivity C-reaction protein and thromboxane B_2, relative to the lower-fat, higher-carbohydrate diet (Wan et al., 2019). Finally, fecal bile acid profiles were measured, as the gut microbiota plays a vital role in the bile acid biotransformation. The higher-fat, lower-carbohydrate diet was associated with a moderate alteration of bile acids, especially unconjugated bile acids and secondary bile acids associated with gut microbiota taxa (Wan et al., 2020). These alterations might confer potentially unfavorable impacts on colonic and host cardiometabolic health in healthy young adults.

Findings of the randomized controlled-feeding trial indicated that, compared with a lower-fat, higher-carbohydrate diet, a higher-fat diet appears to be undesirable owing to unfavorable changes in gut microbiota, fecal metabolomic profiles, and proinflammatory factors for healthy young Chinese adults whose diet is in transition from the traditionally consumed lower-fat, higher-carbohydrate diet to one characterized by an appreciably higher fat content (Fig. 5.1).

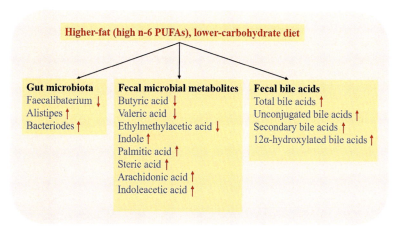

FIG. 5.1 Effects of higher-fat (high n-6 PUFAs), lower-carbohydrate diet on gut microbiota, fecal microbial metabolites, and fecal bile acids in a previously conducted randomized controlled-feeding trial among healthy young Chinese adults.

These findings might also have some relevance in developed countries in which fat intake is already high. However, due to the large variation in dietary habits, and the amount and quality of dietary fats and carbohydrates between different populations, it is of great importance to make dietary recommendations for the general population based on their own evidence. Food sources and environmental factors that influence human cardiometabolic health should also be considered.

5.4 Conclusions

In summary, no specific diet with a fat-to-carbohydrate ratio is the best for the general population from the current evidence. The assessment of the effect of a diet on human health must extend far beyond the amount of macronutrients and quantity. For obese individuals or individuals with cardiometabolic dysfunction, a more specific therapeutic dietary pattern might be needed.

References

Adair, L. S., Gordon-Larsen, P., Du, S. F., Zhang, B., & Popkin, B. M. (2014). The emergence of cardiometabolic disease risk in Chinese children and adults: Consequences of changes in diet, physical activity and obesity. *Obesity Reviews*, *15*(1), 49–59. https://doi.org/10.1111/obr.12123.

Austin, G. L., Ogden, L. G., & Hill, J. O. (2011). Trends in carbohydrate, fat, and protein intakes and association with energy intake in normal-weight, overweight, and obese individuals: 1971-2006. *American Journal of Clinical Nutrition*, *93*(4), 836–843. https://doi.org/10.3945/ajcn.110.000141.

Bhanpuri, N. H., Hallberg, S. J., Williams, P. T., McKenzie, A. L., Ballard, K. D., Campbell, W. W., et al. (2018). Cardiovascular disease risk factor responses to a type 2 diabetes care model including nutritional ketosis induced by sustained carbohydrate restriction at 1 year: An open label, non-randomized, controlled study. *Cardiovascular Diabetology*, *17*(1). https://doi.org/10.1186/s12933-018-0698-8.

Bozzetto, L., Prinster, A., Annuzzi, G., Costagliola, L., Mangione, A., Vitelli, A., et al. (2012). Liver fat is reduced by an isoenergetic MUFA diet in a controlled randomized study in type 2 diabetic patients. *Diabetes Care*, *35*(7), 1429–1435. https://doi.org/10.2337/dc12-0033.

Burlingame, B., Nishida, C., Uauy, R., & Weisell, R. (2009). Fats and fatty acids in human nutrition: Introduction. *Annals of Nutrition and Metabolism*, *55*(1–3), 5–7. https://doi.org/10.1159/000228993.

Carty, C. L., Kooperberg, C., Neuhouser, M. L., Tinker, L., Howard, B., Wactawski-Wende, J., et al. (2011). Low-fat dietary pattern and change in body-composition traits in the Women's Health Initiative Dietary Modification Trial. *American Journal of Clinical Nutrition*, *93*(3), 516–524. https://doi.org/10.3945/ajcn.110.006395.

Dehghan, M., Mente, A., Zhang, X., Swaminathan, S., Li, W., Mohan, V., et al. (2017). Associations of fats and carbohydrate intake with cardiovascular disease and mortality in 18 countries from five continents (PURE): A prospective cohort study. *The Lancet*, *390*(10107), 2050–2062. https://doi.org/10.1016/S0140-6736(17)32252-3.

Du, S. F., Wang, H. J., Zhang, B., Zhai, F. Y., & Popkin, B. M. (2014). China in the period of transition from scarcity and extensive undernutrition to emerging nutrition-related non-communicable diseases, 1949-1992. *Obesity Reviews*, *15*(1), 8–15. https://doi.org/10.1111/obr.12122.

Elmadfa, I., & Kornsteiner, M. (2009). Dietary fat intake—a global perspective. *Annals of Nutrition and Metabolism*, *54*(1), 8–14. https://doi.org/10.1159/000220822.

Forsythe, C. E., Phinney, S. D., Fernandez, M. L., Quann, E. E., Wood, R. J., Bibus, D. M., et al. (2008). Comparison of low fat and low carbohydrate diets on circulating fatty acid composition and markers of inflammation. *Lipids*, *43*(1), 65–77. https://doi.org/10.1007/s11745-007-3132-7.

Ghosh, S., Molcan, E., Decoffe, D., Dai, C., & Gibson, D. L. (2013). Diets rich in n-6 PUFA induce intestinal microbial dysbiosis in aged mice. *British Journal of Nutrition*, *110*(3), 515–523. https://doi.org/10.1017/S0007114512005326.

Goel, M. S., McCarthy, E. P., Phillips, R. S., & Wee, C. C. (2004). Obesity among US immigrant subgroups by duration of residence. *Journal of the American Medical Association*, *292*(23), 2860–2867. https://doi.org/10.1001/jama.292.23.2860.

Halton, T. L., Willett, W. C., Liu, S., Manson, J. A. E., Albert, C. M., Rexrode, K., et al. (2006). Low-carbohydrate-diet score and the risk of coronary heart disease in women. *New England Journal of Medicine*, *355*(19), 1991–2002. https://doi.org/10.1056/NEJMoa055317.

Harika, R. K., Eilander, A., Alssema, M., Osendarp, S. J. M., & Zock, P. L. (2013). Intake of fatty acids in general populations worldwide does not meet dietary recommendations to prevent coronary heart disease: A systematic review of data from 40 countries. *Annals of Nutrition and Metabolism*, *63*(3), 229–238. https://doi.org/10.1159/000355437.

Hjorth, M. F., Zohar, Y., Hill, J. O., & Astrup, A. (2018). Personalized dietary management of overweight and obesity based on measures of insulin and glucose. *Annual Review of Nutrition*, *38*, 245–272. https://doi.org/10.1146/annurev-nutr-082117-051606.

Howard, B. V., Van Horn, L., Hsia, J., Manson, J. A. E., Stefanick, M. L., Wassertheil-Smoller, S., et al. (2006). Low-fat dietary pattern and risk of cardiovascular disease: The Women's Health Initiative randomized controlled dietary modification trial. *Journal of the American Medical Association*, *295*(6), 655–666. https://doi.org/10.1001/jama.295.6.655.

Hu, F. B., Stampfer, M. J., Manson, J. A. E., Rimm, E., Colditz, G. A., Rosner, B. A., et al. (1997). Dietary fat intake and the risk of coronary heart disease in women. *New England Journal of Medicine*, *337*(21), 1491–1499. https://doi.org/10.1056/NEJM199711203372102.

Hulshof, K. F. A. M., Van Erp-Baart, M. A., Anttolainen, M., Becker, W., Church, S. M., Couet, C., et al. (1999). Intake of fatty acids in Western Europe with emphasis on trans fatty acids: The TRANSFAIR study. *European Journal of Clinical Nutrition*, *53*(2), 143–157. https://doi.org/10.1038/sj.ejcn.1600692.

Jakobsen, M. U., O'Reilly, E. J., Heitmann, B. L., Pereira, M. A., Bälter, K., Fraser, G. E., et al. (2009). Major types of dietary fat and risk of coronary heart disease: A pooled analysis of 11 cohort studies. *American Journal of Clinical Nutrition*, *89*(5), 1425–1432. https://doi.org/10.3945/ajcn.2008.27124.

Jenkins, D. J. A., Wong, J. M. W., Kendall, C. W. C., Esfahani, A., Ng, V. W. Y., Leong, T. C. K., et al. (2009). The effect of a plant-based low-carbohydrate (\eco-atkins\) diet on body weight and blood lipid concentrations in hyperlipidemic subjects. *Archives of Internal Medicine*, *169*(11), 1046–1054. https://doi.org/10.1001/archinternmed.2009.115.

Kahn, S. E., Hull, R. L., & Utzschneider, K. M. (2006). Mechanisms linking obesity to insulin resistance and type 2 diabetes. *Nature*, *444*(7121), 840–846. https://doi.org/10.1038/nature05482.

Kaliannan, K., Wang, B., Li, X. Y., Kim, K. J., & Kang, J. X. (2015). A host-microbiome interaction mediates the opposing effects of omega-6 and omega-3 fatty acids on metabolic endotoxemia. *Scientific Reports*, *5*, 11276. https://doi.org/10.1038/srep11276.

Knowler, W. C., Barrett-Connor, E., Fowler, S. E., Hamman, R. F., Lachin, J. M., Walker, E. A., et al. (2002). Reduction in the incidence of type 2 diabetes with lifestyle intervention or metformin. *New England Journal of Medicine*, *346*(6), 393–403. https://doi.org/10.1056/NEJMoa012512.

Kosinski, C., & Jornayvaz, F. R. (2017). Effects of ketogenic diets on cardiovascular risk factors: Evidence from animal and human studies. *Nutrients*, *9*(5). https://doi.org/10.3390/nu9050517.

Levitan, E. B., Cook, N. R., Stampfer, M. J., Ridker, P. M., Rexrode, K. M., Buring, J. E., et al. (2008). Dietary glycemic index, dietary glycemic load, blood lipids, and C-reactive protein. *Metabolism, Clinical and Experimental*, *57*(3), 437–443. https://doi.org/10.1016/j.metabol.2007.11.002.

Li, Y., Hruby, A., Bernstein, A. M., Ley, S. H., Wang, D. D., Chiuve, S. E., et al. (2015). Saturated fats compared with unsaturated fats and sources of carbohydrates in relation to risk of coronary heart disease a prospective cohort study. *Journal of the American College of Cardiology*, *66*(14), 1538–1548. https://doi.org/10.1016/j.jacc.2015.07.055.

Lichtenstein, A. H. (2019). Dietary fat and cardiovascular disease: Ebb and flow over the last half century. *Advances in Nutrition*, *10*(Suppl_4), S332–S339. https://doi.org/10.1093/advances/nmz024.

Livesey, G., Taylor, R., Livesey, H., Buyken, A., Jenkins, D., Augustin, L., et al. (2019). Dietary glycemic index and load and the risk of type 2 diabetes: A systematic review and updated Meta-analyses of prospective cohort studies. *Nutrients*, *11*(6). https://doi.org/10.3390/nu11061280.

Ludwig, D. S., & Ebbeling, C. B. (2018). The carbohydrate-insulin model of obesity: Beyond "calories in, calories out". *JAMA Internal Medicine*, *178*(8), 1098–1103. https://doi.org/10.1001/jamainternmed.2018.2933.

Ludwig, D. S., Willett, W. C., Volek, J. S., & Neuhouser, M. L. (2018). Dietary fat: From foe to friend? *Science*, *362*(6416), 764–770. https://doi.org/10.1126/science.aau2096.

Mansoor, N., Vinknes, K. J., Veierod, M. B., & Retterstol, K. (2016). Effects of low-carbohydrate diets v. low-fat diets on body weight and cardiovascular risk factors a meta-analysis of randomised controlled trials. *British Journal of Nutrition*, *115*(3), 466–479. https://doi.org/10.1017/S0007114515004699.

Mensink, R. P., Zock, P. L., Kester, A. D. M., & Katan, M. B. (2003). Effects of dietary fatty acids and carbohydrates on the ratio of serum total to HDL cholesterol and on serum lipids and apolipoproteins: A meta-analysis of 60 controlled trials. *American Journal of Clinical Nutrition*, *77*(5), 1146–1155. https://doi.org/10.1093/ajcn/77.5.1146.

Mozaffarian, D., Hao, T., Rimm, E. B., Willett, W. C., & Hu, F. B. (2011). Changes in diet and lifestyle and long-term weight gain in women and men. *New England Journal of Medicine*, *364*(25), 2392–2404. https://doi.org/10.1056/NEJMoa1014296.

Nordmann, A. J., Nordmann, A., Briel, M., Keller, U., Yancy, W. S., Brehm, B. J., et al. (2006). Effects of low-carbohydrate vs low-fat diets on weight loss and cardiovascular risk factors: A meta-analysis of randomized controlled trials. *Archives of Internal Medicine*, *166*(3), 285–293. https://doi.org/10.1001/archinte.166.3.285.

Patterson, E., Wall, R., Fitzgerald, G. F., Ross, R. P., & Stanton, C. (2012). Health implications of high dietary omega-6 polyunsaturated fatty acids. *Journal of Nutrition and Metabolism*, *2012*. https://doi.org/10.1155/2012/539426.

Ritenbaugh, C., Patterson, R. E., Chlebowski, R. T., Caan, B., Fels-Tinker, L., Howard, B., et al. (2003). The Women's Health Initiative dietary modification trial: Overview and baseline characteristics of participants. *Annals of Epidemiology*, *13*(9), S87–S97. https://doi.org/10.1016/S1047-2797(03)00044-9.

Rock, C. L., Flatt, S. W., Pakiz, B., Quintana, E. L., Heath, D. D., Rana, B. K., et al. (2016). Effects of diet composition on weight loss, metabolic factors and biomarkers in a 1-year weight loss intervention in obese women examined by baseline insulin resistance status. *Metabolism, Clinical and Experimental*, *65*(11), 1605–1613. https://doi.org/10.1016/j.metabol.2016.07.008.

Roth, G. A., Mensah, G. A., Johnson, C. O., Addolorato, G., Ammirati, E., Baddour, L. M., et al. (2020). Global burden of cardiovascular diseases and risk factors, 1990-2019: Update from the GBD 2019 study. *Journal of the American College of Cardiology*, *76*(25), 2982–3021. https://doi.org/10.1016/j.jacc.2020.11.010.

Shai, I., Schwarzfuchs, D., Henkin, Y., Shahar, D. R., Witkow, S., Greenberg, I., et al. (2008). Weight loss with a low-carbohydrate, Mediterranean, or low-fat diet. *New England Journal of Medicine*, *359*(3), 229–241. https://doi.org/10.1056/NEJMoa0708681.

Shen, X., Fang, A., He, J., Liu, Z., Guo, M., Gao, R., et al. (2017). Trends in dietary fat and fatty acid intakes and related food sources among Chinese adults: A longitudinal study from the China Health and Nutrition Survey (1997-2011). *Public Health Nutrition*, *20*(16), 2927–2936. https://doi.org/10.1017/S1368980017001781.

Siri-Tarino, P. W., Sun, Q., Hu, F. B., & Krauss, R. M. (2010). Meta-analysis of prospective cohort studies evaluating the association of saturated fat with cardiovascular disease. *American Journal of Clinical Nutrition*, *91*(3), 535–546. https://doi.org/10.3945/ajcn.2009.27725.

Sung, H., Ferlay, J., Siegel, R., Laversanne, M., Soerjomataram, I., Jemal, A., et al. (2021). Global cancer statistics 2020: GLOBOCAN estimates of incidence and mortality worldwide for 36 cancers in 185 countries. *CA: a Cancer Journal for Clinicians*, *71*(3), 209–249. https://doi.org/10.3322/caac.21660.

Te, M., Mallard, S., & Mann, J. (2012). Dietary sugars and body weight: Systematic review and meta-analyses of randomised controlled trials and cohort studies. *BMJ*, *346*. https://doi.org/10.1136/bmj.e7492, e7492.

Tobias, D. K., Chen, M., Manson, J. A. E., Ludwig, D. S., Willett, W., & Hu, F. B. (2015). Effect of low-fat diet interventions versus other diet interventions on long-term weight change in adults: A systematic review and meta-analysis. *The Lancet Diabetes and Endocrinology*, *3*(12), 968–979. https://doi.org/10.1016/S2213-8587(15)00367-8.

Volek, J. S., Fernandez, M. L., Feinman, R. D., & Phinney, S. D. (2008). Dietary carbohydrate restriction induces a unique metabolic state positively affecting atherogenic dyslipidemia, fatty acid partitioning, and metabolic syndrome. *Progress in Lipid Research*, *47*(5), 307–318. https://doi.org/10.1016/j.plipres.2008.02.003.

Volek, J. S., Phinney, S. D., Forsythe, C. E., Quann, E. E., Wood, R. J., Puglisi, M. J., et al. (2009). Carbohydrate restriction has a more favorable impact on the metabolic syndrome than a low fat diet. *Lipids*, *44*(4), 297–309. https://doi.org/10.1007/s11745-008-3274-2.

Wan, Y., Wang, F., Yuan, J., Li, J., Jiang, D., Zhang, J., et al. (2017). Effects of macronutrient distribution on weight and related cardiometabolic profile in healthy non-obese Chinese: A 6-month, randomized controlled-feeding trial. *eBioMedicine*, *22*, 200–207. https://doi.org/10.1016/j.ebiom.2017.06.017.

Wan, Y., Wang, F., Yuan, J., Li, J., Jiang, D., Zhang, J., et al. (2019). Effects of dietary fat on gut microbiota and faecal metabolites, and their relationship with cardiometabolic risk factors: A 6-month randomised controlled-feeding trial. *Gut*, *68*(8), 1417–1429. https://doi.org/10.1136/gutjnl-2018-317609.

Wan, Y., Yuan, J., Li, J., Li, H., Zhang, J., Tang, J., et al. (2020). Unconjugated and secondary bile acid profiles in response to higher-fat, lower-carbohydrate diet and associated with related gut microbiota: A 6-month randomized controlled-feeding trial. *Clinical Nutrition*, *39*(2), 395–404. https://doi.org/10.1016/j.clnu.2019.02.037.

Wang, D. D., & Hu, F. B. (2017). Dietary fat and risk of cardiovascular disease: Recent controversies and advances. *Annual Review of Nutrition*, *37*, 423–446. https://doi.org/10.1146/annurev-nutr-071816-064614.

Zhai, F. Y., Du, S. F., Wang, Z. H., Zhang, J. G., Du, W. W., & Popkin, B. M. (2014). Dynamics of the Chinese diet and the role of urbanicity, 1991-2011. *Obesity Reviews*, *15*(1), 16–26. https://doi.org/10.1111/obr.12124.

CHAPTER 6

Dietary lipids and malignant tumor of the digestive system

Canxia He and Xiaohong Zhang

School of Medicine, Ningbo University, Ningbo, China

6.1 Dietary lipids and gastric cancer

Gastric cancer is the fifth most common cancer and the third leading cause of cancer death globally (Smyth, Nilsson, Grabsch, van Grieken, & Lordick, 2020). According to The Global Cancer Statistics 2018, there were 1,033,701 new cases of gastric cancer in the world, with 782,685 deaths (Bray et al., 2018). Gastric cancer is a histologically heterogeneous cancer. Most gastric cancers are adenocarcinomas. According to the Lauren classification system, gastric cancer is classified as intestinal type and diffuse type (Lauren, 1965). Besides that, a group of gastric cancer patients have both intestinal and diffuse types in the gastric cancer specimen, which is classified as a mixed type of gastric cancer (Chen et al., 2016). According to the World Health Organization (WHO) system, gastric cancer is classified as tubular, parietal cell, papillary, micropapillary, mucoepidermoid, mucinous, poorly cohesive, signet ring cell, medullary carcinoma with lymphoid stroma, hepatoid, and Paneth cell type (World Health Organization classification of tumours. Digestive system tumours, 2015). Risk factors for gastric cancer include *Helicobacter pylori* (*H. pylori*) bacteria or Epstein-Barr virus (EBV) infection, atrophic gastritis, intestinal metaplasia, diet, high salt intake, tobacco smoking, alcohol consumption, obesity, racial background, ABO blood group, biological sex, and family history of gastric cancer (Han & Nayoung, 2015). Among all these risk factors, *H. pylori* infection is the most well-described risk factor for noncardial gastric cancer, with nearly 90% of new cases of noncardial gastric cancer attributed to this bacterial infection (Plummer, Franceschi, Vignat, Forman, & De Martel, 2015; Smyth et al., 2020). Inflammation is an important pathogenesis between *H. pylori* and gastric cancer development. Increasing opinion arises that several nutrients and chemicals which have no side effects in long-term administration can suppress inflammation induced by *H. pylori* as well as the gastric carcinogenesis.

6.1.1 Epidemiological evidence of the relationship between dietary lipids and gastric cancer

In a case-control study of 1,464 participants (402 gastric cancer cases and 1,062 controls), a semi-quantitative food frequency questionnaire was utilized to measure dietary PUFAs intake and evaluate the association between PUFAs and the risk of gastric cancer. The result showed a significant inverse association between the intake of marine-derived n-3 PUFA, DHA, and the risk of gastric cancer (Plummer et al., 2015). Results from another case-control study of 179 incident gastric cancer cases and 357 non-cancer controls suggested that gastric cancer risk was not directly associated with dietary intake of n-3 PUFAs; however, the risk was inversely associated with erythrocyte compositions of DHA, especially for well-differentiated adenocarcinomas (Kuriki et al., 2007). However, the findings regarding n-3 PUFAs and the risk of gastric cancer were inconsistent. The results of a systematic review (11 studies) revealed that there were no significant effects of n-3 PUFAs on weight, body mass index, albumin, wound infections, or pneumonia in gastrointestinal cancer patients (Wan et al., 2020). Based on the data from the National Institutes of Health-AARP Diet and Health Study (United States, 1995–2011), long-chain n-3 PUFAs were found to be associated with a 20% decrease in esophageal adenocarcinoma risk; however, no consistent associations were observed for gastric cancer (Zamani et al., 2020). Results from in vitro and in vivo studies suggest anticancer effects of n-3 PUFAs on gastric cancer. In a benzo(*a*)pyrene-induced forestomach tumorigenesis mouse model, mice were fed corn oil (n-6-enriched diet), olein (n-9-enriched diet), *Ziziphus mistol* seed oil (n-3-enriched diet), cod liver oil (n-3-enriched diet), or mixed fat, and the papilloma incidence was reduced in mice fed with *Ziziphus mistol* seed oil or cod liver oil diets in comparison with the olein group. Mice fed with $n-3$-enriched diets (*Ziziphus mistol* seed oil and cod liver oil) showed significant anti-promoting effects. The findings of this study indicated that $n-3$ PUFA-enriched diets exerted a protective effect on benzo(*a*)pyrene-induced forestomach tumorigenesis. Moreover, dietary PUFAs and tumorigenesis appear to be organ specific (Silva, Muñoz, Guzmán, & Evnard, 1995).

6.1.2 Dietary intake of PUFAs and *H. pylori*-induced gastric carcinogenesis

Results from food frequency questionnaires of 389 subjects who received *H. pylori* eradication therapy in Japan showed that a higher intake of n-3 PUFAs was negatively correlated with the success rate of oral eradication therapy for *H. pylori* infection (Ikezaki et al., 2017). Chronic intake of n-3 PUFA-based diet or pills can attenuate *H. pylori*-associated chronic atrophic gastritis and block the progress of gastric adenoma (Lee et al., 2018). In 45 weeks after *H. pylori* infection, wild-type mice indicated both gastric cancer formation and atrophic gastritis, while n-3 PUFA-treated mice did not, suggesting the anti-inflammatory and anticancer effects of n-3 PUFAs in an animal model (Han et al., 2015). DHA has been shown to inhibit *H. pylori* growth in vitro in a dose-dependent manner and colonization in vivo in the gastric mucosa of mice coinciding with decreased inflammation (Correia et al., 2012). DHA altered the expression of *H. pylori* outer membrane proteins associated with stress response and metabolism and modified bacterial lipopolysaccharide phenotype, which ultimately reduced the adhesion of bacteria and the burden of *H. pylori*-related inflammation (Correia et al., 2013). PUFAs inhibit bacterial growth through the disruption of cell membranes, leading to bacterial lysis (Thompson, Cockayne, & Spiller, 1994). Moreover, DHA that is efficiently incorporated into epithelial cells decreases cell membrane cholesterol levels, modulates the lipid profile of the cell membrane, and inhibits *H. pylori* survival (Correia et al., 2014). DHA suppresses *H. pylori* adhesion to gastric cancer cells; reduces the *H. pylori*-enhanced reactive oxygen species (ROS) production; and significantly reduces gastric tumor incidence, number of tumor nodules, and tumor size in mouse model, which is partly attributed to the inhibition of the NF-κB signaling pathway (Su et al., 2019). N-3 PUFAs are beneficial for the prevention of *H. pylori*-associated gastric inflammation by inhibiting pro-inflammatory IL-8 expression (Lee, Lim, Kim, & Kim, 2014). Gastric epithelial cells that were infected with DHA-pretreated *H. pylori* showed a 3-fold reduction in IL-8 production, a decrease in cyclooxygenase-2 (COX-2), and inducible nitric oxide synthase (iNOS) levels (Correia et al., 2013). *Fat-1* transgenic mice overexpress n-3 desaturase, which facilitates the production of n-3 PUFAs from n-6 fatty acids, leading to abundant n-3 PUFAs with reduced levels of n-6 PUFAs in their organs and tissues without a dietary n-3 PUFAs supply. The results showed that *Fat-1* transgenic mice were protected against *H. pylori*-induced inflammation, chronic atrophic gastritis, tumorigenesis, and gastric cancer compared to wild-type mice in a *H. pylori* infection- and high salt diet-induced model of gastric tumorigenesis (Han et al., 2016). Moreover, the expression of inflammatory (COX-2, IL-1β, IL-6) and angiogenic growth factors was significantly decreased in *Fat-1* transgenic mice (Han et al., 2016).

6.1.3 How does dietary lipids influence gastric cancer?

6.1.3.1 Dietary intake of PUFAs and inflammation

Results from a prospective, randomized, double-blind study, in which 99 patients with gastric and colorectal cancer who underwent elective surgery were recruited, suggested that n-3 PUFAs showed an inflammation-attenuating effect (Ma et al., 2015). A meta-analysis, in which nine trials (698 patients in total) were included, suggested that n-3 PUFA when supplemented with fish oil or added to an immunonutrition formula had favorable effects on inflammatory markers (IL-6 and TNF-α) in patients with gastric cancer undergoing surgical procedures (Mocellin, Fernandes, Chagas, & Trindade, 2018). In a prospective, randomized, case-control study, 48 patients who underwent surgery for gastric cancer aged between 29 and 75 years were recruited and randomly divided into two groups. All patients were treated with iso-nitrogen and isocaloric parenteral nutrition support. The intervention group received an n-3 PUFA oil fat emulsion, whereas the control group received soybean oil. The levels of inflammatory markers (IL-6 and TNF-α) were significantly decreased in the intervention group (Wei et al., 2014).

6.1.3.2 PUFAs and cell proliferation and apoptosis

N-3 PUFAs reduce iodoacetamide-induced gastritis in rats by decreasing malondialdehyde (MDA), gastrin, and nitric oxide (NO), and normalizing mucosal glutathione (Mohammed et al., 2012). Erythrocyte composition of DHA was found to be negatively associated with the risk of well-differentiated gastric adenocarcinoma (Kuriki et al., 2007). A n-3 PUFA-rich diet delayed tumor growth in a mouse xenograft model of gastric cancer (Otto et al., 2008). N-3 PUFAs inhibit macrophage-enhanced gastric cancer cell migration, attenuate matrix metalloproteinase (MMP-)10 expression through ERK and STAT3 phosphorylation (Wu et al., 2012), and inhibit the growth of human gastric carcinoma through apoptosis (Wu, Yu, Liu, Kang, & Guo, 2010). N-3 PUFAs are beneficial for preventing oxidative stress-induced apoptosis by inhibiting apoptotic gene expression and DNA fragmentation of gastric epithelial cells (Yu, Kang, Jung, Jun, & Kim, 2009). DHA induces apoptosis of gastric cancer cells by inducing the expression of apoptotic genes (Lee, Lim, & Kim, 2009). Using cisplatin-resistant gastric cancer SNU-601/cis2 cells as a drug-resistant model, DHA induces apoptosis and cell cycle arrest via ROS-, G-protein-coupled receptor 120 (GPR120)-, and C/EBP homologous protein (CHOP)-dependent mechanisms (Shin et al., 2019). GPR120, a receptor of long-chain fatty acids, is expressed in SNU-601/cis2 cells, and knockdown of GPR120 using specific shRNAs alleviated DHA-mediated ROS production, endoplasmic reticulum (ER) stress, and apoptosis (Shin et al., 2019). CHOP, a transcription factor that functions under ER stress conditions, significantly reduced DHA-mediated ROS production (Lee et al., 2013). A combination of docetaxel and DHA was shown to significantly downregulate the expression of matrix metalloproteinases-2, which is known as a metastasis-related gene, in a metastatic gastric cancer cell line (MKN45). Moreover, DHA decreased docetaxel-mediated upregulation of miR-106b in MKN45 cells. The expression level of miR-194 was significantly increased in docetaxel- and DHA-treated cells; however, DHA alone significantly decreased miR-194 expression (Shekari et al., 2020). The n-3 PUFAs (DHA and EPA) inhibited cell viability in a dose-dependent manner, upregulate caspase-3 expression, and induced apoptosis in MKN45 cells through adenosine A1 receptor (ADORA1) (Sheng, Chen, Liu, Li, & Cao, 2016). ADORA1 is a subtype of adenosine receptor and a member of the G-protein-coupled receptors (GPCR) superfamily, which is involved in lipid metabolism and cell death. ADORA1 is linked to Gi protein, which is involved in the inhibition of adenylate cyclase, decreasing intracellular cAMP. Caspases-9 and -3, known as the crucial executioner caspases, are activated by cAMP, followed by apoptosis in cells (Sai et al., 2006). Furthermore, there is a synergistic effect between n-3 PUFAs (DHA and EPA) and cisplatin in MKN45 cells. After the combination of treatment, G0/G1 phase and S phase arrest increased, and the number of apoptotic cells also significantly increased (Sheng et al., 2016).

6.1.3.3 Synergistic anticancer effect of PUFAs and chemotherapeutic agents

The growth inhibitory activities of 5-fluorouracil (5-FU) in gastric carcinoma SGC7901 cells were markedly enhanced when administered in combination with a DHA dose as low as 40μg/mL. Mechanistically, DHA strongly increased the transcription of BAX, a mitochondrial apoptotic gene, whereas it decreased the transcription of FAS, BCL-2, BCL2L12, and caspase-9. DHA and 5-FU alone or in combination markedly suppressed the proliferation of AGS, a human gastric cancer cell line, in a time- and dose-dependent manner. DHA markedly strengthened the antiproliferative effect of 5-FU, decreasing the IC50 by 3.56- to 2.15-fold in an apparent synergy. Combination treatment with DHA and 5-FU resulted in a significantly larger shift toward the G0/G1 phase and subsequent reduction in the S phase. This synergy was also reflected in energy production via the significant downregulation of METC expression in AGS cells (Gao, Liang, Zhao, Li, & Wang, 2016).

6.1.3.4 PUFAs improve chemotherateutic drug resistance

Chemotherapeutic agents, such as cisplatin, have been widely used in many types of cancer therapies, including gastric cancer. However, in many cases, acquired or intrinsic resistance to chemotherapeutic drugs decreases their efficacy. The highly cytotoxic effect of cisplatin is formed in inter- or intra-DNA strands, which interrupts DNA replication and mitosis, severely damages cell proliferation, and induces endoplasmic reticulum stress and cytoplasm-related apoptosis (Sancho-Martinez, Prieto-Garcia, Prieto, Lopez-Novoa, & Lopez-Hernandez, 2008). In a clinical trial, 34 patients were randomly selected and categorized randomly into two groups. Patients in the case group were taking PUFAs along with cisplatin, and those in the control group were under the same chemotherapy protocol without PUFAs. The expressions of caspases-3 and -9 increased significantly in the case group in comparison with those in the control group ($P < 0.0001$). In addition, DNA damage in gastric tissue of patients treated with PUFAs along with cisplatin was also significantly higher than that in the control group ($P = 0.003$) (Dolatkhah et al., 2017). Some studies have reported that n-3 PUFAs improve the chemoresistant effects on treatment. In cisplatin-resistant gastric cancer SNU-601/cis2 cells, DHA treatment induced ROS-, G-protein-coupled receptor 120 (GPR120)-, and CHOP-dependent apoptosis by using antioxidant agents or specific shRNAs (Shin et al., 2019).

6.2 Dietary lipids and liver carcinoma

Liver carcinoma is the sixth most common cancer and fourth most common cause of death from cancer worldwide in 2018, with approximately 841,000 new cases and 782,000 deaths annually (Bray et al., 2018). The incidence and mortality rates are 2–3 times higher among males in most regions; thus, liver carcinoma ranks fifth in terms of global cases and second in terms of deaths for males, with the highest incidence in Eastern Asia, South-Eastern Asia (Mongolia, Cambodia, and Vietnam), and Northern and Western Africa (Egypt, the Gambia, Guinea) (Bray et al., 2018). Primary liver cancer includes hepatocellular carcinoma (HCC; accounting for 75%–85% of cases) and intrahepatic cholangiocarcinoma (accounting for 10%–15% of cases) as well as other rare types (Bray et al., 2018). The most important risk factor in the development of HCC is chronic infection with hepatitis B virus (HBV) or hepatitis C virus (HCV) (Yu & Yuan, 2004). Other reported risk factors for HCC include nonalcoholic fatty liver disease, hereditary hemochromatosis, aflatoxin exposure, heavy alcohol intake, diabetes, and obesity (Forner, Reig, Bruix, & Carcinoma, 2018). The major risk factors vary from region to region. In most high-risk HCC areas, such as China, the key determinants are chronic HBV infection and aflatoxin exposure (Bray et al., 2018).

6.2.1 Epidemiological evidence of the relationship between dietary lipids and liver cancer

In a population-based case-control study with 23,608 cases and 12,395 controls in Hong Kong, China, results showed that liver cancer mortality was associated with a curvilinear reduction of fish intake (Wang et al., 2011). In a population-based prospective cohort study of 90,296 Japanese subjects (aged, 45–74 years), consumption of n-3 PUFA-rich fish and individual n-3 PUFAs, particularly EPA, docosapentaenoic acid (DPA), and DHA, was associated inversely with HCC, in a dose-dependent manner (Sawada et al., 2012). A meta-analysis of 11 observational studies suggested that fish consumption may decrease the risk of HCC risk as much as 35% (Gao et al., 2015). Dietary intake of n-3 PUFA, but not alpha-linolenic acid (ALA), was associated with a lower risk of HCC (Gao et al., 2015). However, in another hospital-based case-control study in Italy in 1999–2002 (188 HCC and 412 cancer-free controls), results showed a strong inverse association between HCC risk and PUFAs, in particular linoleic acid, but not MUFAs or saturated fatty acids (Polesel et al., 2007). The results from a total of 138,483 females and males who participated in the Nurses' Health Study and Health Professionals Follow-up Study showed that the higher intake of n-3 and n-6 PUFAs is associated with lower risk of HCC (Yang et al., 2020). The results from a three-year prospective randomized controlled clinical trial (320 patients) showed that the addition of n-3 PUFA-based parenteral nutrition significantly improved postoperative recovery for cirrhotic patients with liver cancer following hepatectomy, with a significant reduction in overall mortality and length of hospital stay (Zhang et al., 2017). A randomized controlled trial study in which 20 patients with colorectal liver metastasis were randomized to receive a 72-h infusion of parenteral nutrition with or without n-3 PUFAs showed that hepatic colorectal adenocarcinoma metastases had a higher content of n-9 PUFAs and a lower content of n-6 and n-3 PUFAs than liver tissue without tumors (Stephenson et al., 2013). In a prospective randomized controlled clinical trial with 312 cirrhotic patients with liver cancer (155 in the control group and 157 in the treatment group), n-3 PUFA-based parenteral nutrition significantly reduced the morbidity, mortality, and hospital stay compared with the patients in the control group (Yang et al., 2020). In a population-based prospective cohort study in Japan with 90,296 subjects (an average follow-up period of 11.2 years) and a total of 398 HCC cases, the consumption of n-3 PUFA-rich fish and n-3 PUFAs, particularly EPA, DPA, and DHA, was inversely associated with HCC in a dose-dependent manner (Sawada et al., 2012).

6.2.2 How does dietary lipids influence liver cancer?

6.2.2.1 *PUFAs, cell proliferation, and apoptosis*

Results published in 1998 suggested that both EPA and DHA inhibited the growth of hepatocarcinoma. EPA treatment reduced the percentage of proliferating tumor cells labeled with BudR, whereas DHA did not. DHA supplementation doubled the number of cells undergoing apoptosis, whereas EPA treatment was much less effective. These results indicate that the anti-tumor effect of EPA is related mainly to its inhibition of cell proliferation, whereas that of DHA corresponds with its induction of apoptosis (Calviello et al., 1998). EPA inhibited the proliferation of HepG2 cells in a dose-dependent manner and had no significant effect on the viability of humorous liver cells. EPA initially promotes ROS formation, leading to [Ca^{2+}] accumulation and opening of the mitochondrial permeability transition pore (MPTP), cytochrome C and Ca^{2+} efflux to the cytoplasm, and activation of caspases-9 and -3, eventually leading to apoptosis (Zhang et al., 2015). The effect of EPA on inducing apoptosis in HepG2 cells is at least partly through Fas-mediated apoptosis by p53 (Chi, Chen, & Lai, 2004). EPA induced transient nuclear accumulation of p53 protein expression that subsequently upregulated Fas expression. Cells with wild-type p53 may respond to EPA treatment, whereas those with the mutant form of p53 or loss of p53 are resistant to EPA treatment (Chi et al., 2004). DHA could promote apoptosis and inhibit the growth of HepG2 cells, which was probably related to the downregulated expression of β-catenin and c-Myc (Chen, Jiang, & Wang, 2019). The c-Myc regulates up to 10%–15% of human genes involved in cell cycle regulation, development, apoptosis, and metabolism, and its overexpression is a crucial oncogenic mechanism in several cancers, including liver cancer (Bisso et al., 2020). β-Catenin, the primary effector molecule in the Wnt signaling pathway, is known to be aberrantly active in cancers, as it promotes proliferation and prosurvival signals for cancer cell (Anastas & Moon, 2013). In another study, DHA induced time- and dose-dependent apoptosis in HepG2 hepatoma cells by c-Jun N-terminal protein kinase (JNK) activation, followed by an increase in pro-apoptotic Bad and FasL, cytochrome C release, and caspase 3 activity (Lee & Bae, 2007). DHA-mediated apoptosis in E47 cells (HepG2 hepatoma cells transduced with CYP2E1) may be involved in the production of lipid peroxides or reactive oxygen species during the CYP2E1 catalytic cycle, followed by mitochondrial injury and apoptosis. Low dose of n-3 PUFAs generates a less-toxic bile acid pool and prevents the bile acid-induced apoptosis in HepG2 cells. Gene expression analyses of HepG2 cells revealed that EPA and/or DHA reduces the expression of genes involved in toxic bile acids synthesis (cytochrome P450 (CYP)7A1 and 27A1) and uptake (Na^+ taurocholate-cotransporting polypeptide), while upregulates genes encoding metabolic enzymes (sulfotransferase family 2A member 1) and excretion transporters (multidrug resistance protein (MRP) 2, 3) (Cieślak et al., 2018). The addition of α-linolenic acid or EPA to arterial blood inhibits tumor $n-6$ fatty acid uptake, including linoleic acid; its conversion to the mitogen 13-HODE causes hepatoma cell growth inhibition. DHA retarded the proliferation of the human metastatic HCC cell line MHCC97L in a dose-dependent manner, and also induced cell apoptosis. DHA treatment reduced heat shock protein Hsp27 and endoplasmic reticulum-related protein GPR78, oncogene N-myc, as well as COX-2 prostanoid pathways, in addition to the increased expression of superoxide dismutase but with no effect on glutathione synthetase and protein kinase (Lee et al., 2010). EPA inhibited HepG2 cell growth in a dose-dependent manner, starting from 25 μM, and exerted a significant pro-apoptotic effect at 1 μM; arachidonic acid showed the inhibitory effect on cell proliferation and pro-apoptotic effect at 100 μM (Notarnicola et al., 2011). The effect of EPA and arachidonic acid on cell growth and apoptosis is associated with fatty acid synthase and 3-hydroxy-3-methyl-glutaryl coenzyme A reductase (HMG-CoAR) for their downregulation after PUFAs treatment (Notarnicola et al., 2011). Morris hepatoma 3924A cells were grown subcutaneously in rats fed α-linolenic acid-enriched diet, linolenic acid-enriched diet, and control diet. α-Linolenic acid-enriched diet, but not the linoleic acid-enriched diet, induced apoptosis of hepatoma cells (Vecchini et al., 2004). Meanwhile, it was also observed that apoptosis induced by α-linolenic acid-enriched diet correlated with a decrease in arachidonate content in hepatoma cells and decreased cyclooxygenase-2 expression (Vecchini et al., 2004). DHA and EPA inhibited HCC apoptosis through simultaneous inhibition of cyclooxygenase-2 and β-catenin by using human hepatocellular carcinoma cell lines (Hep3B, HepG2, and Huh7). In addition, DHA and EPA, not arachidonic acid, inhibited cell viability in a dose-dependent manner with cleavage of PARP, caspase-3, and caspase-9 in three human HCC cell lines (Hep3B, Huh-7, and HepG2) (Lim, Han, Dai, Shen, & Wu, 2009).

6.2.2.2 PUFAs and cancer stem cells

DHA packaged within low-density lipoprotein (LDL) nanoparticles (LDL-DHA) is effective against cancer stem cells derived from human HCC cell lines and tumor-bearing rats (Reynolds, Mulik, Wen, Dilip, & Corbin, 2014). In addition, these nanoparticles selectively kill malignant rather than normal hepatocytes in vitro (Moss, Mulik, Van Treuren, Kim, & Corbin, 2016). In vivo, rats given LDL-DHA had 3-fold smaller tumors than control rats (Moss et al., 2016). LDL-DHA nanoparticles killed 70–100% of cancer stem cells by inducing lipid peroxidation activity and reactive oxygen species, while DHA and LDL alone had minimal or no cytotoxic effects (Yang, Gong, Sontag, Corbin, & Minuk, 2018). LDL-DHA nanoparticle induced lipid peroxidation activity and reactive oxygen species in cancer stem cells (Yang et al., 2018). After LDL-DHA treatment, both rat and human HCC cells experience pronounced lipid peroxidation, depletion of glutathione, and inactivation of the lipid antioxidant glutathione peroxidase-4 (GPX4) prior to cell death (Ou et al., 2017). LDL-DHA-induced HCC cell death is dependent on apoptotic, necroptotic, or autophagic pathway, which requires the presence of iron. The further results revealed that LDL-DHA-treated HCC tumors experienced ferroptotic cell death characterized by increased levels of tissue lipid hydroperoxides and suppression of GPX4 expression (Ou et al., 2017; Yang et al., 2018). DHA uptake by cells is mainly achieved by membrane-associated fatty acid-binding proteins. The efficacy of such transport is limited and dependent on cell homeostasis. LDL-DHA nanoparticles are transported efficiently through endocytosis. With each endocytosis event, more than 2000 DHA molecules can be transported. Thus, LDL-DHA nanoparticles are expected to transport DHA molecules into cells more efficiently and in larger numbers than membrane-associated DHA alone uptake pathways (Yang et al., 2018).

6.2.2.3 PUFAs and nonalcoholic steatohepatitis associated with hepatocellular carcinoma

In recent years, the prevalence of nonalcoholic steatohepatitis (NASH) has increased rapidly worldwide. NASH is the most severe form of nonalcoholic fatty liver disease and a dominant factor of hepatic cirrhosis and even HCC. Results from a case-control study (9 NASH patients and 9 controls) showed that n-6 PUFA levels within hepatic lipid content were significantly increased in NASH patients (Puri et al., 2007). Results from a population-based prospective cohort of 63,257 Chinese men and women aged 45–74 years enrolled between 1993 and 1998 showed that n-6 PUFA intake displayed a dose-dependent, positive association with HCC risk. Besides that, the higher ratio of n-6 to n-3 PUFAs conferred an increased risk of HCC (Koh et al., 2016). The concentrations of PUFAs in plasma (linolenic acids (α and γ), EPA, DHA, and linoleic acid) were reduced with tumor progression, while linoleic acid was increased in mice with premalignant lesions using a choline-deficient and high trans-fat/sucrose/cholesterol diet-induced NASH-HCC mice models (Vlock, Karanjit, Talmon, & Farazi, 2020). In this model, lower plasma levels of PUFAs occurred with tumor progression and lower levels of PPARα in the tumors. n-3 PUFAs, EPA and DHA prevented the western diet-induced nonalcoholic steatohepatitis and reduced the risk of primary hepatocellular carcinoma (Vlock et al., 2020). In 20-week-old streptozotocin/high-fat diet (STZ/HFD)-treated mice, n-3 PUFA-rich diets alleviated tumor size and numbers significantly. In this study, an increasing number of macrophages in liver tissue with an increased n-3 PUFAs content and the ratio of n-3 to n-6 PUFAs was reported (Liebig, Dannenberger, Vollmar, & Abshagen, 2019). The results from a mice model of NASH showed that dietary DHA is more effective than EPA at attenuating western diet-induced changes in plasma lipids and hepatic injury and at reversing western diet effects on hepatic metabolism, oxidative stress, and fibrosis (Jump, Depner, Tripathy, & Lytle, 2015). In detail, EPA and DHA attenuated the hepatic response to plasma inflammation by downregulating TLRs, CD14, and NF-κB-p50 nuclear abundance (Depner, Philbrick, & Jump, 2013). Besides that, the EPA- and DHA-containing diet significantly lowered western diet-mediated induction of NOX subunits, which are a main source of superoxide and hydrogen peroxide. In hepatic procarcinogen diethylnitrosamine-induced obesity-related HCC mice model, the development of HCC was significantly less in mice fed a high-fat diet supplemented with EPA than in those fed high-fat diet only. In this model, EPA suppressed the activation of pro-tumorigenic IL-6 effector STAT3, which contributed to the inhibition of tumor growth (Depner et al., 2013). These results suggested that high ratio of dietary n-3 to n-6 PUFAs and n-3 PUFAs contents alleviate NAFLD-caused tumorigenesis and tumor growth.

6.2.2.4 Bioactive metabolites of PUFAs and liver cancer

For determining the effect of n-3 PUFA on tumor formation in the diethylnitrosamine-induced liver tumor model, a fat-1 transgenic mouse model was used, which endogenously forms n-3 PUFA from n-6 PUFA in fat-1 mice. In fat-1 mice, the tumor size and number were decreased compared with those of wild-type littermates, and plasma TNF-α concentration and liver cyclooxygenase-2 expression were markedly decreased. n-3 PUFAs suppress liver tumorigenesis, probably through inhibiting lipopolysaccharide-triggered TNF-α formation that is mediated through their hydroxylated metabolites 18-hydroxyeicosapentaenoic acid (18-HEPE) and 17-hydroxydocosahexaenoic acid (17-HDHA). In vitro, 18-HEPE and 17-HDHA could effectively suppress lipopolysaccharide-triggered TNF-α formation in a murine macrophage cell line (Weylandt et al., 2011).

6.3 N-3 PUFAs and colon cancer

Colorectal cancer (CRC) is a major public health problem, ranking as the second most common cancer in females and the third most common in males worldwide (Jemal et al., 2011) with a high mortality rate (Miller, Siegel, Khan, & Jemal, 2018). In the United States, CRC represented approximately 8% of new cancer cases and 8% of all cancer-related deaths in 2015, accounting for 9.2% of all cancer deaths. In Australia, CRC is the second most prevalent type of cancer and third leading cause of cancer-related mortality (Ferlay et al., 2012). In rapidly developing countries, the incidence of and mortality due to CRC rank fifth among all types of malignant tumors (Liu et al., 2019).

6.3.1 Epidemiological evidence of the relationship between dietary n-3 PUFAs and colon cancer

The etiology of CRC is complex and involves both genetic and environmental factors. It has been proven that more than half of CRC cases are potentially preventable through healthy diet and exercise. Dietary fat intake holds the greatest interest among the modifiable factors associated with increased CRC risk. Epidemiological studies have shown that Greenland Eskimo populations consuming a traditional diet rich in n-3 PUFAs had a significantly lower risk for CRC than the Western population (Calviello, Serini, & Piccioni, 2007). A Western-style diet is calorie-dense, characterized by a high intake of fat with a relatively large proportion of n-6 PUFAs and reduced fiber consumption. The replacement of a traditional, high-fiber, low-fat, and low-calorie dietary pattern with a westernized diet induced increased inflammation, thereby increasing the incidence of inflammatory bowel disease (IBD) and colon carcinogenesis (Granci et al., 2013). The n-3 PUFAs have been demonstrated to exert beneficial effects in CRC prevention in both humans and mice and are considered promising "natural" CRC chemoprevention agents. There is substantial epidemiological evidence based on case-control studies indicating that the consumption of diets high in n-3 PUFAs, such as DHA and EPA, protects against colon tumorigenesis compared with the consumption of foods high in n-6 PUFAs (Fernandez, Chatenoud, La Vecchia, Negri, & Franceschi, 1999; Tavani et al., 2003). High consumption of fish rich in n-3 fatty acids is negatively associated with CRC incidence in the Japanese population (Reddy, 2002). Several case-control studies were conducted in Italy and Switzerland between 1991 and 2001 to estimate the role of n-3 PUFA intake in the etiology of cancer. The multivariate odds ratio (OR) for the highest quintile of n-3 PUFAs compared to the lowest quintile for CRC was 0.7, supporting the association between n-3 PUFA intake and reduced colon cancer risk (Tavani et al., 2003). Multiple lines of evidence suggest that not only the amount but also the type and ratio of fatty acids comprising dietary fats have been implicated in the etiology and pathogenesis of colon cancer. A survey of the plasma lipid profiles of patients with cancer showed that a high ratio of dietary n-6 to n-3 PUFAs was associated with an increased risk of cancer development, including colorectal and breast cancer, in Chinese women (Murff et al., 2009). A case-control study of 1,872 subjects clarified a significant dose-dependent decrease in CRC risk for total n-3 PUFA intake and individual EPA or DHA intake (Kim, Sandler, Galanko, Martin, & Sandler, 2010). In a meta-analysis involving 60,627 individuals (1499 CRC cases and 59,128 non-cases), n-3 PUFA composition in colon tissue was shown to be an independent risk factor for CRC, especially EPA and DHA (Yang, Wang, Ren, & Li, 2014). Data from prospective studies also support the protective effect of n-3 PUFAs on CRC. One case-cohort study (Hodge et al., 2015) involving 4205 participants prospectively examined the association between dietary fatty acid intake in Australia and CRC. Plasma phospholipid fatty acid composition was analyzed as a biomarker of fatty acid nutrition, and the positive association of plasma phospholipid saturated fatty acids (SFAs) with CRC risk and the inverse relationship of total n-3 PUFAs and long-chain marine n-3 PUFAs with the risk of CRC were observed. Dietary palmitic acid, MUFAs, and n-6 PUFAs were positively correlated with rectal cancers, while DHA was inversely correlated. A prospective study of US physicians (Hall, Chavarro, Lee, Willett, & Ma, 2008) that documented 500 cases of colorectal cancer over 22 years showed that fish and $n-3$ fatty acid intake were inversely associated with CRC risk. A study based on a cohort of 73,242 Chinese women reported that dietary PUFA and the ratio of n-3 to n-6 PUFAs were negatively associated with CRC risk (Murff et al., 2009). Notarnicola et al. detected the tissue fatty acid profile of patients at several stages of CRC and observed that the ratio of n-6 to n-3 PUFAs in patients with CRC with metastasis was significantly higher than that in those without metastasis (Notarnicola et al., 2018). Oh et al. examined the relationship between dietary n-3 fatty acids and the ratio of n-3 to n-6 with CRC risk among 34,451 US women without colorectal cancer or polyps. During the 18 years of follow-up, 1,719 cases of colorectal adenoma were documented. The results of that study did not support the hypothesis that a high ratio of n-3 to n-6 PUFAs reduces CRC risk but suggested that higher marine n-3 PUFAs intake may reduce the progression of small adenomas to large adenomas (Oh, Willett, Fuchs, & Giovannucci, 2005). Moreover, the protective effect of n-3 PUFAs was observed at both the initiation and post-initiation stages of carcinogenesis. For example, in a phase III double-blind randomized clinical trial on patients with familial adenomatous polyposis, EPA-free fatty acid (2 g daily for 6 months) treatment markedly decreased adenoma numbers and size (West et al., 2010), providing the first definitive evidence of the chemopreventive efficacy of EPA in humans. In a phase II double-blind, randomized, placebo-controlled trial, 2 g of EPA, as free fatty acid (FFA), was administered to patients with advanced CRC undergoing liver surgery. About 30 days of preoperative EPA-FFA intervention reduced vascularity and provided postoperative overall survival benefit (Cockbain et al., 2014). DHA is more flexible than EPA owing to its high level of unsaturation among n-3 PUFAs. DHA is readily incorporated into membrane phospholipids and is incompatible with cholesterol, thus causing the segregation of DHA-containing phospholipids away from cholesterol and a resultant high molecular disorder, which increases membrane characteristics including fluidity (Wassall & Stillwell, 2009). Therefore, it is rational to postulate that DHA and EPA may result in different variations in the physicochemical properties of membrane lipid domains, thereby exerting different antitumor effects. However, to date, the efficacy of DHA and EPA against colon cancer is still not conclusive, although DHA has been shown to be a more powerful tumor-growth inhibitory agent than EPA (Kato et al., 2002).

6.3.2 How do dietary $n-3$ PUFAs influence colon cancer?

6.3.2.1 Immunomodulatory effects of $n-3$ PUFAs

Chronic inflammation plays a decisive role in promoting and accelerating cancer progression. Inflammatory factors promote the growth of tumor cells, perturb their differentiation, and block the apoptosis of cancer cells. Eicosanoids derived from n-6 PUFAs are mainly found in typical foods of westernized diets, such as refined vegetable oils, red and processed meat, and fast foods, which are mainly proinflammatory mediators. In contrast, metabolites produced from n-3 PUFAs (DHA and EPA), mainly found in algal oils and fatty fish, have anti-inflammatory effects. Owing to the close link between inflammation and CRC risk, high intake of long-chain n-3 PUFAs provides biological validity for a chemoprotective role (Cockbain, Toogood, & Hull, 2012). Mechanistically, dietary PUFAs are transported into cells mediated by FAT/CD36, then stored in lipid droplets as triacylglycerides, or incorporated into plasma and mitochondrial membrane lipids, thereby regulating the composition and structure of caveolae/lipid rafts. Phospholipase A_2 (PLA_2) catalyzes the transformation of linoleic acid disassociated from membrane phospholipids into eicosanoid products such as AA, while AA-derived prostaglandins (PGs) through the cyclooxygenase (COX) pathway are closely related to inflammation and carcinogenesis. There are two isoforms of COX, COX-1 and COX-2, of which COX-1 is constitutively expressed in many tissues and cell types, while COX-2 expression is modulated by growth factors, tumor promoters, and cytokines. Overexpression of the COX-2/PGE_2 pathway has been shown to possess a marked pro-carcinogenic action in a series of epithelial malignant tumors (such as breast, colorectum, and urinary bladder cancer). It is widely accepted that the anticarcinogenic action of n-3 PUFAs may in part result from the inhibition of the COX-2/PGE_2 pathway; however, DHA and EPA block the COX-2/PGE_2 pathway by using different strategies. In contrast to DHA, EPA could better compete for AA substrate in the PLA_2 and block COX-2-associated PG formation, thereby suppressing the generation of pro-carcinogenic PGE_2, and inducing the production of alternative prostanoids, such as PGE_3, which inhibits tumor cell growth in vitro and blocks the proliferative effect of PGE_2. DHA inhibits AA metabolic conversion by displacing AA from the sn-2 position of membrane phospholipids with more potent efficacy than EPA, thus inhibiting its PG production. However, both EPA and DHA can efficiently inhibit the expression of COX-2 in cancer cells. 15-Lipoxygenase (15-LOX) mediates the conversion of DHA into 17-hydroperoxydocosahexaenoic acid (17-HpDHA) to a much lower degree via autoxidation. The oxidation of 17-HpDHA by 5-LOX results in the formation of resolvins and protectins, which are a new class of lipid mediators with a potent anti-inflammatory efficacy. These powerful anti-inflammatory mediators (including resolvins and protectins) derived from EPA and DHA compete for fatty acid-metabolizing enzymes with AA, thereby inhibiting the production of AA-derived pro-inflammatory and immunosuppressive eicosanoids such as leukotrienes (LTs) and PGE_2 (Hawcroft, Loadman, Belluzzi, & Hull, 2010). Resolvin E3, the main metabolite of EPA mediated by 15-LOX-1, exerts anti-inflammatory and pro-resolving activities in animals (Isobe et al., 2013). MicroRNAs (miRNAs) are short noncoding RNAs that function as important modulators of carcinogenesis initiation and progression. miR-101 expression is inhibited in colon cancer tissues compared to that in paracancerous tissues and is negatively associated with COX-2 expression. Resolvin E3 was reported to inactivate the COX-2 signaling pathway by promoting the expression of miR-101 in colon cancer. Targeting the EPA/15-LOX-1/

Resolvin E3/miR-101/COX-2 axis signaling pathway is a promising therapeutic strategy for CRC (Cai et al., 2020).

Tumor necrosis factor-α (TNF-α) is a key mediator of the initiation and progression of colitis-associated CRC, since TNF-α activates the canonical NF-κB signaling pathway via a mechanism involving TRADD, RIP, TRAF2, and IKK proteins. NF-κB is activated in response to injury, infection, and inflammation, as indicated by the modulation of iNOS expression, a crucial enzyme mainly upregulated during inflammatory reactions. Elevated expression of iNOS and increased production of NO are commonly observed under some pathophysiological conditions, including acute or chronic inflammation and tumorigenesis. Pro-inflammatory cytokines such as IL-6 can activate the downstream Jak3/Stat3 cascade, thereby enhancing inflammation and promoting the survival of tumor cells. The expression and activities of TNF-α, iNOS, COX-2, and NF-κB are upregulated at the early stages of CRC, as demonstrated by experimental animal models. The n-3 PUFAs inhibit NF-κB activity and thus decrease the generation of pro-inflammatory enzymes and cytokines, such as COX-2, TNF-α, and IL-1β. n-3 PUFA can genetically block CRC development in Apc (min/+) mice (Han et al., 2016). Wild-type C56BL/6 mice, Apc min/+ mice, fat-1 transgenic mice endogenously synthesizing n-3 PUFA, and $Apc^{min/+} \times$ fat-1 double-transgenic mice were used to assess the role of n-3 PUFAs in intestinal polyposis formation in the $Apc^{min/+}$ mouse model. Consequently, n-3 PUFAs significantly suppressed Apc mutation-induced colonic polyposis with prominently inhibited Wnt/β-catenin cascade, COX-2, and PGE_2, but elevated 15-PGDH. In addition, it was found that inflammasome-related substrates, including IL-1β and IL-18, were significantly elevated and caspase-1 was activated in Apc min/+ × fat-1 mice. It was concluded that n-3 PUFAs can block intestinal polyp generation by suppressing Wnt/β-catenin signaling but promoting 15-PGDH and IL-18 production. The effect of EPA in its FFA form (EPA-FFA) on polyps in $Apc^{min/+}$ mice was also assessed. Diets containing EPA-FFA markedly reduced the polyp number and load in both the small intestine and colon after 12 weeks of feeding. In the EPA-FFA groups, COX-2 expression and β-catenin nuclear translocation were significantly inhibited by the replacement of mucosal AA by EPA. In addition, proliferation throughout the intestine significantly decreased, accompanied by increased apoptosis in mice fed the EPA-FFA-enriched diet (Fini et al., 2010). Peroxisome proliferator-activated receptors (PPARs) are a group of ligand-activated nuclear hormone receptors that modulate the expression of multiple genes involved in cellular proliferation and differentiation, fatty acid metabolism, energy homeostasis, immune responses, and inflammation (Akiyama, Meinke, & Berger, 2005). Ligands for PPARα, PPARδ (also known as PPARβ or PPARβ/δ), and PPARγ have been demonstrated to suppress IBD and colon cancer (Akiyama et al., 2005; Zhang & Young, 2002). Ligands for peroxisome proliferator-activated receptors (PPARs) PPARα, PPARδ (also known as PPARβ or PPARβ/δ), and PPARγ have been shown to inhibit IBD and colon carcinogenesis (Daynes & Jones, 2002; Peters, Hollingshead, & Gonzalez, 2008; Tanaka et al., 2001). At nutritionally relevant concentrations, EPA enhanced PPARγ activity in a dose-dependent manner and suppressed growth in human colon cancer HT-29 cells, which was significantly blocked by co-treatment with a PPARγ antagonist, GW9662 (GW), but overexpression of PPARγ resumed it (Allred, Talbert, Southard, Wang, & Kilgore, 2008). EPA also induced the activation of peroxisome proliferator response element (PPRE) reporter in a PPARγ-null cancer cell line, 22Rv1, when co-transfected with plasmids expressing PPARγ1; however, this effect was blocked by GW. Furthermore, EPA promoted the binding of PPARγ1 to DNA sequences containing a

PPRE in HT-29 and 22Rv1 cells, which was not obstructed by co-treatment with acetylsalicylic acid, an inhibitor of COX activity, indicating that PPARγ is the target mediator of EPA action in colon cancer cells and the effect of EPA is independent of the COX pathway. The inhibitory effect of n-3 PUFAs on colitis and CRC, involving the suppression of NF-κB and iNOS activation and reduction of RNS production and expression of transforming growth factor β, was confirmed in fat-1 transgenic mice with endogenous n-3 PUFA synthesis (Hofmanová et al., 2014; Nowak et al., 2007). However, the anti-inflammatory role of dietary n-3 PUFAs in intestinal epithelial cells is not associated with PPARδ (Monk et al., 2012). The activated Wnt/β-catenin signaling pathway is beneficial for cell proliferation and survival; thus, it is activated in more than 90% of human CRC, and DHA has been shown to inhibit Wnt and downstream β-catenin activation, which also underpins the apoptosis-promoting effects of DHA (Narayanan, Narayanan, Simi, & Reddy, 2003). Oxidative stress is a crucial mechanism by which n-3 PUFAs exert antitumor effects. The n-3 PUFAs increase oxidative stress levels in colonocytes, thereby inducing cell apoptosis (Fan et al., 2011). Exogenous PUFAs can induce cancer cell apoptosis by triggering free radical production and lipid peroxidation, but normal cells are not affected (Das, Huang, Begin, Ells, & Horrobin, 1987). DHA is more easily oxidized than EPA due to an additional double bond and is also the most oxidizable fatty acid compared with other common fatty acids present in cells. Therefore, it has been assumed that DHA may play a key role in inhibiting cancer cell growth, particularly by inducing apoptosis (Siddiqui, Harvey, & Stillwell, 2008). The deregulation of the Notch1 signaling cascade, including ligands of the delta-like or jagged families, transmembrane receptors, and transcription factors such as hairy and enhancer of split-1 (HES1), exerts a critical effect in some solid tumors, including CRC (Ranganathan, Weaver, & Capobianco, 2011). Blockage of the Notch1 cascade had a protective effect on CRC formation in the $Apc^{(Min/+)}$ mouse model (van Es et al., 2005). The activation of Notch1 signaling in response to pro-inflammatory stimuli has been observed in CRC (Lin et al., 2013). Epithelial-to-mesenchymal transition (EMT) is a pivotal requirement for tumor progression and enhanced invasiveness, while the release of inflammatory cytokines and overexpression of matrix metalloproteinases (MMPs), especially MMP9, are the master regulators of EMT. Inflammation induces MMP9 expression in CRC cells, which in turn activates the Notch1 pathway. EPA-FFA counteracts the adverse effects of inflammation targeting the Notch1 cascade and promoting cell invasiveness, and blocks inflammatory-driven EMT (Fazio et al., 2016).

6.3.2.2 Fatty acid mediated chemoprevention of mitochondrial apoptosis

Apoptosis, also known as programmed cell death, is a highly conserved cellular process involved in maintaining homeostasis in organisms. The homeostasis of colonic epithelial cells is closely related to the balance between cell proliferation and apoptosis, while enhanced resistance to apoptosis is a prominent feature of cancer cells. N-3 PUFA intervention [EPA (100 mg/d) and DHA (400 mg/d) for 2 years] has been shown to enhance intestinal epithelial cell apoptosis in humans (Cheng et al., 2003). EPA supplementation (2 g/day for 3 months) remarkably induced apoptosis of colonocytes in individuals with colorectal adenomas (Courtney et al., 2007). Exposure to carcinogenic compounds caused abnormalities in nuclear shape and microvilli number, indicating tumor development. Fish oil intervention induced an increase in apoptosis, depicting extensive loss of microvilli along with chromatin condensation under transmission electron microscopy in a dose- and time-dependent manner. The associated ultrastructural alterations in the nucleus and microvilli support the notion that pro-apoptotic regulation is a potential mechanism underlying the beneficial effects of fish oil on colonic tumor establishment (Sharma, Rani, Bhatnagar, & Agnihotri, 2015). In addition, the combination of dietary fish oil with fermentable fiber contributing to the production of butyrate synergistically inhibited colon carcinogenesis, mainly by enhancing apoptosis (Sanders et al., 2004). The mitochondrial apoptosis pathway is a well-known negative modulator of tumorigenesis; thus, targeting mitochondrial apoptotic pathways is an attractive strategy for cancer therapy. There are two important lipids, cholesterol and cardiolipin, in the mitochondrial membrane. Cholesterol loading is required for membrane biogenesis during cell proliferation as an important component of biological membranes, and the enrichment of cholesterol in the mitochondrial membrane renders cells resistant to swelling and apoptosis and is a typical feature of cancer cells. The balance of cholesterol to cardiolipin on the mitochondrial membrane functions as a rheostat to modulate cell death by affecting membrane permeabilization. p21-Ras is an oncogenic guanine nucleotide-binding protein. Approximately 45% of CRCs harbor K-Ras mutations, which induce vigorous antiapoptotic signals and mediate resistance of colon tumor cells to conventional therapy. The effector proteins of Ras include Raf and the MAP kinase pathway, along with the PI3K/Akt/mTOR pathway to promote proliferation and angiogenesis, and inhibit apoptosis, thus acting as seminal hallmarks of cancer. The development of a K-Ras-targeted therapeutic strategy with reduced toxicity is of clinical significance. DHA and EPA have been reported to be incorporated into the membrane phospholipids of colonocytes and mislocalize oncogenic K-Ras from phosphatidic acid (PA)-rich domains into cholesterol-rich but PA-poor domains, thereby disrupting the upregulation of ERK signaling and hyperproliferation of cells induced by K-Ras (Fuentes et al., 2018). DHA inhibits the activation of Ras by blocking its microlocalization to the lipid raft/caveolae (Ma et al., 2004). Cardiolipin inhibits the release of cytochrome C from the mitochondria by anchoring it to the inner mitochondrial membrane. Increased oxidative stress-induced peroxidation of cardiolipin leads to the dissociation of cytochrome C from the mitochondrial membrane and its subsequent release into the cytoplasm, thereby initiating apoptosis. It has been reported that n-3 PUFAs regulate mitochondrial metabolism, promote apoptosis, and thus inhibit carcinogenesis by incorporation into mitochondrial cardiolipins (Agnihotri et al., 2016). Saturated fatty acids promote both aerobic glycolysis and proliferation of tumor cells by modifying the composition of cardiolipin (Cuezva et al., 2002). In addition, n-3 PUFA treatment triggered apoptosis of colon cancer cells via a mitochondrial apoptotic pathway, as evidenced by a series of molecular events, including loss of mitochondrial membrane potential, production of ROS (including superoxide/hydrogen peroxide, and particularly phospholipid hydroperoxides, which damage the mitochondrial permeability transition pore (mtPTP)) (Engel & Evens, 2006), activation of caspases-9 and -3, and increase in the Bax/Bcl2 ratio (Zhang et al., 2015). DHA administration was reported to activate store-operated channels (SOCs), induce a rapid entry of Ca^{2+} through the plasma membrane, and result in mitochondrial Ca^{2+} loading in butyrate-treated immortalized mouse colonocytes (YAMC), which directly or indirectly activates mitochondrial phospholipid hydroperoxides and induces the opening of the permeability transition pore (PTP) and resultant release of pro-apoptotic proteins such as cytochrome C, thereby initiating a distinct intrinsic pro-apoptotic cycle. p53, a well-known tumor suppressor, acts, in part, to suppress the activation of NF-κB, thus inducing apoptosis in human colon cancer cells. In contrast, p53 dysfunction during tumor progression promotes the development of the NF-κB-mediated inflammatory tumor microenvironment (Schwitalla et al., 2013), which is vital for the commitment of stem cells to apoptosis in response to DNA damage. In p53-deficient mice, increased tumor incidence is linked to the loss of acute apoptotic response to the genotoxic carcinogen azoxymethane (AOM) (Davidson et al., 2015), which is a methylating agent that mediates the formation of O^6-methylguanine (O^6-meG) in DNA, causing base mismatches that trigger tumorigenesis in tissues. AOM-induced O^6-methylguanine DNA adducts can be removed by O^6-methylguanine-DNA methyltransferase (MGMT), which is a specific DNA repair protein. Elimination or repair of NA-damaged cells via MGMT is critical for decreasing the risk of carcinomatous changes in cells. The combination of n-3 PUFAs with curcumin expedited the deletion of O6meG by increasing MGMT activity in Lgr5 + colonic stem cells. Dietary fish oil and curcumin also synergistically promote p53 signaling and its downstream Bax level in stem cells responding to AOM exposure and induce apoptosis of damaged Lgr5+ stem cells at the tumor initiation stage, thereby downregulating AOM-induced nuclear β-catenin levels in aberrant crypt foci (Kim et al., 2016). As early as 1979, PUFAs were reported to increase the transport of methotrexate in L1210 leukemia cells by changing the physical and chemical properties of the cell membrane lipid bilayer (Burns, Luttenegger, Dudley, Spector, & Buettner, 1979). The incorporation of n-3 PUFAs into cell membrane phospholipids has been shown to influence the localization of cell surface receptors, including the epidermal growth factor receptor (EGFR). EGFR is overexpressed in 60%–80% of CRC tumors and plays a critical role in CRC initiation and progression, as it modulates cell proliferation and apoptosis through downstream signaling (Cohen, 2003). Eicosapentaenoic acid monoglyceride (MAG-EPA) promotes apoptosis in HCT116 cells and inhibits tumor growth in a xenograft mouse model by suppressing EGFR/AKT pathway activation and reducing VEGF and HIF-1α expression (Morin, Rodríguez, Blier, & Fortin, 2017).

6.3.3 How can n-3 PUFAs enhance sensitization to radiotherapy and chemotherapy?

6.3.3.1 Sensitization to chemotherapy

Rational multidrug combination elicits more effective anticancer activities. The n-3 PUFAs are preferred to chemosensitize tumor cells to antineoplastic agents; in particular, DHA exerts obvious toxic effects on cancer cells, but is less toxic to normal cells (Ding, Liu, Vaught, Palmiter, & Lind, 2006). Therefore, novel strategies have been initiated for colon cancer therapy based on the combined application of prevailing anticancer drugs and small-molecule inhibitors with n-3 PUFAs (Dupertuis, Meguid, & Pichard, 2007).

6.3.3.1.1 N-3 PUFAs and 5-Fluorouracil

5-Fluorouracil (5-FU) is one of the most widely used medicines for the treatment of CRC. DHA was suggested to enhance the therapeutic efficacy of low doses of 5-FU, since serum 5-FU at concentrations lower than that of 5-FU (0.11 μM)-treated patients (Calviello et al., 2005) exhibited antitumor effects. In 2013, Granci et al. confirmed that a fish oil-based lipid emulsion (containing 5 μM of EPA + DHA) effectively increased the pro-apoptotic effect of 1 μM 5-FU on HT-29 cells, in contrast to a soybean oil emulsion. The underlying mechanism is related to the activation of the Bax-dependent apoptotic pathway. A study based on Caco-2 colon cancer cells treated with a combination of 5-FU and fish oil emulsion rich in n-3 PUFAs showed that the combination additively inhibited cell growth, potently decreased cell cycle progression, and induced apoptosis (Jordan & Stein, 2003). Furthermore, blocking the cell cycle in the S-phase (Rani, Vaiphei, & Agnihotri, 2014) also enhanced the inhibitory effect of fish oil and 5-FU combination on the growth of Caco-2 cells. Additionally, n-3 PUFAs significantly augmented the inhibition of cell cycle progression when administered as fish oil in combination with 5-FU (Granci et al., 2013) in a 1,2-dimethyl-hydrazine dihydrochloride/dextran sulfate sodium (DMH/DSS)-induced colon cancer murine model. Furthermore, co-treatment with a fish oil emulsion significantly enhanced the pro-apoptotic and cytotoxic effects of 5-FU, oxaliplatin (OX), and irinotecan (IRI) in HT-29 (Bax$^{+/+}$) cells but not in LS174T (Bax$^{-/-}$) cells. The formation of apoptotic bodies in HT-29 cells and a remarkable increase in mitochondrial membrane depolarization explained the above-mentioned positive effects of combined therapy. Therefore, the co-administration of fish oil emulsions with 5-FU, OX, or IRI is a good strategy to increase the efficacy of standard chemotherapeutic agents via a Bax-dependent mitochondrial pathway (de Segura et al., 2004). It is worth noting that 5-FU is less effective in patients with colon cancer bearing mutant p53. However, DHA intervention can increase the susceptibility of four different human CRC cells to 5-FU by increasing its pro-apoptotic effect regardless of p53 status (Calviello et al., 2005). It should be noted that 5-FU treatment may cause severe side effects such as hematologic depression and gastrointestinal, hepatic, and renal toxicity. Fish oil supplementation is a promising strategy for enhancing the therapeutic efficacy of 5-FU, attenuating its side effects (Granci et al., 2013), and markedly improving the structural and functional abnormalities of these important organs. For instance, dietary DHA treatment was demonstrated to mitigate the lesions caused by 5-FU in the intestinal mucosa of normal rats based on mucosal morphometric data (de Segura et al., 2004).

6.3.3.1.2 N-3 PUFAs and platinum chemotherapeutic drugs

Oxaliplatin is the first platinum-based drug to show clinical activity in CRC. It suppresses the replication and transcription of DNA and induces cell death by covalently bonding with DNA. In addition, oxaliplatin has been shown to induce autophagy and apoptosis in cancer cells. Autophagy is a vital mechanism that maintains cellular homeostasis in response to various stress events, such as starvation and oxidative stress (Zhang et al., 2019). When autophagy is activated, a phagophore engulfs the cytoplasm and organelles and elongates the cell membrane to form a double-membrane autophagosome, which in turn fuses with lysosomes to degrade and recycle the enveloped cell components. Autophagy is most strongly inhibited by the AKT/mammalian target of rapamycin (mTOR) signaling pathway (Kim & Guan, 2015). Sestrin (SESN), a highly conserved metabolic modulator, can be activated and negatively regulate mTOR by stimulating AMP-activated protein kinase (AMPK) under stress conditions, such as DNA damage, starvation, endoplasmic reticulum (ER) stress, and oxidative stress. There are three subtypes of SESN proteins; SESN1, SESN2, and SESN3. SESN2 is the strongest autophagy regulator (Pasha, Eid, Eid, Gorin, & Munusamy, 2017). Due to various side effects associated with oxaliplatin and the antitumor effects of n-3 PUFAs, the combined application of oxaliplatin with DHA was investigated. The results showed that DHA increased oxaliplatin-induced autophagic cell death in CRC cells by triggering ER stress and activating SESN2. It has been proven that the combination of oxaliplatin with DHA promotes the binding of ER stress-related C/EBP homologous protein (CHOP) to the promoter region of SESN2. Thus, the combination of oxaliplatin and DHA is a promising strategy for CRC therapy (-Jeong et al., 2019).

6.3.3.2 N-3 PUFAs and BRD4 inhibitor

Data based on experimental animal models and human clinical trials have shown that the combination of DHA with conventional chemotherapeutic drugs increased the anticancer efficacy of standard chemotherapeutic agents (Jeong et al., 2019; Kim et al., 2016). Bromodomain-containing protein 4 (BRD4), a member of the bromodomain and extra-terminal (BET) family, functions to initiate the transcription of a number of genes like c-Myc by regulating acetylated lysine residues on histones as a chromatin "reader." JQ1 is a proven small-molecule BRD4 inhibitor that competitively binds to the acetyl-lysine recognition motif, thereby reducing oncogene expression and triggering cancer cell apoptosis. The combination of DHA with JQ1 synergistically suppressed cell proliferation by enhancing apoptosis, as indicated by activated apoptosis executors, such as cleaved caspase-3 and its downstream target PARP in human colon cancer cells. The combination of DHA and JQ1 also synergistically blocked the expression of c-Myc and TNF-α-triggered NF-κB activation (Ding, Zhang, & Mei, 2020).

6.3.3.3 N-3 PUFAs and sulindac analogues

Sulindac analogs, a class of nonsteroidal antiinflammatory drugs, are well known for their potent efficiency in decreasing colon cancer risk. DHA treatment synergistically enhanced sulindac-sulfide-induced apoptosis of different colon cancer cells in vitro by inducing caspase-8 activation and PARP cleavage. Moreover, the combination of sulindac and DHA intraperitoneal treatment inhibited the growth of xenograft tumors derived from CRC cells in nude mice than any single agent used alone (Lim et al., 2012).

6.3.3.4 N-3 PUFAs and paclitaxel

Paclitaxel is an anticancer agent commonly used for the treatment of different types of cancers. EPA+DHA treatment significantly enhanced the pro-apoptotic effect of paclitaxel on Caco-2 colon cells (Kuan, Walker, Luo, & Chen, 2011). The covalent binding of DHA to anticancer medicines is a promising therapeutic strategy. DHA-paclitaxel is a conjugate molecule produced by covalently binding DHA to the chemotherapeutic drug paclitaxel. The advantage of covalently binding DHA to paclitaxel is the enhanced cellular uptake of paclitaxel owing to the lipid carrier function of DHA and slow release of paclitaxel inside the cells, rather than the anticancer activities of DHA. Therefore, DHA was used at much lower concentrations and with much longer intervals between administrations as the DHA-paclitaxel conjugate than when combined with concomitant treatments as separate antineoplastic agents. Because the DHA-paclitaxel conjugate can be retained in tumors for long periods at high concentrations and kill residual tumor cells that eventually re-enter the cell cycle, it is capable of inducing complete tumor regression, while paclitaxel alone causes only partial regression. Importantly, the conjugate was less toxic than paclitaxel alone owing to its slow conversion of paclitaxel to cytotoxic metabolites. Similarly, 10-hydroxycamptothecin conjugated with DHA also exerts an enhanced tumor-inhibitory effect (Wang, Li, & Jiang, 2005).

6.3.3.5 N-3 PUFAs ameliorate chemotherapy resistance

It has been shown that the drug transporter protein P-glycoprotein (P-gp) is closely related to the development of multidrug resistance (MDR) during cancer progression, while resistance of tumor cells to conventional anticancer drugs is a major problem for the success of cancer chemotherapy. Both DHA and EPA are capable of downregulating the expression of P-gp (Szakács, Paterson, Ludwig, Booth-Genthe, & Gottesman, 2006). Colon cancer stem-like cells (CSLCs) have also been associated with the acquisition of chemotherapy resistance and tumor relapse. CD133 was used as a marker of CSLCs for the isolation of colon cancer cells. EPA was demonstrated to be actively incorporated into the membrane lipids of the human colorectal adenocarcinoma cell line COLO 320 DM cells and decreased the overall population of cancer cells. EPA reduced CD133 expression and elevated the expression of the colonic epithelial differentiation markers cytokeratin 20 (CK20) and mucin 2 (Muc 2). EPA increased the sensitivity of COLO 320 DM cells to standard-of-care chemotherapies (5-FU and oxaliplatin). EPA treatment did not influence the number of CD133 $^{(+)}$ CSLCs but enhanced the sensitivity of CD133 $^{(+)}$ CSLCs to 5-FU (Flavia, Witte, Elaine, & Paolo, 2013). The combination of dietary fish oil containing EPA plus DHA and pectin, which can be fermented to butyrate by colonic bacteria, upregulated multiple mucosal miRNAs (miR-26b and miR-203) in Lgr5$^+$ stem cells (Shah et al., 2016b), and their target genes were predicted to be PDE4B and transcription factor 4 (TCF4), which are important mediators that exhibit chemoprotective properties (Shah et al., 2016a).

6.3.3.6 Sensitization to radiotherapy

The modulatory effect of $n-3$ and $n-6$ PUFA pretreatment on hyperic photodynamic therapy in HT-29 and HeLa tumor cells was evaluated. Pretreatment with DHA enhanced the cytotoxic effects of photodynamic therapy using hypericin. Moreover, the elevated toxicity of the combined treatment was linked to oxidative stress, as evidenced by accumulated ROS and RNS production, as well as enhanced lipoperoxides (Kello, Mikeš, Jendželovský, Koval, & Fedoročko, 2010). Combined administration of DHA and EPA or the application of conjugated EPA increased the effect of photodynamic therapy or radiation exposure-induced apoptosis in colon cancer cells (Cai et al., 2014). The mechanism for the pro-apoptotic effect of these treatments was proposed to be increased oxidative stress, such as lipid peroxidation, thereby activating the inflammatory response (Manda, Kriesen, Hildebrandt, Fietkau, & Klautke, 2011) and enhancing DNA damage caused by low DNA polymerase expression.

6.3.4 N-3 PUFAs ameliorate cancer cachexia

Cancer anorexia and cachexia, which are very common in cancer patients, are major factors associated with poor prognosis and disease progression. Cachexia manifests as massive weight loss caused by the huge consumption of both adipose tissue and skeletal muscle mass. Clinical trials have revealed the anti-cachexia effects of fish oil as a supplement during radiotherapy or chemotherapy in cancer patients. Compared to individuals who did not receive n-3 PUFAs, cancer patients who received n-3 PUFAs showed an increase in body weight, in particular an increase in lean body mass (Colomer et al., 2007). A fish oil-enriched diet has been reported to suppress the loss of body weight in mice bearing cachexia-inducing colon tumors. Similarly, DHA treatment was demonstrated to obviously inhibit body weight loss triggered by doxorubicin in rodents (Tisdale & Dhesi, 1990). Similarly, DHA treatment was demonstrated to significantly inhibit the doxorubicin-induced body weight loss of rodents (Hajjaji, Couet, Besson, & Bougnoux, 2012). There is evidence supporting that lasting serum inflammatory status mediates the development of cancer-related cachexia (Pajak et al., 2008). High serum levels of inflammatory cytokines such as TNF-α and IL-6 have been identified as markers of the cachectic process and poor prognosis in patients with advanced tumors. Several studies support the notion that an increase in n-3 PUFA consumption may inhibit elevated systemic inflammation and cachexia progression (Szkaradkiewicz et al., 2009). Fish oil administration is capable of protecting cancer patients against the chemotherapy-associated decline in neutrophil numbers and function, as well as cachexia-induced body weight loss. In a randomized, prospective, controlled clinical trial (Mocellin et al., 2013), dietary fish oil supplementation for nine weeks significantly changed the plasma fatty acid profile and decreased CRP values and the CRP/albumin ratio in patients with CRC undergoing chemotherapy. Of note, patients without fish oil intake lost body weight, whereas those consuming fish oil gained weight, although the difference was not significant due to the limited number of patients (only 12 patients). Higher plasma EPA levels were considered the main factor mediating weight gain and lean body mass increase of n-3 PUFA supplementation. EPA in combination with 5-FU not only enhanced the inhibitory effect of 5-FU on tumor growth, but also blocked the progression of cachexia. In a small trial (Trabal, Leyes, Forga, & Maurel, 2010) that enrolled 13 patients receiving standard chemotherapy for stage IV CRC, the beneficial effect of EPA on chemotherapy tolerance was unequivocally demonstrated. EPA-supplemented patients significantly increased their body weight and continued their chemotherapy, while patients receiving only standard chemotherapy interrupted their treatment due to toxic effects, thereby suggesting a positive effect of EPA on the toxicity of standard chemotherapy. The efficacy of either 2.5% or 5% EPA in the form of free fatty acids (EPA-FFA) in the development of polyps in Apc Min/+ animals was evaluated. The results showed that Apc$^{Min/+}$ mice consuming the control diet had cachexia, which was prevented by 12 weeks of dietary EPA-FFA intervention. Mechanistically, the protective effect of EPA on cachexia is related to catabolic suppression through the suppression of adenosine triphosphate (ATP)-dependent proteolytic pathways. Moreover, EPA was reported to elevate the expression of myosin, a skeletal muscle protein, in cachectic mice by repressing 20S proteasome activity by reducing its α-subunits and p42 regulator activity (Stehr & Heller, 2006). Decreased production of active eicosanoids is known to be helpful in improving cachexia associated with tumor-produced proteolytic factors (Deans & Wigmore, 2005). EPA reduced muscle protein degradation in cachectic animals by inhibiting PGE$_2$ release in skeletal muscle. Moreover, EPA exerts anti-lipolytic effects by suppressing the activity of adenylyl cyclase in adipocytes and the resultant formation of cyclic adenosine monophosphate (cAMP) (Tisdale, 1996). It is noteworthy that continuous n-3 PUFAs intake is needed to maintain its anti-cachexia effect. Clinical trials have shown that the ingestion of EPA, DHA, and α-linolenic acid for 6 months caused a remarkable decline in serum IL-1, IL-6, TNF-α, and IFN-α levels in patients with CRC (Purasiri et al., 1994). Notably, the suppressive effects of n-3 PUFAs on inflammatory cytokines were attenuated 3 months after halting fatty acid consumption.

6.4 Conclusion

Malignant tumors of the digestive tract, including hepatic, gastric, and colon cancers, are a major public health problem with high mortality and morbidity rates. A number of epidemiological studies support the negative association of n-3 PUFAs, such as DHA and EPA, with gastrointestinal tumors. The anti-inflammatory, immune-modulatory, and apoptotic actions of n-3 PUFAs dominantly mediate their inhibitory effects on cancer development. Notably, there are some differences in the anticancer efficacy and mechanism of DHA and EPA. Owing to its longer-chain length and great saturation, DHA has a more potent effect on physicochemical properties, such as membrane flexibility and anti-tumor efficacy. In addition, the sensitizing effect of n-3 PUFAs on chemotherapy and radiotherapy of cancer renders them useful in clinical practice. The auxiliary role of n-3 PUFAs in cancer treatment is of interest to clinicians because of their potent anti-cachexia effect. Taken together, n-3 PUFAs are a promising anticancer approach for cancer therapy.

References

Agnihotri, N., Sharma, G., Rani, I., Renuka, & Bhatnagar, A. (2016). Fish oil prevents colon cancer by modulation of structure and function of mitochondria. *Biomedicine and Pharmacotherapy, 82*, 90–97. https://doi.org/10.1016/j.biopha.2016.04.045.

Akiyama, T. E., Meinke, P. T., & Berger, J. P. (2005). PPAR ligands: Potential therapies for metabolic syndrome. *Current Diabetes Reports, 5*(1), 45–52. https://doi.org/10.1007/s11892-005-0067-3.

Allred, C. D., Talbert, D. R., Southard, R. C., Wang, X., & Kilgore, M. W. (2008). PPARgamma1 as a molecular target of eicosapentaenoic acid in human colon cancer (HT-29) cells. *The Journal of Nutrition*, 138(2), 250–256. https://doi.org/10.1093/jn/138.2.250.

Anastas, J. N., & Moon, R. T. (2013). WNT signalling pathways as therapeutic targets in cancer. *Nature Reviews Cancer*, 13(1), 11–26. https://doi.org/10.1038/nrc3419.

Bisso, A., Filipuzzi, M., Gamarra Figueroa, G. P., Brumana, G., Biagioni, F., Doni, M., et al. (2020). Cooperation between MYC and β-catenin in liver tumorigenesis requires Yap/Taz. *Hepatology*, 72(4), 1430–1443. https://doi.org/10.1002/hep.31120.

Bray, F., Ferlay, J., Soerjomataram, I., Siegel, R. L., Torre, L. A., & Jemal, A. (2018). Global cancer statistics 2018: GLOBOCAN estimates of incidence and mortality worldwide for 36 cancers in 185 countries. *CA: a Cancer Journal for Clinicians*, 68(6), 394–424. https://doi.org/10.3322/caac.21492.

Burns, C. P., Luttenegger, D. G., Dudley, D. T., Spector, A. A., & Buettner, G. R. (1979). Effect of modification of plasma membrane fatty acid composition on fluidity and methotrexate transport in L1210 murine leukemia cells 1. *Cancer Research*, 39(5), 1726–1732.

Cai, Y., Liu, J., Cai, S. K., Miao, E. Y., Jia, C. Q., Fan, Y. Z., et al. (2020). Eicosapentaenoic acid's metabolism of 15-LOX-1 promotes the expression of miR-101 thus inhibits Cox2 pathway in colon cancer. *Oncotargets and Therapy*, 13, 5605–5616.

Cai, F., Sorg, O., Granci, V., Lecumberri, E., Miralbell, R., Dupertuis, Y. M., et al. (2014). Interaction of ω-3 polyunsaturated fatty acids with radiation therapy in two different colorectal cancer cell lines. *Clinical Nutrition*, 33(1), 164–170. https://doi.org/10.1016/j.clnu.2013.04.005.

Calviello, G., Di Nicuolo, F., Serini, S., Piccioni, E., Boninsegna, A., Maggiano, N., et al. (2005). Docosahexaenoic acid enhances the susceptibility of human colorectal cancer cells to 5-fluorouracil. *Cancer Chemotherapy and Pharmacology*, 55(1), 12–20. https://doi.org/10.1007/s00280-004-0846-6.

Calviello, G., Palozza, P., Piccioni, E., Maggiano, N., Frattucci, A., Franceschelli, P., et al. (1998). Dietary supplementation with eicosapentaenoic and docosahexaenoic acid inhibits growth of Morris hepatocarcinoma 3924A in rats: Effects on proliferation and apoptosis. *International Journal of Cancer*, 75(5), 699–705. https://doi.org/10.1002/(SICI)1097-0215(19980302)75:5<699::AID-IJC7>3.0.CO;2-U.

Calviello, G., Serini, S., & Piccioni, E. (2007). $n-3$ polyunsaturated fatty acids and the prevention of colorectal cancer: Molecular mechanisms involved. *Current Medicinal Chemistry*, 14(29), 3059–3069. https://doi.org/10.2174/092986707782793934.

Chen, Y. C., Fang, W. L., Wang, R. F., Liu, C. A., Yang, M. H., Lo, S. S., et al. (2016). Clinicopathological variation of Lauren classification in gastric cancer. *Pathology and Oncology Research*, 22(1), 197–202. https://doi.org/10.1007/s12253-015-9996-6.

Chen, Y. J., Jiang, H. T., & Wang, T. F. (2019). Influence of docosahexaenoic acid on proliferation and apoptosis in human HepG2 cell line. *Annals of Clinical and Laboratory Science*, 49(1), 72–78. http://www.annclinlabsci.org.

Cheng, J., Ogawa, K., Kuriki, K., Yokoyama, Y., Kamiya, T., Seno, K., et al. (2003). Increased intake of $n-3$ polyunsaturated fatty acids elevates the level of apoptosis in the normal sigmoid colon of patients polypectomized for adenomas/tumors. *Cancer Letters*, 193(1), 17–24. https://doi.org/10.1016/S0304383502007176.

Chi, T. Y., Chen, G. G., & Lai, P. B. S. (2004). Eicosapentaenoic acid induces fas-mediated apoptosis through a p53-dependent pathway in hepatoma cells. *Cancer Journal*, 10(3), 190–200. https://doi.org/10.1097/00130404-200405000-00009.

Cieślak, A., Trottier, J., Verreault, M., Milkiewicz, P., Vohl, M. C., & Barbier, O. (2018). N-3 polyunsaturated fatty acids stimulate bile acid detoxification in human cell models. *Canadian Journal of Gastroenterology and Hepatology*. https://doi.org/10.1155/2018/6031074.

Cockbain, A. J., Toogood, G. J., & Hull, M. A. (2012). Omega-3 polyunsaturated fatty acids for the treatment and prevention of colorectal cancer. *Gut*, 61(1), 135–149. https://doi.org/10.1136/gut.2010.233718.

Cockbain, A. J., Volpato, M., Race, A. D., Munarini, A., Fazio, C., Belluzzi, A., et al. (2014). Anticolorectal cancer activity of the omega-3 polyunsaturated fatty acid eicosapentaenoic acid. *Gut*, 63(11), 1760–1768. https://doi.org/10.1136/gutjnl-2013-306445.

Cohen, R. B. (2003). Epidermal growth factor receptor as a therapeutic target in colorectal cancer. *Clinical Colorectal Cancer*, 2(4), 246–251. https://doi.org/10.3816/CCC.2003.n.006.

Colomer, R., Moreno-Nogueira, J. M., García-Luna, P. P., García-Peris, P., García-de-Lorenzo, A., Zarazaga, A., et al. (2007). $n-3$ fatty acids, cancer and cachexia: A systematic review of the literature. *British Journal of Nutrition*, 97(5), 823–831. https://doi.org/10.1017/S000711450765795X.

Correia, M., Casal, S., Vinagre, J., Seruca, R., Figueiredo, C., Touati, E., et al. (2014). Helicobacter pylori's cholesterol uptake impacts resistance to docosahexaenoic acid. *International Journal of Medical Microbiology*, 304(3–4), 314–320. https://doi.org/10.1016/j.ijmm.2013.11.018.

Correia, M., Michel, V., Matos, A. A., Carvalho, P., Oliveira, M. J., Ferreira, R. M., et al. (2012). Docosahexaenoic acid inhibits Helicobacter pylori growth in vitro and mice gastric mucosa colonization. *PLoS One*, 7(4).

Correia, M., Michel, V., Osório, H., El Ghachi, M., Bonis, M., Boneca, I. G., et al. (2013). Crosstalk between Helicobacter pylori and gastric epithelial cells is impaired by docosahexaenoic acid. *PLoS One*, 8(4). https://doi.org/10.1371/journal.pone.0060657.

Courtney, E. D., Matthews, S., Finlayson, C., Pierro, D., Belluzzi, A., Roda, E., et al. (2007). Eicosapentaenoic acid (EPA) reduces crypt cell proliferation and increases apoptosis in normal colonic mucosa in subjects with a history of colorectal adenomas. *International Journal of Colorectal Disease*, 22(7), 765–776. https://doi.org/10.1007/s00384-006-0240-4.

Cuezva, J. M., Krajewska, M., de Heredia, M. L., Krajewski, S., Santamaria, G., & Kim, H. (2002). The bioenergetic signature of cancer: a marker of tumor progression. *Cancer Research*, 62, 6674–6681.

Das, U. N., Huang, Y. S., Begin, M. E., Ells, G., & Horrobin, D. F. (1987). Uptake and distribution of cis-unsaturated fatty acids and their effect on free radical generation in normal and tumor cells in vitro. *Free Radical Biology and Medicine*, 3(1), 9–14. https://doi.org/10.1016/0891-5849(87)90033-5.

Davidson, L. A., Callaway, E. S., Kim, E., Weeks, B. R., Fan, Y. Y., Allred, C. D., et al. (2015). Targeted deletion of p53 in Lgr5-expressing intestinal stem cells promotes colon tumorigenesis in a preclinical model of colitis-associated cancer. *Cancer Research*, 75(24), 5392–5397. https://doi.org/10.1158/0008-5472.CAN-15-1706.

Daynes, R. A., & Jones, D. C. (2002). Emerging roles of PPARs in inflammation and immunity. *Nature Reviews Immunology*, 2(10), 748–759. https://doi.org/10.1038/nri912.

de Segura, I. A. G., Valderrábano, S., Vázquez, I., Vallejo-Cremades, M. T., Gómez-García, L., Sánchez, M., et al. (2004). Protective effects of dietary enrichment with docosahexaenoic acid plus protein in 5-fluorouracil-induced intestinal injury in the rat. *European Journal of Gastroenterology and Hepatology*, 16(5), 479–485. https://doi.org/10.1097/00042737-200405000-00008.

Deans, C., & Wigmore, S. J. (2005). Systemic inflammation, cachexia and prognosis in patients with cancer. *Current Opinion in Clinical Nutrition and Metabolic Care*, 8(3), 265–269. https://doi.org/10.1097/01.mco.0000165004.93707.88.

Depner, C. M., Philbrick, K. A., & Jump, D. B. (2013). Docosahexaenoic acid attenuates hepatic inflammation, oxidative stress, and fibrosis without decreasing hepatosteatosis in a Ldlr-/- mouse model of Western diet-induced nonalcoholic steatohepatitis1-3. *Journal of Nutrition*, 143(3), 315–323. https://doi.org/10.3945/jn.112.171322.

Ding, W. Q., Liu, B., Vaught, J. L., Palmiter, R. D., & Lind, S. E. (2006). Clioquinol and docosahexaenoic acid act synergistically to kill tumor cells. *Molecular Cancer Therapeutics*, 5(7), 1864–1872. https://doi.org/10.1158/1535-7163.MCT-06-0067.

Ding, W., Zhang, H., & Mei, G. (2020). Synergistic antitumor activity of DHA and JQ1 in colorectal carcinoma. *European Journal of Pharmacology*, 885. https://doi.org/10.1016/j.ejphar.2020.173500, 173500.

Dolatkhah, H., Movahedian, A., Somi, M. H., Aghaei, M., Samadi, N., Mirza-Aghazade, A., et al. (2017). Effect of PUFAs oral administration on the amount of apoptotic caspases enzymes in gastric cancer patients undergoing chemotherapy. *Anti-Cancer Agents in Medicinal Chemistry*, 17(1), 93–101. https://doi.org/10.2174/1871520616666160520113503.

Dupertuis, Y. M., Meguid, M. M., & Pichard, C. (2007). Colon cancer therapy: New perspectives of nutritional manipulations using polyunsaturated fatty acids. *Current Opinion in Clinical Nutrition and Metabolic Care*, 10(4), 427–432. https://doi.org/10.1097/MCO.0b013e3281e2c9d4.

Engel, R. H., & Evens, A. M. (2006). Oxidative stress and apoptosis: A new treatment paradigm in cancer. *Frontiers in Bioscience*, 11(1), 300–312. https://doi.org/10.2741/1798.

Fan, Y. Y., Ran, Q., Toyokuni, S., Okazaki, Y., Callaway, E. S., Lupton, J. R., et al. (2011). Dietary fish oil promotes colonic apoptosis and mitochondrial proton leak in oxidatively stressed mice. *Cancer Prevention Research*, 4(8), 1267–1274. https://doi.org/10.1158/1940-6207.CAPR-10-0368.

Fazio, C., Piazzi, G., Vitaglione, P., Fogliano, V., Munarini, A., Prossomariti, A., et al. (2016). Inflammation increases NOTCH1 activity via MMP9 and is counteracted by Eicosapentaenoic acid-free fatty acid in colon cancer cells. *Scientific Reports*, 6. https://doi.org/10.1038/srep20670.

Ferlay, J., Soerjomataram, I., Ervik, M., Dikshit, R., Eser, S., Mathers, C., et al. (2012). Cancer incidence and mortality worldwide: Sources, methods and major patterns in GLOBOCAN. *International Journal of Cancer*, 136.

Fernandez, E., Chatenoud, L., La Vecchia, C., Negri, E., & Franceschi, S. (1999). Fish consumption and cancer risk. *American Journal of Clinical Nutrition*, 70(1), 85–90. https://doi.org/10.1093/ajcn/70.1.85.

Fini, L., Piazzi, G., Ceccarelli, C., Daoud, Y., Belluzzi, A., Munarini, A., et al. (2010). Highly purified eicosapentaenoic acid as free fatty acids strongly suppresses polyps in Apc-Min/+ mice. *Clinical Cancer Research*, 16(23), 5703–5711. https://doi.org/10.1158/1078-0432.CCR-10-1990.

Flavia, D. C., Witte, T. R., Elaine, H. W., & Paolo, C. P. (2013). Omega-3 eicosapentaenoic acid decreases CD133 colon cancer stem-like cell marker expression while increasing sensitivity to chemotherapy. *PLoS One*. https://doi.org/10.1371/journal.pone.0069760, e69760.

Forner, A., Reig, M., Bruix, J., & Carcinoma, H. (2018). *Lancet*, 391(10127), 1301–1314.

Fuentes, N. R., Mlih, M., Barhoumi, R., Fan, Y. Y., Hardin, P., Steele, T. J., et al. (2018). Long-chain $n-3$ fatty acids attenuate oncogenic kras-driven proliferation by altering plasma membrane nanoscale proteolipid composition. *Cancer Research*, 78(14), 3899–3912. https://doi.org/10.1158/0008-5472.CAN-18-0324.

Gao, K., Liang, Q., Zhao, Z. H., Li, Y. F., & Wang, S. F. (2016). Synergistic anticancer properties of docosahexaenoic acid and 5-fluorouracil through interference with energy metabolism and cell cycle arrest in human gastric cancer cell line AGS cells. *World Journal of Gastroenterology*, 22(10), 2971–2980. https://doi.org/10.3748/wjg.v22.i10.2971.

Gao, M., Sun, K., Guo, M., Gao, H., Liu, K., Yang, C., et al. (2015). Fish consumption and $n-3$ polyunsaturated fatty acids, and risk of hepatocellular carcinoma: Systematic review and meta-analysis. *Cancer Causes and Control*, 26(3), 367–376. https://doi.org/10.1007/s10552-014-0512-1.

Granci, V., Cai, F., Lecumberri, E., Clerc, A., Dupertuis, Y. M., & Pichard, C. (2013). Colon cancer cell chemosensitisation by fish oil emulsion involves apoptotic mitochondria pathway. *British Journal of Nutrition*, 109(7), 1188–1195. https://doi.org/10.1017/S000711451200308X.

Hajjaji, N., Couet, C., Besson, P., & Bougnoux, P. (2012). DHA effect on chemotherapy-induced body weight loss: An exploratory study in a rodent model of mammary tumors. *Nutrition and Cancer*, 64(7), 1000–1007. https://doi.org/10.1080/01635581.2012.714832.

Hall, M. N., Chavarro, J. E., Lee, I. M., Willett, W. C., & Ma, J. (2008). A 22-year prospective study of fish, $n-3$ fatty acid intake, and colorectal cancer risk in men. *Cancer Epidemiology, Biomarkers and Prevention*, 17(5), 1136–1143. https://doi.org/10.1158/1055-9965.EPI-07-2803.

Han, Y. M., Kim, K. J., Jeong, M., Park, J. M., Go, E. J., Kang, J. X., et al. (2016). Suppressed helicobacter pylori-associated gastric tumorigenesis in Fat-1 transgenic mice producing endogenous ω-3 polyunsaturated fatty acids. *Oncotarget*, 7(41), 66606–66622. https://doi.org/10.18632/oncotarget.11261.

Han, P. Y., & Nayoung, K. (2015). Review of atrophic gastritis and intestinal metaplasia as a premalignant lesion of gastric cancer. *Journal of Cancer Prevention*, 25–40. https://doi.org/10.15430/JCP.2015.20.1.25.

Han, Y. M., Park, J. M., Jeong, M., Yoo, J. H., Kim, W. H., Shin, S. P., et al. (2015). Dietary, non-microbial intervention to prevent Helicobacter pylori-associated gastric diseases. *Annals of Translational Medicine*, 3(9), 122.

Hawcroft, G., Loadman, P. M., Belluzzi, A., & Hull, M. A. (2010). Effect of eicosapentaenoic acid on E-type prostaglandin synthesis and EP4 receptor signaling in human colorectal cancer cells. *Neoplasia*, 12(8), 618–627. https://doi.org/10.1593/neo.10388.

Hodge, A. M., Williamson, E. J., Bassett, J. K., Macinnis, R. J., Giles, G. G., & English, D. R. (2015). Dietary and biomarker estimates of fatty acids and risk of colorectal cancer. *International Journal of Cancer*, 137(5), 1224–1234. https://doi.org/10.1002/ijc.29479.

Hofmanová, J., Straková, N., Vaculová, A. H., Tylichová, Z., Šafaříková, B., Skender, B., et al. (2014). Interaction of dietary fatty acids with tumour necrosis factor family cytokines during colon inflammation and cancer. *Mediators of Inflammation*, 2014. https://doi.org/10.1155/2014/848632.

Ikezaki, H., Furusyo, N., Jacques, P. F., Shimizu, M., Murata, M., Schaefer, E. J., et al. (2017). Higher dietary cholesterol and v-3 fatty acid intakes are associated with a lower success rate of Helicobacter pylori eradication therapy in Japan. *American Journal of Clinical Nutrition*, 106(2), 581–588. https://doi.org/10.3945/ajcn.116.144873.

Isobe, Y., Arita, M., Iwamoto, R., Urabe, D., Todoroki, H., Masuda, K., et al. (2013). Stereochemical assignment and anti-inflammatory properties of the omega-3 lipid mediator resolvin E3. *Journal of Biochemistry*, 153(4), 355–360. https://doi.org/10.1093/jb/mvs151.

Jemal, A., Bray, F., Center, M. M., Ferlay, J., Ward, E., & Forman, D. (2011). Global cancer statistics. *CA: a Cancer Journal for Clinicians*, 61(2), 69–90. https://doi.org/10.3322/caac.20107.

Jeong, S., Kim, D. Y., Kang, S. H., Yun, H. K., Kim, J. L., Kim, B. R., et al. (2019). Docosahexaenoic acid enhances oxaliplatin-induced autophagic cell death via the ER stress/sesn2 pathway in colorectal cancer. *Cancers*, 11(7). https://doi.org/10.3390/cancers11070982.

Jordan, A., & Stein, J. (2003). Effect of an omega-3 fatty acid containing lipid emulsion alone and in combination with 5-fluorouracil (5-FU) on growth of the colon cancer cell line Caco-2. *European Journal of Nutrition*, 42(6), 324–331. https://doi.org/10.1007/s00394-003-0427-1.

Jump, D. B., Depner, C. M., Tripathy, S., & Lytle, K. A. (2015). Potential for dietary omega-3 fatty acids to prevent nonalcoholic fatty liver disease and reduce the risk of primary liver cancer. *Advances in Nutrition*, 6(6), 694–702.

Kato, T., Hancock, R. L., Mohammadpour, H., McGregor, B., Manalo, P., Khaiboullina, S., et al. (2002). Influence of omega-3 fatty acids on the growth of human colon carcinoma in nude mice. *Cancer Letters*, 187(1–2), 169–177. https://doi.org/10.1016/S0304-3835(02)00432-9.

Kello, M., Mikeš, J., Jendželovský, R., Koval, J., & Fedoročko, P. (2010). PUFAs enhance oxidative stress and apoptosis in tumour cells exposed to hypericin-mediated PDT. *Photochemical and Photobiological Sciences*, 9(9), 1244–1251. https://doi.org/10.1039/c0pp00085j.

Kim, E., Davidson, L. A., Zoh, R. S., Hensel, M. E., Salinas, M. L., Patil, B. S., et al. (2016). Rapidly cycling Lgr5(+) stem cells are exquisitely sensitive to extrinsic dietary factors that modulate colon cancer risk. *Cell Death & Disease, 7*(11).

Kim, Y. C., & Guan, K. L. (2015). MTOR: A pharmacologic target for autophagy regulation. *Journal of Clinical Investigation, 125*(1), 25–32. https://doi.org/10.1172/JCI73939.

Kim, S., Sandler, D. P., Galanko, J., Martin, C., & Sandler, R. S. (2010). Intake of polyunsaturated fatty acids and distal large bowel cancer risk in whites and African Americans. *American Journal of Epidemiology, 171*(9), 969–979. https://doi.org/10.1093/aje/kwq032.

Kim, J., Ulu, A., Wan, D., Yang, J., Hammock, B. D., & Weiss, R. H. (2016). Addition of DHA synergistically enhances the efficacy of regorafenib for kidney cancer therapy. *Molecular Cancer Therapeutics, 15*(5), 890–898. https://doi.org/10.1158/1535-7163.MCT-15-0847.

Koh, W. P., Dan, Y. Y., Goh, G. B. B., Jin, A., Wang, R., & Yuan, J. M. (2016). Dietary fatty acids and risk of hepatocellular carcinoma in the Singapore Chinese health study. *Liver International, 36*(6), 893–901. https://doi.org/10.1111/liv.12978.

Kuan, C. Y., Walker, T. H., Luo, P. G., & Chen, C. F. (2011). Long-chain polyunsaturated fatty acids promote paclitaxel cytotoxicity via inhibition of the MDR1 gene in the human colon cancer Caco-2 cell line. *Journal of the American College of Nutrition, 30*(4), 265–273. https://doi.org/10.1080/07315724.2011.10719969.

Kuriki, K., Wakai, K., Matsuo, K., Hiraki, A., Suzuki, T., Yamamura, Y., et al. (2007). Gastric cancer risk and erythrocyte composition of docosahexaenoic acid with anti-inflammatory effects. *Cancer Epidemiology, Biomarkers and Prevention*, 2406–2415. https://doi.org/10.1158/1055-9965.EPI-07-0655.

Lauren, P. (1965). The two histological main types of gastric carcinoma: Diffuse and so-called intestinal-type carcinoma. An attempt at a histo-clinical classification. *Acta Pathologica et Microbiologica Scandinavica, 64*, 31–49.

Lee, M., & Bae, M. (2007). Docosahexaenoic acid induces apoptosis in CYP2E1-containing HepG2 cells by activating the c-Jun N-terminal protein kinase related mitochondrial damage. *Journal of Nutritional Biochemistry, 18*(5), 348–354. https://doi.org/10.1016/j.jnutbio.2006.06.003.

Lee, H. J., Han, Y. M., An, J. M., Kang, E. A., Park, Y. J., Cha, J. Y., et al. (2018). Role of omega-3 polyunsaturated fatty acids in preventing gastrointestinal cancers: Current status and future perspectives. *Expert Review of Anticancer Therapy, 18*(12), 1189–1203. https://doi.org/10.1080/14737140.2018.1524299.

Lee, J. H., Kim, S. H., Oh, S. Y., Lee, S., Lee, H., Lee, H. J., et al. (2013). Third-line docetaxel chemotherapy for recurrent and metastatic gastric cancer. *Korean Journal of Internal Medicine, 28*(3), 314–321. https://doi.org/10.3904/kjim.2013.28.3.314.

Lee, S. E., Lim, J. W., & Kim, H. (2009). Activator protein-1 mediates docosahexaenoic acid-induced apoptosis of human gastric cancer cells. In *Vol. 1171. Annals of the New York academy of sciences* (pp. 163–169). Blackwell Publishing Inc. https://doi.org/10.1111/j.1749-6632.2009.04716.x.

Lee, S. E., Lim, J. W., Kim, J. M., & Kim, H. (2014). Anti-inflammatory mechanism of polyunsaturated fatty acids in helicobacter pylori-infected gastric epithelial cells. *Mediators of Inflammation, 2014*. https://doi.org/10.1155/2014/128919.

Lee, C. Y. K., Sit, W. H., Fan, S. T., Man, K., Jor, I. W. Y., Wong, L. L. Y., et al. (2010). The cell cycle effects of docosahexaenoic acid on human metastatic hepatocellular carcinoma proliferation. *International Journal of Oncology, 36*(4), 991–998. https://doi.org/10.3892/ijo-00000579.

Liebig, M., Dannenberger, D., Vollmar, B., & Abshagen, K. (2019). $n-3$ PUFAs reduce tumor load and improve survival in a NASH-tumor mouse model. *Therapeutic Advances in Chronic Disease, 10*. https://doi.org/10.1177/2040622319872118.

Lim, K., Han, C., Dai, Y., Shen, M., & Wu, T. (2009). Omega-3 polyunsaturated fatty acids inhibit hepatocellular carcinoma cell growth through blocking β-catenin and cyclooxygenase-2. *Molecular Cancer Therapeutics, 8*(11), 3046–3055. https://doi.org/10.1158/1535-7163.MCT-09-0551.

Lim, S. J., Lee, E., Lee, E. H., Kim, S. Y., Cha, J. H., Choi, H., et al. (2012). Docosahexaenoic acid sensitizes colon cancer cells to sulindac sulfide-induced apoptosis. *Oncology Reports, 27*(6), 2023–2030. https://doi.org/10.3892/or.2012.1706.

Lin, J. T., Wang, J. Y., Chen, M. K., Chen, H. C., Chang, T. H., Su, B. W., et al. (2013). Colon cancer mesenchymal stem cells modulate the tumorigenicity of colon cancer through interleukin 6. *Experimental Cell Research, 319*(14), 2216–2229. https://doi.org/10.1016/j.yexcr.2013.06.003.

Liu, F., Tong, T., Huang, D., Yuan, W., Li, D., Lin, J., et al. (2019). Perioperative chemotherapy versus postoperative chemotherapy for locally advanced resectable colon cancer: Protocol for a two-period randomised controlled phase III trial. *BMJ Open, 9*(1).

Ma, D. W. L., Seo, J., Switzer, K. C., Fan, Y. Y., McMurray, D. N., Lupton, J. R., et al. (2004). $n-3$ PUFA and membrane microdomains: A new frontier in bioactive lipid research. *Journal of Nutritional Biochemistry, 15*(11), 700–706. https://doi.org/10.1016/j.jnutbio.2004.08.002.

Ma, C. J., Wu, J. M., Tsai, H. L., Huang, C. W., Lu, C. Y., Sun, L. C., et al. (2015). Prospective double-blind randomized study on the efficacy and safety of an $n-3$ fatty acid enriched intravenous fat emulsion in postsurgical gastric and colorectal cancer patients. *Nutrition Journal, 14*(1). https://doi.org/10.1186/1475-2891-14-9.

Manda, K., Kriesen, S., Hildebrandt, G., Fietkau, R., & Klautke, G. (2011). Omega-3 fatty acid supplementation in cancer therapy: Does eicosapentanoic acid influence the radiosensitivity of tumor cells? *Strahlentherapie und Onkologie, 187*(2), 127–134. https://doi.org/10.1007/s00066-010-2166-6.

Miller, K. D., Siegel, R. L., Khan, R., & Jemal, A. (2018). Cancer statistics. In *Cancer rehabilitation: Principles and practice* (2nd ed., pp. 10–24). Springer Publishing Company. https://www.springerpub.com/cancer-rehabilitation-9780826111388.html.

Mocellin, M. C., Fernandes, R., Chagas, T. R., & Trindade, E. B. S. M. (2018). A meta-analysis of $n-3$ polyunsaturated fatty acids effects on circulating acute-phase protein and cytokines in gastric cancer. *Clinical Nutrition, 37*(3), 840–850. https://doi.org/10.1016/j.clnu.2017.05.008.

Mocellin, M. C., Pastore E Silva, J. D. A., Camargo, C. D. Q., Fabre, M. E. D. S., Gevaerd, S., Naliwaiko, K., et al. (2013). Fish oil decreases C-reactive protein/albumin ratio improving nutritional prognosis and plasma fatty acid profile in colorectal cancer patients. *Lipids, 48*(9), 879–888. https://doi.org/10.1007/s11745-013-3816-0.

Mohammed, A., Janakiram, N. B., Brewer, M., Duff, A., Lightfoot, S., Brush, R. S., et al. (2012). Endogenous $n-3$ polyunsaturated fatty acids delay progression of pancreatic ductal adenocarcinoma in Fat-1-p48Cre/+- LSL-KrasG12D/+mice. *Neoplasia (United States), 14*(12), 1249–1259. https://doi.org/10.1593/neo.121508.

Monk, J. M., Kim, W., Callaway, E., Turk, H. F., Foreman, J. E., Peters, J. M., et al. (2012). Immunomodulatory action of dietary fish oil and targeted deletion of intestinal epithelial cell PPAR δ in inflammation-induced colon carcinogenesis. *American Journal of Physiology - Gastrointestinal and Liver Physiology, 302*(1), G153–G167. https://doi.org/10.1152/ajpgi.00315.2011.

Morin, C., Rodríguez, E., Blier, P. U., & Fortin, S. (2017). Potential application of eicosapentaenoic acid monoacylglyceride in the management of colorectal cancer. *Marine Drugs, 15*(9). https://doi.org/10.3390/md15090283.

Moss, L. R., Mulik, R. S., Van Treuren, T., Kim, S. Y., & Corbin, I. R. (2016). Investigation into the distinct subcellular effects of docosahexaenoic acid loaded low-density lipoprotein nanoparticles in normal and malignant murine liver cells. *Biochimica et Biophysica Acta - General Subjects, 1860*(11), 2363–2376. https://doi.org/10.1016/j.bbagen.2016.07.004.

Murff, H. J., Shu, X. O., Li, H., Dai, Q., Kallianpur, A., Yang, G., et al. (2009). A prospective study of dietary polyunsaturated fatty acids and colorectal cancer risk in Chinese women. *Cancer Epidemiology, Biomarkers and Prevention, 18*(8), 2283–2291. https://doi.org/10.1158/1055-9965.EPI-08-1196.

Narayanan, B. A., Narayanan, N. K., Simi, B., & Reddy, B. S. (2003). Modulation of inducible nitric oxide synthase and related proinflammatory genes by the omega-3 fatty acid docosahexaenoic acid in human colon cancer cells. *Cancer Research, 63*(5), 972–979.

Notarnicola, M., Lorusso, D., Tutino, V., De Nunzio, V., De Leonardis, G., Marangelli, G., et al. (2018). Differential tissue fatty acids profiling between colorectal cancer patients with and without synchronous metastasis. *International Journal of Molecular Sciences, 19*(4). https://doi.org/10.3390/ijms19040962.

Notarnicola, M., Messa, C., Refolo, M. G., Tutino, V., Miccolis, A., & Caruso, M. G. (2011). Polyunsaturated fatty acids reduce fatty acid synthase and hydroxymethyl-glutaryl CoA-reductase gene expression and promote apoptosis in HepG2 cell line. *Lipids in Health and Disease, 10*. https://doi.org/10.1186/1476-511X-10-10.

Nowak, J., Weylandt, K. H., Habbel, P., Wang, J., Dignass, A., Glickman, J. N., et al. (2007). Colitis-associated colon tumorigenesis is suppressed in transgenic mice rich in endogenous $n-3$ fatty acids. *Carcinogenesis, 28*(9), 1991–1995. https://doi.org/10.1093/carcin/bgm166.

Oh, K., Willett, W. C., Fuchs, C. S., & Giovannucci, E. (2005). Dietary marine $n-3$ fatty acids in relation to risk of distal colorectal adenoma in women. *Cancer Epidemiology, Biomarkers and Prevention, 14*(4), 835–841. https://doi.org/10.1158/1055-9965.EPI-04-0545.

Otto, C., Kaemmerer, U., Illert, B., Muehling, B., Pfetzer, N., Wittig, R., et al. (2008). Growth of human gastric cancer cells in nude mice is delayed by a ketogenic diet supplemented with omega-3 fatty acids and medium-chain triglycerides. *BMC Cancer, 8*. https://doi.org/10.1186/1471-2407-8-122.

Ou, W., Mulik, R. S., Anwar, A., McDonald, J. G., He, X., & Corbin, I. R. (2017). Low-density lipoprotein docosahexaenoic acid nanoparticles induce ferroptotic cell death in hepatocellular carcinoma. *Free Radical Biology and Medicine, 112*, 597–607. https://doi.org/10.1016/j.freeradbiomed.2017.09.002.

Pajak, B., Orzechowska, S., Pijet, B., Pijet, M., Pogorzelska, A., Gajkowska, B., et al. (2008). Crossroads of cytokine signaling–the chase to stop muscle cachexia. *Journal of Physiology and Pharmacology, 59*, 251–264.

Pasha, M., Eid, A. H., Eid, A. A., Gorin, Y., & Munusamy, S. (2017). Sestrin2 as a novel biomarker and therapeutic target for various diseases. *Oxidative Medicine and Cellular Longevity, 2017*. https://doi.org/10.1155/2017/3296294.

Peters, J. M., Hollingshead, H. E., & Gonzalez, F. J. (2008). Role of peroxisome-proliferator-activated receptor β/δ (PPARβ/δ) in gastrointestinal tract function and disease. *Clinical Science, 115*(3–4), 107–127. https://doi.org/10.1042/CS20080022.

Plummer, M., Franceschi, S., Vignat, J., Forman, D., & De Martel, C. (2015). Global burden of gastric cancer attributable to pylori. *International Journal of Cancer, 136*(2), 487–490. https://doi.org/10.1002/ijc.28999.

Polesel, J., Talamini, R., Montella, M., Maso, L. D., Crovatto, M., Parpinel, M., et al. (2007). Nutrients intake and the risk of hepatocellular carcinoma in Italy. *European Journal of Cancer, 43*(16), 2381–2387. https://doi.org/10.1016/j.ejca.2007.07.012.

Purasiri, P., Murray, A., Richardson, S., Heys, S. D., Horrobin, D., & Eremin, O. (1994). Modulation of cytokine production in vivo by dietary essential fatty acids in patients with colorectal cancer. *Clinical Science, 87*(6), 711–717. https://doi.org/10.1042/cs0870711.

Puri, P., Baillie, R. A., Wiest, M. M., Mirshahi, F., Choudhury, J., Cheung, O., et al. (2007). A lipidomic analysis of nonalcoholic fatty liver disease. *Hepatology, 46*(4), 1081–1090. https://doi.org/10.1002/hep.21763.

Ranganathan, P., Weaver, K. L., & Capobianco, A. J. (2011). Notch signalling in solid tumours: A little bit of everything but not all the time. *Nature Reviews Cancer, 11*(5), 338–351. https://doi.org/10.1038/nrc3035.

Rani, I., Vaiphei, K., & Agnihotri, N. (2014). Supplementation of fish oil augments efficacy and attenuates toxicity of 5-fluorouracil in 1,2-dimethylhydrazine dihydrochloride/dextran sulfate sodium-induced colon carcinogenesis. *Cancer Chemotherapy and Pharmacology, 74*(2). https://doi.org/10.1007/s00280-014-2497-6.

Reddy, B. S. (2002). Types and amount of dietary fat and colon cancer risk: Prevention by omega-3 fatty acid-rich diets. *Environmental Health and Preventive Medicine, 7*(3), 95–102. https://doi.org/10.1265/ehpm.2002.95.

Reynolds, L., Mulik, R. S., Wen, X., Dilip, A., & Corbin, I. R. (2014). Low-density lipoprotein-mediated delivery of docosahexaenoic acid selectively kills murine liver cancer cells. *Nanomedicine, 9*(14), 2123–2141. https://doi.org/10.2217/NNM.13.187.

Sai, K., Yang, D., Yamamoto, H., Fujikawa, H., Yamamoto, S., Nagata, T., et al. (2006). A1 adenosine receptor signal and AMPK involving caspase-9/-3 activation are responsible for adenosine-induced RCR-1 astrocytoma cell death. *NeuroToxicology, 27*(4), 458–467. https://doi.org/10.1016/j.neuro.2005.12.008.

Sancho-Martinez, S. M., Prieto-Garcia, L., Prieto, M., Lopez-Novoa, J. M., & Lopez-Hernandez, F. J. (2008). Subcellular targets of cisplatin cytotoxicity: An integrated view. *American Journal of Physiology. Renal Physiology, 2012*(1), 44–52.

Sanders, L. M., Henderson, C. E., Hong, M. Y., Barhoumi, R., Burghardt, R. C., Wang, N., et al. (2004). An increase in reactive oxygen species by dietary fish oil coupled with the attenuation of antioxidant defenses by dietary pectin enhances rat colonocyte apoptosis. *Journal of Nutrition, 134*(12), 3233–3238. American Institute of Nutrition https://doi.org/10.1093/jn/134.12.3233.

Sawada, N., Inoue, M., Iwasaki, M., Sasazuki, S., Shimazu, T., Yamaji, T., et al. (2012). Consumption of $n-3$ fatty acids and fish reduces risk of hepatocellular carcinoma. *Gastroenterology, 142*(7), 1468–1475. https://doi.org/10.1053/j.gastro.2012.02.018.

Schwitalla, S., Ziegler, P. K., Horst, D., Becker, V., Kerle, I., Begus-Nahrmann, Y., et al. (2013). Loss of p53 in enterocytes generates an inflammatory microenvironment enabling invasion and lymph node metastasis of carcinogen-induced colorectal tumors. *Cancer Cell, 23*(1), 93–106. https://doi.org/10.1016/j.ccr.2012.11.014.

Shah, M. S., Kim, E., Davidson, L. A., Knight, J. M., Zoh, R. S., Goldsby, J. S., et al. (2016a). Comparative effects of diet and carcinogen on microRNA expression in the stem cell niche of the mouse colonic crypt. *Biochimica et Biophysica Acta - Molecular Basis of Disease, 1862*(1), 121–134. https://doi.org/10.1016/j.bbadis.2015.10.012.

Shah, M. S., Kim, E., Davidson, L. A., Knight, J. M., Zoh, R. S., Goldsby, J. S., et al. (2016b). Data describing the effects of dietary bioactive agents on colonic stem cell microRNA and mRNA expression. *Data in Brief, 6*, 398–404. https://doi.org/10.1016/j.dib.2015.12.026.

Sharma, G., Rani, I., Bhatnagar, A., & Agnihotri, N. (2015). Documentation of ultrastructural changes in nucleus and microvilli by fish oil in experimental colon carcinogenesis. *Ultrastructural Pathology, 39*(5), 351–356. https://doi.org/10.3109/01913123.2015.1048914.

Shekari, N., Javadian, M., Ghasemi, M., Baradaran, B., Darabi, M., & Kazemi, T. (2020). Synergistic beneficial effect of docosahexaenoic acid (DHA) and docetaxel on the expression level of matrix metalloproteinase-2 (MMP-2) and MicroRNA-106b in gastric cancer. *Journal of Gastrointestinal Cancer, 51*(1), 70–75. https://doi.org/10.1007/s12029-019-00205-0.

Sheng, H., Chen, X., Liu, B., Li, P., & Cao, W. (2016). Omega-3 polyunsaturated fatty acids enhance cisplatin efficacy in gastric cancer cells by inducing apoptosis via ADORA1. *Anti-Cancer Agents in Medicinal Chemistry, 16*(9), 1085–1092. https://doi.org/10.2174/1871520616666160330104413.

Shin, J. I., Jeon, Y. J., Lee, S., Lee, Y. G., Kim, J. B., & Lee, K. (2019). G-protein-coupled receptor 120 mediates DHA-induced apoptosis by regulating IP3R, ROS and, ER stress levels in cisplatin-resistant cancer cells. *Molecules and Cells, 42*(3), 252–261. https://doi.org/10.14348/molcells.2019.2440.

Siddiqui, R. A., Harvey, K., & Stillwell, W. (2008). Anticancer properties of oxidation products of docosahexaenoic acid. *Chemistry and Physics of Lipids, 153*(1), 47–56. https://doi.org/10.1016/j.chemphyslip.2008.02.009.

Silva, R. A., Muñoz, S. E., Guzmán, C. A., & Evnard, A. R. E. (1995). Effects of dietary $n-3$, $n-6$ and n-9 polyunsaturated fatty acids on benzo(a)pyrene-induced forestomach tumorigenesis in C57BL6J mice. *Prostaglandins, Leukotrienes and Essential Fatty Acids*, 273–277. https://doi.org/10.1016/0952-3278(95)90127-2.

Smyth, E. C., Nilsson, M., Grabsch, H. I., van Grieken, N. C., & Lordick, F. (2020). Gastric cancer. *The Lancet, 396*(10251), 635–648. https://doi.org/10.1016/S0140-6736(20)31288-5.

Stehr, S. N., & Heller, A. R. (2006). Omega-3 fatty acid effects on biochemical indices following cancer surgery. *Clinica Chimica Acta*, *373*(1–2), 1–8. https://doi.org/10.1016/j.cca.2006.04.024.

Stephenson, J. A., Al-Taan, O., Arshad, A., West, A. L., Calder, P. C., Morgan, B., et al. (2013). Unsaturated fatty acids differ between hepatic colorectal metastases and liver tissue without tumour in humans: Results from a randomised controlled trial of intravenous eicosapentaenoic and docosahexaenoic acids. *Prostaglandins, Leukotrienes, and Essential Fatty Acids*, *88*(6), 405–410. https://doi.org/10.1016/j.plefa.2013.04.002.

Su, T., Li, F., Guan, J., Liu, L., Huang, P., Wang, Y., et al. (2019). Artemisinin and its derivatives prevent Helicobacter pylori-induced gastric carcinogenesis via inhibition of NF-κB signaling. *Phytomedicine*, *63*. https://doi.org/10.1016/j.phymed.2019.152968.

Szakács, G., Paterson, J. K., Ludwig, J. A., Booth-Genthe, C., & Gottesman, M. M. (2006). Targeting multidrug resistance in cancer. *Nature Reviews Drug Discovery*, *5*(3), 219–234. https://doi.org/10.1038/nrd1984.

Szkaradkiewicz, A., Marciniak, R., Chudzicka-Strugała, I., Wasilewska, A., Drews, M., Majewski, P., et al. (2009). Proinflammatory cytokines and IL-10 in inflammatory bowel disease and colorectal cancer patients. *Archivum Immunologiae et Therapiae Experimentalis*, *57*(4), 291–294. https://doi.org/10.1007/s00005-009-0031-z.

Tanaka, T., Kohno, H., Yoshitani, S., Okumura, A., Murakami, A., & Hosokawa, M. (2001). Ligands for peroxisome proliferator-activated receptors alpha and gamma inhibit chemically induced colitis and formation of aberrant crypt foci in rats. *Cancer Research*, *61*(6), 2424–2428.

Tavani, A., Pelucchi, C., Parpinel, M., Negri, E., Franceschi, S., Levi, F., et al. (2003). n−3 polyunsaturated fatty acid intake and cancer risk in Italy and Switzerland. *International Journal of Cancer*, *105*(1), 113–116. https://doi.org/10.1002/ijc.11018.

Thompson, L., Cockayne, A., & Spiller, R. C. (1994). Inhibitory effect of polyunsaturated fatty acids on the growth of helicobacter pylori: A possible explanation of the effect of diet on peptic ulceration. *Gut*, *35*(11), 1557–1561. https://doi.org/10.1136/gut.35.11.1557.

Tisdale, M. J. (1996). Inhibition of lipolysis and muscle protein degradation by EPA in cancer cachexia. *Nutrition*, *12*(1), S31–S33. https://doi.org/10.1016/0899-9007(95)00066-6.

Tisdale, M. J., & Dhesi, J. K. (1990). Inhibition of weight loss by ω-3 fatty acids in an experimental cachexia model. *Cancer Research*, *50*(16), 5022–5026.

Trabal, J., Leyes, P., Forga, M., & Maurel, J. (2010). Potential usefulness of an EPA-enriched nutritional supplement on chemotherapy tolerability in cancer patients without overt malnutrition. *Nutrición Hospitalaria*, *25*(5), 736–740. https://doi.org/10.3305/nh.2010.25.5.4616.

van Es, J. H., van Gijn, M. E., Riccio, O., van den Born, M., Vooijs, M., Begthel, H., et al. (2005). Notch/gamma-secretase inhibition turns proliferative cells in intestinal crypts and adenomas into goblet cells. *Nature*, *435*(7044), 959–963.

Vecchini, A., Ceccarelli, V., Susta, F., Caligiana, P., Orvietani, P., Binaglia, L., et al. (2004). Dietary α-linolenic acid reduces COX-2 expression and induces apoptosis of hepatoma cells. *Journal of Lipid Research*, *45*(2), 308–316. https://doi.org/10.1194/jlr.M300396-JLR200.

Vlock, E. M., Karanjit, S., Talmon, G., & Farazi, P. A. (2020). Reduction of polyunsaturated fatty acids with tumor progression in a lean non-alcoholic steatohepatitis- associated hepatocellular carcinoma mouse model. *Journal of Cancer*, *11*(19), 5536–5546. https://doi.org/10.7150/jca.48495.

Wan, G. Y., Zheng, L. Y., Li, H. Q., Yuan, H., Xue, H., & Zhang, X. Y. (2020). Effects of enteral nutritional rich in n−3 polyunsaturated fatty acids on the nutritional status of gastrointestinal cancer patients: A systematic review and meta-analysis. *European Journal of Clinical Nutrition*, *74*(2), 220–230. https://doi.org/10.1038/s41430-019-0527-5.

Wang, M. P., Thomas, G. N., Ho, S. Y., Lai, H. K., Mak, K. H., & Lam, T. H. (2011). Fish consumption and mortality in Hong Kong Chinese-the LIMOR study. *Annals of Epidemiology*, *21*(3), 164–169. https://doi.org/10.1016/j.annepidem.2010.10.010.

Wang, Y., Li, L., & Jiang, W. (2005). Synthesis and evaluation of a DHA and 10-hydroxycamptothecin conjugate. *Bioorganic & Medicinal Chemistry*, *13*, 5592–5599. https://doi.org/10.1016/j.bmc.2005.06.039.

Wassall, S. R., & Stillwell, W. (2009). Polyunsaturated fatty acid-cholesterol interactions: Domain formation in membranes. *Biochimica et Biophysica Acta - Biomembranes*, *1788*(1), 24–32. https://doi.org/10.1016/j.bbamem.2008.10.011.

Wei, Z., Wang, W., Chen, J., Yang, D., Yan, R., & Cai, Q. (2014). A prospective, randomized, controlled study of ω-3 fish oil fat emulsion-based parenteral nutrition for patients following surgical resection of gastric tumors. *Nutrition Journal*, *13*(1). https://doi.org/10.1186/1475-2891-13-25.

West, N. J., Clark, S. K., Phillips, R. K. S., Hutchinson, J. M., Leicester, R. J., Belluzzi, A., et al. (2010). Eicosapentaenoic acid reduces rectal polyp number and size in familial adenomatous polyposis. *Gut*, *59*(7), 918–925. https://doi.org/10.1136/gut.2009.200642.

Weylandt, K. H., Krause, L. F., Gomolka, B., Chiu, C. Y., Bilal, S., Nadolny, A., et al. (2011). Suppressed liver tumorigenesis in fat-1 mice with elevated omega-3 fatty acids is associated with increased omega-3 derived lipid mediators and reduced TNF-α. *Carcinogenesis*, *32*(6), 897–903. https://doi.org/10.1093/carcin/bgr049.

World Health Organization classification of tumours. Digestive system tumours. (2015).

Wu, M. H., Tsai, Y. T., Hua, K. T., Chang, K. C., Kuo, M. L., & Lin, M. T. (2012). Eicosapentaenoic acid and docosahexaenoic acid inhibit macrophage-induced gastric cancer cell migration by attenuating the expression of matrix metalloproteinase 10. *Journal of Nutritional Biochemistry*, *23*(11), 1434–1439. https://doi.org/10.1016/j.jnutbio.2011.09.004.

Wu, Q., Yu, J. C., Liu, Y. Q., Kang, W. M., & Guo, W. D. (2010). Effect of combination of docosahexaenoic acid and fluorouracil on human gastric carcinoma cell strain MGC803. *Acta Academiae Medicinae Sinicae*, *32*(1), 65–70. https://doi.org/10.3881/j.issn.1000-503X.2010.01.016.

Yang, J., Gong, Y., Sontag, D. P., Corbin, I., & Minuk, G. Y. (2018). Effects of low-density lipoprotein docosahexaenoic acid nanoparticles on cancer stem cells isolated from human hepatoma cell lines. *Molecular Biology Reports*, *45*(5), 1023–1036. https://doi.org/10.1007/s11033-018-4252-2.

Yang, W., Sui, J., Ma, Y., Simon, T. G., Petrick, J. L., Lai, M., et al. (2020). High dietary intake of vegetable or polyunsaturated fats is associated with reduced risk of hepatocellular carcinoma. *Clinical Gastroenterology and Hepatology : The Official Clinical Practice Journal of the American Gastroenterological Association*, *18*(12), 2775–2783.

Yang, B., Wang, F. L., Ren, X. L., & Li, D. (2014). Biospecimen long-chain $N-3$ PUFA and risk of colorectal cancer: A meta-analysis of data from 60, 627 individuals. *PLoS One*, *9*(11). https://doi.org/10.1371/journal.pone.0110574.

Yu, J. H., Kang, S. G., Jung, U. Y., Jun, C. H., & Kim, H. (2009). Effects of omega-3 fatty acids on apoptosis of human gastric epithelial cells exposed to silica-immobilized glucose oxidase. In *Vol. 1171. Annals of the New York academy of sciences* (pp. 359–364). Blackwell Publishing Inc. https://doi.org/10.1111/j.1749-6632.2009.04703.x.

Yu, M. C., & Yuan, J. M. (2004). Environmental factors and risk for hepatocellular carcinoma. *Gastroenterology*, *127*(5), S72–S78. W.B. Saunders https://doi.org/10.1016/j.gastro.2004.09.018.

Zamani, S. A., McClain, K. M., Graubard, B. I., Liao, L. M., Abnet, C. C., Cook, M. B., et al. (2020). Dietary polyunsaturated fat intake in relation to head and neck, esophageal, and gastric cancer incidence in the National Institutes of Health-AARP diet and health study. *American Journal of Epidemiology*, *189*(10), 1096–1113. https://doi.org/10.1093/aje/kwaa024.

Zhang, Y., Han, L., Qi, W., Cheng, D., Ma, X., Hou, L., et al. (2015). Eicosapentaenoic acid (EPA) induced apoptosis in HepG2 cells through ROS-Ca2+-JNK mitochondrial pathways. *Biochemical and Biophysical Research Communications*, *456*(4), 926–932. https://doi.org/10.1016/j.bbrc.2014.12.036.

Zhang, L., Qiang, P. F., Yu, J. T., Miao, Y. M., Chen, Z. Q., Qu, J., et al. (2019). Identification of compound CA-5f as a novel late-stage autophagy inhibitor with potent anti-tumor effect against non-small cell lung cancer. *Autophagy*, *15*(3), 391–406. https://doi.org/10.1080/15548627.2018.1511503.

Zhang, B., Wei, G., Li, R., Wang, Y., Yu, J., Wang, R., et al. (2017). $n-3$ fatty acid-based parenteral nutrition improves postoperative recovery for cirrhotic patients with liver cancer: A randomized controlled clinical trial. *Clinical Nutrition*, *36*(5), 1239–1244. https://doi.org/10.1016/j.clnu.2016.08.002.

Zhang, X., & Young, H. A. (2002). PPAR and immune system—what do we know? *International Immunopharmacology*, *2*(8), 1029–1044. https://doi.org/10.1016/S1567-5769(02)00057-7.

Zhang, C., Yu, H., Shen, Y., Ni, X., Shen, S., & Das, U. N. (2015). Polyunsaturated fatty acids trigger apoptosis of colon cancer cells through a mitochondrial pathway. *Archives of Medical Science*, *11*(5), 1081–1094. https://doi.org/10.5114/aoms.2015.54865.

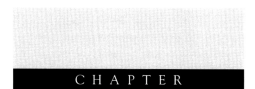

CHAPTER 7

Dietary lipids and breast cancer

Jiaomei Li

Department of Nutrition and Food Hygiene, Zhejiang Chinese Medical University, Hangzhou, China

7.1 Introduction

Breast cancer is the most commonly diagnosed cancer and the second leading cause of cancer death among women worldwide, accounting for 25% of the total cancer cases and 15% of cancer deaths in 2012 (Torre et al., 2012). Clinically, breast cancer is a heterogeneous disease, primarily grouped into four subtypes, namely, luminal A, luminal B, triple negative (or basal-like), and HER2-overexpressing. These subtypes are varied widely in morphological appearance, tumor phenotype, gene expression, and prognosis (Barnard, Boeke, & Tamimi, 2015; Wörmann, 2017). Several factors have been identified as risk factors associated with elevated breast cancer risk, such as older age (>65 years), late menopause (>55 years), infertility, hormonal treatment, obesity, no history of breastfeeding, and giving birth to a child (Sun et al., 2017; Zare, Haem, Lankarani, Heydari, & Barooti, 2013). Current treatments, such as surgery, systemic therapy, and radiation therapy, can effectively improve the survival rate of breast cancer, but they always come together with adverse events and the patients always have risk of recurrence. Thus, alternate strategies to reduce initial cancer risk as well as to improve long-term disease-free survival are urgently required.

Epidemiological studies have showed that a healthy diet and lifestyle pattern has a protective effect on the prevention of breast cancer (Hardefeldt, Penninkilampi, Edirimanne, & Eslick, 2018; Harvie, Howell, & Evans, 2015; Scoccianti, Lauby-Secretan, Bello, Chajes, & Romieu, 2014). High consumption of vegetables, fruits, poultry, and fish as well as low consumption of refined food, sweets, red meat, and high-fat dairy products, might improve the overall survival and prognosis of women with early stage breast cancer (Kwan et al., 2009). Nutritional counseling and supplementation with some specific dietary constituents might be helpful to enhance therapeutic efficacy and limit drug-induced side effects (De Cicco et al., 2019). Thus, nutritional intervention might be considered as an integral part of the preventive and therapeutic approach for breast cancer disease.

Dietary lipid is one of the most intensively studied nutritional factors associated with breast cancer (MacLean et al., 2006; Park, Kolonel, Henderson, & Wilkens, 2012). The relationship between dietary lipids and breast cancer in terms of incidence, treatment, and recurrence was reviewed in this chapter, including the effect of dietary fat exposure with different amount and in different period and with some specific fatty acids, such as EPA and/or

DHA, on the development of breast cancer. In addition, the potential mechanisms by which dietary lipid regulate the breast cancer risk were investigated.

7.2 Epidemiological evidence regarding dietary lipids intake and breast cancer

7.2.1 Effect of total amount of fat intake

During recent years, several dietary intervention trials have evaluated the relationship between total amount of dietary lipid and breast cancer development. A randomized controlled trial, called as the Women's Health Initiative Dietary Modification Trial, enrolled 48,835 postmenopausal women in the United States and investigated whether a low-fat dietary pattern can decrease breast cancer risk. Participants were randomized into low-fat diet (20% energy from fat) and usual dietary fat intake groups (38% energy from fat). The results showed that the low-fat diet decreased the risk of breast cancer by approximately 9% after an 8.1-year follow-up. And the reduction was greater among women who had a habitual high-fat diet at baseline (Prentice et al., 2006).

Another multicenter randomized controlled trial based on 2437 postmenopausal women with resected early stage breast cancer and receiving conventional cancer management was conducted to evaluate the effect of reduced dietary fat on relapse-free survival rate of breast cancer patients. The hazard ratio of relapse events in the low-fat dietary group (20.3% energy from fat) was 0.76 (95% CI: 0.60–0.98) compared with that of the control group (29.2% energy from fat). The recurrence rate decreased to 9.9% in low-fat dietary group from 12.4% in the control group after 60 months of follow-up (Chlebowski et al., 2006). Additionally, the low-fat dietary intervention has a greater influence on relapse-free survival rate in women with estrogen receptor-negative subtype (HR=0.58; 95% CI: 0.37–0.91) than in women with estrogen receptor-positive subtype (HR=0.85; 95% CI: 0.63–1.14). Low-fat dietary pattern also resulted in a significant reduction in body weight by approximately 6 pounds. As body weight is inversely associated with breast cancer risk, a reduction in dietary fat ratio might have a protective effect on the risk of breast cancer recurrence.

However, evidences regarding total fat intake and the development of breast cancer are not always consistent. A multiinstitutional randomized controlled trial, enrolling 3088 women previously treated for early stage breast cancer, was conducted to assess the effect of a dietary pattern low in fat as well as high in vegetables, fruits, and fiber on prognosis following treatment. Compared with the control group, the intervention group decreased energy intake from fat by 13% for 4 years and increased servings of vegetable, fruit, and fiber by 65%, 25%, and 30%, respectively. Over the mean 7.3-year follow-up, no significant changes were observed in terms of breast cancer recurrence (HR=0.96; 95% CI: 0.80–1.14) and mortality (HR=0.91; 95% CI: 0.72–1.15) between intervention and control groups (Pierce et al., 2007). In the Life After Cancer Epidemiology Cohort study, the association between dairy intake and recurrence and mortality of breast cancer was conducted in 1893 women who were diagnosed with early stage invasive breast cancer. After a median follow-up of 11.8 years, overall dairy intake showed no correlation with breast cancer-specific outcomes. However, further analysis indicated that high-fat dairy intake was positively associated with breast cancer mortality (HR=1.2; 95% CI: 0.82–1.77) and showed no significant association with breast cancer recurrence (Kroenke, Kwan, Sweeney, Castillo, & Caan, 2013). A meta-analysis based on 15 prospective cohort studies showed no difference in breast cancer-specific mortality for women in the highest compared with the lowest categories of total fat intake (HR=1.14; 95% CI: 0.86–1.52) (Brennan, Woodside, Lunny, Cardwell, &

Cantwell, 2017). The inconsistent result might be attributed to the confounding factors, such as heterogeneity of breast cancer, difference in age, and population of patients.

7.2.2 Effect of different fatty acid types

Dietary lipids contain a mixture of various fatty acids, such as trans fatty acids, monounsaturated fatty acids, saturated fatty acids, and polyunsaturated fatty acids (PUFA). Various types of fatty acids in diet play different roles in breast cancer development. However, studies focusing on the effect of the specific individual fatty acid on breast cancer are quite limited.

Generally, saturated, monounsaturated, and trans fatty acids have been found to increase the risk of breast cancer, whereas specific PUFA such as n-3 PUFA are indicated to exert an anticancer activity (Boyd et al., 2003; Brennan et al., 2017). A meta-analysis based on 3 cohort and 7 case-control studies showed that total monounsaturated fatty acids, palmitic acid (C16:0) and oleic acid (C18:1n-9), were all positively associated with breast cancer risk. Total saturated fatty acid showed a significant association with an increased breast cancer risk only in postmenopausal women (Saadatian-Elahi, Norat, Goudable, & Riboli, 2004). As to breast cancer mortality, saturated fatty acid intake shows a significantly negative impact upon breast cancer survival (HR = 1.51; 95% CI: 1.09–2.09) (Brennan et al., 2017). A positive association between dietary cholesterol intake and breast cancer risk is also observed in a meta-analysis involving 6 cohort and 3 case-control studies (Li, Yang, Zhang, & Jiang, 2016).

Different subtypes of breast cancer respond to dietary fatty acids diversely. A recent heterogeneous cohort study with 10,062 breast cancer patients showed that high saturated fat were significantly associated with an increased risk of ER^+PR^+ (HR = 1.2; 95% CI: 1.00–1.45) and $HER2^-$ subtypes (HR = 1.04; 95% CI: 1.00–1.09), whereas not ER^-PR^- subtype (Sieri et al., 2014). These results suggest that saturated fat might be involved in the etiology of receptor-positive breast cancer subtype.

7.2.3 Effect of timing of dietary lipids exposure

Substantial evidence indicated that not only the types and amount of dietary fat, but also the time when the diet is consumed may determine their influence on breast cancer development. It can partly explain the controversy regarding dietary fat exposures and breast cancer. As we all know, the breast undergoes extensive changes during the whole life of a woman, mainly in the period associated with dramatic hormonal alteration, such as in utero, puberty, pregnancy, lactation, and menopause (Hilakivi-Clarke et al., 2005). All these periods play an important role in the development of mammary gland structure, from initial appearance to mature. For example, mammary gland may be more sensitive to dietary fat exposures during pregnancy as it undergoes extensive proliferation and differentiation in this period.

A meta-analysis of fat intake and breast cancer risk showed that high fat and PUFA intake after menopausal were significantly associated with breast cancer risk, while in premenopausal women, there was no significant relation observed between intake of all fat types and breast cancer (Turner, 2011). It was proposed that the years before the first child was given birth are the most important period determining breast cancer risk in future basing on a mathematical model (Colditz & Frazier, 1995). As the virtual lack of reliable information on childhood dietary fat exposure in women who develop breast cancer, it is difficult to address the possible link between dietary fat intake during childhood and later breast cancer risk in humans. Animal studies have consistently proved that perinatal, prepubertal, or pubertal exposures to dietary fat have an effect on breast cancer risk in later life (Hilakivi-Clarke et al., 2005; Li et al.,

2018). Thus, epidemiological studies covering the dietary information from the fetal period to the menopausal period are needed to comprehensively investigate the association between dietary fat intake and breast cancer development.

7.3 Effects of n-3 PUFA on breast cancer development

7.3.1 Epidemiological evidence regarding n-3 PUFA intake and breast cancer

Polyunsaturated fatty acids mainly consist of two families: n-3 PUFA and n-6 PUFA. They are both essential fatty acids for human health and cannot be interconverted between them. Linoleic acid (LA, C18:2n-6) and arachidonic acid (AA, C20:4n-6) are the most common n-6 PUFA types, whereas α-linolenic acid (ALA, C18:3n-3), eicosapentaenoic acid (EPA, C20:5n-3) and docosahexaenoic acid (DHA, C22:6n-3) are the mainly n-3 PUFA types in diet. Substantial results from laboratory investigations suggest that n-3 PUFA is the most promising type of fatty acids to protect against the initiation and early stage of breast cancer, while n-6 PUFA shows the opposite effect (AL-Jawadi et al., 2018; Brown et al., 2020). The recommended ratio of n-6 to n-3 PUFA is 1:1 to 3:1, while the current Western diet always contains excessive amount of n-6 PUFA, leading to a very high ratio of n-6 to n-3 PUFA (16:1 or higher) (Simopoulos, 2002). Hence, the lack of n-3 PUFA in diet may be associated with the increasing morbidity of breast cancer in Western countries.

Nevertheless, results from cohort studies about the relationship between n-3 PUFA and breast cancer remain contentious. Several large prospective cohort studies have investigated the association between n-3 PUFA and risk of developing breast cancer, suggesting an inverse association between them. For instance, in the Japan Collaborative Cohort study (Wakai et al., 2005), a significant reduction of breast cancer incidence was observed in women with the highest intake of n-3 PUFA or fish fat (RR = 0.63; 95% CI: 0.38–1.03). Similar results were also obtained in the Singapore Chinese Health study (Gago-Dominguez, Yuan, Sun, Lee, & Yu, 2003), which enrolled 359,298 Singapore women (RR = 0.74; 95% CI: 0.58–0.94). However, there are still some cohort studies that are less consistent and somewhat contradictory. A prospective cohort study including 23,693 postmenopausal women explored the association between total fish intake and breast cancer morbidity, suggesting that the intake of fish was positively associated with breast cancer incidence rate, especially to estrogen receptor-positive subtype (Stripp et al., 2003). Another cohort study including 310,671 women found no association between fish intake and breast cancer risk (Engeset et al., 2006). Most null conclusions were obtained from studies based on European populations, and it might be associated with the relatively low content of n-3 PUFA in their habitual dietary. To summarize the association between dietary intake of n-3 PUFA and breast cancer incidence, a meta-analysis based on 21 independent prospective cohort studies was conducted and found that n-3 PUFA was associated with a 14% reduction in breast cancer risk, which provided a robust and solid evidence of the protective effect of n-3 PUFA on breast cancer risk (Zheng, Hu, Zhao, Yang, & Li, 2013).

The dietary n-3 PUFA and fish consumption included in the above cohort studies was mostly obtained relying on self-reported food frequency questionnaires and might be influenced by errors and bias from dietary recall. It is so difficult to obtain an absolutely accurate and comprehensive data about the intake of individual food and fatty acids that the inconsistent result from different cohort studies seems reasonable. In contrast to dietary estimates, biomarker measurements of n-3 PUFA are free of recall bias or memory errors. Thus, it can provide relatively unbiased assessments of n-3 PUFA exposure. The most common human biospecimens for the determination of n-3 PUFA biomarker are circulating blood (serum, plasma, and erythrocyte) and adipose tissue (Katan, Deslypere, Van Birgelen, Penders, & Zegwaard, 1997). Several case-control studies have been conducted to investigate the relationship between biomarkers of n-3 PUFA and breast cancer risk.

In a case-control study in the United States, breast adipose tissue was collected from 73 breast cancer patients and 74 controls, and n-3 PUFA level in the tissue was determined as a biomarker of the past qualitative dietary intake of fatty acids. The results showed that both EPA and DHA have a protective effect on breast cancer risk. In addition, high n-6 PUFA level and ratio of n-6 to n-3 PUFA both contribute to the high risk of breast cancer (Bagga, Anders, Wang, & Glaspy, 2002). Another case-control study conducted in Japan showed that breast cancer risk was inversely associated with contents of EPA (OR=0.27; 95% CI: 0.14–0.51), DHA (OR=0.06; 95% CI: 0.02–0.16), and total n-3 PUFA (OR=0.11; 95% CI: 0.05–0.24) as assessed in erythrocyte membrane (Kuriki et al., 2007). These results were consistent with a recent meta-analysis, showing that biomarkers of n-3 PUFA were linearly associated with a lower risk of breast cancer, and circulating EPA and DHA reduced breast cancer risk in a dose-response manner (Yang et al., 2019). Although it is hard to ascertain whether it is excess n-6 PUFA or scarce n-3 PUFA that is the causal driver of breast cancer, these studies emphasize the potential value of n-3 PUFA as an effective agent against breast cancer as n-6 PUFAs are adequate almost in all populations.

To date, few human intervention studies have investigated the effect of n-3 PUFA on the prevention or treatment of breast cancer. One randomized controlled trial assessed the effect of combined n-3 PUFA and raloxifene administration on breast cancer risk of postmenopausal women (Signori et al., 2012). After intervention of 2 years, even though the ratio of n-6 to n-3 PUFA in plasma was significantly decreased, none of the biomarkers associated with breast cancer were affected. However in the subset analysis, a decrease in breast density, a validated biomarker of breast cancer risk, was significantly associated with the increased DHA in plasma, but only in participants with BMI $\geq$29, suggesting that the obese women may selectively benefit from n-3 PUFA administration (Sandhu et al., 2016).

Interestingly, EPA and DHA supplementations are effective in reducing common side effects induced by chemotherapy. A small randomized pilot trial indicated that n-3 PUFA (EPA+DHA=4g/day for 3months) effectively inhibited bone resorption in postmenopausal breast cancer survivors receiving aromatase inhibitors therapy (Hutchins-Wiese et al., 2014). Another randomized controlled trial demonstrated that n-3 PUFA significantly reduced aromatase inhibitor-associated arthralgia in postmenopausal obese patients with stage I-III breast cancer (Shen et al., 2018). In addition, a small randomized trial, conducted on 20 breast cancer patients receiving paclitaxel therapy, suggested that EPA (0.19g/day) and DHA (1.04g/day) effectively lower the incidence of paclitaxel-induced peripheral neuropathy from 60% to 30% (OR=0.3; 95% CI: 0.10–0.88) (Ghoreishi et al., 2012).

Last but not the least, n-3 PUFAs are associated with the decreased breast cancer recurrence. A large cohort of 3081 individuals with early stage breast cancer showed that higher intake of marine fatty acids (EPA+DHA) was associated with a reduction in breast cancer recurrence (HR=0.72; 95% CI: 0.57–0.90) as well as overall mortality (HR=0.59; 95% CI: 0.43–0.82) after a median follow-up of 7.3 years (Patterson et al., 2011). Therefore, these studies provide evidence for using n-3 PUFA as an effective nutritional intervention method in the prevention, treatment, and prognosis of breast cancer to enhance conventional therapeutics and reduce the cancer risk and recurrence (Table 7.1).

7.3.2 Mechanisms mediating the effect of n-3 PUFA on breast cancer

Mounting studies have shown that dietary n-3 PUFAs inhibit the initiation and progression of breast cancer. The mechanisms have been explored for several decades. It is not allowed for epidemiological studies to analyze specific molecular changes in cell during the tumor initiation and progression in the mammary gland. Thus, several potential mechanisms through which n-3 PUFAs affect carcinogenesis are proposed always based on animal models and cell lines.

Inhibiting the biosynthesis of arachidonic acid-derived eicosanoid by n-3 PUFA is the most salient mechanism (Fig. 7.1). Generally, an important function of both n-3 and n-6 PUFA is related to their conversion to eicosanoids, which are usually involved in immune modulation, inflammatory response, cell growth, and cell differentiation (Calder, 2017; Schunck, Konkel, Fischer, & Weylandt, 2018). The eicosanoids generated from n-6 PUFA are of the 2-series prostaglandins and the 4-series leukotrienes, such as PGE_2, leukotriene B_4, thromboxane A_2, and 12-hydroxyeicosatetraenoic acid. They always show proinflammatory effects and are positively linked to carcinogenesis. However, eicosanoids produced from n-3 PUFA are of the 3-series prostaglandins and the 5-series leukotrienes, always showing antiinflammatory effects (Calder, 2001). In addition, n-3 PUFA competes with n-6 PUFA for desaturases and elongases, and shows greater affinities than n-6 PUFA for the enzymes (Larsson, Kumlin, Ingelman-Sundberg, & Wolk, 2004). Thus, a higher intake of n-3 PUFA inhibits the desaturation and elongation of LA to AA, thus reducing the production of AA-derived eicosanoids.

Another mechanism involved in the protective effect of n-3 PUFAs on breast cancer is their influence on the activity of transcription factor and expression of genes associated with cell growth, apoptosis, differentiation, and metastasis. Cell proliferation and apoptosis are two fundamental processes integral to carcinogenesis (Goldar, Khaniani, Derakhshan, & Baradaran, 2015). Substantial evidences have shown the function of n-3 PUFA in inhibiting the expression of some growth factors, including human epidermal growth factor receptor-2 (HER-2) (Yee et al., 2013), insulin-like growth factor 1 (IGF-1R) (Liu & Ma, 2014), and epidermal growth factor receptor (EGFR) (Corsetto et al., 2011); in reducing proliferation by activating transcription factor PPARγ (Jump, 2002); and in promoting apoptosis by the inhibition of PI3K/Akt, NF-κB pathway and lowering Bcl-2/Bax ratio (Daak et al., 2015; Zhuang et al., 2017).

Traditional concept about the potential mechanisms of the protective effect of n-3 PUFA on breast cancer also includes alteration of estrogen metabolism, which leads to the reduced growth of estrogen-stimulated cell (Noble et al., 1997). In addition, n-3 PUFA can change the membrane fluidity and decrease the insulin sensitivity (Rogers et al., 2010), and increase or decrease the production of free radicals and reactive oxygen species (Calder, 2001). All these changes are partly contributed to the anticancer effect of n-3 PUFA (Fig. 7.2).

In recent years, epigenetics has emerged as a glaring discipline showing an important role in a number of fundamental processes associated with cancer development, such as gene transcription, cell cycle, migration, survival, and metabolism (Sapienza & Issa, 2016; Toh, Lim, & Chow, 2017). Generally, epigenetic events include histone modification, DNA methylation, and gene expression regulated by non-coding RNA. Epigenetics modification plays a crucial role in disease occurrence and pathogenesis of cancer and possesses an

TABLE 7.1 Summary of the effect of n-3 PUFA or fish fat intake on breast cancer development.

Study design	Included sample/study	Country	Time of follow-up/intervention	Method of assessment	Key outcomes	References
Cohort	26,291 women; 129 BC cases	Japan	7.6 year	FFQ	BC incidence was reduced in women with the highest quartile of n-3 PUFA (RR=0.50; 95% CI: 0.30–0.85) or fish fat (RR=0.56; 95% CI: 0.33–0.94).	Wakai et al. (2005)
Cohort	359,298 women; 342 BC cases	Singapore	5.1 year	FFQ	Relative to the lowest quartile of intake, individuals in the higher three quartiles reduced BC risk by 26% (RR=0.74; 95% CI: 0.58–0.94).	Gago-Dominguez et al. (2003)
Cohort	23,693 postmenopausal women, 424 BC cases	Denmark	4.8 year	FFQ	Higher fish intake was associated with higher BC incidence (RR=1.13; 95% CI: 1.03–1.23).	Stripp et al. (2003)
Cohort	310,671 women; 4776 BC cases	10 European countries	6.4 year	FFQ	No significant association between fish intake and BC risk (HR=1.01; 95% CI: 0.99–1.02).	Engeset et al. (2006)
Cohort	3081 early stage BC patients	United States	7.3-year	24-h dietary recalls	N-3 PUFA (EPA+DHA) was inversely associated with BC recurrence (HR=0.72; 95% CI: 0.57–0.90) and overall mortality (HR=0.59; 95% CI: 0.43–0.82).	Patterson et al. (2011)
Case-control	73 BC patients; 74 healthy controls	United States	—	Breast adipose tissue	EPA and DHA have a protective effect on BC risk (OR=0.91; 95% CI: 0.84–1.00).	Bagga et al. (2002)
Case-control	241 BC patients; 88 benign breast carcinoma patients	France	—	Breast adipose tissue	ALA (OR=0.39; 95% CI: 0.19–0.78) and DHA (OR=0.31; 95% CI: 0.13–0.75) have a protective effect on BC risk.	Maillard et al. (2002)
Case-control	103 BC patients; 309 healthy controls	Japan	—	Erythrocyte membrane	EPA (OR=0.27; 95% CI: 0.14–0.51), DHA (OR=0.06; 95% CI: 0.02–0.16), and total n-3 PUFA (OR=0.11; 95% CI: 0.05–0.24) were inversely associated with BC risk.	Kuriki et al. (2007)

Continued

TABLE 7.1 Summary of the effect of n-3 PUFA or fish fat intake on breast cancer development—cont'd

Study design	Included sample/study	Country	Time of follow-up/intervention	Method of assessment	Key outcomes	References
Meta-analysis	21 cohort studies	—	—	FFQ or tissue biomarker	N-3 PUFA was associated with a 14% reduction in BC risk (RR=0.86; 95% CI: 0.78–0.94).	Zheng et al. (2013)
Meta-analysis	13 cohort and 11 case-control studies	—	—	circulating blood or breast adipose tissue	N-3 PUFAs were associated with lower BC risk (RR=0.84; 95% CI: 0.74–0.96)	Yang et al. (2019)
RCT	46 BC patients	United States	2 year	Serum	N-3 PUFA affected none of the biomarkers associated with breast cancer.	Signori et al. (2012)
RCT	266 healthy postmenopausal women	United States	2 year	Plasma	DHA was inversely associated with absolute breast density in participants with BMI > 29 kg/m^2.	Sandhu et al. (2016)
RCT	69 BC patients	Iran	1 month	Serum	EPA (0.19 g/day) and DHA (1.04 g/day) lower the incidence of paclitaxel-induced peripheral neuropathy from 60% to 30%.	Ghoreishi et al. (2012)
RCT	38 postmenopausal BC survivors	United States	3 month	Serum	N-3 PUFA inhibited aromatase inhibitor-associated bone resorption in BC patients.	Hutchins-Wiese et al. (2014)
RCT	249 postmenopausal obese patients with stage I-III BC	United States	6 month	Serum	N-3 PUFA reduced aromatase inhibitor-associated arthralgia in patients with BMI ≥30 kg/m^2.	Shen et al. (2018)

PUFA, polyunsaturated fatty acid; BC, breast cancer; FFQ, food frequency questionnaire; RR, relative risk for highest with the lowest category; HR, hazard ratio; OR, odds ratio; ALA, α-linolenic acid; EPA, eicosapentaenoic acid; DHA, docosahexaenoic acid; BMI, body mass index; RCT, randomized controlled trial.

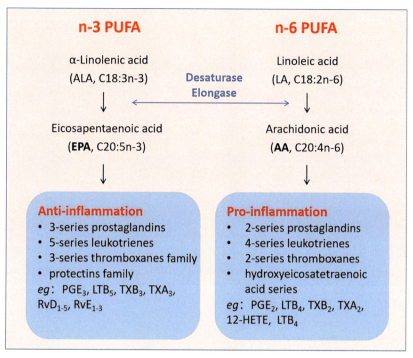

FIG. 7.1 Overview of the metabolism of n-3 PUFA and n-6 PUFA into eicosanoids involved in inflammation and carcinogenesis. Eicosanoids from n-3 PUFA have an antiinflammatory effect, while eicosanoids from n-6 PUFA show a proinflammatory effect. *PUFA*, polyunsaturated fatty acids; *PGE*, prostaglandin; *LT*, leukotrienes; *TX*, thromboxane; *HETE*, hydroxyeicosatetraenoic acid; *Rv*, resolvin.

enormous potential being applied for the prevention and management of certain carcinomas and diseases (Nebbioso, Tambaro, Dell'Aversana, & Altucci, 2018). However, the evidence focusing on the epigenetics as the mechanisms of anticancer effect of n-3 PUFA is limited. Long non-coding RNA (lncRNA) regulation is one of the most common ways of epigenetic modification. An animal experiment with transgenic *fat-1* mice model investigated the effects of maternal n-3 PUFAs on lncRNA changes in offspring and explored how these changes significantly reduced the offspring's susceptibility to breast cancer. The result showed that endogenously synthetic n-3 PUFA in mother significantly decreased 45 lncRNAs and increased 53 lncRNAs expression in the mammary gland of offspring. The changes in lncRNA were associated with the changes of mRNA in multiple oncogenic signaling pathways, especially Jak-STAT, NF-κB, and MAPK pathways (Li et al., 2019).

Another mechanism proposed in recent years, which is responsible for an anticancer effect of n-3 PUFA, is related to the regulation of gut microbiota. Gut microbiota is a complex microbial ecosystem that plays a crucial role in regulating host metabolism, immune system, and many key physiological pathways (Human Microbiome Project Consortium, 2012). Most of available data indicate that the onset of breast cancer is related to bacterial dysbiosis in the microenvironment of both gut and breast tissues. Changes in the composition and function of several taxa may contribute to breast cancer development and progression. One of the most prominent effects of gut microbiota is the regulation of hormone metabolism, which is

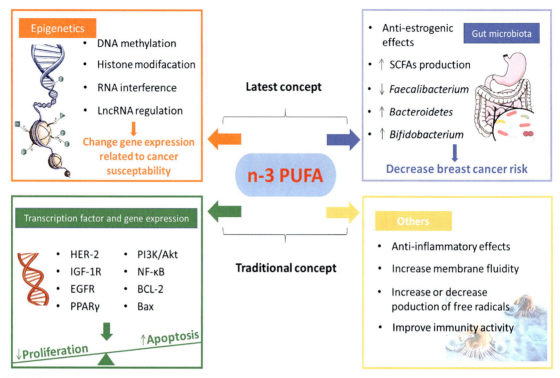

FIG. 7.2 Potential mechanisms involved in the protective effect of n-3 PUFA on breast cancer. *PUFA*, polyunsaturated fatty acid; *LncRNA*, long-noncoding RNA; *SCFAs*, short-chain fatty acids; *HER-2*, human epidermal growth factor receptor-2; *IGF-1*, insulin-like growth factor 1; *EGFR*, epidermal growth factor receptor; *PPAR*, peroxisome proliferator-activated receptors; *NF-κB*, nuclear factor kappa-B.

an important risk factor in breast cancer development, especially in postmenopausal women (Laborda-Illanes et al., 2020). It has been shown that dietary habits can create an interindividual variation in gut microbiota (Flint, Duncan, & Louis, 2017). Among many factors that could affect the gut microbiota, n-3 PUFA has received considerable attention. The common positive changes in gut microbiota after n-3 PUFA supplementation include a reduction in *Faecalibacterium*, an increase in *Bacteroidetes* and butyrate-producing bacteria, which are always in disorder in breast cancer patients (Costantini, Molinari, Farinon, & Merendino, 2017).

However, to date, the studies concerning the links among gut microbiota, n-3 PUFA intake, and breast cancer development are quite limited. A cross-sectional study was conducted to assess the link between blood PUFA and gut microbiota composition in breast cancer patients. The results showed that DHA level was positively associated with the abundance of phylum Actinobacteria and genus *Bifidobacterium*, and EPA level was positively associated with the abundance of phylum *Bacteroidetes* (Horigome et al., 2019). An animal experiment investigated the effect of maternal n-3 PUFA on gut microbiota of offspring and breast cancer risk in adulthood. The result showed that relative abundances of *Akkermansia*, *Lactobacillus*, and *Mucispirillum* were significantly higher in 7-week-old offspring of n-3 PUFA group, whereas the maternal n-6 PUFA diet was associated with decreased abundances of *Lactobacillus*, *Bifidobacterium*, and *Barnesiella* in adult offspring (Li et al., 2021). Further studies are required to gain an insight into the mechanism of anticancer property of n-3 PUFA in terms of gut microbiota.

7.4 Conclusions

The association between breast cancer and dietary lipids has been reviewed in this chapter. It is well established that amount and type of dietary fat both have an effect on breast cancer development, including incidence, treatment, recurrence, and prognosis. Most epidemiological studies show that high-fat diet and low n-3 PUFA diet both have an inverse effect on breast cancer development. The traditional concept of mechanism associated with the anticancer effect of n-3 PUFA mainly involves suppressing biosynthesis of proinflammatory eicosanoid, influencing signaling transcriptional pathway to balance the proliferation and apoptosis. Some novel mechanisms were also proposed, such as the regulation of epigenetics and gut microbiota by n-3 PUFA. Based on these findings, breast cancer patients and women with high breast cancer risk should be encouraged to improve their dietary fat habits before, during, and after treatment, in order to reduce the cancer risk and have better quality of life and long-term survival.

References

AL-Jawadi, A., Moussa, H., Ramalingam, L., Dharamawardhane, S., Gollahon, L., Gunaratne, P., et al. (2018). Protective properties of n-3 fatty acids and implications in obesity-associated breast cancer. *Journal of Nutritional Biochemistry*, 53, 1–8. https://doi.org/10.1016/j.jnutbio.2017.09.018.

Bagga, D., Anders, K. H., Wang, H. J., & Glaspy, J. A. (2002). Long-chain n-3-to-n-6 polyunsaturated fatty acid ratios in breast adipose tissue from women with and without breast cancer. *Nutrition and Cancer*, 42(2), 180–185. https://doi.org/10.1207/S15327914NC422_5.

Barnard, M. E., Boeke, C. E., & Tamimi, R. M. (2015). Established breast cancer risk factors and risk of intrinsic tumor subtypes. *Biochimica et Biophysica Acta, Reviews on Cancer*, 1856(1), 73–85. https://doi.org/10.1016/j.bbcan.2015.06.002.

Boyd, N. F., Stone, J., Vogt, K. N., Connelly, B. S., Martin, L. J., & Minkin, S. (2003). Dietary fat and breast cancer risk revisited: A meta-analysis of the published literature. *British Journal of Cancer*, 89(9), 1672–1685. https://doi.org/10.1038/sj.bjc.6601314.

Brennan, S. F., Woodside, J. V., Lunny, P. M., Cardwell, C. R., & Cantwell, M. M. (2017). Dietary fat and breast cancer mortality: A systematic review and meta-analysis. *Critical Reviews in Food Science and Nutrition*, 57(10), 1999–2008. https://doi.org/10.1080/10408398.2012.724481.

Brown, I., Lee, J., Sneddon, A. A., Cascio, M. G., Pertwee, R. G., Wahle, K. W. J., et al. (2020). Anticancer effects of n-3 EPA and DHA and their endocannabinoid derivatives on breast cancer cell growth and invasion. *Prostaglandins, Leukotrienes, and Essential Fatty Acids*, 156. https://doi.org/10.1016/j.plefa.2019.102024.

Calder, P. C. (2001). Omega 3 polyunsaturated fatty acids, inflammation and immunity. *World Review of Nutrition and Dietetics*, 88, 109–116.

Calder, P. C. (2017). Omega-3 fatty acids and inflammatory processes: From molecules to man. *Biochemical Society Transactions*, 45(5), 1105–1115. https://doi.org/10.1042/BST20160474.

Chlebowski, R. T., Blackburn, G. L., Thomson, C. A., Nixon, D. W., Shapiro, A., Hoy, M. K., et al. (2006). Dietary fat reduction and breast cancer outcome: Interim efficacy results from the women's intervention nutrition study. *Journal of the National Cancer Institute*, 98(24), 1767–1776. https://doi.org/10.1093/jnci/djj494.

Colditz, G. A., & Frazier, A. L. (1995). Models of breast cancer show that risk is set by events of early life: Prevention efforts must shift focus. *Cancer Epidemiology, Biomarkers & Prevention*, 4(5), 567–571.

Corsetto, P. A., Montorfano, G., Zava, S., Jovenitti, I. E., Cremona, A., & Rizzo, A. M. (2011). Effects of n-3 PUFAs on breast cancer cells through their incorporation in plasma membrane. *Lipids in Health and Disease*, 10. https://doi.org/10.1186/1476-511X-10-73.

Costantini, L., Molinari, R., Farinon, B., & Merendino, N. (2017). Impact of omega-3 fatty acids on the gut microbiota. *International Journal of Molecular Sciences*, 18(12). https://doi.org/10.3390/ijms18122645.

Daak, A. A., Elderdery, A. Y., Elbashir, L. M., Mariniello, K., Mills, J., Scarlett, G., et al. (2015). Omega 3 (n-3) fatty acids down-regulate nuclear factor-kappa B (NF-κB) gene and blood cell adhesion molecule expression in patients with homozygous sickle cell disease. *Blood Cells, Molecules, and Diseases, 55*(1), 48–55. https://doi.org/10.1016/j.bcmd.2015.03.014.

De Cicco, P., Catani, M. V., Gasperi, V., Sibilano, M., Quaglietta, M., & Savini, I. (2019). Nutrition and breast cancer: A literature review on prevention, treatment and recurrence. *Nutrients, 11*(7). https://doi.org/10.3390/nu11071514.

Engeset, D., Alsaker, E., Lund, E., Welch, A., Khaw, K. T., Clavel-Chapelon, F., et al. (2006). Fish consumption and breast cancer risk. The European Prospective Investigation into Cancer and Nutrition (EPIC). *International Journal of Cancer, 119*(1), 175–182. https://doi.org/10.1002/ijc.21819.

Flint, H. J., Duncan, S. H., & Louis, P. (2017). The impact of nutrition on intestinal bacterial communities. *Current Opinion in Microbiology, 38*, 59–65. https://doi.org/10.1016/j.mib.2017.04.005.

Gago-Dominguez, M., Yuan, J. M., Sun, C. L., Lee, H. P., & Yu, M. C. (2003). Opposing effects of dietary n-3 and n-6 fatty acids on mammary carcinogenesis: The Singapore Chinese Health Study. *British Journal of Cancer, 89*(9), 1686–1692. https://doi.org/10.1038/sj.bjc.6601340.

Ghoreishi, Z., Esfahani, A., Djazayeri, A., Djalali, M., Golestan, B., Ayromlou, H., et al. (2012). Omega-3 fatty acids are protective against paclitaxel-induced peripheral neuropathy: A randomized double-blind placebo controlled trial. *BMC Cancer, 12*. https://doi.org/10.1186/1471-2407-12-355.

Goldar, S., Khaniani, M. S., Derakhshan, S. M., & Baradaran, B. (2015). Molecular mechanisms of apoptosis and roles in cancer development and treatment. *Asian Pacific Journal of Cancer Prevention, 16*(6), 2129–2144. https://doi.org/10.7314/APJCP.2015.16.6.2129.

Hardefeldt, P. J., Penninkilampi, R., Edirimanne, S., & Eslick, G. D. (2018). Physical activity and weight loss reduce the risk of breast cancer: A meta-analysis of 139 prospective and retrospective studies. *Clinical Breast Cancer, 18*(4), e601–e612. https://doi.org/10.1016/j.clbc.2017.10.010.

Harvie, M., Howell, A., & Evans, D. G. (2015). Can diet and lifestyle prevent breast cancer: What is the evidence? *American Society of Clinical Oncology Educational Book*, 66–73.

Hilakivi-Clarke, L., Olivo, S. E., Shajahan, A., Khan, G., Zhu, Y., Zwart, A., et al. (2005). Mechanisms mediating the effects of prepubertal (n-3) polyunsaturated fatty acid diet on breast cancer risk in rats. *Journal of Nutrition, 135*(12). https://doi.org/10.1093/jn/135.12.2946s. American Institute of Nutrition.

Horigome, A., Okubo, R., Hamazaki, K., Kinoshita, T., Katsumata, N., Uezono, Y., et al. (2019). Association between blood omega-3 polyunsaturated fatty acids and the gut microbiota among breast cancer survivors. *Beneficial Microbes, 10*(7), 751–758. https://doi.org/10.3920/BM2019.0034.

Human Microbiome Project Consortium. (2012). Structure, function and diversity of the healthy human microbiome. *Nature, 486*(7402), 207–214.

Hutchins-Wiese, H. L., Picho, K., Watkins, B. A., Li, Y., Tannenbaum, S., Claffey, K., et al. (2014). High-dose eicosapentaenoic acid and docosahexaenoic acid supplementation reduces bone resorption in postmenopausal breast cancer survivors on aromatase inhibitors: A pilot study. *Nutrition and Cancer, 66*(1), 68–76. https://doi.org/10.1080/01635581.2014.847964.

Jump, D. B. (2002). The biochemistry of n-3 polyunsaturated fatty acids. *Journal of Biological Chemistry, 277*(11), 8755–8758. https://doi.org/10.1074/jbc.R100062200.

Katan, M. B., Deslypere, J. P., Van Birgelen, A. P. J. M., Penders, M., & Zegwaard, M. (1997). Kinetics of the incorporation of dietary fatty acids into serum cholesteryl esters, erythrocyte membranes, and adipose tissue: An 18-month controlled study. *Journal of Lipid Research, 38*(10), 2012–2022.

Kroenke, C. H., Kwan, M. L., Sweeney, C., Castillo, A., & Caan, B. J. (2013). High-and low-fat dairy intake, recurrence, and mortality after breast cancer diagnosis. *Journal of the National Cancer Institute, 105*(9), 616–623. https://doi.org/10.1093/jnci/djt027.

Kuriki, K., Hirose, K., Wakai, K., Matsuo, K., Ito, H., Suzuki, T., et al. (2007). Breast cancer risk and erythrocyte compositions of n-3 highly unsaturated fatty acids in Japanese. *International Journal of Cancer, 121*(2), 377–385. https://doi.org/10.1002/ijc.22682.

Kwan, M. L., Weltzien, E., Kushi, L. H., Castillo, A., Slattery, M. L., & Caan, B. J. (2009). Dietary patterns and breast cancer recurrence and survival among women with early-stage breast cancer. *Journal of Clinical Oncology, 27*(6), 919–926. https://doi.org/10.1200/JCO.2008.19.4035.

Laborda-Illanes, A., Sanchez-Alcoholado, L., Dominguez-Recio, M. E., Jimenez-Rodriguez, B., Lavado, R., Comino-Méndez, I., et al. (2020). Breast and gut microbiota action mechanisms in breast cancer pathogenesis and treatment. *Cancers, 12*(9), 1–27. https://doi.org/10.3390/cancers12092465.

Larsson, S. C., Kumlin, M., Ingelman-Sundberg, M., & Wolk, A. (2004). Dietary long-chain n-3 fatty acids for the prevention of cancer: A review of potential mechanisms. *American Journal of Clinical Nutrition, 79*(6), 935–945. https://doi.org/10.1093/ajcn/79.6.935.

Li, J. M., Li, K. L., Gao, J. L., Guo, X. F., Lu, M. Q., Li, Z. H., et al. (2018). Maternal exposure to an n-3 polyunsaturated fatty acid diet decreases mammary cancer risk of female offspring in adulthood. *Food & Function*, 9(11), 5768–5777. https://doi.org/10.1039/c8fo01006d.

Li, J. M., Li, K. L., Gao, J. L., Guo, X. F., Lu, M. Q., Li, Z. H., et al. (2019). Endogenously synthesized n-3 polyunsaturated fatty acids in pregnant fat-1 mice decreases mammary cancer risk of female offspring by regulating expression of long noncoding RNAs. *Molecular Nutrition & Food Research*, 63(6). https://doi.org/10.1002/mnfr.201801150.

Li, C., Yang, L., Zhang, D., & Jiang, W. (2016). Systematic review and meta-analysis suggest that dietary cholesterol intake increases risk of breast cancer. *Nutrition Research*, 36(7), 627–635. https://doi.org/10.1016/j.nutres.2016.04.009.

Li, J. M., Wan, Y., Zheng, Z. H., Zhang, H. Q., Li, Y., Guo, X. F., et al. (2021). Maternal n-3 polyunsaturated fatty acids restructure gut microbiota of offspring mice and decrease their susceptibility to mammary gland cancer. *Food & Function*, 12(17), 8154–8168. https://doi.org/10.1039/d1fo00906k.

Liu, J., & Ma, D. W. L. (2014). The role of n-3 polyunsaturated fatty acids in the prevention and treatment of breast cancer. *Nutrients*, 6(11), 5184–5223. https://doi.org/10.3390/nu6115184.

MacLean, C. H., Newberry, S. J., Mojica, W. A., Khanna, P., Issa, A. M., Suttorp, M. J., et al. (2006). Effects of omega-3 fatty acids on cancer risk: A systematic review. *Journal of the American Medical Association*, 295(4), 403–415. https://doi.org/10.1001/jama.295.4.403.

Maillard, V., Bougnoux, P., Ferrari, P., Jourdan, M. L., Pinault, M., Lavillonnière, F., et al. (2002). N-3 and N-6 fatty acids in breast adipose tissue and relative risk of breast cancer in a case-control study in Tours. *International Journal of Cancer*, 98(1), 78–83. https://doi.org/10.1002/ijc.10130.

Nebbioso, A., Tambaro, F. P., Dell'Aversana, C., & Altucci, L. (2018). Cancer epigenetics: Moving forward. *PLoS Genetics*, 14(6). https://doi.org/10.1371/journal.pgen.1007362.

Noble, L. S., Takayama, K., Zeitoun, K. M., Putman, J. M., Johns, D. A., Hinshelwood, M. M., et al. (1997). Prostaglandin E2 stimulates aromatase expression in endometriosis-derived stromal cells. *Journal of Clinical Endocrinology and Metabolism*, 82(2), 600–606. https://doi.org/10.1210/jc.82.2.600.

Park, S. Y., Kolonel, L. N., Henderson, B. E., & Wilkens, L. R. (2012). Dietary fat and breast cancer in postmenopausal women according to ethnicity and hormone receptor status: The multiethnic cohort study. *Cancer Prevention Research*, 5(2), 216–228. https://doi.org/10.1158/1940-6207.CAPR-11-0260.

Patterson, R. E., Flatt, S. W., Newman, V. A., Natarajan, L., Rock, C. L., Thomson, C. A., et al. (2011). Marine fatty acid intake is associated with breast cancer prognosis. *Journal of Nutrition*, 141(2), 201–206. https://doi.org/10.3945/jn.110.128777.

Pierce, J. P., Natarajan, L., Caan, B. J., Parker, B. A., Greenberg, E. R., Flatt, S. W., et al. (2007). Influence of a diet very high in vegetables, fruit, and fiber and low in fat on prognosis following treatment for breast cancer: The Women's Healthy Eating and Living (WHEL) randomized trial. *Journal of the American Medical Association*, 298(3), 289–298. https://doi.org/10.1001/jama.298.3.289.

Prentice, R. L., Caan, B., Chlebowski, R. T., Patterson, R., Kuller, L. H., Ockene, J. K., et al. (2006). Low-fat dietary pattern and risk of invasive breast cancer: The Women's Health Initiative randomized controlled dietary modification trial. *Journal of the American Medical Association*, 295(6), 629–642. https://doi.org/10.1001/jama.295.6.629.

Rogers, K. R., Kikawa, K. D., Mouradian, M., Hernandez, K., McKinnon, K. M., Ahwah, S. M., et al. (2010). Docosahexaenoic acid alters epidermal growth factor receptor-related signaling by disrupting its lipid raft association. *Carcinogenesis*, 31(9), 1523–1530. https://doi.org/10.1093/carcin/bgq111.

Saadatian-Elahi, M., Norat, T., Goudable, J., & Riboli, E. (2004). Biomarkers of dietary fatty acid intake and the risk of breast cancer: A meta-analysis. *International Journal of Cancer*, 111(4), 584–591. https://doi.org/10.1002/ijc.20284.

Sandhu, N., Schetter, S. E., Liao, J., Hartman, T. J., Richie, J. P., McGinley, J., et al. (2016). Influence of obesity on breast density reduction by omega-3 fatty acids: Evidence from a randomized clinical trial. *Cancer Prevention Research*, 9(4), 275–282. https://doi.org/10.1158/1940-6207.CAPR-15-0235.

Sapienza, C., & Issa, J. P. (2016). Diet, nutrition, and cancer epigenetics. *Annual Review of Nutrition*, 36, 665–681. https://doi.org/10.1146/annurev-nutr-121415-112634.

Schunck, W. H., Konkel, A., Fischer, R., & Weylandt, K. H. (2018). Therapeutic potential of omega-3 fatty acid-derived epoxyeicosanoids in cardiovascular and inflammatory diseases. *Pharmacology and Therapeutics*, 183, 177–204. https://doi.org/10.1016/j.pharmthera.2017.10.016.

Scoccianti, C., Lauby-Secretan, B., Bello, P. Y., Chajes, V., & Romieu, I. (2014). Female breast cancer and alcohol consumption: A review of the literature. *American Journal of Preventive Medicine*, 46(3), S16–S25. https://doi.org/10.1016/j.amepre.2013.10.031.

Shen, S., Unger, J. M., Crew, K. D., Till, C., Greenlee, H., Gralow, J., et al. (2018). Omega-3 fatty acid use for obese breast cancer patients with aromatase inhibitor-related arthralgia (SWOG S0927). *Breast Cancer Research and Treatment, 172*(3), 603–610. https://doi.org/10.1007/s10549-018-4946-0.

Sieri, S., Chiodini, P., Agnoli, C., Pala, V., Berrino, F., Trichopoulou, A., et al. (2014). Dietary fat intake and development of specific breast cancer subtypes. *Journal of the National Cancer Institute, 106*(5). https://doi.org/10.1093/jnci/dju068.

Signori, C., Dubrock, C., Richie, J. P., Prokopczyk, B., Demers, L. M., Hamilton, C., et al. (2012). Administration of omega-3 fatty acids and Raloxifene to women at high risk of breast cancer: Interim feasibility and biomarkers analysis from a clinical trial. *European Journal of Clinical Nutrition, 66*(8), 878–884. https://doi.org/10.1038/ejcn.2012.60.

Simopoulos, A. P. (2002). The importance of the ratio of omega-6/omega-3 essential fatty acids. *Biomedicine and Pharmacotherapy, 56*(8), 365–379. https://doi.org/10.1016/S0753-3322(02)00253-6.

Stripp, C., Overvad, K., Christensen, J., Thomsen, B. L., Olsen, A., Møller, S., et al. (2003). Fish intake is positively associated with breast cancer incidence rate. *Journal of Nutrition, 133*(11), 3664–3669. https://doi.org/10.1093/jn/133.11.3664.

Sun, Y. S., Zhao, Z., Yang, Z. N., Xu, F., Lu, H. J., Zhu, Z. Y., et al. (2017). Risk factors and preventions of breast cancer. *International Journal of Biological Sciences, 13*(11), 1387–1397. https://doi.org/10.7150/ijbs.21635.

Toh, T. B., Lim, J. J., & Chow, E. K. H. (2017). Epigenetics in cancer stem cells. *Molecular Cancer, 16*(1). https://doi.org/10.1186/s12943-017-0596-9.

Torre, L., Bray, F., Siegel, R., Ferlay, J., Lortet-Tieulent, J., & Jemal, A. (2012). Global cancer statistics. *CA: A Cancer Journal for Clinicians, 65*(65), 87–108.

Turner, L. B. (2011). A meta-analysis of fat intake, reproduction, and breast cancer risk: An evolutionary perspective. *American Journal of Human Biology, 23*(5), 601–608. https://doi.org/10.1002/ajhb.21176.

Wakai, K., Tamakoshi, K., Date, C., Fukui, M., Suzuki, S., Lin, Y., et al. (2005). Dietary intakes of fat and fatty acids and risk of breast cancer: A prospective study in Japan. *Cancer Science, 96*(9), 590–599. https://doi.org/10.1111/j.1349-7006.2005.00084.x.

Wörmann, B. (2017). Brustkrebs: Grundlagen, früherkennung, diagnostik und therapie. *Medizinische Monatsschrift für Pharmazeuten, 40*(2), 55–64. http://www.medmopharm.de/archiv/artikel/2017/02/3170.html.

Yang, B., Ren, X. L., Wang, Z. Y., Wang, L., Zhao, F., Guo, X. J., et al. (2019). Biomarker of long-chain n-3 fatty acid intake and breast cancer: Accumulative evidence from an updated meta-analysis of epidemiological studies. *Critical Reviews in Food Science and Nutrition, 59*(19), 3152–3164. https://doi.org/10.1080/10408398.2018.1485133.

Yee, L. D., Agarwal, D., Rosol, T. J., Lehman, A., Tian, M., Hatton, J., et al. (2013). The inhibition of early stages of HER-2/neu-mediated mammary carcinogenesis by dietary n-3 PUFAs. *Molecular Nutrition & Food Research, 57*(2), 320–327. https://doi.org/10.1002/mnfr.201200445.

Zare, N., Haem, E., Lankarani, K. B., Heydari, S. T., & Barooti, E. (2013). Breast cancer risk factors in a defined population: Weighted logistic regression approach for rare events. *Journal of Breast Cancer, 16*(2), 214–219. https://doi.org/10.4048/jbc.2013.16.2.214.

Zheng, J. S., Hu, X.-J., Zhao, Y.-M., Yang, J., & Li, D. (2013). Intake of fish and marine n-3 polyunsaturated fatty acids and risk of breast cancer: Meta-analysis of data from 21 independent prospective cohort studies. *BMJ*, f3706. https://doi.org/10.1136/bmj.f3706.

Zhuang, J. Y., Chen, Z. Y., Zhang, T., Tang, D. P., Jiang, X. Y., & Zhuang, Z. H. (2017). Effects of different ratio of n-6/n-3 polyunsaturated fatty acids on the PI3K/Akt pathway in rats with reflux esophagitis. *Medical Science Monitor, 23*, 542–547. https://doi.org/10.12659/MSM.898131.

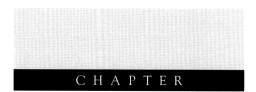

CHAPTER 8

Marine lipids and diabetes

Yunyi Tian and Ju-Sheng Zheng

School of Life Sciences, Westlake University, Hangzhou, China

8.1 Introduction

Diabetes is one of the most common chronic diseases among adults worldwide. There are over 450 million people worldwide living with diabetes in 2019, and this number is projected to rise to over 700 million by 2045 (Global Report on Diabetes, 2016; IDF Diabetes Atlas, 2019). Type 2 diabetes (T2D), accounting for over 90% of diabetes cases, has become one of the foremost public health concerns confronting the world as a major risk factor for blindness, cardiovascular disease (CVD), stroke, kidney failure, and lower limb amputation (Global Report on Diabetes, 2016). Environmental factors including diet play important roles in the onset, development, and progression of T2D and the related phenotypes.

The research interest in the effect of marine n-3 polyunsaturated fatty acids (PUFAs) on cardiometabolic health originated from epidemiological studies in Greenland Inuits, who had a lower prevalence of coronary heart disease (CHD) and a higher consumption of fish and marine n-3 PUFAs, compared with Scandinavian control participants (Bang, Dyerberg, & Hjørne, 1976). Therefore, the observation of a lower CHD prevalence in Greenland Inuits was attributed to the Eskimo diet with high contents of fish. Similar associations between high fish consumption and mortality from CHD were found in Japanese and Alaskans (Nakamura et al., 2003; Newman, Middaugh, Propst, & Rogers, 1993). In addition, prospective cohort studies and clinical trials have demonstrated the protective effects of fish and fish oil, abundant in n-3 PUFAs, on cardiometabolic health (Hu et al., 2002; Leaf et al., 1994). In vitro and in vivo studies have demonstrated that diets rich in n-3 PUFAs could modulate the metabolism of bioactive eicosanoids arising from long-chain fatty acids and reduce atherogenesis and thrombosis (Endo & Arita, 2016).

Dietary marine n-3 PUFAs, including eicosapentaenoic acid (EPA, 20:5n-3), docosahexaenoic acid (DHA, 22:6n-3), and docosapentaenoic acid (DPA, 22:5n-3), are usually from fish or seafood sources. These fatty acids are "essential fatty acids" since humans cannot synthesize them and must therefore introduce them with diets. Marine n-3 PUFAs are fundamental components of phospholipids in cell membranes and can be metabolized through reactions catalyzed by cyclooxygenases and lipoxygenases to eicosanoids (Cholewski, Tomczykowa, & Tomczyk, 2018).

Marine n-3 PUFAs are postulated to be beneficial for the prevention of T2D (Jeppesen, Schiller, & Schulze, 2013). The potential mechanisms are summarized in Fig. 8.1. Marine n-3 PUFAs could modulate inflammatory pathways and metabolize to prostaglandins (PGE$_3$), thromboxanes (TXA$_3$), and leukotrienes (LTB$_5$) associated with improved immunocompetence, which exerts anti-inflammatory and anticoagulant effects (Raffaele & Antonella, 2004). In addition to the anti-inflammatory properties, marine n-3 PUFAs can also influence cell growth and differentiation through the activation of peroxisome proliferator-activated receptors; thereafter, marine n-3 PUFAs could reduce the expression of genes involved in lipid synthesis and potentially affect insulin sensitivity via adiponectin (Haluzik & Haluzik, 2006; Jacobo-Cejudo et al., 2017; Sawada et al., 2016; Seo, Blaner, & Deckelbaum, 2005). The enhancement of lipid oxidation and thermogenesis by dietary marine n-3 PUFAs could improve glucose uptake and glycogen synthesis, as well as glycogen storage in the skeletal muscle (De Caterina, Madonna, Bertolotto, & Schmidt, 2007).

In this chapter, we will give a brief introduction to the health effects of marine n-3 PUFAs on glucose metabolism in humans. We will introduce the epidemiological evidence assessing the cross-sectional and prospective association between dietary marine n-3 PUFA intake or blood biomarkers and the T2D risk and evaluate the clinical evidence about the effect of marine n-3 PUFA supplements on blood lipids and glycemic traits (Table 8.1).

8.2 Marine n-3 PUFAs and T2D prevention

Habitual fish intake was associated with a lower risk of glucose intolerance in a cross-sectional study among an elderly cohort

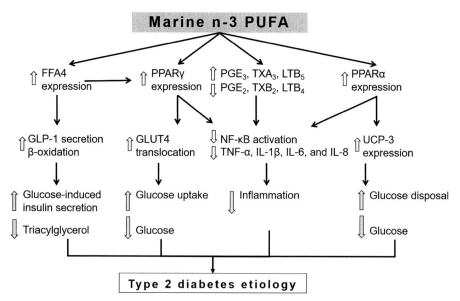

FIG. 8.1 Potential mechanisms underlying the link between marine n-3 fatty acids and type 2 diabetes. *FFA4*, free fatty acid receptor 4; *GLP-1*, glucagon-like peptide-1; *PPARγ*, peroxisome proliferator-activated receptor γ; *GLUT4*, glucose transporter-4; *PGE$_3$*, prostaglandin E$_3$; *TXA$_3$*, thromboxane A$_3$; *LTB$_5$*, leukotriene B$_5$; *PGE$_2$*, prostaglandin E$_2$; *TXB$_2$*, thromboxane B$_2$; *LTB$_4$*, leukotriene B$_4$; *NFκB*, nuclear factor κB; *TNF-α*, tumor necrosis factor-α; *IL-1β*, interleukin-1 β; *IL-6*, interleukin-6; *IL-8*, interleukin-8; *PPARα*, peroxisome proliferator-activated receptor α; *UCP3*, uncoupling protein 3.

TABLE 8.1 Selected key meta-analyses or prospective studies on marine lipids and T2D.

Study	Total number of incident T2D cases	Study design	Exposure	Main findings
Prospective cohort evidence				
Zheng, Huang, Yang, Fu, and Li (2012) (PMID: 22984522)	21,530 T2D cases	Meta-analysis of 11 prospective cohorts	Dietary marine n-3 PUFA intake	Dietary marine n-3 PUFA was inversely associated with T2D risk among Asian populations, but positively associated with T2D risk among Western populations
Neuenschwander et al. (2020) (PMID: 33264277)	24,396 T2D cases	Meta-analysis of 16 prospective cohorts	Dietary marine n-3 PUFA intake	Dietary marine n-3 PUFA was inversely associated with T2D risk among Asian populations, but positively associated with T2D risk among US populations
Forouhi et al. (2016) (PMID: 27434045)	2499 T2D cases	Meta-analysis of 9 prospective cohorts	Plasma phospholipid n-3 PUFA biomarkers	Plasma phospholipid EPA or DHA was not associated with T2D, but DPA was inversely associated with T2D
Forouhi et al. (2016) (PMID: 27434045)	12,131 T2D cases	Case-cohort study based on the European Prospective Investigation into Cancer and Nutrition–InterAct study from eight European countries	Plasma phospholipid n-3 PUFA biomarkers	Plasma phospholipid EPA or DHA was not associated with T2D risk, but DPA was marginally inversely associated with lower risk of T2D in the European cohort
Zheng et al. (2019) (PMID: 30309708)	213 T2D cases	A community-based prospective cohort study in the urban area of southern China (Guangzhou Nutrition and Health Study)	Erythrocyte membrane fatty acids	Erythrocyte DPA and EPA were inversely associated with T2D risk in Chinese populations, while there was no association for erythrocyte DHA
Trial evidence				
Chen, Yu, and Shao (2015) (PMID: 26431431)	1209 T2D cases	Meta-analysis of 20 clinical trials. Outcome: triacylglycerol, total cholesterol, HbA1c, fasting glucose, postprandial plasma glucose, fasting insulin, BMI, body weight	Marine n-3 PUFA supplements	Marine n-3 PUFA supplements significantly decrease triacylglycerol, but not any glycemic traits Higher ratio of EPA/DHA non-significantly decreases plasma insulin, HbA1c, total cholesterol, triacylglycerol and BMI
Brown et al. (2019) (PMID: 31434641)	2196 T2D cases	Meta-analysis of 66 clinical trials. Outcomes: diagnosis of T2D, HbA1c, fasting insulin, fasting glucose	Marine n-3 PUFA supplements	Marine n-3 PUFA intervention has no effect on the T2D incidence or any glycemic traits

Abbreviations: *BMI*, Body mass index; *DHA*, docosahexaenoic acid; *DPA*, docosapentaenoic acid; *EPA*, eicosapentaenoic acid; *PUFA*, polyunsaturated fatty acid; *T2D*, type 2 diabetes.

(Feskens, Bowles, & Kromhout, 1991) and in the Finnish and Dutch prospective cohorts of the Seven Countries Study (Feskens et al., 1995). Another ecological study with data from 41 countries suggested that higher fish and seafood intake was associated with a lower T2D risk (Nkondjock & Receveur, 2003). These early studies lead to the hypothesis that higher fish and marine n-3 PUFA intake may help T2D prevention. However, as revealed in several meta-analyses of prospective studies, the prospective associations of marine n-3 PUFAs with T2D incidence were quite inconsistent for cohorts from different geographic regions (Wu et al., 2012; Zheng et al., 2012). In general, marine n-3 PUFAs were inversely associated with T2D risk in studies from Asian populations, while a positive association in US populations and a null association in European populations were observed.

Blood marine n-3 PUFA biomarkers could provide objective assessment of dietary marine n-3 PUFA intake and are therefore applied widely in epidemiological studies. With the world's largest blood fatty acid database (Forouhi et al., 2016) in the European Prospective Investigation into Cancer and Nutrition (EPIC)-InterAct study (with 12,132 incident T2D cases and 15,919 subcohort participants), researchers measured plasma phospholipid fatty acid composition and investigated the prospective association of the marine n-3 PUFA biomarkers with incident T2D. They found that marine EPA or DHA was not associated with T2D, but DPA was associated with lower risk of T2D in the European cohort. A meta-analysis based on the nine cohort studies (all based on participants with European ancestry) assessing PUFA biomarkers and T2D incidence produced similar results as the EPIC-InterAct study (Forouhi et al., 2016). In addition to the above biomarker studies in Europeans, the prospective association of marine n-3 PUFA biomarkers with T2D was examined in a Chinese population, suggesting an inverse association with T2D for erythrocyte EPA, but not for other individual marine n-3 PUFAs (Zheng et al., 2019). Taken together, there is no convincing evidence suggesting the prospective association of marine n-3 PUFAs with T2D in epidemiological studies, while some evidence indicates that marine n-3 PUFAs may be beneficial in Asian populations.

Nutrigenetics, or gene-diet interaction, may provide new insight to interpret the heterogeneity in epidemiological studies, given the different genetic and dietary backgrounds in different populations and among the people of different ethnicities. Using genome-wide genotype-n-3 PUFA biomarker interaction analysis, researchers found that DPA had a significant genotype-by-environment interaction (GxE) variance contribution to total phenotypic variance of insulin resistance and fasting insulin, demonstrating that erythrocyte n-3 PUFA contributed a significant GxE variance to diabetes-related traits at a genome-wide level (Zheng et al., 2014). Other studies also found that marine n-3 PUFAs may have interaction with specific genetic variants to modulate T2D risk or related traits (Zheng et al., 2013, 2015).

8.3 Marine n-3 PUFAs and T2D management

8.3.1 Marine n-3 PUFAs and blood lipids

A large proportion of mortality and morbidity among patients with T2D is caused by cardiovascular complications (Leon & Maddox, 2015). The high prevalence of cardiovascular risk factors, including dyslipidemia, chronic low-grade inflammation and oxidative stress, and insulin resistance, increases the risk of coronary artery blockage, chronic heart failure, and stroke in patients with T2D (Halter et al., 2014; Patel et al., 2016). Therefore, it is of great interest and importance to examine whether the evidence supports a beneficial effect of marine n-3 PUFA supplementation on cardiovascular risk factors, such as blood lipids, among T2D patients.

The effects of dietary marine n-3 PUFAs on blood lipids have been investigated extensively in many prior randomized controlled trials (RCTs), summarized in several systematic reviews and meta-analyses (Chen et al., 2015; Hartweg, Perera, & Montori, 2008; Montori, Farmer, Wollan, & Dinneen, 2000). In patients with T2D, for every increase in 1 g/day dose of n-3 PUFA, an increase by 0.14 mmoL/L and a decrease by 0.36 mmoL/L were observed for low-density lipoprotein (LDL) cholesterol and serum triacylglycerol (TAG), respectively. The dose–response relationship was unclear in patients with type 1 diabetes (De Caterina et al., 2007). The most recent meta-analyses reported a significant reduction in TAG levels from 0.24 mmol/L to 0.56 mmol/L with EPA and DHA supplementation compared to the control group (Chen et al., 2015; Hartweg et al., 2008 ; Montori et al., 2000). In two meta-analyses, marine n-3 PUFA supplementation resulted in decreased TAG and increased LDL cholesterol levels, mainly ascribed to a reduced hepatic synthesis of very-low-density lipoprotein (VLDL) (Hartweg et al., 2008; Montori et al., 2000). In addition, subgroup analyses in these two meta-analyses also highlighted the TAG-lowering effect and the elevation in LDL cholesterol with marine n-3 PUFA supplementation in hypertriglyceridemic patients. One RCT evaluated the kinetics of the effects of n-3 PUFAs on apolipoprotein B (ApoB) metabolism in viscerally obese participants with insulin resistance, and the study concluded that marine n-3 PUFAs lowered the plasma concentrations of TAG by decreasing VLDL ApoB production without altering the catabolism of ApoB-containing lipoproteins or chylomicron remnants (Chan et al., 2003). The possible explanation is the formation of smaller VLDLs resulting from the hepatic secretion of TAG-poor VLDLs and an enhanced activity of lipoprotein lipase toward n-3 PUFA-enriched TAG. Smaller VLDLs are then transformed into less atherogenic LDLs that are less susceptible to oxidative modifications and slowly cleared from the circulation (De Caterina et al., 2007).

Regarding high-density lipoprotein (HDL) cholesterol, overall, no effects of marine n-3 PUFA supplementation have been reported among patients with T2D, but increased HDL cholesterol levels have been observed compared with subjects whose diets were enriched in MUFAs (predominant olive oil) (Baldassarre et al., 2006; Rivellese et al., 2003; Sanders et al., 2011). A meta-analysis of 60 RCTs reported that, by replacing carbohydrates with PUFAs, when the dietary SFA remained constant, a substantial decrease in total HDL cholesterol and LDL cholesterol plasma levels was observed (Mensink, Zock, Kester, & Katan, 2003). The most recent meta-analysis, including a total of 12 RCTs, concluded that fish oil supplements increased HDL cholesterol levels, but without changing any of the glycemic traits among patients with T2D (Gao et al., 2020).

Evidence from trials suggests the potential interaction of genetic variations with marine n-3 PUFAs on blood lipids. For example, genetic variants in CD36, NOS3, and PPARG had significant interactions with marine n-3 PUFAs on blood lipids in clinical trials (Corella & Ordovás, 2012; Zheng et al., 2018). However, more replications in large-scale trials or prospective cohort studies are needed to confirm these interactions.

Taken together, there is evidence supporting the effect of marine n-3 PUFAs on reducing blood TAG levels in T2D patients, while the results for other blood lipids are still inconsistent, with some evidence showing improved HDL cholesterol after marine n-3 PUFA intervention. Genetic variation may affect the association between marine n-3 PUFA and blood lipids among T2D patients.

8.3.2 Marine n-3 PUFAs and weight management

Marine n-3 PUFAs in hypocaloric diets have also been studied for their efficacy in weight management interventions. One RCT conducted in postmenopausal women with T2D reported that a two-month moderate marine n-3 PUFA

(1.08 g/d EPA and 0.72 g/d DHA) supplementation had no effect on body weight but significantly reduced total fat mass and adipocyte size in subcutaneous abdominal adipose tissue by 3.5% and 6%, respectively, compared to placebo groups (Kabir et al., 2007). A meta-analysis reported that marine n-3 PUFA intervention, however, had no significant effect on body weight regardless of the EPA/DHA dosage or study duration compared with the control group among T2D patients (Chen et al., 2015).

8.3.3 Marine n-3 PUFAs and glycemic control

Marine n-3 PUFA supplementation was postulated to improve glycemic control based on early epidemiological work suggesting an inverse relationship between fish intake and glucose intolerance (Feskens et al., 1991). Animal studies have provided potential mechanisms for epidemiological observations: improved hepatic insulin sensitivity through hepatic fatty acid oxidation and reducing lipogenesis, direct and indirect anti-inflammatory effects and associated improvements in insulin sensitivity in various tissues, modulation of incretin hormones involved in glucose-stimulated insulin secretion (Flachs, Rossmeisl, & Kopecky, 2014; Kuda et al., 2009; Matsuura et al., 2004; Rossi et al., 2005; Wu et al., 2012).

A recent meta-analysis of 20 RCTs among 1,209 patients with established T2D documented no significant effects of marine n-3 PUFA supplementation (0.52–3.89 g/day EPA and up to 3.69 g/day of DHA, duration ranged 2–48 weeks) in reducing fasting blood glucose (19 of 20 studies included), postprandial plasma glucose (3 of 20 studies included), fasting insulin (17 of 20 studies included), or HbA1c levels (10 of 20 studies included) compared to the control group (Chen et al., 2015). Another recent meta-analysis of 66 clinical trials involving 2196 T2D cases also suggested that marine n-3 PUFA supplementation did not have an effect on T2D incidence or any glycemic traits (Brown et al., 2019). Similarly, an earlier Cochrane review of 23 RCTs including 1075 T2D patients reported that marine n-3 PUFA supplementation (1.08–5.20 g/day EPA and 0.3–4.8 g/day of DHA, duration ranged 2–32 weeks) did not significantly affect HbA1c (15 of 23 studies included), fasting glucose (16 of 23 studies included), or fasting insulin levels (6 of 23 studies included) (Hartweg et al., 2008). To conclude, there is no evidence supporting the effect of marine n-3 PUFAs on glycemic control among T2D patients.

Ingestion of both EPA and DHA has been demonstrated to suppress hepatic lipogenesis and glucose production, reduce the hepatic output of TAG, enhance ketogenesis, and induce fatty acid oxidation in both the liver and the skeletal muscle (De Caterina et al., 2007; Julius, 2003). Substitution of 3.4% total energy of SFAs with marine n-3 PUFAs was reported to partially prevent high-fat-diet-induced insulin resistance in mice (Lanza et al., 2013). A potential mechanism may be the increased mRNA expression of insulin-stimulated glucose transporter-4 and insulin receptor substrate-1 in the skeletal muscle. Therefore, marine n-3 PUFAs have been proposed as a potential nutritional therapeutical against insulin resistance in humans. However, currently, there is no clear consensus on the use of marine n-3 PUFA supplements for individuals with insulin resistance or T2D although preclinical studies have suggested beneficial effects on insulin sensitivity and glucose intolerance (De Castro et al., 2015; Lanza et al., 2013; Liu et al., 2013; Poudyal, Panchal, Ward, & Brown, 2013).

Most observational studies use homeostasis model assessment (HOMA-IR) to assess insulin resistance, and some studies demonstrated an inverse association between marine n-3 PUFAs and the index of insulin resistance in healthy and pre-diabetes individuals (Ebbesson, Risica, Ebbesson, Kennish, & Tejero, 2005; Thorseng et al., 2009; Zhou, Kubow, Dewailly, Julien, &

Egeland, 2009). Results from a six-month RCT among 31 insulin-resistant and overweight patients demonstrated no change in insulin-stimulated peripheral glucose disposal or insulin secretion with 3.9 g/day EPA and DHA supplementation (Lalia et al., 2015). RCTs using intravenous glucose tolerance test to assess insulin sensitivity with a general intake of 3–4 g/day EPA and DHA reported no changes in insulin sensitivity (Spencer et al., 2013). Therefore, the above meta-analyses of RCTs failed to support the protective effects of EPA or DHA on insulin sensitivity.

8.4 Marine n-3 PUFAs and gestational diabetes

Gestational diabetes is the most common metabolic complication during pregnancy. Healthy diets and lifestyles are key for the prevention and treatment of gestational diabetes. Among dietary factors, the role of marine n-3 PUFAs in the development of gestational diabetes is less clear, and related studies are sparse. A prospective study involving 107 gestational diabetes patients and 214 controls suggested that marine n-3 PUFA biomarkers may be inversely associated with insulin resistance biomarkers, but not gestational diabetes (Zhu et al., 2019). One RCT based on a cohort of 2399 pregnant women <21 wk. gestation did not find evidence that DHA supplementation could reduce the incidence of gestation diabetes (Zhou et al., 2012). Therefore, the role of marine n-3 PUFAs in gestational diabetes is still unclear so far.

8.5 Conclusion

To conclude, there is evidence from preclinical studies supporting the beneficial effects of marine n-3 PUFAs on glucose metabolism and T2D prevention. However, in human cohorts or clinical trials, whether marine n-3 PUFAs could help prevent T2D risk or help glycemic control in T2D patients is still unclear. There is weak evidence supporting the potentially beneficial association of marine n-3 PUFAs with a lower risk of T2D in Asian but not Western populations. Possible explanations for the conflicting evidence in humans may be due to different study designs, varied study durations/follow-up time, different dosages, or ethnicities. Clinical data support the potentially beneficial effect of marine n-3 PUFA supplements on blood TAG levels among T2D patients. Future work could take the nutrigenetics or gut microbiome into account as an additional angle to understand the relationship between marine n-3 PUFAs and T2D development or management.

References

Baldassarre, D., Amato, M., Eligini, S., Barbieri, S. S., Mussoni, L., Frigerio, B., et al. (2006). Effect of n-3 fatty acids on carotid atherosclerosis and haemostasis in patients with combined hyperlipoproteinemia: A double-blind pilot study in primary prevention. *Annals of Medicine, 38*(5), 367–375. https://doi.org/10.1080/07853890600852880.

Bang, H. O., Dyerberg, J., & Hjørne, N. (1976). The composition of food consumed by Greenland Eskimos. *Acta Medica Scandinavica, 200*(1–6), 69–73. https://doi.org/10.1111/j.0954-6820.1976.tb08198.x.

Brown, T., Brainard, J., Song, F., Wang, X., Abdelhamid, A., & Hoope, L. (2019). Omega-3, omega-6, and total dietary polyunsaturated fat for prevention and treatment of type 2 diabetes mellitus: Systematic review and meta-analysis of randomised controlled trials. *BMJ, 366*, l4697.

Chan, D. C., Watts, G. F., Mori, T. A., Barrett, P. H. R., Redgrave, T. G., & Beilin, L. J. (2003). Randomized controlled trial of the effect of n-3 fatty acid supplementation on the metabolism of apolipoprotein B-100 and chylomicron remnants in men with visceral obesity. *American Journal of Clinical Nutrition, 77*(2), 300–307. https://doi.org/10.1093/ajcn/77.2.300.

Chen, C., Yu, X., & Shao, S. (2015). Effects of Omega-3 fatty acid supplementation on glucose control and lipid levels in type 2 diabetes: A meta-analysis. *PLoS One*. https://doi.org/10.1371/journal.pone.0139565, e0139565.

Cholewski, M., Tomczykowa, M., & Tomczyk, M. (2018). A comprehensive review of chemistry, sources and bioavailability of Omega-3 fatty acids. *Nutrients, 10*, 1662.

Corella, D., & Ordovás, J. M. (2012). Interactions between dietary n-3 fatty acids and genetic variants and risk of disease. *British Journal of Nutrition*, 107(2), S271–S283. https://doi.org/10.1017/S0007114512001651.

De Castro, G. S., Deminice, R., Simões-Ambrosio, L. M. C., Calder, P. C., Jordão, A. A., & Vannucchi, H. (2015). Dietary docosahexaenoic acid and eicosapentaenoic acid influence liver triacylglycerol and insulin resistance in rats fed a high-fructose diet. *Marine Drugs*, 13(4), 1864–1881. https://doi.org/10.3390/md13041864.

De Caterina, R., Madonna, R., Bertolotto, A., & Schmidt, E. B. (2007). n-3 fatty acids in the treatment of diabetic patients: Biological rationale and clinical data. *Diabetes Care*, 30(4), 1012–1026. https://doi.org/10.2337/dc06-1332.

Ebbesson, S. O. E., Risica, P. M., Ebbesson, L. O. E., Kennish, J. M., & Tejero, M. E. (2005). Omega-3 fatty acids improve glucose tolerance and components of the metabolic syndrome in Alaskan Eskimos: The Alaska Siberia project. *International Journal of Circumpolar Health*, 64(4), 396–408. https://doi.org/10.3402/ijch.v64i4.18016.

Endo, J., & Arita, M. (2016). Cardioprotective mechanism of omega-3 polyunsaturated fatty acids. *Journal of Cardiology*, 67(1), 22–27. https://doi.org/10.1016/j.jjcc.2015.08.002.

Feskens, E. J. M., Bowles, C. H., & Kromhout, D. (1991). Inverse association between fish intake and risk of glucose intolerance in normoglycemic elderly men and women. *Diabetes Care*, 14(11), 935–941. https://doi.org/10.2337/diacare.14.11.935.

Feskens, E. J. M., Virtanen, S. M., Räsänen, L., Tuomilehto, J., Stengård, J., Pekkanen, J., et al. (1995). Dietary factors determining diabetes and impaired glucose tolerance: A 20-year follow-up of the Finnish and Dutch cohorts of the Seven Countries Study. *Diabetes Care*, 18(8), 1104–1112. https://doi.org/10.2337/diacare.18.8.1104.

Flachs, P. M., Rossmeisl, M., & Kopecky, J. (2014). The effect of n-3 fatty acids on glucose homeostasis and insulin sensitivity. *Physiological Research*, 63, S93.

Forouhi, N. G., Imamura, F., Sharp, S. J., Koulman, A., Schulze, M. B., Zheng, J., et al. (2016). Association of Plasma Phospholipid n-3 and n-6 polyunsaturated fatty acids with type 2 diabetes: The EPIC-InterAct Case-Cohort Study. *PLoS Medicine*, 13(7). https://doi.org/10.1371/journal.pmed.1002094.

Gao, C., Liu, Y., Gan, Y., Bao, W., Peng, X., Xing, Q., et al. (2020). Effects of fish oil supplementation on glucose control and lipid levels among patients with type 2 diabetes mellitus: A meta-analysis of randomized controlled trials. *Lipids in Health and Disease*, 19(1). https://doi.org/10.1186/s12944-020-01214-w.

Global Report on Diabetes (2016) World Health Organization. https://www.who.int/publications/i/item/9789241565257.

Halter, J. B., Musi, N., Horne, F. M. F., Crandall, J. P., Goldberg, A., Harkless, L., et al. (2014). Diabetes and cardiovascular disease in older adults: Current status and future directions. *Diabetes*, 63(8), 2578–2589. https://doi.org/10.2337/db14-0020.

Haluzik, M., & Haluzik, M. (2006). PPAR-alpha and insulin sensitivity. *Physiological Research*, 55(2), 115–122.

Hartweg, J., Perera, R., & Montori, V. (2008). Cochrane database syst rev: Omega-3 polyunsaturated fatty acids (PUFA) for type 2 diabetes mellitus. *Alternative Medicine Review*, 13(2), 171–172.

Hu, F. B., Bronner, L., Willett, W. C., Stampfer, M. J., Rexrode, K. M., Albert, C. M., et al. (2002). Fish and omega-3 fatty acid intake and risk of coronary heart disease in women. *Journal of the American Medical Association*, 287(14), 1815–1821. https://doi.org/10.1001/jama.287.14.1815.

IDF Diabetes Atlas. (2019). *International Diabetes Federation*. https://www.diabetesatlas.org/en/.

Jacobo-Cejudo, M. G., Valdés-Ramos, R., Guadarrama-López, A. L., Pardo-Morales, R. V., Martínez-Carrillo, B. E., & Harbige, L. S. (2017). Effect of n-3 polyunsaturated fatty acid supplementation on metabolic and inflammatory biomarkers in type 2 diabetes mellitus patients. *Nutrients*, 9(6), 1–11. https://doi.org/10.3390/nu9060573.

Jeppesen, C., Schiller, K., & Schulze, M. B. (2013). Omega-3 and omega-6 fatty acids and type 2 diabetes. *Current Diabetes Reports*, 13(2), 279–288. https://doi.org/10.1007/s11892-012-0362-8.

Julius, U. (2003). Influence of plasma free fatty acids on lipoprotein synthesis and diabetic dyslipidemia. *Experimental and Clinical Endocrinology and Diabetes*, 111(5), 246–250. https://doi.org/10.1055/s-2003-41284.

Kabir, M., Skurnik, G., Naour, N., Pechtner, V., Meugnier, E., Rome, S., et al. (2007). Treatment for 2 mo with n-3 polyunsaturated fatty acids reduces adiposity and some atherogenic factors but does not improve insulin sensitivity in women with type 2 diabetes: A randomized controlled study. *American Journal of Clinical Nutrition*, 86(6), 1670–1679. https://doi.org/10.1093/ajcn/86.6.1670.

Kuda, O., Jelenik, T., Jilkova, Z., Flachs, P., Rossmeisl, M., Hensler, M., et al. (2009). N-3 Fatty acids and rosiglitazone improve insulin sensitivity through additive stimulatory effects on muscle glycogen synthesis in mice fed a high-fat diet. *Diabetologia*, 52(5), 941–951. https://doi.org/10.1007/s00125-009-1305-z.

Lalia, A. Z., Johnson, M. L., Jensen, M. D., Hames, K. C., Port, J. D., & Lanza, I. R. (2015). Effects of dietary n-3 fatty acids on hepatic and peripheral insulin sensitivity in insulin-resistant humans. *Diabetes Care*, 38(7), 1228–1237. https://doi.org/10.2337/dc14-3101.

Lanza, I., Blachnio-Zabielska, A., Johnson, M., Schimke, J., Jakaitis, D., Lebrasseur, N., et al. (2013). Influence of fish oil on skeletal muscle mitochondrial energetics and lipid metabolites during high-fat diet. *American Journal of Physiology. Endocrinology and Metabolism*, E1391–E1403. https://doi.org/10.1152/ajpendo.00584.2012.

Leaf, A., Jorgensen, M. B., Jacobs, A. K., Cote, G., Schoenfeld, D. A., Scheer, J., et al. (1994). Do fish oils prevent restenosis after coronary angioplasty? *Circulation*, *90*(5), 2248–2257. https://doi.org/10.1161/01.CIR.90.5.2248.

Leon, B., & Maddox, T. M. (2015). Diabetes and cardiovascular disease: Epidemiology, biological mechanisms, treatment recommendations and future research. *World Journal of Diabetes*, *1246*. https://doi.org/10.4239/wjd.v6.i13.1246.

Liu, X., Xue, Y., Liu, C., Lou, Q., Wang, J., Yanagita, T., et al. (2013). Eicosapentaenoic acid-enriched phospholipid ameliorates insulin resistance and lipid metabolism in diet-induced-obese mice. *Lipids in Health and Disease*, *12*(1). https://doi.org/10.1186/1476-511X-12-109.

Matsuura, B., Kanno, S., Minami, H., Tsubouchi, E., Iwai, M., Matsui, H., et al. (2004). Effects of antihyperlipidemic agents on hepatic insulin sensitivity in perfused Goto-Kakizaki rat liver. *Journal of Gastroenterology*, *39*(4), 339–345. https://doi.org/10.1007/s00535-003-1300-y.

Mensink, R. P., Zock, P. L., Kester, A. D. M., & Katan, M. B. (2003). Effects of dietary fatty acids and carbohydrates on the ratio of serum total to HDL cholesterol and on serum lipids and apolipoproteins: A meta-analysis of 60 controlled trials. *American Journal of Clinical Nutrition*, *77*(5), 1146–1155. https://doi.org/10.1093/ajcn/77.5.1146.

Montori, V. M., Farmer, A., Wollan, P. C., & Dinneen, S. F. (2000). Fish oil supplementation in type 2 diabetes: A quantitative systematic review. *Diabetes Care*, *23*(9), 1407–1415. https://doi.org/10.2337/diacare.23.9.1407.

Nakamura, T., Azuma, A., Kuribayashi, T., Sugihara, H., Okuda, S., & Nakagawa, M. (2003). Serum fatty acid levels, dietary style and coronary heart disease in three neighbouring areas in Japan: The Kumihama study. *British Journal of Nutrition*, *89*(2), 267–272. https://doi.org/10.1079/BJN2002787.

Neuenschwander, M., Barbaresko, J., Pischke, C. R., Iser, N., Beckhaus, J., Schwingshackl, L., & Schlesinger, S. (2020). Intake of dietary fats and fatty acids and the incidence of type 2 diabetes: A systematic review and dose-response meta-analysis of prospective observational studies. *PLoS Medicine*, *17*(12), e1003347. https://doi.org/10.1371/journal.pmed.1003347.

Newman, W. P., Middaugh, J. P., Propst, M. T., & Rogers, D. R. (1993). Atherosclerosis in Alaska natives and non-natives. *The Lancet*, *341*(8852), 1056–1057. https://doi.org/10.1016/0140-6736(93)92413-N.

Nkondjock, A., & Receveur, O. (2003). Fish-seafood consumption, obesity, and risk of type 2 diabetes: An ecological study. *Diabetes & Metabolism*, *29*(6), 635–642. https://doi.org/10.1016/S1262-3636(07)70080-0.

Patel, T. P., Rawal, K., Bagchi, A. K., Akolkar, G., Bernardes, N., Dias, D. D. S., et al. (2016). Insulin resistance: An additional risk factor in the pathogenesis of cardiovascular disease in type 2 diabetes. *Heart Failure Reviews*, *21*(1), 11–23. https://doi.org/10.1007/s10741-015-9515-6.

Poudyal, H., Panchal, S. K., Ward, L. C., & Brown, L. (2013). Effects of ALA, EPA and DHA in high-carbohydrate, high-fat diet-induced metabolic syndrome in rats. *Journal of Nutritional Biochemistry*, *24*(6), 1041–1052. https://doi.org/10.1016/j.jnutbio.2012.07.014.

Raffaele, D. C., & Antonella, Z. (2004). From asthma to atherosclerosis—5-lipoxygenase, leukotrienes, and inflammation. *New England Journal of Medicine*, *350*, 4–7. https://doi.org/10.1056/NEJMp038190.

Rivellese, A. A., Maffettone, A., Vessby, B., Uusitupa, M., Hermansen, K., Berglund, L., et al. (2003). Effects of dietary saturated, monounsaturated and n-3 fatty acids on fasting lipoproteins, LDL size and post-prandial lipid metabolism in healthy subjects. *Atherosclerosis*, *167*(1), 149–158. https://doi.org/10.1016/S0021-9150(02)00424-0.

Rossi, A. S., Lombardo, Y. B., Lacorte, J. M., Chicco, A. G., Rouault, C., Slama, G., et al. (2005). Dietary fish oil positively regulates plasma leptin and adiponectin levels in sucrose-fed, insulin-resistant rats. *American Journal of Physiology—Regulatory, Integrative and Comparative Physiology*, *289*(2), R486–R494. https://doi.org/10.1152/ajpregu.00846.2004.

Sanders, T. A. B., Hall, W. L., Maniou, Z., Lewis, F., Seed, P. T., & Chowienczyk, P. J. (2011). Effect of low doses of long-chain n-3 PUFAs on endothelial function and arterial stiffness: A randomized controlled trial. *American Journal of Clinical Nutrition*, *94*(4), 973–980. https://doi.org/10.3945/ajcn.111.018036.

Sawada, T., Tsubata, H., Hashimoto, N., Takabe, M., Miyata, T., Aoki, K., et al. (2016). Effects of 6-month eicosapentaenoic acid treatment on postprandial hyperglycemia, hyperlipidemia, insulin secretion ability, and concomitant endothelial dysfunction among newly-diagnosed impaired glucose metabolism patients with coronary artery disease. An open label, single blinded, prospective randomized controlled trial. *Cardiovascular Diabetology*, *15*(1). https://doi.org/10.1186/s12933-016-0437-y.

Seo, T., Blaner, W. S., & Deckelbaum, R. J. (2005). Omega-3 fatty acids: Molecular approaches to optimal biological outcomes. *Current Opinion in Lipidology*, *16*(1), 11–18. https://doi.org/10.1097/00041433-200502000-00004.

Spencer, M., Finlin, B. S., Unal, R., Zhu, B., Morris, A. J., Shipp, L. R., et al. (2013). Omega-3 fatty acids reduce adipose tissue macrophages in human subjects with insulin resistance. *Diabetes*, *62*(5), 1709–1717. https://doi.org/10.2337/db12-1042.

Thorseng, T., Witte, D. R., Vistisen, D., Borch-Johnsen, K., Bjerregaard, P., & Jørgensen, M. E. (2009). The association between n-3 fatty acids in erythrocyte membranes and insulin resistance: The inuit health in transition study. *International Journal of Circumpolar Health*, *68*(4), 327–336. https://doi.org/10.3402/ijch.v68i4.17373.

Wu, J. H. Y., Micha, R., Imamura, F., Pan, A., Biggs, M. L., Ajaz, O., et al. (2012). Omega-3 fatty acids and incident type 2 diabetes: A systematic review and meta-analysis. *British Journal of Nutrition*, *107*(2), S214–S227. https://doi.org/10.1017/S0007114512001602.

Zheng, J. S., Arnett, D. K., Parnell, L. D., Lee, Y. C., Ma, Y., Smith, C. E., et al. (2013). Genetic variants at PSMD3 interact with dietary fat and carbohydrate to modulate insulin resistance1-3. *Journal of Nutrition*, *143*(3), 354–361. https://doi.org/10.3945/jn.112.168401.

Zheng, J. S., Chen, J., Wang, L., Yang, H., Fang, L., Yu, Y., et al. (2018). Replication of a gene-diet interaction at CD36, NOS3 and PPARG in response to omega-3 fatty acid supplements on blood lipids: A double-blind randomized controlled trial. *eBioMedicine*, *31*, 150–156. https://doi.org/10.1016/j.ebiom.2018.04.012.

Zheng, J. S., Huang, T., Li, K., Chen, Y., Xie, H., Xu, D., et al. (2015). Modulation of the association between the PEPD variant and the risk of type 2 diabetes by n-3 fatty acids in Chinese Hans. *Journal of Nutrigenetics and Nutrigenomics*, *8*(1), 36–43. https://doi.org/10.1159/000381348.

Zheng, J. S., Huang, T., Yang, J., Fu, Y. Q., & Li, D. (2012). Marine N-3 polyunsaturated fatty acids are inversely associated with risk of type 2 diabetes in Asians: A systematic review and meta-analysis. *PLoS One*, *7*(9). https://doi.org/10.1371/journal.pone.0044525.

Zheng, J. S., Lai, C. Q., Parnell, L. D., Lee, Y. C., Shen, J., Smith, C. E., et al. (2014). Genome-wide interaction of genotype by erythrocyte n-3 fatty acids contributes to phenotypic variance of diabetes-related traits. *BMC Genomics*, *15*(1). https://doi.org/10.1186/1471-2164-15-781.

Zheng, J. S., Lin, J. S., Dong, H. L., Zeng, F. F., Li, D., Song, Y., et al. (2019). Association of erythrocyte n-3 polyunsaturated fatty acids with incident type 2 diabetes in a Chinese population. *Clinical Nutrition*, *38*(5), 2195–2201. https://doi.org/10.1016/j.clnu.2018.09.018.

Zhou, Y. E., Kubow, S., Dewailly, E., Julien, P., & Egeland, G. M. (2009). Decreased activity of desaturase 5 in association with obesity and insulin resistance aggravates declining long-chain n-3 fatty acid status in Cree undergoing dietary transition. *British Journal of Nutrition*, *102*(6), 888–894. https://doi.org/10.1017/S0007114509301609.

Zhou, S. J., Yelland, L., McPhee, A., Quinlivan, J., Gibson, R., & Makrides, M. (2012). Fish-oil supplementation in pregnancy does not reduce the risk of gestational diabetes or preeclampsia. *American Journal of Clinical Nutrition*, *95*(6), 1378–1384. https://doi.org/10.3945/ajcn.111.033217.

Zhu, Y., Li, M., Rahman, M. L., Hinkle, S. N., Wu, J., Weir, N. L., et al. (2019). Plasma phospholipid n-3 and n-6 polyunsaturated fatty acids in relation to cardiometabolic markers and gestational diabetes: A longitudinal study within the prospective NICHD Fetal Growth Studies. *PLoS Medicine*, *16*(9). https://doi.org/10.1371/journal.pmed.1002910.

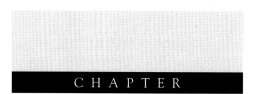

Lipids and nonalcoholic fatty liver disease

Xiao-fei Guo[a,b] and Wen-Jun Ma[a,b]

[a]Institute of Nutrition & Health, Qingdao University, Qingdao, China [b]School of Public Health, Qingdao University, Qingdao, China

9.1 Introduction

As the most common form of chronic liver diseases, nonalcoholic fatty disease (NAFLD) consists of a wide spectrum of conditions, ranging from isolated hepatic steatosis to nonalcoholic steatohepatitis (NASH), fibrosis, cirrhosis, and hepatocellular carcinoma (Guo, Yang, Tang, & Li, 2018). It is regulated by numerous mechanisms such as dietary pattern, metabolic, genetic, environmental, and gut microbial factors. The presence of steatosis is an indispensable step to developing NASH accompanied by inflammatory infiltration, cellular injury, and subsequently liver fibrosis (Jorgensen, 2003; Rinella, 2015).

Increased triacylglycerol (TAG) deposition in the liver indicates an input/output imbalance of hepatic free fatty acid (FFA) metabolism. During the fed state, adipose tissue insulin resistance induces an increase in FFA delivery to the liver (Donnelly et al., 2005; Sanyal et al., 2001). Additionally, the de novo lipogenesis driven by hyperinsulinemia has been increased (Lambert, Ramos-Roman, Browning, & Parks, 2014). Compensatory production of very low density lipoprotein (VLDL) secretion is insufficient to improve the excess formation of TAG (Fabbrini et al., 2008). In the early stage, the accumulated TAG in steatosis appears to be relatively inert; however, hepatocellular injury is driven by lipotoxicity from FFAs and their derivatives. Due to excess accumulation of fat in the liver, visceral adipose tissue induces multiple signaling pathways that change lipid and glucose metabolism and induces hepatic fat accumulation and a pro-inflammatory milieu, contributing to hepatocellular injury, increased fibrosis, and hepatic architectural distortion (Rotman & Sanyal, 2017). Because of the burden of this disease, it is a challenge for public health to manage and treat NAFLD.

In recent years, the remarkable progress in understanding the pathogenesis of NAFLD has promoted an explosion of medical therapies with respect to fat accumulation and injury pathways. Generally, targets of upcoming therapies for NAFLD have been grouped into four groups: (1) medications with a primary metabolic target reducing fat accumulation in the liver; (2) medications focusing on endoplasmic reticulum stress, oxidative stress, inflammation, and injury components of NASH; (3) medications with a primary gut target modulating the interaction between gut microbiome and liver; and (4) antifibrotics, targeting to decrease the progressive fibrosis and resultant complications (Rotman & Sanyal, 2017).

Current estimates suggest that the prevalence of NAFLD is 10% in children and affects as high as 30% of adults in Western countries (Rinella, 2015; Welsh, Karpen, & Vos, 2013; Younossi et al., 2016). With the changes in lifestyle and dietary patterns, the prevalence of NAFLD has reached as high as 25% around the world (Younossi et al., 2016). The patients with NAFLD are asymptomatic at the beginning. However, increasing studies indicate that NAFLD is positively associated with noncommunicable diseases, including type 2 diabetes mellitus (T2DM) (Chitturi et al., 2002) and cardiovascular diseases (CVD) (Hamaguchi et al., 2007; Targher & Arcaro, 2007). Lifestyle interventions are a feasible and practical treatment option for NAFLD, and weight loss is a pivotal goal to improve historical features of NAFLD. In addition, drug treatment, such as thiazolidinediones, has been shown to improve historical features of NAFLD. Considering that poor adherence to lifestyle modifications and adverse effects of pharmacotherapy, it is necessary and urgent to identify an effective and therapeutic approach in the management and treatment of NAFLD. To date, substantial evidence has paid increasing attention to dietary and nutritional inventions. Of these, n-3 polyunsaturated fatty acids (PUFAs) of marine origin have received extensive research, due to their ability to improve glucose and lipid metabolism and inflammation (Calder, 2012; Carpentier, Portois, & Malaisse, 2006).

9.2 Fatty acids and NAFLD

To the best of our knowledge, there is no prospective cohort study investigating the association of circulating and/or liver fatty acid composition with NAFLD. Several case–control studies have suggested that a significantly higher composition of n-3 PUFA (especially DHA) in healthy subjects in comparison to patients with NAFLD (Araya et al., 2004; Elizondo et al., 2008; Kishino et al., 2011; Lou et al., 2014; Pettinelli et al., 2009; Zheng, Xu, Huang, Yu, & Li, 2012; Zhu et al., 2010), whereas the other studies have indicated opposite or null associations (Parker et al., 2015; Spahis et al., 2015; Walle et al., 2016). Of the 10 case–control studies, three studies reported fatty acid composition in the liver (Araya et al., 2004; Elizondo et al., 2008; Pettinelli et al., 2009), and eight studies reported the circulating composition of fatty acid (Araya et al., 2004; Kishino et al., 2011; Lou et al., 2014; Parker et al., 2015; Pettinelli et al., 2009; Spahis et al., 2015; Walle et al., 2016; Zheng et al., 2016; Zhu et al., 2010). Meanwhile, one study reported fatty acid composition in both the blood and liver tissue (Table 9.1) (Elizondo et al., 2008). Case–control studies demonstrated that blood and liver DHA composition (weighted mean difference (WMD): 3.42; 95%CI: 2.03, 4.07) was significantly higher in healthy subjects in comparison with NAFLD patients, whereas the composition of C16:1 (WMD: −0.62; 95%CI: −1.01, −0.24), C18:0 (WMD: −2.69; 95%CI: −5.31, −0.07), C18:1 (WMD: −1.66; 95%CI: −2.82, −0.50), saturated fatty acids (WMD: −2.29; 95%CI: −3.53, −1.05), and monounsaturated fatty acids (WMD: −1.92; 95%CI: −3.16, −0.69) was significantly lower in the controls compared with cases (Guo et al., 2018).

Considering that diagnosis of NAFLD is time-consuming and costly, including liver biopsy, magnetic resonance imaging (MRI), and ultrasound, and no prospective cohort study up to date has investigated the relationship between circulating fatty acid and/or liver fatty acid composition and risk of developing NAFLD. Thus, case–control studies were conducted to investigate these associations. The summary estimate suggested that circulating and liver compositions of docosahexaenoic acid (DHA) were significantly lower in the cases compared with controls, whereas the

TABLE 9.1 Characteristics of the 10 eligible case–control studies in the present meta-analysis.

First author	Country	No. (case/control)	Gender (F/M); mean age, year	Biospecimen	Individual n-3 PUFA	Cases vs. controls
Araya	Chile	30 (19/11)	NR	Liver	EPA DHA	0.14±0.03 vs. 0.39±0.09 1.26±0.41 vs. 6.76±0.82
Elizondo	Chile	20 (12/8)	NR; 42.2±10.2	Blood cell phospholipids Liver phospholipids	EPA DPA DHA EPA DPA DHA	2.87±1.56 vs. 2.61±1.55 2.16±1.66 vs. 7.12±2.26 7.37±3.18 vs. 15.2±2.3 2.04±0.79 vs. 4.8±2.5 3.14±2.21 vs. 6.53±1.33 4.58±2.21 vs. 15.1±1.9
Kishino	Japan	33 (14/19)	(18/15); 59.21±14.00	Serum	EPA DPA DHA	1.6±0.9 vs. 2.6±1.1 0.5±0.1 vs. 0.7±0.1 3.5±1.1 vs. 4.7±1.1
Lou	China	87 (45/42)	(31/56); 57.0±7.9	Serum phospholipids	EPA DPA DHA	1.80±0.75 vs. 2.47±0.94 0.84±0.32 vs. 0.92±0.4 4.14±1.44 vs. 6.44±1.26
Parker	Australia	80 (30/50)	(24/56); 38.8±11.6	Erythrocyte	EPA DHA	2.5±1.1 vs. 2.2±1.4 6.5±1.1 vs. 6.2±1.4
Pettinelli	Chile	19 (11/8)	(13/6); 35.9±12.2	Liver	EPA DHA	1.36±1.39 vs. 1.3±1.05 7.9±4.31 vs. 18.5±4.81
Spahis	Canada	54 (21/33)	NR; 14.17±0.66	Plasma	EPA DPA DHA	0.62±0.06 vs. 0.28±0.01 0.37±0.02 vs. 0.27±0.01 1.29±0.1 vs. 0.82±0.05
Walle	Finland	92 (53/39)	(28/64); 46.8±8.7	Serum phospholipids	EPA DPA DHA	1.56±0.78 vs. 1.64±0.73 1.13±0.19 vs. 1.24±0.16 6.25±1.27 vs. 6.42±1.42
Zheng	China	200 (100/100)	(62/138); 44.17±11.76	Plasma phospholipids	EPA DPA DHA	1.50±0.56 vs. 1.48±0.56 0.81±0.28 vs. 0.79±0.31 5.45±1.07 vs. 5.79±1.15
Zhu	China	87 (45/42)	(31/56); 57.0±7.9	Serum phospholipids	EPA DPA DHA	1.80±0.75 vs.2.47±0.94 0.84±0.32 vs.0.92±0.4 4.14±1.44 vs.6.44±1.26

Abbreviations: *DHA*, docosahexaenoic acid; *DPA*, docosapentaenoic acid; *EPA*, eicosapentaenoic acid; *F*, female; *M*, male; *no.*, number of subjects; *NR*, none reported.

compositions of saturated and monounsaturated fatty acids were significantly higher in the cases compared with controls. The meta-analysis of case–control studies provided a hypothesis that supplemental n-3 PUFA might be favorable in the management and treatment of NAFLD. Therefore, a meta-analysis of randomized controlled trials (RCTs) was included to illuminate whether n-3 supplementation was favorable for therapy of NAFLD. A total of 11 independent RCTs were included to investigate supplemental n-3 PUFA on biomarkers of NAFLD (Table 9.2) (Argo et al., 2015; Capanni et al., 2006; Chen et al., 2008; Cussons, Watts, Mori, & Stuckey, 2009; Dasarathy et al., 2015; Janczyk et al., 2015; Li et al., 2015; Qin et al., 2015; Scorletti et al., 2014; Sofi et al., 2010; Spadaro et al., 2008). One study explored the effect of caloric restriction (30%) with and without fish oil supplementation (2g per day for 6 months) (Spadaro et al., 2008). Compared with the pretreatment BMI, it was decreased by 6.3% in the group receiving fish oil supplementation and by 2.9% in the control group at the end of this trial. Besides, supplementation with n-3 PUFA showed a significant reduction in concentrations of alanine aminotransferase (ALT), glutamyl transpeptidase (GGT), and TAG (Spadaro et al., 2008). In another study, liver steatosis improved by more than 60% after fish oil intervention (1 g per day for 12 months); however, liver steatosis did not change as determined by ultrasound in the control group. Accordingly, supplementation with fish oil significantly reduced the serum concentrations of ALT, GGT, and TAG (Capanni et al., 2006).

A randomized cross-over study was conducted to investigate fish oil intervention on biomarkers of NAFLD patients with polycystic ovary syndrome (PCOS). The patients received fish oil (4g per day) and olive oil (4g per day) for 8 weeks with a washout period of 8 weeks. The results showed that supplementation with fish oil significantly decreased liver fat content (18.2 vs. 14.8%) as determined by magnetic resonance spectroscopy (Cussons et al., 2009). On the contrary, a prospective, randomized, double-blind placebo-controlled trial was conducted on nonalcoholic steatohepatitis with T2DM. The patients were randomized to consume fish oil (2.16g per day eicosapentaenoic acid (EPA) and 1.44g per day DHA, respectively) or placebo containing corn oil. After 48 weeks of intervention, hepatic steatosis and the activity score were improved significantly, but were unchanged in the fish oil group with hepatic histology and biochemical indicators. Given the small number of participants ($n=37$), the results of this study should be explained with caution (Dasarathy et al., 2015). A 15- to 18-month randomized double-blinded placebo trial was implemented to investigate whether highly purified DHA+EPA (1.84g per day EPA and 1.52g per day DHA) could decrease liver fat and improve liver fibrosis biomarker scores. After intervention, the composition of DHA increased 1% in the red blood cells and was associated with a 3.3% decrease in hepatic fat as determined by magnetic resonance spectroscopy. A 6% DHA increment was associated with a 20% reduction in hepatic fat. However, there was a nonsignificant association between circulating EPA and liver fat content. The data support that DHA might be a biomarker indicating NAFLD (Scorletti et al., 2014). In a one-year randomized, double-blind, and placebo-controlled trial, n-3 PUFA (EPA 1.05g per day and DHA 0.75g per day) supplementation significantly reduced liver fat but not nonalcoholic steatohepatitis activity score. Additionally, the patients who received n-3 PUFA showed a significant reduction in body weight, and the effects of weight loss and n-3 PUFA intervention were synergistical for the reduction in liver fat content. However, insulin sensitivity and serum ALT concentration were unchanged in patients' supplementation with n-3 PUFA (Argo et al., 2015). A limited trial

TABLE 9.2 Characteristics of the 11 independent RCTs in the present meta-analysis.

First author	Country	No. (control/intervention)	Gender (F/M); mean age, year	Health status	Duration	Study design	Does n-3 PUFA supplementation per day	Control	Method of diagnosis
Argo	USA	34 (17/17)	(21/13); 46.8±11.9	NASH	12 months	Parallel	3 g (1.05 g EPA and 0.75 g DHA)	Placebo (soybean oil)	Liver biopsy
Capanni	Italy	56 (14/42)	(24/32); 61.0±12.5	NAFLD	12 months	Parallel	1 g (0.375 g EPA and 0.625 g DHA)	No treatment	Ultrasound
Chen	China	31 (16/15)	(16/15); 46	NAFLD	24 weeks	Parallel	5 g n-3 PUFA	Placebo	Elevated transaminases
Cussons	Australia	24 (12/12)	(12/0); 35.3±6.7	Premenopausal women with PCOS	8 weeks	Crossover	4 g (2.24 g DHA and 1.08 g EPA)	Placebo (olive oil)	MRI
Dasarathy	USA	37 (19/18)	(29/8); 50.6±9.8	NAHS subjects with diabetes	48 weeks	Parallel	3.6 g (2.16 g EPA and 1.44 g DHA)	Placebo (corn oil)	Liver biopsy
Li	China	78 (39/39)	(8/70); 51.9±7.8	NASH	6 months	Parallel	50 mL into daily diet	Placebo (saline)	Undetailed
Janczyk	Poland	64 (30/34)	(9/55); 13.0±3.0	NAFLD	6 months	Parallel	0.45–1.3 g n-3 PUFA	Placebo (sunflower oil)	Ultrasound
Qin	China	70 (34/36)	(19/51); 45.2±10.7	NAFLD subjects with hyperlipidemia	3 months	Parallel	4 g (0.728 g EPA and 0.516 g DHA)	Placebo (corn oil)	Ultrasound
Scorletti	UK	95 (48/47)	(40/55); 51.3±10.7	NAFLD	15–18 months	Parallel	4 g (1.84 g EPA and 1.52 g DHA)	Placebo (olive oil)	Ultrasound, MRI, or CT
Sofi	Italy	11 (5/6)	(2/9); 54.5±4.9	NAFLD	12 months	Parallel	0.83 g (0.47 g EPA and 0.24 g DHA)	Placebo (olive oil)	Ultrasound
Spadaro	Italy	36 (18/18)	(17/19); 50.7±11.3	NAFLD	6 months	Parallel	2 g n-3 PUFA	No placebo	Ultrasound

Abbreviations: *MRI*, magnetic resonance imaging; *NALFD*, nonalcoholic liver fatty disease; *CT*, computed tomography scan; *NASH*, nonalcoholic steatohepatitis.

focused on children with NAFLD. In a randomized, double-blind, placebo-controlled trial, supplementation with algal oil rich in EPA and DHA was investigated in overweight/obese children with NAFLD diagnosed by ultrasound. The intervention and the placebo groups also received nutritional counseling as part of treatment. No significant differences were observed between the groups with respect to insulin resistance and serum ALT and lipid profiles. Supplementation with n-3 PUFA significantly decreased the concentrations of aspartate aminotransferase (AST) and GGT and increased circulating adiponectin in comparison with the placebo group (Janczyk et al., 2015). Similarity, Sofi et al. reported the effectiveness of one-year of n-3 PUFA intervention in patients with NAFLD. The results demonstrated that n-3 PUFA supplementation significantly reduced the concentrations of ALT, AST, GGT, and TAG at the end of this trial. Furthermore, the patients who received n-3 PUFA had a significant increase in concentrations of adiponectin (Sofi et al., 2010). Up to now, there have been three RCTs investigating whether n-3 PUFA supplementation was favorable for improving NAFLD in China. One study reported that n-3 PUFA intervention significantly decreased concentrations of TAG, ALT, and AST compared with the control group after 6 months of intervention. Simultaneously, supplemental n-3 PUFA profoundly improved steatosis grade, necro-inflammatory grade, fibrosis stage, and ballooning score in comparison with the control group, suggesting that n-3 supplementation had beneficial roles in offsetting NASH progression (Li et al., 2015). Another RCT involved 46 NAFLD patients. The patients were randomized to consume n-3 PUFA (low dose, $n=15$; high dose $n=15$) or placebo ($n=16$) for a period of 24 weeks. The results demonstrated that a higher dose of n-3 PUFA intervention had a positive role in improving ultrasound scores and decreasing serum TAG levels. However, there was no significant difference with respect to ALT and GGT levels before and after treatment (Chen et al., 2008). Qin et al. investigated where n-3 PUFA supplementation had benefits in NAFLD patients associated with hyperlipidemia through a double-blind, randomized clinical trial (Qin et al., 2015). Supplemental n-3 PUFA significantly reduced the concentrations of total cholesterol, glucose, ALT, AST, and TAG. Besides, n-3 PUFA intervention significantly decreased the concentrations of fibroblast growth factors 21, while increasing the adiponectin levels (Qin et al., 2015). These trials demonstrated that n-3 PUFA intervention had inconsistent results with respect to biomarkers of NAFLD. Therefore, a meta-analysis of RCTs was implemented to illuminate whether n-3 PUFA intervention has favorable effects in NAFLD patients. Of the inclusive studies, 10 RCTs reported n-3 PUFA intervention on ALT concentrations. Supplemental n-3 PUFA significantly reduced the concentrations of ALT (-7.53 U/L; 95%CI: -9.98, -5.08; $P<0.001$), with nonsignificant between-study heterogeneity ($I^2=0.0\%$, $P=0.846$) (Guo et al., 2018). Eight RCTs investigated supplemental n-3 PUFA on AST concentrations, and the pooled effect was -7.10 U/L (95%CI, -11.67, -2.52 U/L, $P=0.002$), with a significant between-study heterogeneity ($I^2=83.4\%$, $P<0.001$) (Guo et al., 2018). Only four RCTs provided available data regarding liver fat content, and the summary estimated mean change was marginally significant (-5.11%; 95%CI: -10.24, 0.02; $P=0.051$), with a significant between-study heterogeneity ($I^2=72.1\%$, $P=0.013$) (Guo et al., 2018). The summary estimated mean difference in TAG concentrations was pooled in 11 RCTs, and supplemental n-3 PUFA showed a significant reduction in concentrations of TAG (-36.15 mg/dL; 95%CI: -49.15, -23.18 mg/dL, $P<0.001$), with a significant between-study heterogeneity ($I^2=51.0\%$, $P=0.026$) (Guo et al., 2018).

9.3 Factors affecting NAFLD on biomarkers of NAFLD

Supplementation of n-3 PUFA exerted a significant reduction in ALT concentrations in NAFLD patients whose mean age was >50 years (−8.09 U/L; 95%CI: −10.73, −5.46 U/L; $I^2 = 0.00\%$), but not in patients whose mean age was ≤50 years. In addition, the trials with Jadad score <4 significantly decreased the concentrations of ALT (−8.07 U/L; 95%CI: −10.69, −5.45 U/L; $I^2 = 0.00\%$), but not in trials with Jadad score ≥4 (Guo et al., 2018). On the contrary, supplemental n-3 PUFA significantly reduced the concentration of AST in mean age of subjects ≤50 years (−8.88 U/L; 95%CI: −13.85, −3.91 U/L; $I^2 = 76.3\%$), but not in mean age of patients >50 years (Guo et al., 2018). Similarly, supplemental n-3 PUFA significantly reduced the concentrations of TAG in the trials with Jadad score <4 (−40.38 mg/dL; 95%CI: −52.21, −28.55 mg/dL; $I^2 = 25.8\%$), but not in trials with Jadad score ≥4. Therefore, the quality of the trials was responsible for the n-3 PUFA on biomarkers of NAFLD (Guo et al., 2018). Supplementation with n-3 PUFA showed a higher reduction in TAG concentrations in mean age of patients >50 years (−42.65 mg/dL; 95%CI: −61.81, −23.49 mg/dL; $I^2 = 50.7\%$), compared with the mean age of patients ≤50 years (−24.71 mg/dL; 95%CI: −36.70, −12.73 mg/dL; $I^2 = 0.00\%$) (Guo et al., 2018). The trials with Jadad score <4 exerted a significant reduction in ALT, AST, and TAG concentrations, but not in high-quality studies. The reason is that only four trials were regarded as high-quality studies (Argo et al., 2015; Dasarathy et al., 2015; Janczyk et al., 2015; Qin et al., 2015); thus, the statistical power of the summary estimate was insufficient. Furthermore, two RCTs with EPA plus DHA intervention were less than 1.5 g per day (Janczyk et al., 2015; Qin et al., 2015). Therefore, the summary estimates were not significant on the basis of high-quality trials. Intervention with n-3 PUFA >3 g per day did not exert significant reduction in serum concentrations of ALT and AST. Considering that the duration of n-3 PUFA supplementation also played a pivotal role in treatment of NAFLD, a longer duration with a higher dose would have significant reductions in ALT and AST concentrations. Based on the present study, the optimal dose of n-3 PUFA intervention could not be obtained. However, the present study provided strong evidence that a longer duration of DHA intervention would have favorable benefits in treatment of NAFLD.

9.4 Dose–response relationship between n-3 PUFA intake and biomarkers

Dose–response analysis showed that one gram per day increment of EPA+DHA was associated with a 3.14 U/L reduction in ALT concentration (95%CI; −5.25, −1.02 U/L; P for trend = 0.004). There was a nonsignificant association between the dose of supplemental n-3 PUFA and AST concentration using meta-regression analysis, but a significant linear association was detected. One gram per day increment of EPA+DHA exerted a 2.43 U/L reduction in AST (95%CI: −3.90, −0.90 U/L; P for trend = 0.001). Meanwhile, one gram per day increment of EPA+DHA was associated with a 2.74% reduction in liver fat content (95%CI: −4.32, −1.16%; P for trend <0.001) and a 9.95 mg/dL reduction in TAG concentration (95%CI: −14.47, −5.48 mg/dL; P for trend <0.001). There were seven trials which were available for dose–response analysis to evaluate EPA or DHA intervention on biomarkers of NAFLD. DHA supplementation had superior benefits in the management and treatment of NAFLD. Docosapentaenoic acid (DPA, C22:5n-3) is an intermediary of EPA and DHA; it was unclear whether its supplementation has favorable benefits in NAFLD patients. It has been reported that supplemental seal oil, which is rich in DPA, could improve circulating ALT and lipid profiles in patients with NAFLD (Zhu, Liu, Chen, Huang, & Zhang, 2008). Given that the patients received drug therapy during sea oil supplementation, the trial was excluded for data synthesis in the present meta-analysis. Further studies are warranted to investigate DPA supplementation in patients with NAFLD.

9.5 The underlying mechanisms why n-3 PUFAs protect against NAFLD

Insulin resistance is a crucial factor for the initiation and development of NAFLD, contributing to increased hepatic de novo lipogenesis and impaired lipolysis. With the release of free fatty acids, they would be accumulated as TAG in the liver, resulting in lipotoxicity, mitochondrial dysfunction, inflammatory cascades, and fibrogenesis (Cusi, 2009; Peverill, Powell, & Skoien, 2014). The underlying mechanisms why n-3 PUFA supplementation could improve NAFLD have been summarized as follows (Fig. 9.1): (1) n-3 PUFA could decrease TAG synthesis and increase lipid oxidation in the liver. As the ligands of n-3 PUFA, the activation of peroxisome activation receptor (PPAR)-α would enhance fatty acid oxidation in mitochondria and inhibit TAG synthesis in the liver. Furthermore, the enzymes responsible for lipogenesis, namely fatty acid synthase and acetyl-CoA carboxylase, are regulated by sterol regulatory element-binding protein (SREBP)-1c (Scorletti & Byrne, 2013). In the cell and animal models, they have shown that n-3 PUFA could inhibit the expression level of SREBP-1c and that might be involved in the activation of AMP-activated protein kinase (AMPK) through n-3 PUFA (Guo, Gao, Li, & Li, 2017; Musso, Gambino, & Cassader, 2009; Takeuchi et al., 2010). In addition, the phosphorylation of AMPK would be in favor of insulin sensitivity and lipid metabolism (Lorente-Cebrián, Bustos, Marti, Martinez, & Moreno-Aliaga, 2009). (2) From a nongenomic perspective, n-3 PUFA might contribute to improvement in the fluidity of cell membranes. The adequate fluidity of cell membrane could improve the functions of surface receptors and the efficiency of the signal transduction pathway (Salem Jr, Litman, Kim, & Gawrisch, 2001). With the improvement of membrane fluidity, the numbers of insulin receptors would be increased, and the translocation of glucose transporter-4 (GLUT4) would be improved for glucose transport into the cytoplasm (Bugianesi, McCullough, & Marchesini, 2005). Additionally, appropriate fluidity of cell membrane, which would boost the activity of tyrosine kinase, facilitates phosphorylation of insulin receptor substrate-1 and substrate-2 for insulin signaling transduction (Ficková et al., 1994; Gormaz, Rodrigo, Videla, & Beems, 2010). (3) Anti-inflammatory activities of n-3 PUFA are another possible mechanism. TAG accumulation in the liver is accompanied with the recruitment of macrophages, inducing the generation of pro-inflammatory cytokines, including monocyte chemoattractant protein-1 (MCP-1), interleukin-1β (IL-1β), IL-6, and tumor necrosis factor-α (TNF-α). The increased expression of inflammatory cytokines would accelerate the initiation and progression of NAFLD, ranging from hepatic steatosis, steatohepatitis, and fibrosis (Du Plessis et al., 2015). On the contrary, the production of adiponectin from adipose tissue has anti-inflammatory functions (Neschen et al., 2006; Scorletti & Byrne, 2013). A meta-analysis of case–control studies has shown that the NAFDL patients had a significantly lower circulating adiponectin concentration in comparison with healthy subjects (Polyzos, Toulis, Goulis, Zavos, & Kountouras, 2011). Administration of n-3 PUFA could increase adiponectin section through a PPAR-γ-dependent pathway (Neschen et al., 2006). Meanwhile, the toll-like receptor-4/nuclear factor-κB signaling pathway could be inhibited through n-3 PUFA supplementation, contributing to decrease in the

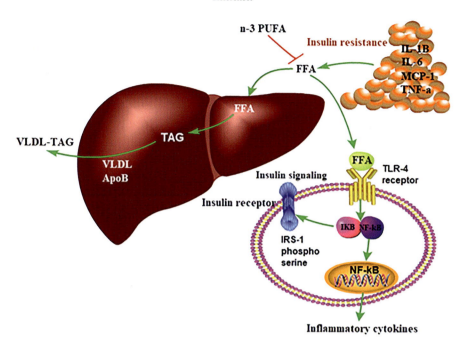

FIG. 9.1 The underlying mechanisms for n-3 PUFA supplementation improving NAFLD. Supplementation with n-3 PUFA exert on lipid and lipoprotein metabolism. Reduced VLDL production in the liver largely results from a decreased availability of FFA released from adipose stores, together with the suppression of lipogenic genes and the induction of genes involved in fatty acid oxidation. n-3 PUFA is able to regulate metabolism and other cell and tissue responses, including adipocyte differentiation and inflammation. The activated TLR-4 signaling pathway by FFA also be suppressed by n-3 PUFAs, inhibiting proinflammatory cascades to induce NAFLD. Abbreviations: *n-3 PUFA*, n-3 polyunsaturated fatty acid; *FFA*, free fatty acid; *Apo B*, apolipoprotein B; *TAG*, triacylglycerol; *TLR-4*, toll-like receptor 4; *IKK*, inhibitor of NF-κB kinase; *NF-κB*, nuclear factor-καρρα B; *IκB*, inhibitor of κB; *IRS-1*, insulin receptor substrate-1; *NAFLD*, nonalcoholic fatty liver disease; *VLDL*, very-low-density lipoprotein.

expression of inflammatory cytokines (Guo et al., 2017; Puglisi, Hasty, & Saraswathi, 2011). Besides, EPA- and DHA-derived three-series prostaglandins and thromboxanes and five-series leukotrienes have anti-inflammatory effects to inhibit the production of inflammatory cytokines (Le, Meisel, De Meijer, Gura, & Puder, 2009). Finally, n-3 PUFA intervention could ameliorate NAFLD by reducing TAG synthesis, improving fluidity of cell membrane, and inhibiting the production of pro-inflammatory cytokines.

In summary, the present study demonstrates strong evidence that supplemental n-3 PUFA significantly improves the circulating levels of ALT, AST, and TAG and marginally reduces liver fat content. The findings of this study will have significant implications in the treatment and management of NAFLD. Meanwhile, well-designed RCTs with a large simple size are warranted to be implemented to obtain the optimal dose and duration of n-3 PUFA supplementation for therapy of NAFLD.

References

Araya, J., Rodrigo, R., Videla, L. A., Thielemann, L., Orellana, M., Pettinelli, P., et al. (2004). Increase in long-chain polyunsaturated fatty acid n - 6/n - 3 ratio in relation to hepatic steatosis in patients with nonalcoholic fatty liver disease. *Clinical Science*, 106(6), 635–643. https://doi.org/10.1042/cs20030326.

Argo, C. K., Patrie, J. T., Lackner, C., Henry, T. D., De Lange, E. E., Weltman, A. L., et al. (2015). Effects of n-3 fish oil on metabolic and histological parameters in NASH: A double-blind, randomized, placebo-controlled trial. *Journal of Hepatology, 62*(1), 190–197. https://doi.org/10.1016/j.jhep.2014.08.036.

Bugianesi, E., McCullough, A. J., & Marchesini, G. (2005). Insulin resistance: A metabolic pathway to chronic liver disease. *Hepatology, 42*(5), 987–1000. https://doi.org/10.1002/hep.20920.

Calder, P. C. (2012). Mechanisms of action of (n-3) fatty acids. *The Journal of Nutrition, 142*(3), 592s–599s. https://doi.org/10.3945/jn.111.155259.

Capanni, M., Calella, F., Biagini, M. R., Genise, S., Raimondi, L., Bedogni, G., et al. (2006). Prolonged n-3 polyunsaturated fatty acid supplementation ameliorates hepatic steatosis in patients with non-alcoholic fatty liver disease: A pilot study. *Alimentary Pharmacology & Therapeutics, 23*(8), 1143–1151. https://doi.org/10.1111/j.1365-2036.2006.02885.x.

Carpentier, Y. A., Portois, L., & Malaisse, W. J. (2006). n-3 fatty acids and the metabolic syndrome. *The American Journal of Clinical Nutrition, 83*(6 Suppl), 1499s–1504s. https://doi.org/10.1093/ajcn/83.6.1499S.

Chen, R., Guo, Q., Zhu, W., Xie, Q., Wang, H., & Cai, W. (2008). Therapeutic efficacy of ω-3 polyunsaturated fatty acid capsule in treatment of patients with non-alcoholic fatty liver disease. *World Chinese Journal of Digestology, 18*, 2002–2006.

Chitturi, S., Abeygunasekera, S., Farrell, G. C., Holmes-Walker, J., Hui, J. M., Fung, C., et al. (2002). NASH and insulin resistance: Insulin hypersecretion and specific association with the insulin resistance syndrome. *Hepatology, 35*(2), 373–379. https://doi.org/10.1053/jhep.2002.30692.

Cusi, K. (2009). Role of insulin resistance and lipotoxicity in non-alcoholic steatohepatitis. *Clinics in Liver Disease, 13*(4), 545–563. https://doi.org/10.1016/j.cld.2009.07.009.

Cussons, A. J., Watts, G. F., Mori, T. A., & Stuckey, B. G. (2009). Omega-3 fatty acid supplementation decreases liver fat content in polycystic ovary syndrome: A randomized controlled trial employing proton magnetic resonance spectroscopy. *The Journal of Clinical Endocrinology and Metabolism, 94*(10), 3842–3848. https://doi.org/10.1210/jc.2009-0870.

Dasarathy, S., Dasarathy, J., Khiyami, A., Yerian, L., Hawkins, C., Sargent, R., et al. (2015). Double-blind randomized placebo-controlled clinical trial of omega 3 fatty acids for the treatment of diabetic patients with nonalcoholic steatohepatitis. *Journal of Clinical Gastroenterology, 49*(2), 137–144. https://doi.org/10.1097/mcg.0000000000000099.

Donnelly, K. L., Smith, G. I., Schwarzenberg, S. J., Jessurun, J., Boldt, M. D., & Parks, E. J. (2005). Sources of fatty acids stored in liver and secreted via lipoproteins in patients with nonalcoholic fatty liver disease. *The Journal of Clinical Investigation, 115*(5), 1343–1351. https://doi.org/10.1172/jci23621.

Du Plessis, J., Van Pelt, J., Korf, H., Mathieu, C., Van der Schueren, B., Lannoo, M., et al. (2015). Association of adipose tissue inflammation with histologic severity of nonalcoholic fatty liver disease. *Gastroenterology, 149*(3). https://doi.org/10.1053/j.gastro.2015.05.044. 635–648. e614.

Elizondo, A., Araya, J., Rodrigo, R., Signorini, C., Sgherri, C., Comporti, M., et al. (2008). Effects of weight loss on liver and erythrocyte polyunsaturated fatty acid pattern and oxidative stress status in obese patients with nonalcoholic fatty liver disease. *Biological Research, 41*(1), 59–68.

Fabbrini, E., Mohammed, B. S., Magkos, F., Korenblat, K. M., Patterson, B. W., & Klein, S. (2008). Alterations in adipose tissue and hepatic lipid kinetics in obese men and women with nonalcoholic fatty liver disease. *Gastroenterology, 134*(2), 424–431. https://doi.org/10.1053/j.gastro.2007.11.038.

Ficková, M., Hubert, P., Klimes, I., Staedel, C., Cremel, G., Bohov, P., et al. (1994). Dietary fish oil and olive oil improve the liver insulin receptor tyrosine kinase activity in high sucrose fed rats. *Endocrine Regulations, 28*(4), 187–197.

Gormaz, J. G., Rodrigo, R., Videla, L. A., & Beems, M. (2010). Biosynthesis and bioavailability of long-chain polyunsaturated fatty acids in non-alcoholic fatty liver disease. *Progress in Lipid Research, 49*(4), 407–419. https://doi.org/10.1016/j.plipres.2010.05.003.

Guo, X. F., Gao, J. L., Li, J. M., & Li, D. (2017). Fat-1 mice prevent high-fat plus high-sugar diet-induced non-alcoholic fatty liver disease. *Food & Function, 8*(11), 4053–4061. https://doi.org/10.1039/c7fo01050h.

Guo, X. F., Yang, B., Tang, J., & Li, D. (2018). Fatty acid and non-alcoholic fatty liver disease: Meta-analyses of case-control and randomized controlled trials. *Clinical Nutrition, 37*(1), 113–122. https://doi.org/10.1016/j.clnu.2017.01.003.

Hamaguchi, M., Kojima, T., Takeda, N., Nagata, C., Takeda, J., Sarui, H., et al. (2007). Nonalcoholic fatty liver disease is a novel predictor of cardiovascular disease. *World Journal of Gastroenterology, 13*(10), 1579–1584. https://doi.org/10.3748/wjg.v13.i10.1579.

Janczyk, W., Lebensztejn, D., Wierzbicka-Rucińska, A., Mazur, A., Neuhoff-Murawska, J., Matusik, P., et al. (2015). Omega-3 fatty acids therapy in children with non-alcoholic fatty liver disease: A randomized controlled trial. *The Journal of Pediatrics, 166*(6). https://doi.org/10.1016/j.jpeds.2015.01.056. 1358–1363.e1351-1353.

Jorgensen, R. A. (2003). Nonalcoholic fatty liver disease. *Gastroenterology Nursing, 26*(4), 150–154. quiz 154–155 https://doi.org/10.1097/00001610-200307000-00003.

Kishino, T., Ohnishi, H., Ohtsuka, K., Matsushima, S., Urata, T., Watanabe, K., et al. (2011). Low concentrations of serum n-3 polyunsaturated fatty acids in non-alcoholic fatty liver disease patients with liver injury. *Clinical Chemistry and Laboratory Medicine*, 49(1), 159–162. https://doi.org/10.1515/cclm.2011.020.

Lambert, J. E., Ramos-Roman, M. A., Browning, J. D., & Parks, E. J. (2014). Increased de novo lipogenesis is a distinct characteristic of individuals with nonalcoholic fatty liver disease. *Gastroenterology*, 146(3), 726–735. https://doi.org/10.1053/j.gastro.2013.11.049.

Le, H. D., Meisel, J. A., De Meijer, V. E., Gura, K. M., & Puder, M. (2009). The essentiality of arachidonic acid and docosahexaenoic acid. *Prostaglandins, Leukotrienes, and Essential Fatty Acids*, 81(2–3), 165–170. https://doi.org/10.1016/j.plefa.2009.05.020.

Li, Y. H., Yang, L. H., Sha, K. H., Liu, T. G., Zhang, L. G., & Liu, X. X. (2015). Efficacy of poly-unsaturated fatty acid therapy on patients with nonalcoholic steatohepatitis. *World Journal of Gastroenterology*, 21(22), 7008–7013. https://doi.org/10.3748/wjg.v21.i22.7008.

Lorente-Cebrián, S., Bustos, M., Marti, A., Martinez, J. A., & Moreno-Aliaga, M. (2009). Eicosapentaenoic acid stimulates AMP-activated protein kinase and increases visfatin secretion in cultured murine adipocytes. *Clinical Science (London, England)*, 117(6), 243–249. https://doi.org/10.1042/cs20090020.

Lou, D. J., Zhu, Q. Q., Si, X. W., Guan, L. L., You, Q. Y., Yu, Z. M., et al. (2014). Serum phospholipid omega-3 polyunsaturated fatty acids and insulin resistance in type 2 diabetes mellitus and non-alcoholic fatty liver disease. *Journal of Diabetes and its Complications*, 28(5), 711–714. https://doi.org/10.1016/j.jdiacomp.2014.04.008.

Musso, G., Gambino, R., & Cassader, M. (2009). Recent insights into hepatic lipid metabolism in non-alcoholic fatty liver disease (NAFLD). *Progress in Lipid Research*, 48(1), 1–26. https://doi.org/10.1016/j.plipres.2008.08.001.

Neschen, S., Morino, K., Rossbacher, J. C., Pongratz, R. L., Cline, G. W., Sono, S., et al. (2006). Fish oil regulates adiponectin secretion by a peroxisome proliferator-activated receptor-gamma-dependent mechanism in mice. *Diabetes*, 55(4), 924–928. https://doi.org/10.2337/diabetes.55.04.06.db05-0985.

Parker, H. M., O'Connor, H. T., Keating, S. E., Cohn, J. S., Garg, M. L., Caterson, I. D., et al. (2015). Efficacy of the Omega-3 index in predicting non-alcoholic fatty liver disease in overweight and obese adults: A pilot study. *The British Journal of Nutrition*, 114(5), 780–787. https://doi.org/10.1017/s0007114515002305.

Pettinelli, P., Del Pozo, T., Araya, J., Rodrigo, R., Araya, A. V., Smok, G., et al. (2009). Enhancement in liver SREBP-1c/PPAR-alpha ratio and steatosis in obese patients: Correlations with insulin resistance and n-3 long-chain polyunsaturated fatty acid depletion. *Biochimica et Biophysica Acta*, 1792(11), 1080–1086. https://doi.org/10.1016/j.bbadis.2009.08.015.

Peverill, W., Powell, L. W., & Skoien, R. (2014). Evolving concepts in the pathogenesis of NASH: Beyond steatosis and inflammation. *International Journal of Molecular Sciences*, 15(5), 8591–8638. https://doi.org/10.3390/ijms15058591.

Polyzos, S. A., Toulis, K. A., Goulis, D. G., Zavos, C., & Kountouras, J. (2011). Serum total adiponectin in nonalcoholic fatty liver disease: A systematic review and meta-analysis. *Metabolism*, 60(3), 313–326. https://doi.org/10.1016/j.metabol.2010.09.003.

Puglisi, M. J., Hasty, A. H., & Saraswathi, V. (2011). The role of adipose tissue in mediating the beneficial effects of dietary fish oil. *The Journal of Nutritional Biochemistry*, 22(2), 101–108. https://doi.org/10.1016/j.jnutbio.2010.07.003.

Qin, Y., Zhou, Y., Chen, S. H., Zhao, X. L., Ran, L., Zeng, X. L., et al. (2015). Fish oil supplements lower serum lipids and glucose in correlation with a reduction in plasma fibroblast growth factor 21 and prostaglandin E2 in nonalcoholic fatty liver disease associated with hyperlipidemia: A randomized clinical trial. *PLoS One*, 10(7). https://doi.org/10.1371/journal.pone.0133496, e0133496.

Rinella, M. E. (2015). Nonalcoholic fatty liver disease: A systematic review. *JAMA*, 313(22), 2263–2273. https://doi.org/10.1001/jama.2015.5370.

Rotman, Y., & Sanyal, A. J. (2017). Current and upcoming pharmacotherapy for non-alcoholic fatty liver disease. *Gut*, 66(1), 180–190. https://doi.org/10.1136/gutjnl-2016-312431.

Salem, N., Jr., Litman, B., Kim, H. Y., & Gawrisch, K. (2001). Mechanisms of action of docosahexaenoic acid in the nervous system. *Lipids*, 36(9), 945–959. https://doi.org/10.1007/s11745-001-0805-6.

Sanyal, A. J., Campbell-Sargent, C., Mirshahi, F., Rizzo, W. B., Contos, M. J., Sterling, R. K., et al. (2001). Nonalcoholic steatohepatitis: Association of insulin resistance and mitochondrial abnormalities. *Gastroenterology*, 120(5), 1183–1192. https://doi.org/10.1053/gast.2001.23256.

Scorletti, E., Bhatia, L., McCormick, K. G., Clough, G. F., Nash, K., Hodson, L., et al. (2014). Effects of purified eicosapentaenoic and docosahexaenoic acids in nonalcoholic fatty liver disease: Results from the welcome* study. *Hepatology*, 60(4), 1211–1221. https://doi.org/10.1002/hep.27289.

Scorletti, E., & Byrne, C. D. (2013). Omega-3 fatty acids, hepatic lipid metabolism, and nonalcoholic fatty liver disease. *Annual Review of Nutrition*, 33, 231–248. https://doi.org/10.1146/annurev-nutr-071812-161230.

Sofi, F., Giangrandi, I., Cesari, F., Corsani, I., Abbate, R., Gensini, G. F., et al. (2010). Effects of a 1-year dietary intervention with n-3 polyunsaturated fatty acid-enriched olive oil on non-alcoholic fatty liver disease patients: A preliminary study. *International Journal of Food Sciences and Nutrition*, 61(8), 792–802. https://doi.org/10.3109/09637486.2010.487480.

Spadaro, L., Magliocco, O., Spampinato, D., Piro, S., Oliveri, C., Alagona, C., et al. (2008). Effects of n-3 polyunsaturated fatty acids in subjects with nonalcoholic fatty liver disease. *Digestive and Liver Disease*, *40*(3), 194–199. https://doi.org/10.1016/j.dld.2007.10.003.

Spahis, S., Alvarez, F., Dubois, J., Ahmed, N., Peretti, N., & Levy, E. (2015). Plasma fatty acid composition in French-Canadian children with non-alcoholic fatty liver disease: Effect of n-3 PUFA supplementation. *Prostaglandins, Leukotrienes, and Essential Fatty Acids*, *99*, 25–34. https://doi.org/10.1016/j.plefa.2015.04.010.

Takeuchi, Y., Yahagi, N., Izumida, Y., Nishi, M., Kubota, M., Teraoka, Y., et al. (2010). Polyunsaturated fatty acids selectively suppress sterol regulatory element-binding protein-1 through proteolytic processing and autoloop regulatory circuit. *The Journal of Biological Chemistry*, *285*(15), 11681–11691. https://doi.org/10.1074/jbc.M109.096107.

Targher, G., & Arcaro, G. (2007). Non-alcoholic fatty liver disease and increased risk of cardiovascular disease. *Atherosclerosis*, *191*(2), 235–240. https://doi.org/10.1016/j.atherosclerosis.2006.08.021.

Walle, P., Takkunen, M., Männistö, M., Vaittinen, M., Lankinen, M., Kärjä, V., et al. (2016). Fatty acid metabolism is altered in non-alcoholic steatohepatitis independent of obesity. *Metabolism*, *65*(5), 655–666. https://doi.org/10.1016/j.metabol.2016.01.011.

Welsh, J. A., Karpen, S., & Vos, M. B. (2013). Increasing prevalence of nonalcoholic fatty liver disease among United States adolescents, 1988-1994 to 2007-2010. *The Journal of Pediatrics*, *162*(3), 496–500. https://doi.org/10.1016/j.jpeds.2012.08.043.

Younossi, Z. M., Koenig, A. B., Abdelatif, D., Fazel, Y., Henry, L., & Wymer, M. (2016). Global epidemiology of nonalcoholic fatty liver disease-Meta-analytic assessment of prevalence, incidence, and outcomes. *Hepatology*, *64*(1), 73–84. https://doi.org/10.1002/hep.28431.

Zheng, J. S., Lin, M., Imamura, F., Cai, W., Wang, L., Feng, J. P., et al. (2016). Serum metabolomics profiles in response to n-3 fatty acids in Chinese patients with type 2 diabetes: A double-blind randomised controlled trial. *Scientific Reports*, *6*, 29522. https://doi.org/10.1038/srep29522.

Zheng, J. S., Xu, A., Huang, T., Yu, X., & Li, D. (2012). Low docosahexaenoic acid content in plasma phospholipids is associated with increased non-alcoholic fatty liver disease in China. *Lipids*, *47*(6), 549–556. https://doi.org/10.1007/s11745-012-3671-4.

Zhu, F. S., Liu, S., Chen, X. M., Huang, Z. G., & Zhang, D. W. (2008). Effects of n-3 polyunsaturated fatty acids from seal oils on nonalcoholic fatty liver disease associated with hyperlipidemia. *World Journal of Gastroenterology*, *14*(41), 6395–6400. https://doi.org/10.3748/wjg.14.6395.

Zhu, Q., Lou, D., Si, X., Guan, L., You, Q., Yu, Z., et al. (2010). Serum omega-3 polyunsaturated fatty acid and insulin resistance in type 2 diabetes mellitus and non-alcoholic fatty liver disease. *Zhonghua Nei Ke Za Zhi*, *49*(4), 305–308.

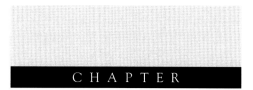

10

Dietary lipids and pulmonary diseases

Zuquan Zou

Beilun District Center for Disease Control and Prevention, Ningbo, Zhejiang, China

10.1 Pulmonary diseases

Pulmonary diseases include a wide spectrum of both neoplastic and nonneoplastic diseases which lead to pulmonary hypofunction. Lung cancer, the neoplastic pulmonary disease, is a major cause of the cancer-related deaths worldwide, and non-small-cell lung cancer alone accounts for a toll of around 85%. Due to the symptom-free nature of early-stage lung cancer, the majority of patients are diagnosed with advanced stage lung cancer. Five-year survival rate is about 5.2% in patients with advanced stage lung cancer with poor prognosis. In 2016, it was estimated that lung cancer has a global prevalence about 2.8 million cases. Lung cancer is the sixth leading causes of death accounting for 1.708 million deaths in 2016. Several risk factors have been correlated with and used as predictors of lung cancer risk. Cigarette smoking is the most dominant risk factor for lung cancer, but additional risk factors such as age, sex, race/ethnicity, family history of lung cancer, chronic obstructive pulmonary disease (COPD), emphysema, radon, and occupational exposure also induce the initiation, development, and progression of lung cancer. However, in the past decades, incidence and mortality rates have begun a continuous decline, particularly in men. These trends parallel changes in the cigarette consumption, the major risk factor for developing lung cancer (Vos et al., 2017).

Nonneoplastic pulmonary diseases include COPD, asthma, pneumonia, and idiopathic pulmonary fibrosis. COPD is defined by the World Health Organization as a common, preventable, and treatable disease that is characterized by persistent respiratory symptoms and an accelerated decline in lung function that is due to airway and/or alveolar abnormalities usually caused by long-term exposure to toxic gas and particles. COPD remains a major public health problem and is a major cause of death and disability worldwide. In 2016, it was estimated globally that there were 251 million COPD individuals (Vogelmeier et al., 2017). COPD has similar symptoms with lung cancer such as cough, shortness of breath, fatigue, and potential weight loss. The main risk factors for development of COPD include exposure to cigarette smoking, work places, or environmental exposure to toxic substances or pollutants (Maurer, 2010). Among these risk factors, cigarette smoking is the single most important causative factor of COPD, and as smoking rates continue to increase in South-East Asia, the burden of COPD will increase for future decades despite medical intervention.

Asthma was defined by an expert panel of the National Institutes of Health as an obstructive airway disease in which the inflammation leads to recurrent symptom of wheezing, breathlessness, chest tightness, and cough in susceptible populations. Patients often have following symptoms such as wheezing, shortness of breath, and sense of suppression in the chest and cough, with or without sputum production. Some patients also are troubled by chest tightness, substernal pressure, chest pain, and nocturnal awakenings. The symptoms are characterized by episodic and of sudden onset (Subbarao, Mandhane, & Sears, 2009; Toop, 1985). The prevalence of asthma is increasing worldwide and remains poorly understood and difficult to manage. The susceptible population is children aged from 1 to 4 years (approximately 900 in 100,000 population) (Duksal, Becerir, Ergin, Akcay, & Guler, 2014; Mattiuzzi & Lippi, 2020). A variety of "triggers" can cause asthma symptoms. Some of common triggers include viral or bacterial infections and respiratory irritants, such as smoking, cold air, laughter, and activation of emotions. Patients may be completely asymptomatic before asthmatic attacks.

Pneumonia is an inflammatory process within the pulmonary parenchyma caused by infectious agents including virus and bacterium that influence normal pulmonary function. Characteristically, the pneumonia patients suffer from symptoms such as cough and shortness of breath. Risk factors for the development of pneumonia include older age, a lot of cigarette smoking, inhalation of dust, alcoholism, asthma, immunosuppression, institutionalization, dementia, seizure disorder, congestive heart failure, peripheral vascular disease, and COPD.

Idiopathic pulmonary fibrosis is a chronic fibrotic interstitial lung disease of unknown etiology and a median survival of 3–6 years after initial diagnosis with a variable clinical course. It more commonly occurs in patients of age range from 50 to 70 years. Prevalence was estimated to be 227.2 per 100,000 among those 75 year or older. A histologic feature of usual interstitial pneumonia is the presence of fibroblastic foci seen in the majority of patients with idiopathic pulmonary fibrosis. This disease is also characterized by parenchymal fibrosis and excess collagen deposition.

10.2 Dietary lipids and clinically manifest asthma

Asthma is characterized by persistent airway inflammation in the absence of significant triggers. Currently, there are contrasting results in observational studies that n-3 polyunsaturated fatty acids (n-3 PUFA) are efficacious in lung function such as forced expiratory volume in the first second (FEV1), respiratory symptoms, or asthma control. Barros et al. showed that higher intakes of n-3 PUFAs, alpha-linolenic acid (ALA), and saturated fatty acids (SFAs) (data ascertained by questionnaire) were associated with good asthma control, whereas a higher ratio of n-6/n-3 PUFA increased the risk for uncontrolled asthma (Barros et al., 2011). In addition, no association between antioxidant vitamins and minerals and controlled asthma was observed. Two studies from Australia reported that dietary fish intake protected against asthma prevalence in children. It was very important because these studies did not depend solely on questionnaire data, but also included an estimation of airway responsiveness. Peat et al. reported that children eating fish more than once a week improved airway responsiveness than did children rarely eating fish (Peat, Salome, & Woolcock, 1992). Intake of fresh fish, and particularly oily fish, showed protective effects against wheeze and asthma (Hodge et al., 1998). Supplementation with n-3 PUFA-rich fish oil in pregnant women decreased the risk of persistent wheeze and asthma in their offspring. It was found that supplement of fish oil in the third trimester of pregnancy was associated with a reduced risk of asthma or nonatopic persistent wheeze in their offspring (Bisgaard et al., 2016). It was also found by Nwaru et al. that high maternal intake of butter and butter spreads and higher ratio of n-6/n-3 PUFAs during pregnancy were linked with an increased risk of allergic rhinitis in their offspring by 5 years of age (Nwaru et al., 2012). A 20-y follow-up cohort of 4162 Americans (age 18–30 y) without a history of asthma showed that intake of n-3 PUFAs was inversely longitudinally associated with asthma incidence in American young adults (Li et al., 2013). In agreement, serum phospholipid levels of DHA, one of n-3 PUFAs, were associated with improved lung function in men but not women. Dihomo-gama-linolenic acid, one of n-6 PUFA and palmitoleic acids and monosaturated fatty acids (MUFAs), were negatively associated with lung function in men but not in women (Kompauer et al., 2008). In agreement with the pro-asthma function of palmitoleic acid observed by Kompauer et al., Rodriguez-Rodriguez et al. in a pediatric study found that palmitoleic acid as well as butter intake was significantly associated with current asthma (Rodríguez-Rodríguez et al., 2010). In addition, in this study, it is shown that SFAs such as myristic acids exert pro-asthma effects, which was not in line with the findings of Barros et al., who demonstrated that SFAs were associated with good asthma control. Scott et al. suggested that plasma SFA and MUFA can be used as important predictors of neutrophilic airway inflammation in asthma (Scott, Gibson, Garg, & Wood, 2011). However, Nakamura et al. demonstrated that no association was observed between asthma diagnosis and any type of fatty acid intake (Nakamura et al., 2013). Furthermore, Broadfield et al. found that n-3 PUFA promoted asthma and n-6 PUFAs reduced the risk of asthma (Broadfield et al., 2004). In agreement with the findings of Broadfield et al., McKeever et al. observed that n-3 PUFA intake is not protective against asthma. High n-6 PUFA intake is associated with reduction of FEV1, notably in smokers. It was even found that consumption of n-3 PUFA and n-6 PUFA is significantly associated with increased prevalence of wheeze (McKeever et al., 2008). The inconsistency of observational studies may be largely explained that fatty acid consumption is estimated by food frequency questionnaires or plasma or cell membrane fatty acid levels. Therefore, it is difficult to calculate the actual levels of fatty acids ingested by the subjects (Table 10.1).

Similarly, there are conflicting results about the prevention of asthma of n-3 PUFA in clinical studies. Fish oil supplementation improved the lung function and decreased the sputum pro-inflammatory mediators compared with placebo and normal diets (Mickleborough et al., 2006). Fish oil supplementation during late pregnancy reduced the risk of asthma and allergic asthma in offspring (Olsen et al., 2008). However, it also was observed that n-3 PUFAs are less efficacious in asthma treatment. For example, a short-term dietary supplementation with n-3 PUFA was not associated with changes in exhaled NO levels, asthma control, or lung function in women with stable asthma (Moreira et al., 2007). Plasma levels of n-3 PUFAs or n-6 PUFAs were not associated with wheeze, eczema, or atopy at age 5 years (Almqvist et al., 2007). Dietary enrichment of n-3 PUFA over 6 months increased the plasma levels of these fatty acids and reduced the stimulated tumor necrosis factor alpha production, but had no effect on the clinical severity of asthma in children aged 8–12 years (Hodge et al., 1998) (Table 10.1). Therefore, the authors found insufficient evidence to change clinical outcomes of asthmatic patients. Considering that asthma is a complex syndrome comprised of diseases with different clinical phenotypes, select asthmatic patients could benefit from taking n-3 PUFA supplements.

10.3 Dietary lipids and pneumonia

It has been known that PUFA regulates inflammation and immunity and 19%–22% of the energy for dietary PUFA (Kris-Etherton

TABLE 10.1 Randomized control trials on fatty acid exposure and pulmonary diseases.

References	Clinical condition	Treatment and length	Primary outcome
Bisgaard et al. (2016)	Wheeze and asthma in their offspring	Treatment group: 736 pregnant women at 24 weeks of gestation received 2.4 g n-3 PUFA (fish oil) per day until delivery; control group: olive oil	n-3 PUFA reduced infection risk of the lower respiratory tract ($P = .033$, CI, 0.58–0.98) and had no effects on asthma exacerbation, eczema, or allergic sensitization
Mickleborough, Lindley, Ionescu, and Fly (2006)	Exercise-induced bronchoconstriction (EIB) in asthmatic patients	Treatment group: 3.2 g EPA and 2.0 DHA (fish oil diet) for 3 weeks; control group: normal diet and placebo diet	Fish oil supplementation improved pulmonary function such as the severity of EIB ($P < .05$). The normal diet (1024; CI, 978–1070), placebo diet (1045.1; CI, 997–1093), and fish oil diet (328.3; 95% CI, 315–342)
Olsen et al. (2008)	Asthma in their offspring	Treatment group: 266 pregnant women at week 30 received 2.7 n-3 PUFA (fish oil capsule) until delivery; control group: olive oil capsule and no oil capsule	The hazard rate of asthma was reduced by 63% (95% CI: 8%, 85%; $P = .03$), and the hazard rate of allergic asthma was reduced by 87% (95% CI: 40%, 97%; $P = .01$) in the fish oil compared with the olive oil group
Moreira et al. (2007)	Asthma	Treatment group: 2 fish oil capsules (455 mg EPA and 325 mg DHA) plus 10 mg vitamin E each, taken once daily for 2 weeks; the placebo group received two capsules of amide daily	Short-term dietary supplementation with n-3 PUFAs in women with stable asthma was not associated with statistically significant changes in FeNO, asthma control, or lung function
Almqvist et al. (2007)	Childhood asthma	Treatment group: 500 mg fish oil capsule (37% n-3 PUFAs); control group: control diet in Australian population	Plasma levels of n-3 or n-6 PUFAs were not associated with wheeze, eczema, or atopy at age 5 years
Hodge et al. (1998)	Childhood asthma	Treatment group: The n-3 group received the maxEPA capsule (0.18 g EPA and 0.12 g DHA), to give a total of 1.2 g n-3 PUFAs per day; placebo capsule (0.45 g safflower, 0.45 palm and 0.1 g olive oil)	n-3 PUFA supplement over 6 months increased plasma levels of these fatty acids, reduced stimulated TNF-α production, but had no effect on the clinical severity of childhood asthma

TABLE 10.1 Randomized control trials on fatty acid exposure and pulmonary diseases.—cont'd

References	Clinical condition	Treatment and length	Primary outcome
Broekhuizen, Wouters, Creutzberg, Weling-Scheepers, and Schols (2005)	Functional status chronic obstructive pulmonary disease (COPD)	Treatment group: Patients received nine capsules daily for 8 weeks, each capsule containing 1 g of either a blend of PUFA or placebo. The daily dosage of PUFA consisted of 3.4 g fatty acids (400 mg stearidonic acid (18:4n-3), 760 mg gamma-linolenic acid (GLA, 18:3n-6), 1200 mg alpha-linolenic acid (18:3n-3), 700 mg EPA, and 340 DHA); the placebo capsules contained 80% palm oil and 20% sunflower oil.	The peak load of the incremental exercise test increased more in the PUFA group than in the placebo group (difference in increase 9.7W (95% CI 2.5–17.0), $P=.009$); the duration of the constant work rate test increased more in patients receiving PUFA (difference in increase 4.3 min (95% CI 0.6–7.9), $P=.023$)
De Vizia et al. (2003)	Cystic fibrosis	Patients took 1 g capsule contained 400 mg EPA, 200 mg DHA, and 10 mg vitamin E for 8 months	n-3 PUFA supplementation significantly decreased serum immunoglobulin G (IgG) and of alpha-1 antitrypsin ($P<.05$) concentrations. n-3 PUFA intervention showed mild but significant improvement of forced expiratory volume (FEV)-1 from 61% ±19% to 57% ±19% of predicted values ($P<.05$)
Olveira et al. (2010)	Cystic fibrosis	Patients received 6 daily capsules of synerbiol for 12 months. Each capsule contained EPA (54 mg), DHA (36 mg), LIN (80 mg), GLA (43 mg), and vitamin E (10 mg)	Low-dose supplements of n-3 and gamma-linolenic fatty acids over a long period (1 year) appears to improve pulmonary status (lung function, respiratory exacerbations, and antibiotic consumption)
Panchaud et al. (2006)	Cystic fibrosis	Patients received PUFA supplementation for 6 months. The volume of supplementation was determined according to patients' weight (570–1710 mg of PUFA mixture); the placebo (placebo) was the same liquid dietary supplement without the PUFA mixture	EPA levels in neutrophil membranes increased following supplement of n-3 PUFAs. EPA supplementation for 6 months did not produce significant changes either in anthropometric parameters or in pulmonary function parameters (FEV1, FVC)

Continued

TABLE 10.1 Randomized control trials on fatty acid exposure and pulmonary diseases.—cont'd

References	Clinical condition	Treatment and length	Primary outcome
Van Der Meij et al. (2012)	Lung cancer	Treatment group: Patients received oral nutritional supplement containing (n-3) fatty acids (2.0 g EPA+0.9 g DHA/d) for 5 weeks; Control group: an isocaloric control oral nutritional supplement without EPA and DHA	The intervention group had a better weight maintenance than the control group (B=1.3 and 1.7 kg, respectively; $P<.05$), a better FFM maintenance after (B=1.5 and 1.9 kg, respectively; $P<.05$), a reduced REE (B=−16.7% of predicted; $P=.01$)
Sánchez-Lara et al. (2014)	Non-small-cell lung cancer	Patients with advanced NSCLC were randomized to receive diet plus oral nutritional supplement containing EPA (ONS-EPA) or only isocaloric diet	Patients receiving the ONS-EPA gained 1.6±5 kg of lean body mass (LBM) compared with a loss of −2.0±6 kg in the control ($P=.01$). Fatigue, loss of appetite, and neuropathy decreased in the ONS-EPA group ($P \leq .05$). There was no difference in response rate or overall survival between groups
Finocchiaro et al. (2012)	Non-small-cell lung cancer	The n-3 group was provided with a daily dose of four capsules containing 510 mg of EPA and 340 mg of DHA, for 66 d; the placebo group with a daily dose of four capsules containing 850 mg of placebo (olive oil)	A significant increase of body weight in the n-3 group at T3v. T0 was observed. C-reactive protein and IL-6 levels differed significantly between the n-3 and placebo groups at T3 and progressively decreased during chemotherapy in the n-3 group

et al., 2000). Increasing intakes of n-3 PUFA reduce inflammation associated with autoimmune diseases, and increased intakes of n-3 and n-6 PUFAs decrease the incidence and duration of infections in children. In the Health Professionals Cohort, 38,378 male participants aged 44–79 years at the outset, during 10 years of follow-up, pneumonia risk was decreased by 31% for every 1-g/d increase in ALA intake. Intakes of EPA and DHA were not significantly associated with pneumonia risk, suggesting that higher intakes of ALA may reduce pneumonia risk (Merchant, Curhan, Rimm, Willett, & Fawzi, 2005). Similarly, Alperovich et al. also investigated the association between fatty acid intake and the risk of community-acquired pneumonia. In the Nurses' Health Study II cohort, 83,165 women aged from 27 to 44 y in 1991, palmitic acid intake increased pneumonia risk, whereas oleic acid (OA) intake was inversely associated with the risk of pneumonia. No significant associations were observed for LA, ALA, or DHA alone. It suggests that high dietary intakes of palmitic acid and possibly DHA and EPA may increase the risk of community-acquired pneumonia in women, whereas higher OA intake may reduce the risk (Alperovich, Neuman, Willett, & Curhan, 2007). Although there are conflicting results in fatty acid dietary interventions of pneumonia, it is important to determine whether specific fatty acids can be used as therapeutic agents to treat pneumonia patients.

10.4 Dietary lipids and chronic obstructive pulmonary disease

Dietary intake is associated with the risk of and progression of chronic obstructive pulmonary disease (COPD). In particular, dietary fatty acids have attracted specific attention for their immunomodulating roles. However, results on the association between fatty acids and COPD are conflicting. Low dietary intake of n-3 PUFA may be a novel reversible risk factor for chronic inflammation and subsequent pulmonary functional decline, in COPD patients, through different mechanisms via cell surface and intracellular receptors controlling inflammatory cell signaling and related gene expression (Deckelbaum, Worgall, & Toru, 2006). Epidemiological evidences (cross-sectional and prospective cohort studies) consistently demonstrate an inverse association between n-3 PUFA intake and inflammation status across different populations including COPD patients (de Batlle et al., 2012). The National Health and Nutrition Examination Survey (NHANES) study showed a protective effect of fish consumption in chronic bronchitis (Schwartz & Weiss, 1994). Furthermore, smoking-related COPD, including bronchitis, emphysema, and spirometrically detected COPD, was inversely associated with the combined supplementation of EPA and DHA in a quantity-dependent fashion in a cross-sectional analysis (Shahar et al., 1994). In the cross-sectional population-based Monitoring Project on Risk Factors and Health in the Netherlands-European Prospective Investigation into Cancer and Nutrition (MORGEN-EPIC) study, it was found that COPD prevalence was correlated negatively with the intake of docosapentaenoic acid (n-3) and docosapentaenoic acid (n-6) and positively with eicosadienoic acid (n-6), eicosatrienoic acid (n-6), arachidonic acid (ARA; n-6), and docosatetraenoic acid (n-6) (McKeever et al., 2008). It was also found that inverse associations existed between dietary PUFA intake and COPD prevalence for Japanese adults, together with significant dose-effect relationship for the breathlessness symptom (Hirayama et al., 2010). These findings demonstrated that the traditional Japanese diet, with a high intake of fish, but a relatively low intake of red meat, may improve lung health and protect against the harmful effects of cigarette. PUFA supplement containing a total dose of

3.4 g PUFA (400 mg stearidonic acid; 760 mg GLA; 1200 mg ALA; 700 mg EPA; 340 mg DHA) was only beneficial to exercise capacity, but not significantly improved pulmonary function and systemic inflammation in COPD patients (Broekhuizen et al., 2005). According to a cross-sectional study of 13,820 adults in the Netherlands, compared with all other (n-6) and (n-3) fatty acids, increased dietary intake of docosapentaenoic acid (n-6) significantly improved lung function (McKeever et al., 2008). Meanwhile, a population-based cohort survey undertaken in seven countries reported a negative relationship between COPD mortality and the supplementation of EPA and DHA, but not total (n-6) and total (n-3) PUFA (Tabak et al., 1998). Further research is required to ascertain the effect of PUFA on COPD and respiratory symptoms and to determine whether increased intakes of PUFA can decrease the COPD mortality rate.

10.5 Dietary lipids and pulmonary fibrosis

It has been found that patients with cystic fibrosis transmembrane conductance regulator mutations had significantly lower levels of LA and DHA in the serum phospholipid than healthy controls (Strandvik, Gronowitz, Enlund, Martinsson, & Wahlström, 2001). The ratio of ARA/DHA was increased in patients with mutations in the cystic fibrosis transmembrane conductance regulator gene (Freedman et al., 2004). Essential fatty acid deficiency, in particularly LA and DHA content, was observed in patients with cystic fibrosis despite an adequate nutritional therapy (Aldámiz-Echevarría et al., 2009). Several clinical trials have suggested that supplementation with PUFA has beneficial effects on lung diseases in patient with cystic fibrosis. Supplementation with fish oil for 4 and 8 months in patients with cystic fibrosis led to an increase in DHA level and a progressive decrease of ARA in erythrocyte membrane phospholipids. Pulmonary function testing showed mild but significant improvement of FEV1 with a decreased inflammation (De Vizia et al., 2003). One-year course of low-dose dietary supplements with a mixture of fatty acids (324 mg of EPA, 216 mg of DHA, 480 mg of LA, and 258 mg of gamma-linolenic acid/day) in adult patients with cystic fibrosis increased serum levels of DHA, total n-3 PUFA, and LA, and more favorable profiles were seen in monoenoic acids, ARA, and the ARA/DHA ratio. Moreover, low-dose supplementation of n-3 PUFA and gamma-linolenic acid over a long period improved pulmonary status (lung function, respiratory exacerbations, and antibiotic consumption) and inflammatory and anthropometric parameters (Olveira et al., 2010). A case–control study found that intake of SFA, MUFA, n-6 PUFA, and meat was independently associated with an increased risk of idiopathic pulmonary fibrosis, whereas intake of cholesterol, n-3 PUFA, fish, eggs, and dairy products was not related to the risk, suggesting that consumption of SFA and meat may increase the risk of idiopathic pulmonary fibrosis (Miyake et al., 2006). However, a double-blind, randomized, crossover without a washout period, and placebo-controlled study with 17 young patients with cystic fibrosis reported that EPA levels in neutrophil membranes increased following supplement of n-3 PUFA for two 6 months (390–1170 mg/day) (Panchaud et al., 2006). It was found that EPA supplementation for 6 months did not produce significant changes either in anthropometric parameters or in pulmonary function parameters (FEV1, FVC). An observational study found that there was no relation of plasma fatty acid composition with pulmonary function, which may be due to essential fatty acid deficiency, particularly in LA and DHA content, despite an adequate nutritional therapy. In this sense, it remains to demonstrate whether supplementation with n-3 PUFA to patients will improve n-3 PUFA deficiency and benefit patients with pulmonary fibrosis (Aldámiz-Echevarría et al., 2009).

10.6 Dietary lipids and lung cancer

The topic about whether n-3 PUFAs help to prevent someone from developing lung cancer is still disputed. Cod liver oil supplements (rich in n-3 PUFA and vitamin A) showed lower risk of lung cancer in 25,956 men and 25,496 women of aged 16–56 years from Norwegian Health Screening between 1977 and 1983, while increased intake of MUFA and PUFA showed an increased risk of lung cancer (Veierød, Laake, & Thelle, 1997). Dietary intake of total PUFA and the ratio of n-6/n-3 PUFA were inversely associated with the risk of lung cancer, highlighting the important role of PUFA intakes against lung cancer from two population-based cohort studies, with a total of 121,970 participants (65,076 women and 56,894 men) (Luu et al., 2018). A recent pooling study with data from 17 case–control and three cohort studies comprising 8,799 cases of lung cancer and 17,072 noncases demonstrated that high supplementation of PUFA was associated with reduced lung cancer risk (Song, Su, Wang, Zhou, & Guo, 2014). However, MacLean et al. found that there was no relationship between n-3 PUFA intake and the incidence of lung cancer (MacLean et al., 2006). A meta-analysis of eight prospective cohort studies (two US, two Japanese, and four European cohorts) also concluded that high PUFA intake was not significantly correlated with the risk of lung cancer (Zhang, Lu, Yu, Gao, & Zhou, 2014). Plasma n-3 PUFAs were lower in lung cancer patients compared with healthy controls, and this difference did not reach statistical significance (Zuijdgeest-Van Leeuwen et al., 2002). These contradicting results shown above suggest that more research is needed to ascertain the association between n-3 PUFA intakes and lung cancer incidence.

Increasing evidences show that n-3 PUFA supplement exerts a beneficial effect on patients with lung cancer. Chemotherapy generally leads patients to suffer from nausea, vomiting, diarrhea, and other ailments, which impair patient nutritional status and overall well-being. It has been demonstrated that about 45%–69% of lung cancer patients suffer from malnutrition associated with adverse reaction to chemotherapy and other cancer therapies (Kiss, Krishnasamy, & Isenring, 2014). Lung cancer patients experience sarcopenia during chemotherapy. Additionally, patients suffering from sarcopenia have been determined to have a low plasma concentration of n-3 PUFA (Murphy, Mourtzakis, Chu, Reiman, & Mazurak, 2010). In general, n-3 PUFA from fish oil has been shown to maintain body weight and improve overall quality of life for lung cancer patients undergoing chemotherapy. Forty patients with stage III NSCLC were randomized to receive two cans per day of a protein- and energy-dense oral nutritional supplement containing n-3 PUFA (2.02 g eicosapentaenoic acid + 0.92 g docosahexaenoic acid per day) or an isocaloric control supplement, during multimodality treatment, n-3 PUFA supplement decreased anorexia, muscle degradation and weight loss in cancer patients, and improve an overall quality of life (Van Der Meij et al., 2012). Serum albumin levels were significantly decreased after surgery. However, patients with an n-3 PUFA-rich diet showed a statistically significant amelioration in albumin loss (Kaya et al., 2016). Nutritional supplements containing EPA promote energy and protein intake accompanied with decreasing fatigue and neuropathy in NSCLC patients who undergo chemotherapy (Sánchez-Lara et al., 2014). Therefore, n-3 PUFA intake shows a promising strategy to benefit patients in post-surgery recovery. Chemoradiotherapy is often accompanied with many severe side effects including nausea, vomiting, poor appetite, anorexia, anemia, and weight loss. These side effects often result in a poor nutritional status and quality of life. It can also lead to treatment-related morbidity and mortality. If this condition cannot be improved in time, it may lead to cancer cachexia. Continual EPA and DHA supplementation can benefit the cachectic therapy in lung cancer patients (Finocchiaro et al., 2012). Supplementation of n-3 PUFA may beneficially affect nutritional status, quality of life, and the physical activity of NSCLC patients who receive multimodality treatment (Kaya et al., 2016).

10.7 How do dietary lipids influence pulmonary diseases?

It is well known that lipids and their mediators are involved in the processes of initiation and resolution of chronic and acute inflammation (Serhan & Levy, 2018). Therefore, lipid mediator lipidomics is an actively developing scientific field. Fatty acids and their metabolites play a crucial role in regulating the persistence and the resolution of inflammation in chronic respiratory diseases. n-3 and n-6 PUFA-derived lipid mediators are closely interrelated with these processes.

10.7.1 The n-6 PUFA-derived pro- and anti-inflammatory lipid mediators

The fatty acid profiles of cell membrane phospholipids have important roles in cell structure and cell function. The fatty acid composition of membrane phospholipids influences the fluidity of the membrane, which in turn modifies the activities and interactions between integral proteins and membrane phospholipids. In addition, some lipid mediators are produced by phospholipases acting on membrane phospholipids upon cellular activation and are substrates of lipid second messengers in signal transduction. Fatty acids can alter intracellular and extracellular signaling pathways via modulation of membrane order, lipid rafts, second messengers, and eicosanoids, which ultimately affect cell function.

ARA is a precursor of parent compounds for production of bioactive eicosanoids. Indeed, ARA is typically the major n-6 PUFA in the membranes of cells involved in inflammation progress in humans. ARA can be converted to eicosanoid mediators as a substrate for cyclooxygenase (COX), lipoxygenase (LOX), and cytochrome P450 enzymes (Saini & Keum, 2018). For example, prostaglandin E_2 (PGE_2) is commonly considered a potent pro-inflammatory lipid mediator and is implicated in several inflammatory diseases including pulmonary diseases. The four-series LTs are also involved in a number of pro-inflammatory processes. Leukotriene B_4 (LTB_4) is a secondary chemoattractant secreted by neutrophils in response to primary chemoattractants such as formyl peptides and plays an important role in initiating inflammation process. LTC_4, LTD_4, and LTE_4, which are produced by mast cells, eosinophils and basophils, also promote inflammatory processes through effecting arteriole and bronchoconstriction and increasing vascular permeability, mucus production, hypersensitivity, and skin dilation. It has been reported that n-3 PUFA incorporated in neutrophil membranes with supplement of n-3 PUFA for two 6 months resulted in a decrease in the ratio of LTB_4/LTB_5, suggesting that, in such conditions, neutrophils may produce less pro-inflammatory lipid mediators derived from the ARA pathway (Panchaud et al., 2006). Supplementation of the diet with EPA (2.7g/day) for 6weeks also reduced LTB_4 levels in the airways, followed by a decrease in the exposure of circulating neutrophils to LTB_4 (Lawrence & Sorrell, 1994; Lawrence & Sorrell, 1993). In addition, EPA supplement led to a significant decrease in sputum and improvements in Schwachman score in patients with cystic fibrosis (Lawrence & Sorrell, 1993). In another study, patients with cystic fibrosis received n-3 ethyl ester concentrate from menhaden oil for 6weeks (100–131mg/kg/day, mean 112.8), and EPA and DHA were incorporated into platelet phospholipids and reduced serum LTB_4 levels

(Kurlandsky, Bennink, Webb, Ulrich, & Baer, 1994), although no statistically significant differences were found in Shwachman-Brasfield scores and FEV1.

It is noteworthy that not all ARA-derived eicosanoids act as pro-inflammatory lipid mediators and that some n-6-derived lipid mediators seem to be vital in inflammation resolution. For example, PGE_2 is generally regarded as being a potent pro-inflammatory mediator; however, it is noteworthy that PGE_2 was shown to function as an anti-inflammatory lipid mediator in certain settings. For example, it also acts as an inhibitor of the production of classical pro-inflammatory cytokines such as tumor necrosis factor (TNF)-α. Furthermore, through induction of 15-LOX, PGE_2 induces the production of lipoxins (LXs) such as LXA_4, which plays a temporal role in inflammation resolution upon acute inflammatory response (Gewirtz et al., 2002). Lipoxins are produced in response to cell–cell interactions. LXA_4 blocks leukocyte migration and activation through several underlying mechanisms including inhibition of transendothelial and transepithelial migration and azurophilic degranulation. LXA_4 administration decreased pulmonary inflammation levels and airway hyperreactivity in a murine model of asthma (Levy et al., 2002). It has been shown that a decrease of LXA_4 relative to cysteinyl leukotrienes in blood, induced sputum, bronchoalveolar lavage fluid, and exhaled breath condensates is correlated with the persistence of inflammation in severe asthma (Planagumà et al., 2008). Besides asthmatic individuals, moderate-to-severe COPD patients also show decreased levels of LXA_4 in exhaled breath condensates (Genehr et al., 2012).

10.7.2 The n-3 PUFA-derived anti-inflammatory lipid mediators

Interest in n-3 PUFA has escalated in recent years because of their vital roles in health promotion and the reduction of disease risk. EPA and ARA are precursors of prostaglandins and leukotrienes. Functional antagonism exists between the prostaglandins and leukotrienes derived from EPA and those derived from ARA. The n-3 PUFA is generally regarded to possess potential antiinflammation. Following dietary enrichment with n-3 PUFA, they partially replace n-6 PUFA especially ARA in cell membranes and shift metabolism away from potent pro-inflammatory ARA-derived eicosanoids toward n-3 PUFA-derived anti-inflammatory lipid mediators. As a result, there is a reduction of PGE_2 metabolites; a decreased production of TXA_2, a potent platelet aggregator, and vasoconstrictor; and a decrease in LTB_4, an inducer of leukocyte chemotaxis, and adherence. On the contrary, PGE_3 metabolites, TXA_3, a weak platelet aggregator and a weak vasoconstrictor; prostacyclin I_3 (PGI_3), a potential vasodilator and inhibitor of platelet aggregation; and LTB_5, a potential chemotactic agent for neutrophils, have been found to increase (Fig. 10.1).

In addition, in active inflammation resolution, these resolving lipids are produced by successive conversion enzymes from ARA (LXA_4), EPA (resolvin E-series), or DHA (resolvin D-series, maresins, or protectins) (Arita et al., 2007). RvE1 and RvE2 are the major members of the E-series resolvins. Resolvins and protectins exhibit potent anti-inflammatory actions. It has been described in a number of reports that RvE1 exerts a powerful protective effect against airway inflammation, particularly in asthma (Haworth, Cernadas, Yang, Serhan, & Levy, 2008). RvD are produced from DHA with the participation of 15- and 5-lipoxygenase (LOX). Currently, six types of RvD (RvD1, RvD2, RvD3, RvD4, RvD5, and RvD6) are known to synthesize from the intermediate product 17S-hydroperoxy-DHA. Reduced mucosal levels of DHA were observed in asthma and cystic fibrosis, which would adversely affect the production of DHA-derived specialized pro-resolving mediators such as D-series resolvins, maresins, and protectins (Freedman et al.,

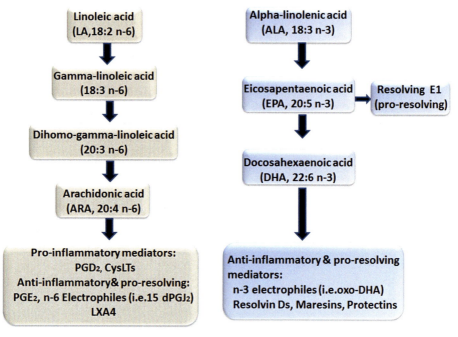

FIG. 10.1   Lipid mediators derived from n-6 and n-3 PUFA.

2004). The 17S-hydroxy-4Z,7Z,10Z,13Z,15E,19Z-DHA (17R/S-HDHA), RvD1, and RvD2 levels significantly increased in human blood with oral n-3 PUFA supplementation. The peroral administration of n-3 PUFA combined with low doses of aspirin promoted the conversion of EPA and DHA to RvD (Serhan & Levy, 2018). Recent studies have shown good prospects for using of RvD3 and aspirin-triggered (AT)-RvD3 in pulmonology (Colby et al., 2016). DHA is converted resolving exudates into another new family of mediators named protectins. Protectins are also involved in protective activity in inflammation resolution. Protectin D1 has the most potential anti-inflammation activity. The other natural protectin D isomers have different double-bond configurations and are less capable of attenuating neutrophil recruitment and inflammation. The presence of PD1 in the airways of normal human subjects has been documented in condensates of exhaled breath, whereas decreased PD1 levels below the detection limit in severe and uncontrolled asthma were observed (Levy et al., 2007). Decreased levels of PD1 and 15-HETE, a 15-lipoxygenase metabolite of ARA, were observed, by stimulated peripheral blood eosinophils from patients with severe asthma, suggesting an impaired activity of 15-LOX in severe asthma (Miyata et al., 2013). Interestingly, in asthmatic patients, it was found that decreased protectin D1 potentially reduces both airway inflammation and hyperreactivity (Levy et al., 2007). Therefore, it suggests that pro-resolution lipid mediators may have roles in both physiologic and pathophysiologic processes in specific tissues. Maresins are biosynthesized from DHA and newly described macrophage-derived mediators of inflammation (Serhan et al., 2009). Maresins are lipids produced by macrophages via initial lipoxygenation at the carbon 14 position of DHA by the insertion of molecular oxygen followed by epoxidation and oxygen incorporation at the carbon 7 position from a molecule of H_2O, producing a

13S, 14S-epoxide-maresin intermediate which is enzymatically converted to maresin family members maresin 1, maresin 2, and maresin conjugate in tissue regeneration.

Maresin 1 as a specialized pro-resolving lipid mediator produced during the resolution of airway inflammation associated with acute and repetitive exposure to organic dust by activating protein kinase C (PKC) isoforms α and ε; inhibiting neutrophil infiltration; and reducing IL-6, TNF-α, and chemokine C-X-C motif ligand 1 levels (Romano et al., 1993). Maresin 1 also exhibits novel mechanisms in inflammation resolution, which can block pro-inflammatory mediator production by LTA_4 hydrolase and can impede arachidonate conversion by human 12-LOX, rather than merely terminating the recruitment of phagocytes. These studies suggest maresins can be used as promising new therapeutic agents for treating pulmonary inflammation-related diseases.

In addition, n-3 PUFA supplementation during pregnancy was associated with an increase in specialized pro-resolving mediator precursors including 18-HEPE derived from EPA and 17-HDHA derived from DHA in the offspring at birth (See et al., 2017). The level of EPA was decreased by twofold and the ratio of ARA/EPA was increased by threefold in COPD patients (Novgorodtseva et al., 2013). Meantime, an increase of LA-derived lipid mediators was observed in a female-dominated subphenotype of COPD (Balgoma et al., 2016). These studies have shown that chronic respiratory disease development is correlated with the disturbance of the fatty acid composition in erythrocyte membranes or serum and the unbalanced ratio between precursors of pro- and antiinflammatory lipid mediators (Fig. 10.1).

10.7.3 Polyunsaturated fatty acids and immunity regulation

The immune system, including its inflammatory components, is fundamental to host defense against pathogenic invaders by activation of T cells with clonal expansion (proliferation) and release of cytokines that perform effector cell functions such as antibody production and killing cell activity. Inappropriate immunologic activity, including inflammation, is tightly associated with many common human disorders. The earliest research on the role of fatty acids on immunity started in the 1970s by comparing the effects of SFA and LA (Meade & Mertin, 1978). The immunity regulatory role of fatty acids involved modifications of membrane order and modulation of eicosanoid production, both driven by alterations of the fatty acid composition of the phospholipids within membranes of inflammatory and immune cells. The first study about effects of n-3 PUFA on inflammation and immunity was reported in the 1980s (Leslie et al., 1985); to this day, the effects of n-3 PUFA on aspects of inflammation and immunity have been extensively investigated. The n-3 PUFA has been demonstrated to influence the functions of a range of cell types including T cells and other immune cells, to modulate the expression levels of key cell surface membrane proteins, and to regulate the production of reactive oxygen species, eicosanoids, and cytokines (Kew et al., 2003; Yaqoob, Newsholme, & Calder, 1995).

Modulation of the immune response varies according to fatty acid type. SFAs such as palmitate elicit a more potent effect on toll-like receptor 2 (TLR2) activation than unsaturated fatty acids, while n-3 PUFAs are inhibitory or show no effect. In asthma, several studies have demonstrated a reduction in inflammation due to n-3 PUFA supplementation, including a decrease in LTB_4 (Broughton, Johnson, Pace, Liebman, & Kleppinger, 1997), TBX_2 (Picado et al., 1988), and TNF-a (Hodge et al., 1998). EPA supplement did not alter neutrophil or monocyte phagocytosis, monocyte respiratory burst, or the production of inflammatory cytokines by mononuclear cells in the young or older men. EPA treatment resulted in a dose-dependent reduction in neutrophil respiratory burst only in the older men (Rees et al., 2006).

In a placebo-controlled, double-blind, parallel study with a total of 150 healthy men and women aged 25–72 years also observed that supplementation of 9.5 g ALA/d or 1.7 g EPA +DHA/d does not impact the functional activity of neutrophils, monocytes, or lymphocytes, although the fatty acid profiles of mononuclear cells were altered (Kew et al., 2003). In this sense, although there is a strongly held belief that dietary PUFA significantly affects human health, in part by regulating the immune system, the data from human clinical trials with patients suffering from inflammatory or immune-mediated diseases fail to support that PUFAs are efficacious at altering the clinical outcomes of these diseases. Accounting for that inherent (genetic) variation affects individual responsiveness to nutrient modulation of immune and inflammatory responses, future studies in this field should focus on identifying and clarifying genotype-PUFA response interactions at the level of the immune system.

10.8 Conclusion

Dietary lipids play a crucial role in the development and resolution of inflammation relevant to the pathophysiology of pulmonary diseases. Although results from epidemiologic studies and RCT are conflicting between fatty acid consumption and the outcomes of pulmonary diseases, there is emerging need to understand the physiology and molecular basis of dietary lipids and determine whether specific fatty acids can be used as adjuvant therapeutic agents in treating pulmonary diseases or, more importantly, to determine which type of pulmonary diseases would gain the greatest benefit.

References

Aldámiz-Echevarría, L., José, A. P., Fernando, A., Javier, E., Amaia, S., Sergio, L., et al. (2009). Persistence of essential fatty acid deficiency in cystic fibrosis despite nutritional therapy. *Pediatric Research*, 66(5), 585–589. https://doi.org/10.1203/PDR.0b013e3181b4e8d3.

Almqvist, C., Garden, F., Xuan, W., Mihrshahi, S., Leeder, S. R., Oddy, W., et al. (2007). Omega-3 and omega-6 fatty acid exposure from early life does not affect atopy and asthma at age 5 years. *Journal of Allergy and Clinical Immunology*, 119(6), 1438–1444. https://doi.org/10.1016/j.jaci.2007.01.046.

Alperovich, M., Neuman, M. I., Willett, W. C., & Curhan, G. C. (2007). Fatty acid intake and the risk of community-acquired pneumonia in U.S. women. *Nutrition*, 23(3), 196–202. https://doi.org/10.1016/j.nut.2006.11.007.

Arita, M., Ohira, T., Sun, Y. P., Elangovan, S., Chiang, N., & Serhan, C. N. (2007). Resolvin E1 selectively interacts with leukotriene B4 receptor BLT1 and ChemR23 to regulate inflammation. *Journal of Immunology*, 178(6), 3912–3917. https://doi.org/10.4049/jimmunol.178.6.3912.

Balgoma, D., Yang, M., Sjödin, M., Snowden, S., Karimi, R., Levänen, B., et al. (2016). Linoleic acid-derived lipid mediators increase in a female-dominated subphenotype of COPD. *European Respiratory Journal*, 47(6), 1645–1656. https://doi.org/10.1183/13993003.01080-2015.

Barros, R., Moreira, A., Fonseca, J., Delgado, L., Graça Castel-Branco, M., Haahtela, T., et al. (2011). Dietary intake of α-linolenic acid and low ratio of n-6:n-3 PUFA are associated with decreased exhaled NO and improved asthma control. *British Journal of Nutrition*, 106(3), 441–450. https://doi.org/10.1017/S0007114511000328.

de Batlle, J., Sauleda, J., Balcells, E., Gómez, F. P., Méndez, M., Rodriguez, E., et al. (2012). Association between Ω3 and Ω6 fatty acid intakes and serum inflammatory markers in COPD. *Journal of Nutritional Biochemistry*, 23(7), 817–821. https://doi.org/10.1016/j.jnutbio.2011.04.005.

Bisgaard, H., Stokholm, J., Chawes, B. L., Vissing, N. H., Bjarnadóttir, E., Schoos, A. M. M., et al. (2016). Fish oil-derived fatty acids in pregnancy and wheeze and asthma in offspring. *New England Journal of Medicine*, 375(26), 2530–2539. https://doi.org/10.1056/NEJMoa1503734.

Broadfield, E. C., McKeever, T. M., Whitehurst, A., Lewis, S. A., Lawson, N., Britton, J., et al. (2004). A case-control study of dietary and erythrocyte membrane fatty acids in asthma. *Clinical and Experimental Allergy*, 34(8), 1232–1236. https://doi.org/10.1111/j.1365-2222.2004.02032.x.

Broekhuizen, R., Wouters, E. F. M., Creutzberg, E. C., Weling-Scheepers, C. A. P. M., & Schols, A. M. W. J. (2005). Polyunsaturated fatty acids improve exercise capacity in chronic obstructive pulmonary disease. *Thorax*, 60(5), 376–382. https://doi.org/10.1136/thx.2004.030858.

Broughton, K. S., Johnson, C. S., Pace, B. K., Liebman, M., & Kleppinger, K. M. (1997). Reduced asthma symptoms with n-3 fatty acid ingestion are related to 5-series leukotriene production. *American Journal of Clinical Nutrition*,

65(4), 1011–1017. https://doi.org/10.1093/ajcn/65.4.1011.

Colby, J. K., Abdulnour, R. E. E., Sham, H. P., Dalli, J., Colas, R. A., Winkler, J. W., et al. (2016). Resolvin D3 and aspirin-triggered resolvin D3 are protective for injured epithelia. *American Journal of Pathology, 186*(7), 1801–1813. https://doi.org/10.1016/j.ajpath.2016.03.011.

De Vizia, B., Raia, V., Spano, C., Pavlidis, C., Coruzzo, A., & Alessio, M. (2003). Effect of an 8-month treatment with ω-3 fatty acids (eicosapentaenoic and docosahexaenoic) in patients with cystic fibrosis. *Journal of Parenteral and Enteral Nutrition, 27*(1), 52–57. https://doi.org/10.1177/014860710302700152.

Deckelbaum, R. J., Worgall, T. S., & Toru, S. (2006). n-3 Fatty acids and gene expression. *American Journal of Clinical Nutrition, 6*, 1520S–1525S. https://doi.org/10.1093/ajcn/83.6.1520S.

Duksal, F., Becerir, T., Ergin, A., Akcay, A., & Guler, N. (2014). The prevalence of asthma diagnosis and symptoms is still increasing in early adolescents in Turkey. *Allergology International, 63*(2), 189–197. https://doi.org/10.2332/allergolint.13-OA-0612.

Finocchiaro, C., Segre, O., Fadda, M., Monge, T., Scigliano, M., Schena, M., et al. (2012). Effect of n-3 fatty acids on patients with advanced lung cancer: A double-blind, placebo-controlled study. *British Journal of Nutrition, 108*(2), 327–333. https://doi.org/10.1017/S0007114511005551.

Freedman, S. D., Blanco, P. G., Zaman, M. M., Shea, J. C., Ollero, M., Hopper, I. K., et al. (2004). Association of cystic fibrosis with abnormalities in fatty acid metabolism. *New England Journal of Medicine, 350*(6), 560–569. https://doi.org/10.1056/NEJMoa021218.

Genehr, F. L., Martin, P., Tadday, R. M., Frances, S., Mayer, B., Chapman, K. R., et al. (2012). Profile of eicosanoids in breath condensate in asthma and COPD. *Journal of Breath Research*, 026001. https://doi.org/10.1088/1752-7155/6/2/026001.

Gewirtz, A. T., Collier-Hyams, L. S., Young, A. N., Kucharzik, T., Guilford, W. J., Parkinson, J. F., et al. (2002). Lipoxin A4 analogs attenuate induction of intestinal epithelial proinflammatory gene expression and reduce the severity of dextran sodium sulfate-induced colitis. *Journal of Immunology, 168*(10), 5260–5267. https://doi.org/10.4049/jimmunol.168.10.5260.

Haworth, O., Cernadas, M., Yang, R., Serhan, C. N., & Levy, B. D. (2008). Resolvin E1 regulates interleukin 23, interferon-γ and lipoxin A4 to promote the resolution of allergic airway inflammation. *Nature Immunology, 9*(8), 873–879. https://doi.org/10.1038/ni.1627.

Hirayama, F., Lee, A. H., Binns, C. W., Hiramatsu, N., Mori, M., & Nishimura, K. (2010). Dietary intake of isoflavones and polyunsaturated fatty acids associated with lung function, breathlessness and the prevalence of chronic obstructive pulmonary disease: Possible protective effect of traditional Japanese diet. *Molecular Nutrition & Food Research, 54*(7), 909–917. https://doi.org/10.1002/mnfr.200900316.

Hodge, L., Salome, C. M., Hughes, J. M., Liu-Brennan, D., Rimmer, J., Allman, M., et al. (1998). Effect of dietary intake of omega-3 and omega-6 fatty acids on severity of asthma in children. *European Respiratory Journal, 11*(2), 361–365. https://doi.org/10.1183/09031936.98.11020361.

Kaya, S. O., Akcam, T. I., Ceylan, K. C., Samancllar, O., Ozturk, O., & Usluer, O. (2016). Is preoperative protein-rich nutrition effective on postoperative outcome in non-small cell lung cancer surgery? A prospective randomized study. *Journal of Cardiothoracic Surgery, 11*(1). https://doi.org/10.1186/s13019-016-0407-1.

Kew, S., Banerjee, T., Minihane, A. M., Finnegan, Y. E., Muggli, R., Albers, R., et al. (2003). Lack of effect of foods enriched with plant- or marine-derived n-3 fatty acids on human immune function. *American Journal of Clinical Nutrition, 77*(5), 1287–1295. https://doi.org/10.1093/ajcn/77.5.1287.

Kiss, N. K., Krishnasamy, M., & Isenring, E. A. (2014). The effect of nutrition intervention in lung cancer patients undergoing chemotherapy and/or radiotherapy: A systematic review. *Nutrition and Cancer, 66*(1), 47–56. https://doi.org/10.1080/01635581.2014.847966.

Kompauer, I., Demmelmair, H., Koletzko, B., Bolte, G., Linseisen, J., & Heinrich, J. (2008). Association of fatty acids in serum phospholipids with lung function and bronchial hyperresponsiveness in adults. *European Journal of Epidemiology, 23*(3), 175–190. https://doi.org/10.1007/s10654-007-9218-y.

Kris-Etherton, P. M., Taylor, D. S., Yu-Poth, S., Huth, P., Moriarty, K., Fishell, V., et al. (2000). Polyunsaturated fatty acids in the food chain in the United States. *American Journal of Clinical Nutrition, 71*(1). https://doi.org/10.1093/ajcn/71.1.179s. American Society for Nutrition.

Kurlandsky, L. E., Bennik, M. R., Webb, P. M., Ulrich, P. J., & Baer, L. J. (1994). The absorption and effect of dietary supplementation with omega-3 fatty acids on serum leukotriene B4, in patients with cystic fibrosis. *Pediatric Pulmonology, 18*(4), 211–217. https://doi.org/10.1002/ppul.1950180404.

Lawrence, R., & Sorrell, T. (1993). Eicosapentaenoic acid in cystic fibrosis: Evidence of a pathogenetic role for leukotriene B4. *The Lancet, 342*(8869), 465–469. https://doi.org/10.1016/0140-6736(93)91594-C.

Lawrence, R. H., & Sorrell, T. C. (1994). Eicosapentaenoic acid modulates neutrophil leukotriene B4 receptor expression in cystic fibrosis. *Clinical and Experimental Immunology, 98*(1), 12–16. https://doi.org/10.1111/j.1365-2249.1994.tb06599.x.

Leslie, C. A., Gonnerman, W. A., David Ullman, M., Hayes, K. C., Franzblau, C., & Cathcart, E. S. (1985). Dietary fish oil modulates macrophage fatty acids and decreases arthritis susceptibility in mice. *Journal of Experimental Medicine*, *162*(4), 1336–1349. https://doi.org/10.1084/jem.162.4.1336.

Levy, B. D., De Sanctis, G. T., Devchand, P. R., Kim, E., Ackerman, K., Schmidt, B. A., et al. (2002). Multi-pronged inhibition of airway hyper-responsiveness and inflammation by lipoxin A4. *Nature Medicine*, *8*(9), 1018–1023. https://doi.org/10.1038/nm748.

Levy, B. D., Kohli, P., Gotlinger, K., Haworth, O., Hong, S., Kazani, S., et al. (2007). Protectin D1 is generated in asthma and dampens airway inflammation and hyperresponsiveness. *Journal of Immunology*, *178*(1), 496–502. https://doi.org/10.4049/jimmunol.178.1.496.

Li, J., Xun, P., Zamora, D., Sood, A., Liu, K., Daviglus, M., et al. (2013). Intakes of long-chain omega-3 (n-3) PUFAs and fish in relation to incidence of asthma among American young adults: The CARDIA study. *American Journal of Clinical Nutrition*, *97*(1), 173–178. https://doi.org/10.3945/ajcn.112.041145.

Luu, H. N., Cai, H., Murff, H. J., Xiang, Y. B., Cai, Q., Li, H., et al. (2018). A prospective study of dietary polyunsaturated fatty acids intake and lung cancer risk. *International Journal of Cancer*, *143*(9), 2225–2237. https://doi.org/10.1002/ijc.31608.

MacLean, C. H., Newberry, S. J., Mojica, W. A., Khanna, P., Issa, A. M., Suttorp, M. J., et al. (2006). Effects of omega-3 fatty acids on cancer risk: A systematic review. *Journal of the American Medical Association*, *295*(4), 403–415. https://doi.org/10.1001/jama.295.4.403.

Mattiuzzi, C., & Lippi, G. (2020). Worldwide asthma epidemiology: Insights from the Global Health Data Exchange database. In *Vol. 10. International Forum of Allergy and Rhinology* (pp. 75–80). https://doi.org/10.1002/alr.22464. 1.

Maurer, J. R. (2010). The natural history of chronic airflow obstruction revisited: An analysis of the Framingham offspring cohort. In *Yearbook of Pulmonary Disease* (pp. 80–82). https://doi.org/10.1016/s8756-3452(09)79330-2.

McKeever, T. M., Lewis, S. A., Cassano, P. A., Ocké, M., Burney, P., Britton, J., et al. (2008). The relation between dietary intake of individual fatty acids, FEV 1 and respiratory disease in Dutch adults. *Thorax*, *63*(3), 208–214. https://doi.org/10.1136/thx.2007.090399.

Meade, C. J., & Mertin, J. (1978). Fatty acids and immunity. *Advances in Lipid Research*, *16*, 127–165. https://doi.org/10.1016/b978-0-12-024916-9.50008-1.

Merchant, A. T., Curhan, G. C., Rimm, E. B., Willett, W. C., & Fawzi, W. W. (2005). Intake of n-6 and n-3 fatty acids and fish and risk of community-acquired pneumonia in US men. *American Journal of Clinical Nutrition*, *82*(3), 668–674. https://doi.org/10.1093/ajcn/82.3.668.

Mickleborough, T. D., Lindley, M. R., Ionescu, A. A., & Fly, A. D. (2006). Protective effect of fish oil supplementation on exercise-induced bronchoconstriction in asthma. *Chest*, *129*(1), 39–49. https://doi.org/10.1378/chest.129.1.39.

Miyake, Y., Sasaki, S., Yokoyama, T., Chida, K., Azuma, A., Suda, T., et al. (2006). Dietary fat and meat intake and idiopathic pulmonary fibrosis: A case-control study in Japan. *The International Journal of Tuberculosis and Lung Disease*, *10*(3), 333–339.

Miyata, J., Fukunaga, K., Iwamoto, R., Isobe, Y., Niimi, K., Takamiya, R., et al. (2013). Dysregulated synthesis of protectin D1 in eosinophils from patients with severe asthma. *Journal of Allergy and Clinical Immunology*, *131*(2), 353–e2. https://doi.org/10.1016/j.jaci.2012.07.048.

Moreira, A., Moreira, P., Delgado, L., Fonseca, J., Teixeira, V., Padrão, P., et al. (2007). Pilot study of the effects of n-3 polyunsaturated fatty acids on exhaled nitric oxide in patients with stable asthma. *Journal of Investigational Allergology and Clinical Immunology*, *17*(5), 309–313. http://www.jiaci.org/issues/vol17issue05/5.pdf.

Murphy, R. A., Mourtzakis, M., Chu, Q. S., Reiman, T., & Mazurak, V. C. (2010). Skeletal muscle depletion is associated with reduced plasma (n-3) fatty acids in non-small cell lung cancer patients. *Journal of Nutrition*, *140*(9), 1602–1606. https://doi.org/10.3945/jn.110.123521.

Nakamura, K., Wada, K., Sahashi, Y., Tamai, Y., Tsuji, M., Watanabe, K., et al. (2013). Associations of intake of antioxidant vitamins and fatty acids with asthma in preschool children. *Public Health Nutrition*, *16*(11), 2040–2045. https://doi.org/10.1017/S1368980012004363.

Novgorodtseva, T. P., Denisenko, Y. K., Zhukova, N. V., Antonyuk, M. V., Knyshova, V. V., & Gvozdenko, T. A. (2013). Modification of the fatty acid composition of the erythrocyte membrane in patients with chronic respiratory diseases. *Lipids in Health and Disease*, *12*(1). https://doi.org/10.1186/1476-511X-12-117.

Nwaru, B. I., Erkkola, M., Lumia, M., Kronberg-Kippilä, C., Ahonen, S., Kaila, M., et al. (2012). Maternal intake of fatty acids during pregnancy and allergies in the offspring. *British Journal of Nutrition*, *108*(4), 720–732. https://doi.org/10.1017/S0007114511005940.

Olsen, S. F., Østerdal, M. L., Salvig, J. D., Mortensen, L. M., Rytter, D., Secher, N. J., et al. (2008). Fish oil intake compared with olive oil intake in late pregnancy and asthma in the offspring: 16 y of registry-based follow-up from a randomized controlled trial. *American Journal of Clinical Nutrition*, *88*(1), 167–175. https://doi.org/10.1093/ajcn/88.1.167.

Olveira, G., Olveira, C., Acosta, E., Espíldora, F., Garrido-Sánchez, L., García-Escobar, E., et al. (2010). La suplementación con ácidos grasos mejora parámetros respiratorios, inflamatorios y nutricionales en adultos con fibrosis quística. *Archivos de Bronconeumología*, *46*(2), 70–77. https://doi.org/10.1016/S1579-2129(10)70018-5.

Panchaud, A., Sauty, A., Kernen, Y., Decosterd, L. A., Buclin, T., Boulat, O., et al. (2006). Biological effects of a dietary omega-3 polyunsaturated fatty acids supplementation in cystic fibrosis patients: A randomized, crossover placebo-controlled trial. *Clinical Nutrition*, 25(3), 418–427. https://doi.org/10.1016/j.clnu.2005.10.011.

Peat, J. K., Salome, C. M., & Woolcock, A. J. (1992). Factors associated with bronchial hyperresponsiveness in Australian adults and children. *European Respiratory Journal*, 5(8), 921–929.

Picado, C., Castillo, J. A., Schinca, N., Pujades, M., Ordinas, A., Coronas, A., et al. (1988). Effects of a fish oil enriched diet on apirin intolerant asthmatic patients: A pilot study. *Thorax*, 43(2), 93–97. https://doi.org/10.1136/thx.43.2.93.

Planagumà, A., Kazani, S., Marigowda, G., Haworth, O., Mariani, T. J., Israel, E., et al. (2008). Airway lipoxin A4 generation and lipoxin A4 receptor expression are decreased in severe asthma. *American Journal of Respiratory and Critical Care Medicine*, 178(6), 574–582. https://doi.org/10.1164/rccm.200801-061OC.

Rees, D., Miles, E. A., Banerjee, T., Wells, S. J., Roynette, C. E., Wahle, K. W. J., et al. (2006). Dose-related effects of eicosapentaenoic acid on innate immune function in healthy humans: A comparison of young and older men. *American Journal of Clinical Nutrition*, 83(2), 331–342. https://doi.org/10.1093/ajcn/83.2.331.

Rodríguez-Rodríguez, E., Perea, J. M., Jiménez, A. I., Rodríguez-Rodríguez, P., López-Sobaler, A. M., & Ortega, R. M. (2010). Fat intake and asthma in Spanish schoolchildren. *European Journal of Clinical Nutrition*, 64(10), 1065–1071. https://doi.org/10.1038/ejcn.2010.127.

Romano, M., Chen, X. S., Takahashi, Y., Yamamoto, S., Funk, C. D., & Serhan, C. N. (1993). Lipoxin synthase activity of human platelet 12-lipoxygenase. *Biochemical Journal*, 296(1), 127–133. https://doi.org/10.1042/bj2960127.

Saini, R. K., & Keum, Y. S. (2018). Omega-3 and omega-6 polyunsaturated fatty acids: Dietary sources, metabolism, and significance—A review. *Life Sciences*, 203, 255–267. https://doi.org/10.1016/j.lfs.2018.04.049.

Sánchez-Lara, K., Turcott, J. G., Juárez-Hernández, E., Nuñez-Valencia, C., Villanueva, G., Guevara, P., et al. (2014). Effects of an oral nutritional supplement containing eicosapentaenoic acid on nutritional and clinical outcomes in patients with advanced non-small cell lung cancer: RANDOMISED trial. *Clinical Nutrition*, 33(6), 1017–1023. https://doi.org/10.1016/j.clnu.2014.03.006.

Schwartz, J., & Weiss, S. T. (1994). The relationship of dietary fish intake to level of pulmonary function in the first National Health and Nutrition Survey (NHANES I). *European Respiratory Journal*, 7(10), 1821–1824. https://doi.org/10.1183/09031936.94.07101821.

Scott, H. A., Gibson, P. G., Garg, M. L., & Wood, L. G. (2011). Airway inflammation is augmented by obesity and fatty acids in asthma. *European Respiratory Journal*, 38(3), 594–602. https://doi.org/10.1183/09031936.00139810.

See, V. H. L., Mas, E., Prescott, S. L., Beilin, L. J., Burrows, S., Barden, A. E., et al. (2017). Effects of prenatal n-3 fatty acid supplementation on offspring resolvins at birth and 12 years of age: A double-blind, randomised controlled clinical trial. *British Journal of Nutrition*, 118(11), 971–980. https://doi.org/10.1017/S0007114517002914.

Serhan, C. N., & Levy, B. D. (2018). Resolvins in inflammation: Emergence of the pro-resolving superfamily of mediators. *Journal of Clinical Investigation*, 128(7), 2657–2669. https://doi.org/10.1172/JCI97943.

Serhan, C. N., Yang, R., Martinod, K., Kasuga, K., Pillai, P. S., Porter, T. F., et al. (2009). Maresins: Novel macrophage mediators with potent antiinflammatory and proresolving actions. *Journal of Experimental Medicine*, 206(1), 15–23. https://doi.org/10.1084/jem.20081880.

Shahar, E., Folsom, A. R., Melnick, S. L., Tockman, M. S., Comstock, G. W., Gennaro, V., et al. (1994). Dietary n-3 polyunsaturated fatty acids and smoking-related chronic obstructive pulmonary disease. *New England Journal of Medicine*, 331(4), 228–233. https://doi.org/10.1056/NEJM199407283310403.

Song, J., Su, H., Wang, B. L., Zhou, Y. Y., & Guo, L. L. (2014). Fish consumption and lung cancer risk: Systematic review and meta-analysis. *Nutrition and Cancer*, 66(4), 539–549. https://doi.org/10.1080/01635581.2014.894102.

Strandvik, B., Gronowitz, E., Enlund, F., Martinsson, T., & Wahlström, J. (2001). Essential fatty acid deficiency in relation to genotype in patients with cystic fibrosis. *Journal of Pediatrics*, 139(5), 650–655. https://doi.org/10.1067/mpd.2001.118890.

Subbarao, P., Mandhane, P. J., & Sears, M. R. (2009). Asthma: Epidemiology, etiology and risk factors. *CMAJ*, 181(9), E181–E190. https://doi.org/10.1503/cmaj.080612.

Tabak, C., Feskens, E. J. M., Heederik, D., Kromhout, D., Menotti, A., & Blackburn, H. W. (1998). Fruit and fish consumption: A possible explanation for population differences in COPD mortality (The Seven Countries Study). *European Journal of Clinical Nutrition*, 52(11), 819–825. https://doi.org/10.1038/sj.ejcn.1600653.

Toop, L. J. (1985). Active approach to recognising asthma in general practice. *BMJ*, 290(6482), 1629–1631. https://doi.org/10.1136/bmj.290.6482.1629.

Van Der Meij, B. S., Langius, J. A. E., Spreeuwenberg, M. D., Slootmaker, S. M., Paul, M. A., Smit, E. F., et al. (2012). Oral nutritional supplements containing n-3 polyunsaturated fatty acids affect quality of life and functional status in lung cancer patients during multimodality treatment:

An RCT. *European Journal of Clinical Nutrition*, *66*(3), 399–404. https://doi.org/10.1038/ejcn.2011.214.

Veierød, M. B., Laake, P., & Thelle, D. S. (1997). Dietary fat intake and risk of lung cancer: A prospective study of 51,452 Norwegian men and women. *European Journal of Cancer Prevention*, *6*(6), 540–549. https://doi.org/10.1097/00008469-199712000-00009.

Vogelmeier, C. F., Criner, G. J., Martínez, F. J., Anzueto, A., Barnes, P. J., Bourbeau, J., et al. (2017). Informe 2017 de la Iniciativa Global para el Diagnóstico, Tratamiento y Prevención de la Enfermedad Pulmonar Obstructiva Crónica: Resumen Ejecutivo de GOLD. *Archivos de Bronconeumología*, *53*(3), 128–149. https://doi.org/10.1016/j.arbr.2017.02.001.

Vos, T., Abajobir, A. A., Abate, K. H., Abbafati, C., Abbas, K. M., Abd-Allah, F., et al. (2017). Global, regional, and national incidence, prevalence, and years lived with disability for 328 diseases and injuries for 195 countries, 1990–2016: A systematic analysis for the Global Burden of Disease Study 2016. *The Lancet*, *390*(10100), 1211–1259. https://doi.org/10.1016/S0140-6736(17)32154-2.

Yaqoob, P., Newsholme, E. A., & Calder, P. C. (1995). Influence of cell culture conditions on diet-induced changes in lymphocyte fatty acid composition. *Biochimica et Biophysica Acta (BBA)/Lipids and Lipid Metabolism*, *1255*(3), 333–340. https://doi.org/10.1016/0005-2760(94)00251-S.

Zhang, Y. F., Lu, J., Yu, F. F., Gao, H. F., & Zhou, Y. H. (2014). Polyunsaturated fatty acid intake and risk of lung cancer: A meta-analysis of prospective studies. *PLoS One*, *9*(6). https://doi.org/10.1371/journal.pone.0099637.

Zuijdgeest-Van Leeuwen, S. D., Van Der Heijden, M. S., Rietveld, T., Van Den Berg, J. W., Tilanus, H. W., Burgers, J. A., et al. (2002). Fatty acid composition of plasma lipids in patients with pancreatic, lung and oesophageal cancer in comparison with healthy subjects. *Clinical Nutrition*, *21*(3), 225–230. https://doi.org/10.1054/clnu.2001.0530.

CHAPTER 11

Dietary lipids and hypertension

Xiang Hu[a,b] and Bo Yang[b]

[a]Department of Endocrine and Metabolic Diseases, The First Affiliated Hospital of Wenzhou Medical University, Wenzhou, China [b]Institute of Lipids Medicine & School of Public Health and Management, Wenzhou Medical University, Wenzhou, China

11.1 Introduction

Hypertension defined as a systolic blood pressure (SBP) value ≥140 mmHg and/or diastolic BP (DBP) ≥90 mmHg has resulted in a high medical burden for the major chronic noncommunicable disease, affecting more than one billion people worldwide. As one of the major modifiable risk factors of cardiovascular diseases (CVD) responsible for nearly 10 million deaths per year, hypertension ranked as the largest contributor to global attributable deaths, disability-adjusted life-years. Given the large proportion of the world's adult population with high BP, which is estimated to increase to 29% by 2025, the World Health Organization declared hypertension as a global public health crisis in 2013.

Efforts to reduce the prevalence of hypertension have been concentrated on nonpharmacologic interventions that lower BP. As an important modifiable risk factor for hypertension, dietary modifications have been recommended by the Working Group on Primary Prevention of Hypertension of the United States, traced back to 1993. Again, the recent guidelines by the American Heart Association emphasized the role of dietary modifications in the prevention and management of hypertension. The Dietary Approaches to Stop Hypertension (DASH) trails established a diet pattern rich in fruits, vegetables, and low-fat dairy foods, as well as with reduced saturated fatty acids (SFAs) and total fat that can substantially lower BP. In addition to DASH diets, which ranked as the most effective dietary approach in reducing BP, Mediterranean diet and Paleolithic diet also showed beneficial effects on BP, suggesting that the monounsaturated fatty acids (MUFAs) from vegetable source and $n-3$ polyunsaturated fatty acids (PUFAs) from marine source might play an important role in the prevention of hypertension (Schwingshackl et al., 2019). Furthermore, regarding CVD risks, the 2015 to 2020 Dietary Guidelines for Americans recommend consuming less than 10% of calories from SFA for the general population and replacing SFA with unsaturated fat (US Department of Agriculture, 2015). Later, the American Heart Association advised strongly that reduction in the consumption of SFA and replacement of it with unsaturated fats, especially PUFA, will reduce the incident CVD (Sacks et al., 2017).

However, it remains to be unclear whether the effects of dietary lipids, including SFA, MUFA, and PUFA, on the prevention and management of hypertension would be diverse in individuals with different healthy status. The present section is to analyze, interpret, discuss, and summarize the results of meta-analyses of observational studies and randomized clinical trials, as well as the evidence based on the epidemiological studies of large sample-sized cohorts, providing an overview of the associations between different components of dietary lipids and hypertension in healthy population and populations with hypertension or other cardio-metabolic diseases.

11.2 General background on the relationship between lipids and hypertension

11.2.1 Clinical epidemiological traits of hypertension based on global data

The prevalence of hypertension varied from approximately 20% to 50% in adults. Previously, hypertension was more prevalent in economically developed countries than developing countries, with a prevalence of 37.3% versus 22.9% in 2010 (Mittal & Singh, 2010). However, the absolute numbers of patients affected by hypertension are considerably higher in the developing countries. Furthermore, rapid globalization and urbanization lead to huge changes in lifestyle, more stressful social environments, and longer life expectancy, accelerating the increase in the prevalence of hypertension in developing countries, which has been coming closer to those in developed countries (Mittal & Singh, 2010; Pereira, Lunet, Azevedo, & Barros, 2009).

For most of the economically developed countries, the trends in prevalence of hypertension have increased during these decades. In the United States, based on the data from the National Health and Nutrition Examination Survey, the prevalence of hypertension was 31.3% in 1999–2000 (Fields et al., 2004), which increased to as high as 48.8% in 2007–2014 (Li, Chen, & Zhang, 2019). In Italy, hypertension was a recorded diagnosis in 25.9% of patients in 2013 (Tocci et al., 2017). This prevalence was higher than that reported in the previous analysis (19.3%), which was from the same database extracted in 2005 (Filippi et al., 2009). In Japan, one of the developed Asian countries, prevalent hypertension has reached as high as 45% in 1990 (Sekikawa & Hayakawa, 2004), which rose slightly (48.9%) in 2010 (Satoh et al., 2017), but remained stable in some other countries. In the United Kingdom, for instance, the prevalence of hypertension was 25.3%, 27.8%, and 26.9% in 1998, 2003, and 2006, respectively (MacDonald & Morant, 2008).

Over the last 30 years, the world has witnessed the sustained and rapid economy, of developing Asian countries, which indirectly contributed to a heavier health burden of CVD and its major contributing factors, e.g., hypertension, obesity, hyperlipidemia (Wang, 2016). Particularly, this influence brought by economic development and population growth was more pronounced in China and India, the two most populous countries in Asia (Wang, 2016). In China, 23.2% of the adult population suffered from hypertension, and another 41.3% had pre-hypertension according to the Chinese guidelines from 2012 to 2014 (Wang et al., 2018). The prevalence of hypertension increased rapidly from 2014 to 2017, reaching 44.7% according to the data from 1.7 million adults in a population-based screening study (Lu et al., 2017). In India, the prevalence of hypertension declined from 29.8% (1950–2013) to 25.3% (2012–2014) (Anchala et al., 2014; Geldsetzer et al., 2018), but both of them remained more than one fourth. Additionally, owing to rapid population growth and aging, the burden of hypertension has also become heavier in Africa. The overall pooled prevalence of hypertension increased from 19.7% (1990) to 27.4% (2000) to 30.8% (2010) (Adeloye & Basquill, 2014).

Furthermore, prevalent hypertension varied between populations with different demographic characteristics. Because of the progressive increase in BP with age, the prevalence of hypertension is higher in the elderly population, which is present in both genders, different ethnic groups, and most industrialized countries (Hajjar & Kotchen, 2003; Vasan et al., 2002; Whelton, He, & Muntner, 2004; Wolf-Maier et al., 2003), but not in some nonindustrialized countries with a low dietary salt intake (Abbasnezhad et al., 2020; Elliott et al., 1996; Oliver, Cohen, & Neel, 1975). There is little difference in prevalence of hypertension between men and women. Nevertheless, this association with gender might be modified by age and region. The prevalence of hypertension in women is lower than that in men at a younger age, while it is higher than for men at older age, which might be attributed to the steeper increase in BP in women after menopause (Kannel, Wolf, McGee, McNamara, & Castelli, 1981). The established market economies, Latin America and the Caribbean, and China have a higher prevalence of hypertension in men, while the Middle Eastern crescent, Sub-Saharan Africa, and India have higher prevalence of hypertension in women (Kearney et al., 2005).

Given the high frequency of high BP worldwide, the management of hypertension should not only be focused on an increase in awareness and treatment of this condition, but should also exert efforts on primary prevention, such as encouraging the changes in diet patterns among the general population.

11.2.2 Essential lipids and their metabolites in the context of hypertension

Dietary pattern is one of the critical modifiable risk factors for hypertension. Unlike the well-established effects of salt intake, dietary potassium, and alcohol consumption, the roles of dietary fat and of individual fatty acids (FA) in the context of high BP remain controversial. According to the number of the double bonds present in their hydrocarbon chains, FAs are classified into three groups: saturated fatty acids (SFAs), monounsaturated fatty acids (MUFA), and polyunsaturated fatty acids (PUFA) (Lorente-Cebrián et al., 2013). The main SFA in diets includes palmitic acid (16:0) and stearic acid (18:0), which represent 15%–20% and 5%–10% of total circulating FAs, respectively (Grynberg, 2005). The characteristic FA composition in plasma derived from a saturated fat diet, manifested as an increase in palmitic acid and a decrease in linoleic acid (18:2 n-6), was observed in hypertensive patients (Zheng et al., 1999).

The relevance of unsaturated FA, especially PUFA, for human health has increased growing interest in recent decades. The families of n-3 and n-6 FA, with the first of the double bonds in the cis configuration starting from the third and sixth carbon atom, are essential for humans, which cannot be synthesized de novo and therefore should be supplied in diet (Ratnayake & Galli, 2009). The desaturation and elongation reactions of n-3 and n-6 PUFAs share the common enzymatic pathways to generate arachidonic acid (AA, 20:4 n-6), eicosapentaenoic acid (EPA, $20:5n-3$), and docosahexaenoic acid (DHA, 22:6n-3). These metabolites are precursors of prostaglandins and leukotrienes, which mediate the regulation of vasoconstriction, platelet aggregation, and synthesis of inflammatory mediators (Ratnayake & Galli, 2009). Since the metabolic conversions and corresponding physiological effects of n-3 PUFA and n-6 PUFA compete, antagonize, and interfere with each other, a disbalance between n-3 and n-6 PUFAs in vivo would result in an unfavorable impact on the levels of BP (Biscione, Pignalberi, Totteri, Messina, & Altamura, 2007; Cabo, Alonso, & Mata, 2012). Compared to the diet enriched in SFA, diets with a high intake of PUFA and MUFA contribute to lower levels of BP. The effect of n-3 PUFA is mild in cohorts with different metabolic characteristics, which are pronounced in elderly and hypertensive individuals. In addition, patients with dyslipidemia, diabetes, and hypertension can benefit from the consumption of n-3 PUFA with a lower cardiovascular risk to prevent an increase in BP (Cabo et al., 2012; Lahoz et al., 1997). Among the individual n-3 PUFAs, DHA may be more principal and favorable in the reduction of BP (Mori, Bao, Burke, Puddey, & Beilin, 1999). Regular dietary intake of $n-6$ PUFA exerts the opposite effect on BP between healthy individuals and those with diabetes, which can contribute to the prevention of hypertension or increased risk of hypertension (Nakamura et al., 2018). A lower ratio of n-3:n-6 PUFAs is associated with present hypertension, while this association disappears after adjustment of age and gender (Chen, Sun, & Zhang, 2019).

11.2.3 Lipid medical implications in prevention and management of hypertension

With an unfavorable effect on cholesterol metabolism, SFA is widely recognized as a risk factor of CVD. Given the growing basic evidence supporting the contribution of a highly saturated diet to the progressive increase in SBP, the specific effects of SFA on hypertension in humans, which is difficult to be distinguished from the influence of excess consumption of total fat, however, have not yet been fully understood. Dietary Approaches to Stop Hypertension (DASH) recommended a diet rich in fruits, vegetables, and low-fat dairy foods and with reduced SFA and total fat for the prevention of hypertension (Appel et al., 1997), which was confirmed to be effective in reducing both SBP and DBP in adults (Saneei, Salehi-Abargouei, Esmaillzadeh, & Azadbakht, 2014). However, when replacing nonfat and low-fat dairy with full-fat dairy products and reducing sugars, the modified DASH diet with more liberal total and saturated fat intake was as effective as the standard DASH diet in lowering BP (Chiu et al., 2016). Additionally, because FAs are contained in large amounts of cell membranes to affect cellular functions, the contents of SFA, PUFA, and SFA/PUFA ratio in cell membranes and plasma might be related to the incidence of hypertension (Colussi, Catena, Novello, Bertin, & Sechi, 2017), with a high SFA:PUFA ratio in relation to a high risk of hypertension.

Although the findings about the influence of MUFA on hypertension are limited and inconsistent to some extent, a conclusion can be drawn that MUFA from vegetable sources rather than animal sources, especially from olive oil, have small but apparent effects on BP, contributing to the primary prevention of hypertension in the general population (Alonso, Ruiz-Gutierrez, & Martínez-González, 2006). This favorable influence might be stronger and more significant in DBP, but not in SBP (Miura et al., 2013).

Dietary n-3 PUFAs serves as an important health care intervention in the current climate of globalization, whereas their benefits in the management of cardiovascular risk varied among different ethnic groups and limited to cultures with a very high consumption of n-3 PUFA (Patel, Tracey, Hughes, & Lip, 2010; Wyrwoll, Mark, Mori, Puddey, & Waddell, 2006). Diet intake of n-3 PUFA is inversely associated with BP, with a small estimated effect size in healthy individuals (Ueshima et al., 2007). This influence is enhanced in patients with hypertension, showing a significant reduction in both SBP and DBP, and further a lower risk of stroke and ischemic CVD (Campbell, Dickinson, Critchley, Ford, & Bradburn, 2013). A high-dose of n-3 PUFA (≥ 3 g/day) is clinically effective in BP reductions in hypertensive individuals without treatment (Appel, Miller, Seidler, & Whelton, 1993). Nevertheless, long-term dietary intake of n-3 PUFA is failed to be associated with incident hypertension in middle-aged and elderly men, which might be due to the insufficient intake of n-3 PUFA in daily diets (Matsumoto, Yoruk, Wang, Gaziano, & Sesso, 2019). Notably, postnatal dietary supplementation with n-3 PUFA might even be able to prevent hypertension in offspring.

Therefore, in the aspect of hypertension, a lower level of SFA and higher levels of MUFA (from vegetable sources) and PUFA, along with a smaller ratio of SFA:PUFA and an appropriate ratio of n-3:n-6 (about 1/5), are recommended for the prevention and management of high BP.

11.3 Meta-analytic evidence based on dietary intervention studies

To date, there are numerous intervention studies on the effects of dietary lipids (dietary fat or individual fatty acids) on BP in the general population or in CVD patients, including hypertension. Given that the evidence based on meta-analyses has been ranked to be highest among all of the individual population-based epidemiological studies, we summarized the meta-analytic evidence based on the intervention studies with dietary lipids (Table 11.1).

11.3.1 Dietary supplements of lipids for blood pressure in the general/health population

Given the limited data focused on the intervention of dietary fat on BP in a healthy population, the findings were mostly provided by meta-analysis among individuals without health restrictions, including those with and without slightly elevated BP. DASH diet is featured by lower total fat and SFA used to prevent hypertension. The effects of the DASH diet on cardiovascular risk factors were determined by a meta-analysis of randomized controlled trials (RCT), enrolling 1,917 participants with or without comorbidities. With the duration of interventions ranging from 2 to 24 weeks, the DASH diet was found to result in significant decreases in SBP and DBP (Siervo et al., 2015). The meta-analysis conducted in children and adolescents aged 2–19 years found that reduced SFA had significant effects on DBP (a decrease in DBP by 1.45 mmHg) rather than SBP (Morenga & Montez, 2017). Nevertheless, a recent meta-analysis included 15 RCT to assess the effect of reducing SFA intake on mortality and cardiovascular morbidity. The results showed that compared to the usual diet, SFA reduction exerted no effect on either SBP or DBP (Hooper et al., 2020).

A meta-analysis of intervention studies compared the effects on blood pressure of different diets rich in carbohydrate and MUFA. High MUFA diets seemed to be associated with slightly lower BP than high-carbohydrate diets. However, when the study was limited to randomized crossover studies, the difference in BP between these two types of diets was no longer significant. Therefore, although given the magnitude of the difference observed, dietary recommendations may not be justified altering the carbohydrate and MUFA content of the diet in the management of hypertension (Shah, Adams-Huet, & Garg, 2007). Another meta-analysis of 14 randomized clinical trials, of which all had a follow-up period of more than 3 weeks, also provided the evidence that in the context of low SFAs, isocaloric substitution of a high-carbohydrate diet for a high-MUFA diet did not demonstrate a greater reduction in BP (Elena et al., 2019). Nevertheless, using 12% of total energy consumption (TEC) as the cut-off proportion set by the Dietary Guidelines for Americans, dietary regimens with a high amount of MUFA contribute to significant decreases in SBP by 2.26 mmHg and DBP by 1.15 mmHg compared to that with a low amount of MUFA (differentiated to be low fat diets, low or high glycemic index diets, high PUFA diets, high-protein diets, or controlled diets with total fat content ≥30% of TEC and/or SFA ≥10% of TEC) (Schwingshackl, Strasser, & Hoffmann, 2011). The Mediterranean-style diet is another well-known dietary pattern with CVD benefits. For Mediterranean-style diet, a high MUFA/SFA ratio is one of the key components required to achieve its definition. In healthy adults and

TABLE 11.1 Major meta-analytic evidence of interventional trials on effects of dietary total fat and individual fatty acids on blood pressure

Population		Intervention					BP, mmHg	
Health status	Age and gender	Fat subtypes	Diet/supplement	Amount or dose	Duration	Comparator	SBP	DBP
Health/general population	29–60y and both	Total fat	DASH diet	Low fat	2–24 wks	Typical diet/ health diet	5.2↓	2.6↓
	2–19y and both >18y and both	SFA	SFA reduction	7.7–13.3% TEC significantly lower than control	5 wks–19 yrs >2 yrs	higher SFA intake or usual diet	No effect	1.45↓ ns.
	24–62y and both	MUFA	High-MUFA diet	>12% TEC	3–24 wks	High-carbohydrate diet	No effect	No effect
	55y (median) & both		High-MUFA diet		6–48 mons	Low-MUFA diet	2.26↓	1.15↓
	44–71y & both	MUFA/SFA	Mediterranean diet (high MUFA/SFA ratio)		3–24 mons	no or minimal intervention	2.99↓	2.0↓
	51–61y & both				3–12 mons	Traditional low-fat diet	1.5↓	0.26↓ ns.
	20–54y and both	PUFA	fish intake/fish oil	$n-3$ PUFA 2.4–6.5 g/d (mean)	3–24 wks	Placebo	no effect to 1.25↓	no effect to 1.14↓
	25–57y and both			Fish oil: 3–12g/d (0.8–4.86g/d EPA + DHA with ratio of 0.25–5)	8–78 wks			
	46y (mean) and both			Fish oil: 0.2–15.0 g/d (mean: 4.1 g/d)	3–52 wks			
	18–90y and both			EPA +DHA:3.8g/d (mean)	69 days (mean)			

Condition	Age/sex	Factor	Diet/Intervention	Dose	Duration	Control		
Hypertension	24–71y and both	Total fat	Low fat diet	<30% TEC	3–48 mons	Usual diet	2.32↓	1.27↓
			DASH diet	Low fat			7.38↓	4.37↓
		MUFA/SFA	Mediterranean diet				4.07↓	2.81↓
	18–80y and both	n−3 PUFA	Fish intake/fish oil	2–15g/d (mean)	4–12wks	Placebo	2.56–5.5↓	1.47–3.5↓
	42–61y and both			0.05–50g/d (0.013–13.33g/d EPA+DHA with ratio of 1.43–3)	8–24wks;			
	46y (mean) and both			0.2–15.0g/d (mean: 4.1g/d)	3–52 wks			
	18–90y& both			EPA+DHA: 3.8g/d (mean)	69 days (mean)			
				>3g/d (mean)	<3 mons			
Diabetes	42–57y and both	Total fat	Low-fat diet	<30% TEC	4–22wks	Usual diet	5.72↓	5.53↓
	52–62y and both		High-fat diet	>30% of TEC	1–6yrs	Low-fat diet	No effect	1.30↓
	45–74y & both	MUFA	high-MUFA diet	10–49%TEC	2–52wks	high-carbohydrate-diet	2.31↓	No effect
	20–54y and both	n−3 PUFA	Fish intake/fish oil supplementation	1.7–10g/d EPA+DHA with different EPA/DHA ratios	4–24wks	Vegetable oils including olive, safflower, and corn oils	No effect	No effect to 2↓
	40–75y and both			1.2–4.8g/d EPA+DHA and 1.8g/d EPA	6–108wks			
	33–70y and both			0.4–18g/d EPA+DHA with different EPA/DHA ratios	2–108wks			

Continued

TABLE 11.1 Major meta-analytic evidence of interventional trials on effects of dietary total fat and individual fatty acids on blood pressure—cont'd

Population			Intervention				BP, mmHg	
Health status	Age and gender	Fat subtypes	Diet/supplement	Amount or dose	Duration	Comparator	SBP	DBP
Hypercholesterolemia	18–60y and both	n−3 PUFA	Fish intake/fish oil	EPA+DHA with different EPA/DHA ratios 1.7–6.0g/d (mean)	4–12wks	Placebo	4.4↓	1.1↓ ns.
ASCVD	52–73y and both	n−3 PUFA	Fish oil	3–6g/d (mean)	4–16wks	Placebo	6.3↓ ns.	2.9↓ ns.
	21–74y and both		Purified fish oil or EPA and DHA	0.18–15g/d EPA+DHA with different EPA/DHA ratios	4–240wks	Placebo/control	2.195↓	1.08↓
	<60y and men	n−6 PUFA	Soya oil/safflower oil	15–21.9%TEC	4–4.3yrs	Usual diets	No effect	No effect

DASH, Dietary Approaches to Stop Hypertension; DBP, diastolic blood pressure; DHA, docosahexaenoic acid, 22:5n-3; EPA, eicosapentaenoic acid, 20:5n-3; MUFA, monounsaturated fatty acids; ns.: no statistical significance; PUFA, polyunsaturated fatty acids; SBP, systolic blood pressure; SFA, saturated fatty acids; TEC, total energy consumption. Diet compositions: DASH diet: high intake of fruits and vegetables, low-fat dairy products, and whole grains, and low in sodium; Mediterranean diet: high consumption of fruit, vegetables, olive oil, legumes, cereals, fish, and moderate intake of red wine during meals; placebo, vegetable oils including olive, safflower, and corn/SFA mixed.

adults at high CVD risk, there was moderate-quality evidence supporting that Mediterranean dietary intervention rich in high MUFA and low SFA contributed to reductions in SBP by 2.99 mmHg and DBP by 2.0 mmHg (Rees et al., 2019).

The antihypertensive effect of fish oil, which is enriched in mare n-3 PUFA (EPA plus DHA), was mild, even absent, in normal populations. The effects of n-3 PUFA at an overall mean dose of 4.2 g/d on BP were close to zero in a population with normal BP (Morris, Sacks, & Rosner, 1993). Similarly, taking fish oil capsules for a minimum of 8 weeks cannot affect BP levels in participants with less than 140/85 mmHg, and the findings remain not to be reached a significant BP reduction in respect of the different components of n-3 PUFAs (EPA, DHA, and EPA + DHA with their multiple ratios) (Campbell et al., 2013). However, a previous meta-analysis reported that fish oil supplement reduced the BP among normal populations (reducing SBP/DBP by 1.21/1.14 mmHg), although the reductions were not as much as those among hypertensive populations. Additionally, a larger BP sensitivity to fish oil was more likely to appear in women and at an older age (Campbell et al., 2013). The latest meta-analysis explored the effect of EPA + DHA, without upper dose limits and including food sources, on blood pressure in non-hospitalized and normotensive adults and found small but significant reductions in both SBP and DBP, decreasing by 1.25 mmHg and 0.62 mmHg, respectively (Miller, Van Elswyk, & Alexander, 2014).

11.3.2 Dietary supplements of lipids on blood pressure in patients with cardiometabolic disorder

In patients with hypertension or prehypertension, a low-fat dietary approach with less than 30% fat of total energy intake and DASH diet were significantly effective in reducing SBP and DBP. The Mediterranean diet with high consumption of fruit, vegetables, olive oil, legumes, cereals, fish, and moderate intake of red wine during meals, and Nordic diets with whole-grain products, abundant use of berries, fruit and vegetables, rapeseed oil, three fish meals per week, low-fat dairy products, and avoidance of sugar-sweetened products, demonstrate the superiority of lowering DBP compared to low-fat diet, suggesting the important role of fish and vegetable oil in the regulation of BP (Schwingshackl et al., 2019). The low fat diets remained to be effective in reducing SBP and DBP by 5.72 mmHg and 5.53 mmHg in patients with diabetes (Abbasnezhad et al., 2020; Schwingshackl et al., 2019). However, in pre-diabetics and patients with established type 2 diabetes, DBP was decreased in subjects following high-fat diets (provide >30% of TEC in the form of fat, including usual diet with SFA content >10% of TEC, low carbohydrate diet with <50-g carbohydrates/day, and MUFA diet with MUFA content >12% TEC) compared to those following low fat diets (provide ≤30% of TEC in the form of fat), and SBP did not differ between subjects with high fat and low fat diets (Schwingshackl & Hoffmann, 2014).

A meta-analysis of 24 intervention trials made comparisons between diets with a high MUFA pattern and a high carbohydrate pattern in patients with diabetes. The amount of MUFA contained in high MUFA diets was more than twice as the amount of MUFA in high carbohydrate diets. The diet rich in MUFA can improve metabolic risk factors among patients with diabetes. This comparison of high MUFA diets with high carbohydrate diets results in a significant reduction in SBP but not DBP. When comparing high MUFA to high carbohydrate diets, SBP was decreased by 2.31 mmHg, along with favorable effects in metabolism of glucose and lipids (Qian, Korat, Malik, & Hu, 2016).

High doses of n-3 PUFA, generally more than 3 g/d, can contribute to reductions in BP among hypertensive patients. A meta-analysis of 6 clinical trials observed that supplementation of n-3 PUFA could lead to decreases in SBP by 5.5 mmHg and DBP by 3.5 mmHg in patients with untreated hypertension. The magnitude of this effect was associated with the higher BP at baseline rather than the higher dose of supplemental n-3 PUFAs (Appel et al., 1993). In the meantime, another meta-analysis reported that the estimated effect of n-3 PUFA in a stable hypertensive population was to reduce 4.5 mmHg in SBP and 2.5 mmHg in DBP, which was significantly different from the healthy individuals for SBP but not DBP. In addition, a dose-response effect of n-3 PUFA in BP was observed among the hypertensive individuals, which, however, was not evident when the supplemental dose was restricted to 2 to 6 g/d. The BP-lowering effects were confirmed in a larger meta-analysis of 36 intervention studies in which 50% of the trial population was hypertensive. The reduction in SBP and DBP remained to be larger in hypertensive individuals compared to normotensive individuals after adjustment of age, gender, study design, baseline blood pressure, and dose of fish oil. Similarly, the decrease in BP during intervention was associated with the baseline SBP (decreasing 0.11 mmHg BP per unit) instead of the intake dose of fish oil (Geleijnse, Giltay, Grobbee, Donders, & Kok, 2002). A recent meta-analysis among predominantly middle-aged patients with moderately elevated hypertension revealed a statistically significant reduction in SBP by 2.56 mmHg and DBP by 1.47 mmHg, given the supplementation of n-3 PUFA for more than 8 weeks, with no evidence of a dose-dependent response. Notably, this study drew a conclusion that the effect on lowering BP was significant, though small, and this fact was associated with relatively low-dose intake of n-3 PUFA rather than high-dose intake (Campbell et al., 2013). The comprehensive meta-analysis examined the effect of n-3 PUFA on BP, without upper dose limits and including food sources. The BP-lowering effects were stronger in untreated hypertensive individuals compared to healthy individuals, with a reduction in SBP by 4.51 mmHg and in DBP by 3.05 mmHg, and the pattern of dose-response between n-3 PUFA and BP remains unclear (Miller et al., 2014).

The beneficial effect of n-3 PUFA on BP was small and unapparent for patients with diabetes in an early meta-analysis of three studies (Rees et al., 2019). Later, a meta-analysis of 12 randomized controlled trials performed a comparison of intake of n-3 PUFA with placebo in type 2 diabetes. The mean treatment duration was 8.5 weeks and the mean dose of n-3 PUFA supplementation was 4.3 g/day. DBP, rather than SBP, showed a significant reduction by about 2 mmHg with the supplementation of n-3 PUFA (Hartweg, Farmer, Holman, & Neil, 2007). Further meta-analysis updated the findings with 7 newly published studies, in which the mean dose of n-3 PUFA was 2.4 g/d, and found no association between supplementation of n-3 PUFA and reduction in both of SBP and DBP (Hartweg, Farmer, Holman, & Neil, 2009), suggesting that BP might not benefit from n-3 PUFA supplements at lower dose, even though their cardioprotective effects were definitive in patients with diabetes. A recent meta-analysis including 2674 adults also failed to find the effects of n-3 PUFA supplement (dose: 0.40–18.00 g; duration: 2–104 weeks) on SBP or DBP (O'Mahoney et al., 2018).

For hypercholesterolemic patients, supplementation of n-3 PUFA exerted a strengthened effect on SBP (reduced by 4.4 mmHg), which was significantly greater than the effect for healthy individuals (Morris et al., 1993). For patients with atherosclerotic cardiovascular disease (ASCVD), reductions in BP with supplementation of n-3 PUFA were observed. However, they did not reach statistical significance (Morris et al., 1993). The effects of α-linolenic acid (ALA, 18:3n-3), a kind of plant n-3 PUFA which is a precursor of DHA and EPA, were analyzed among patients with hypercholesterolemia or cardiovascular risks. However, even with contributions to lower concentration of fibrinogen and fasting glucose, both of which are established cardiovascular risk factors, α-linolenic acid showed little effects on BP (Wendland, Farmer, Glasziou, & Neil, 2006). A recent meta-analysis included 171 studies in final quantitative synthesis to quantify the effect of supplementation of n-3 PUFA (EPA and DHA) on CVD risk factors. For the participants with different healthy statuses, who varied from healthy individuals, to those with cardio-metabolic diseases, and even those having received heart transplant recipient or myocardial graft procedure, the supplementations of EPA and/or DHA lead to decreases in SBP by 2.195 mmHg and DBP by 1.08 mmHg (AbuMweis, Jew, Tayyem, & Agraib, 2018). Based on the limited data on BP, there were evident effects of n-6 PUFA on neither SBP nor DBP in individuals with low (no specific CVD risk factors), moderate (established CVD risk factors), to high (existing CVD) risk of CVD (Hooper et al., 2018). For patients with current use of statins, high-PUFA diets reduced both SBP and DBP after 4-weeks, however, low-ratio (n-6:n-3=1.7:1) diets showed no significant superiority to high-ratio (n-6:n-3=30:1) diets (Lee et al., 2012).

11.4 Evidence based on the relevant epidemiological studies

Given the limited meta-analytic evidence based on the relevant epidemiological studies, a series of major evidence to date on the relationship between dietary lipids and high BP in individual population-based cohort, case-control, and cross-sectional epidemiological studies are summarized in Table 11.2.

11.4.1 Longitudinal cohort-based relationship of dietary lipids with high blood pressure

Based on data from prospective cohort studies, in which food-frequency questionnaires were mostly used to collect the information about dairy intake, a dose-response meta-analysis revealed that low fat dairy was linearly and inversely associated with incident hypertension, with a 4% lower risk of hypertension per 200 g/d, which was not interfered with age and BMI. While there was no significant association of high-fat dairy with incidence of hypertension (Lee et al., 2012), this longitudinal association of dairy consumption with hypertension was confirmed and pronounced by another meta-analysis which showed the outcome of elevated blood pressure, defined as SBP ≥130 mmHg and/or DBP ≥85 mmHg. With the length of follow-up ranging from 2 to 15 years, this meta-analysis resulted in a decrease in risk of elevated blood pressure by 16% in subjects consuming high amounts of low-fat dairy foods (Ralston, Lee, Truby, Palermo, & Walker, 2012).

A relevant meta-analysis of 8 prospective cohort studies with a median follow-up duration ranging from 3 to 20 years demonstrated that circulating n-3 PUFA, a biomarker of diet intake of n-3 PUFA, was significantly associated with a lower risk of elevated BP, although the evidence was not strong enough to support the association between dietary consumption of fish or n-3 PUFA with reduced incidence of elevated BP (Yang et al., 2016). The possibility of interactive impacts on BP for populations with different background consumption of marine food and genetic characteristics response to individual n-3 PUFAs cannot be excluded. For example, the Chinese population has undergone a rapid transition in food patterns and disease profiles during the past decades. According to a longitudinal study by the China Health and Nutrition Survey from 1997 to 2011, Chinese adults consumed more vegetable oils, but fewer animal fats, leading to increases in MUFA and PUFA intakes with a low percentage of energy from SFA (Shen et al., 2017). Although less consumption of fish and seafood resulted in low EPA and DHA intakes of about 20 mg/d, more than 60% of the Chinese population showed an increasing or stabilized level of Mediterranean diet adherence

TABLE 11.2 Major epidemiological evidence on the association of dietary fat or individual fatty acids with hypertension risk or blood pressure

Author, year (y)	Design	Case/ participants	Age, gender	Follow-up duration (median)	Baseline measurement Fat subtypes, assessment	Exposure range	OR/RR (95% CI)	Outcomes SBP changes (Coef. or mean)	DBP changes (Coef. or mean)
Yang, Shi, Li, Yang, & Li, 2016	Meta-analysis	20,497/56,204	39–70y, Both	3–20years	EPA+DHA (g/d), FFQ	The highest vs. the lowest categories	0.80 (0.58–1.10)[a]	ND	
					Circulating PL LC n-3 PUFA (%), GLC		0.67 (0.55–0.83)[a]		
					Circulating PL EPA (%), GLC		0.53 (0.35–0.78)[a]		
					Circulating PL DHA (%), GLC		0.64 (0.45–0.89)[a]		
Gao et al., 2018	Longitudinal	1109/6586	≥18y, Both	2–4years	High-MUFA, 24-h recalls	The highest vs. the lowest MD adherence score	0.17 (0.09–0.32)[a]	Coef.: −8.44[a]	Coef.: −3.64[a]
Zeng et al., 2014	Longitudinal	NG/1477	40–75y, Both	3years	Erythrocyte SFA (%), GC	The highest vs. the lowest quartile	ND	Mean change per yr: 0.148	Mean change per yr: −0.109
					Erythrocyte MUFA (%), GC			0.366	0.201
					Erythrocyte PUFA (%), GC			−0.514	−0.111
					Erythrocyte n-3 PUFA (%), GC			−0.851[a]	−0.363[a]
					Erythrocyte n-6 PUFA (%), GC			−0.232	0.032
					n-3:n-6 PUFA ratio			−0.923[a]	−0.500[a]
					PUFA:SFA ratio			−0.231	−0.013
Zec et al. (2019)	Longitudinal	195/300	>30y, both	10years	Plasma PL EPA (%), GC	The highest vs. the lowest tertiles	1.46 (1.03, 2.08)[a]	Coef.: 2.92	Coef.: 1.94
					Plasma PL DPA (%), GC		1.01 (0.70, 1.46)	−2.11	−1.86
					Plasma PL DHA (%), GC		1.01 (0.70, 1.46)	−2.21	−1.50
					Plasma PL Dihomo-γ-linolenic acid (%), GC		1.33 (0.93, 1.92)	−1.59	−1.19
					Plasma PL AA (%), GC		0.85 (0.60, 1.21)	−3.81[a]	−3.82[a]

Study	Design	Cases/Total	Age, Sex	Exposure, Method	Comparison	Outcome/Estimate (95% CI)	Additional estimates
Huang, Shou, Cai, Wahlqvist, & Li, 2012	cross-sectional	214/1154	48.6y (mean), both	Plasma PL SFA (%), GLC	Hypertension: upper vs. lower median	2.01 (1.05–2.98)[a]	Coef.: 0.459 for HP and 0.087 for NP	Coef.: −0.085 for HP and 0.082 for NP
				Plasma PL MUFA (%), GLC		0.67 (0.45–1.22)	0.319 for HP and −0.071 for NP	0.580[a] for HP and −0.011 for NP
				Plasma PL PUFA (%), GLC	BP: per 1-unit increase	1.03 (0.38–2.16)	0.031 for HP and −0.037 for NP	−0.522[a] for HP and −0.069 for NP
				Plasma PL n-3 PUFA (%), GLC		0.43 (0.29–1.19)[a]	−0.102 for HP and 0.072 for NP	−0.392[a] for HP and −0.080 for NP
				Plasma PL n-6 PUFA (%), GLC		0.56 (0.21–2.17)	0.076 for HP and −0.067 for NP	−0.434 for HP and −0.033 for NP
				n-3:n-6 PUFA		0.48 (0.12–1.86)[a]	−0.309 for HP and 0.080 for NP	−0.360 for HP and −0.065 for NP
Yang et al., 2016	Cross-sectional	748/2447	35–79y, both	Serum n-6 PUFA pattern, GLC	The top vs. the bottom tertiles	ND	Adjusted BP mean: 131.11 vs. 123.80[b]	Adjusted BP mean: 82.58 vs. 80.33
				Serum n-3 PUFA pattern, GLC			126.40 vs.127.80	79.84 vs. 82.99[b]
				D6D Component, GLC	The highest vs. the lowest quartile	1.42 (1.00–2.09)[a]	ND	
				SCD-2 Component, GLC		1.42 (0.93–2.17)		
				D5D Component, GLC		0.68 (0.46–0.98)[a]		
Chen et al., 2019	Cross-sectional	8976/18434	>18y, both	n-3 PUFA (mg/kg/day), 24-h recall	The highest vs. the lowest tertiles	0.58 (0.49–0.68)[a]	ND	
				n-6 PUFA (mg/kg/day), 24-h recall		0.53 (0.45–0.63)[a]		
				n-6:n-3 PUFA		0.92 (0.80–1.06)		
Nakamura et al., 2018	Cross-sectional	350/633	>40y, both	Total n-6 PUFA (g/1000 kcal), BDHQ	The highest vs. the lowest categories	0.88 (0.77–1.01) (HbA1c ≥6.5%: 3.62 (1.02–12.84)[a]	ND	
				LA (g/1000 kcal), BDHQ	The highest vs. the lowest categories	0.88 (0.77–1.02) HbA1c ≥6.5%: 3.98 (1.05–15.13)[a] HbA1c <6.5%: 0.86 (0.74–0.99)[a]		

Continued

TABLE 11.2 Major epidemiological evidence on the association of dietary fat or individual fatty acids with hypertension risk or blood pressure—cont'd

Author, year (y)	Design	Case/ participants gender	Age, gender	Follow-up duration (median)	Baseline measurement Fat subtypes, assessment	Exposure range	OR/RR (95% CI)	SBP changes (Coef. or mean)	DBP changes (Coef. or mean)
O'Sullivan et al., 2012	Cross-sectional	NG/814	13–15y, both		Total fat (g/d), 3-day food record	The highest vs. the lowest categories	ND	Coef.: 0.054 for girl and −0.122[a] for boy	Coef.: 0.023 for girl and −0.028 for boy
					Total PUFA (g/d), 3-day diet record			−0.045 for girl and −0.146[a] for boy	0.054 for girl and −0.140 for boy
					Total n-3 PUFA (g/d), 3-day food record			−0.005 for girl and −0.124[a] for boy	−0.027 for girl and −0.057 for boy
					ALA (g/d), 3-day food record			−0.004 for girl and −0.088 for boy	0.014 for girl and 0.017 for boy
					EPA (g/d), 3-day food record			−0.017 for girl and −0.108[a] for boy	−0.040 for girl and −0.147[a] for boy
					DPA (g/d), 3-day food record			−0.054 for girl and −0.022 for boy	−0.047 for girl and −0.090 for boy
					DHA (g/d), 3-day food record			−0.008 for girl and −0.100 for boy	−0.079 for girl and −0.137[a] for boy
					Total n-6 PUFA (g/d), 3-day food record			−0.006 for girl and −0.114[a] for boy	0.118 for girl and −0.026 for boy
					LA (g/d), 3-day food record			−0.006 for girl and −0.114[a] for boy	0.119 for girl and −0.020 for boy
					AA (g/d), 3-day food record			−0.004 for girl and −0.007 for boy	0.018 for girl and −0.120[a] for boy
					n-6:n-3 PUFA			−0.033 for girl and 0.042 for boy	0.098 for girl and 0.065 for boy

Ueshima et al., 2007	Cross-sectional	1009/4680	40–59y, both	n-3 PUFA (%), 24-h recall	Higher by two Standard Deviations	ND	Coef.: −0.55[a]	Coef.: −0.57[a]
				Linolenic acid (%), 24-h recall			−0.60[a]	−0.50[a]
				EPA + DHA (%), 24-h recall			−0.03[a]	−0.28[a]

[a] Statistically significant.
[b] Statistically significant for trend.

AA: arachidonic acid, 20:4n-6; ALA: a-linoleic acid, 18:3n-3; BDHQ, brief self-administered diet history questionnaire; Coef., coefficient value; DHA, docosahexaenoic acid, 22:6n-3; DPA, docosapentaenoic acid, 22:6n-3; D5D, Δ(5)-desaturase, 20:4n-6/20:3n-6; D6D, Δ(6)-desaturase, 18:3n-6/18:2n-6; EPA, eicosapentaenoic acid, 20:5n-3; FFQ, food frequency questionnaire; GC: gas chromatography; g/d, gram per day; GLC, gas-liquid chromatography; HbA1c, glycated hemoglobin; LA, linoleic acid; LC long-chain; MD, Mediterranean diet; MUFA, monounsaturated fatty acid; HP, hypertensive population; ND, no report; NP, normotensive population; OR, odds ratio; PL, phospholipids; PUFA, polyunsaturated fatty acid; RR, risk ratio; n-3; SCD-1, 16:1n-7/16:0; SCD-2, 18:1n-9/18:0; Mediterranean diet: high consumption of fruit, vegetables, olive oil, legumes, cereals, fish, and moderate intake of red wine during meals; High n-6 PUFA pattern: serum 14:0, 16:0, 16:1n-7, 18:2n-6, 18:3n-6, 20:3n-6; high n-3 PUFA pattern: serum 20:5n-3, 22:5n-3, 22:6n-3, 18:1n-9; D6D Component: higher positive loadings from serum 16:0, 16:1n-7, 18:3n-6, 20:3n-6, 22:5n-3, SCD-1 and D6D and a negative loading from 18:2n-6; SCD-2 Component: higher positive loadings from 18:2n-9 and negative loadings from 18:3n-3 and 18:0; D5D Component: higher loadings from serum 20:5n-3, 20:4n-6, 22:6n-3 and D5D.

(MDA). Moreover, a lower risk of developing hypertension was associated with initially high or increasingly higher MDA levels (Gao et al., 2018). In the Japanese general population for 24 years, a high level of n-3 PUFA intake was independently associated with the lower risk of total CVD mortality (Miyagawa et al., 2014).

Additionally, it is well-known that the blood (serum, plasma, or erythrocyte) content of FA is an objective and accurate biomarker reflecting short- to mid-term internal exposure to dietary intake of FA and its metabolism in vivo. A community-based prospective cohort of Chinese individuals aged 40–75 years was followed up from 2008 to 2010 and showed that higher erythrocyte contents of n-3 PUFAs were marginally associated with lower increases in SBP and DBP. In terms of different subtypes of n-3 PUFA, it was observed that higher levels of very long-chain n–3 PUFAs, including 20:5n-3, 22:5n-3, and 22:6n-3 PUFAs, were significantly associated with less increase in SBP. Among them, however, only 20:5n-3 PUFAs were inversely associated with an increase in DBP (Zeng et al., 2014). Urbanization has taken place in sub-Saharan Africa since 1980, followed by nutritional transition with increased consumption of energy-dense food, which contributed to the high prevalence of hypertension. A recently published research followed FA status in black South Africans for 10 years and determined the longitudinal associations between individual PUFA and hypertension. The results showed that individual plasma n-6 PUFA was inversely associated with BP, whereas EPA was adversely associated with hypertension (Zec et al., 2019).

11.4.2 Case-control or cross-sectional studies on the relationship between dietary lipids and high blood pressure

A Japanese cross-sectional study of the rural population demonstrated an inverse relationship between high consumption of specific SFA, such as total SFA, C14:0, C15:0, C16:0, C17:0, C18:0, and C20:0, and the presence of hypertension, which was pronounced in the elderly population. SFA, which is used to be considered unhealthy in the cardiovascular field because of its negative effects on cholesterol metabolism, might contribute to the prevention and treatment of hypertension in the elderly population through regular consumption (Nakamura et al., 2019).

There is some evidence among the Chinese population in terms of blood FA. In the cross-sectional analyses enrolling 1834 middle-aged and elderly Chinese individuals, the erythrocyte SFA content was positively associated with BP, while PUFAs, no matter total PUFA or its subtypes (n-3 PUFA and n-6 PUFA), and the PUFA-to-SFA ratio were inversely and independently associated with SBP and DBP (Zeng et al., 2014). Another cross sectional study conducted in eastern China obtained similar findings supporting the positive association of plasma phospholipid SFA with hypertension, as well as the inverse associations of plasma phospholipid n-3 PUFA and n-3:n-6 PUFA ratio with hypertension (Huang et al., 2012). In a recent cross-sectional study, low serum linoleic acid/ high SFA pattern was negatively associated with SBP and the high n-3 PUFA pattern was inversely associated with DBP. Hence, the serum FA pattern is beneficial because of the low proportions of 14:0, 16:0, 16:1 n-7, and 18:3n-6, as well as high 18:2n-6 and 22:6n-3 is beneficial for BP control in Chinese population. Subsequently, Yang and his co-researchers further investigated the associations of serum FAs and related Δ-desaturase with hypertension. The results showed that an interquartile increase in Δ(5)-desaturase (D5D) and Δ(6)-desaturase (D6D) was associated with a 26% decrease and 32% increase in the risk of hypertension, respectively. Individuals with higher scores of the D5D component, which mainly comprised higher positive loadings from 20:5n-3, 20:4n-6, 22:6n-3, and D5D, were more likely to develop hypertension (Yang et al., 2016).

By contrast, a cross-sectional study conducted in the American general population of 18,434 participants revealed that higher dietary intakes of n-3 and n-6 PUFA were associated with lower odds ratios of hypertension after adjustment of age, gender, race, educational level, income, recreational activity, work activity, drinking status, smoking status, diabetes, and total energy intake. Furthermore, there was a nonlinear negative and L-shaped association of the dose of n-3 PUFA and n-6 PUFA with the presence of hypertension. The prevalence of hypertension decreased with increases in doses of n-3 PUFA and n-6 PUFA, but will reach a plateau when the n-3 PUFA and n-6 PUFA intakes exceed certain doses (Chen et al., 2019). The International Study of Macro- and Micronutrients and Blood Pressure (INTERMAP), an international cross-sectional epidemiological study of 17 population-based samples in China, Japan, United Kingdom, and United States, showed that dietary total n-3 PUFA was associated with decreases in SBP by 0.4–0.6 mmHg and DBP by 0.5–0.6 mmHg, respectively (Ueshima et al., 2007). In terms of DHA and EPA, either summed or separately, ingested either from total food or only fish/shellfish and their products, this inverse relationship with BP remains similar.

This beneficial effect of PUFA on hypertension has become controversial among patients with diabetes. For the middle-aged and elderly Japanese population, the intake of n-6 PUFA was inversely correlated with the presence of hypertension in subjects with HbA1c < 6.5%. On the contrary, in subjects with HbA1c ≥ 6.5%, the association between n-6 PUFA intake and the presence of hypertension was significantly positive. It is suggested that regular intake of n-6 PUFA may contribute to the prevention and treatment of hypertension in a normoglycemic population, which, however, might predispose the subjects with diabetes to the development of hypertension (Nakamura et al., 2018). In adolescents, the inverse association between intakes of PUFA and blood pressure (both of SBP and DBP) was only found in boys rather than girls. Additionally, for long chain n-3 PUFA, the blood pressure decreased with an increase in EPA instead of DHA (O'Sullivan et al., 2012).

11.5 Biological mechanisms for the antihypertensive effects of dietary n-3 lipids

The hypothesis that supplemental n-3 PUFAs confer antihypertensive efficacy is biologically plausible. Coronary benefits of supplemental n-3 PUFAs are currently consistent with data from laboratory investigations, animal experiments, and small trials with intermediate cardiovascular endpoints in humans, which suggest that n-3 PUFAs have a variety of positive effects on blood pressure levels through mechanistic actions in endothelial function, vascular reactivity, antiinflammatory response, renin-angiotensin aldosterone system (RAAS), eicosanoid pathway, and gut-brain axis that is believed to convey cardiovascular protections related to reduced risk of CVD (Fig. 11.1).

11.5.1 Endothelial function and vascular reactivity

The n-3 fatty acids may affect blood pressure by altering arterial compliance. BP is strongly influenced by arterial compliance, which, in turn, is influenced by endothelial function. N-3 PUFA is demonstrated to improve endothelial function, no matter whether the endothelium is damaged or not. Endothelial function is commonly assessed in vivo by the production of endothelial nitric oxide (eNO) mediated by the activation of eNO synthase (eNOS). Diet enriched in n-3 PUFA stimulated an increase in the expression of eNOS in the level of mRNA and protein, leading to the upregulation of eNOS-cyclic guanosine monophosphate (cGMP) pathway with increased levels of nitric oxide

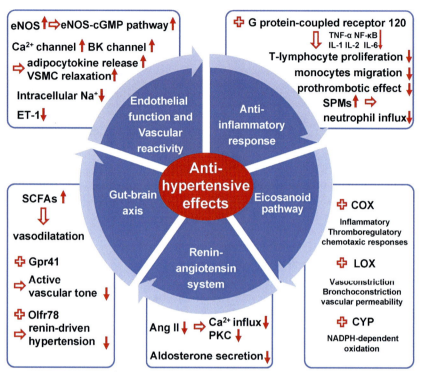

FIG. 11.1 Biological mechanisms for the antihypertensive effects of dietary n-3 lipids. *From Biological mechanisms for the antihypertensive effects of dietary n-3 lipids. (2021). Wenzhou Medical University.*

and cGMP by 90% and 100%, respectively. The increase in nitric oxide contributed to the blood vessel relaxation and antioxidation of low-density lipoprotein (López et al., 2004). EPA induced the translocation of eNOS to the cytosol and its dissociation from caveolin, which is colocalized with EPA in the cell membrane at a resting state, with a Ca^{2+} independent activation (Omura et al., 2001).

The metabolic pathway of the cytochrome P450 epoxygenases might be another mechanism responsible for the endothelium-mediated vasodilatation induced by n-3 PUFA. The epoxides generated from this system could activate the calcium- and voltage-activated potassium channels to hyperpolarize vascular smooth muscle cells (VSMC) and their function on perivascular adipocytes to stimulate the release of adiponectin (Hoshi et al., 2013; Sukumar et al., 2012). Both the relaxation of VSMC and stimulation of adipocytokine release contributed to the potent vasodilatation and blood pressure reduction.

Endothelin-1 (ET1), mainly synthesized and released from endothelial cells, is a potent vasoconstrictor and pressor substance to exert a wide variety of biological effects. EPA was able to suppress the basal and insulin-enhanced ET-1 production in a dose-dependent manner by its inhibition of ET-1 mRNA production, which is very likely to contribute to the vasorelaxant and hypotensive effects of VFA (Chisaki et al., 2003). Additionally, supplementation of EPA could not only increase the membrane EPA content but also decrease the intracellular sodium concentration, suggesting that the effects of EPA on blood pressure might be mediated by the alteration in the activities of the membrane sodium transport systems (Miyajima, Tsujino, Saito, & Yokoyama, 2001). Supplementation of n-3 PUFA also has regenerative properties on the vascular endothelium independent of eNOS genotype. Supplementation of n-3 PUFA favored the maintenance of endothelial integrity with an increase in endothelial progenitor cells and a decrease in endothelial microparticles (Wu, Mayneris-Perxachs, Lovegrove, Todd, & Yaqoob, 2014).

Meta-analyses provided additional clinical evidence supporting the effects of n-3 PUFA on endothelial function. Daily supplementation of n-3 PUFA at a dose ranging from 0.45 to 4.5 g/d significantly improved endothelial function manifested by an increase in flow-mediated dilation by 2.30%. This effect was significant in individuals with cardiovascular disease or its risk factor profiles at baseline rather than in healthy individuals, and enhanced in individuals with higher doses of n-3 PUFA compared to those with lower dose (Wang et al., 2012). Evidence from another meta-analysis also suggested a possible role of n-3 PUFA intake in improving endothelial function with improved flow-mediated dilation. Nevertheless, in this study, individuals with normal blood glucose and lower DBP were more likely to benefit from the supplementation of n-3 PUFA with remarkable improvement of endothelial function (Xin, Wei, & Li, 2012).

11.5.2 Anti-inflammatory response

Growing evidence supports an important relationship between inflammation and hypertension. N-3 PUFA is involved in some inflammatory pathways that are responsible for the progression of atherogenesis, contributing to the pathological process of hypertension. The supplementation of n-3 PUFA, even at a low dose of 2.4 g/day, is capable of reducing the production of pro-inflammatory mediators, including tumor necrosis factor-α (TNF-α), interleukin-1, and interleukin-6 from mononuclear cells under endotoxin stimulation. Furthermore, n-3 PUFA suppressed the generation of interleukin-2 and T-lymphocyte proliferation, inhibited the expression of adhesion molecules to prevent monocytes from migrating to the vascular wall, and attenuated the prothrombotic effect of platelet activating factor (Meydani et al., 1991). Further study discovered that G protein-coupled receptor 120 served as a receptor/sensor of n-3 PUFA to mediate broad anti-inflammatory effects in macrophages. Proinflammatory transcription factors, including activator protein-1 that activated production of TNF-α and nuclear factor kappa B that regulated the expression of proinflammatory cytokines and adhesion molecules, were down-regulated by n-3 PUFA via binding to the G protein-coupled receptor 120 (Oh et al., 2010). Moreover, this suppression of nuclear factor kappa B via G protein-coupled receptor 120, and the stimulation of autophagy involving essential autophagy protein ATG7, were two distinct mechanisms underlying the inhibiting effect of n-3 PUFA on inflammasomes activation induced by infection, host-molecules of injured cells, and cardiovascular risk-related molecules (Williams-Bey et al., 2014).

In addition, the acute inflammatory response is divided into initiation and resolution, and the latter is recognized to be a passive process. N-3 PUFA can be used to resolve inflammatory exudates to produce specialized pro-resolving mediators (SPMs), which function as agonists to prevent further neutrophil influx, the activation of nonphlogistic responses by macrophages, as well as the resolution process, leading to a reduction in the magnitude and duration of inflammation (Serhan, 2014).

11.5.3 Renin-angiotensin system

The renin-angiotensin aldosterone system (RAAS) is a hormonal cascade that is involved in the regulation of arterial pressure, tissue perfusion, and extracellular volume. Combined with its receptors, especially the type 1 receptor, angiotensin (Ang) II serves as the primary effector of a variety of well-recognized physiological and pathophysiological effects of RAAS, including vasoconstriction, cardiac hypertrophy, hypertension, sodium reabsorption, as well as aldosterone biosynthesis and release (Li, Zhang, & Zhuo, 2017). Treatment of hypertensive patients with fish oil enriched in DHA and EPA (2:3, 500 mg) shows a hypotensive effect on SBP, which is accompanied by a decrease in plasma concentrations of Ang II. It is suggested that there is an involvement of RAAS in the mechanism underlying the antihypertensive effects of dietary n-3 PUFA (Yang et al., 2019). Acute exposure of vascular smooth muscle cells to EPA, even with low concentrations of 10 to 30 μmol/L, can not only decrease the amount of calcium available for release but also inhibit the release of calcium from inositol trisphosphate-sensitive stores in the sarcoplasmic reticulum as well as extracellular sources in response to Ang II. In addition to its effects on calcium influx, EPA is also capable of the inhibition of protein kinase C stimulated by Ang II. The inhibition of these mediators, calcium and protein kinase C by EPA may be responsible for the favorable effects of EPA on BP (Nyby, Hori, Ormsby, Gabrielian, & Tuck, 2003). Aldosterone is another effector in RAAS that regulates blood pressure via its control of sodium and water reabsorption, as well as its powerful vasoconstrictor effect (Xanthakis & Vasan, 2013). N-3 PUFA appears to suppress the secretion of aldosterone compared to physiological stimuli such as Ang II. This effect may be related to changes in intracellular signal transduction, alterations in plasma viscosity, or an inhibition of angiotensin converting enzyme (Cabo et al., 2012).

11.5.4 Eicosanoid pathway

N-3 PUFAs are substrates for cyclooxygenases (COX), lipoxygenases (LOX), or cytochrome P450 monooxygenases (CYP). As the key enzyme for the conversion of AA to prostaglandins, COX products give rise to prostanoids and thromboxanes, and thus modulate thromboregulatory, inflammatory, and chemotaxic responses (DuBois et al., 1998; Hwang, 2000). Stimulating the insertion of molecular oxygen into AA, LOX is involved in the first step to forming leukotrienes and hydroxyeicosatetraenoic acid, and further takes a part in vascular permeability, vasoconstriction, and bronchoconstriction. Although n-3 PUFA is a weaker substrate for COX and LOX reactions compared to n-6 PUFA, binding n-3 PUFA to COX-1 exposes a strained configuration to misalign carbon 13 with respect to Tyr-385, of which the residue leads to a 7-fold reduction in oxygenation efficiency relative to n-6 PUFA (Hwang, 2000). Since the AA is the precursor of the 2-series pro-inflammatory and pro-thrombotic eicosanoids (prostaglandins, leukotriene, and thromboxane), EPA could directly compete with AA for COX and LOX pathways, generating 3-series eicosanoid derivatives with less pro-inflammatory and pro-thrombotic actions than those derived from AA. In addition, CYP catalyzes the NADPH-dependent oxidation of fatty acids, including n-3 PUFA that was converted to both epoxy and hydroxy fatty acids. CYP-eicosanoid formation is known as the "third branch of the AA cascade," and this mechanism may also be alternative and important in cells in the absence of COX or LOX (Oliw & Sprecher, 1991).

11.5.5 Gut-brain axis

Supplementation of 4-g of EPA and DHA for 8 weeks, no matter as a nutraceutical in the form of capsules or as functional drink, induced a reversible increase in several short-chain fatty acids (SCFAs)-producing bacteria, including

Bifidobacterium, Roseburia, and Lactobacillus (Watson et al., 2018). SCFAs bind to the metabolite-sensing receptors to trigger intracellular signaling, which is widely expressed in diverse organs/tissues, including sympathetic ganglia, endothelial cells, epithelial cells, renal juxtaglomerular apparatus, and smooth muscle cells (Li, Su, Zhou, & Yao, 2014; Nøhr et al., 2015; Pluznick et al., 2013). Acting as vasodilators, SCFAs reduce BP in a dose-dependent manner when applied systemically. Moreover, SCFAs exert physiological actions through binding with host G protein-coupled receptors as ligands, of which G protein-coupled receptor 41 (Gpr41) and olfactory receptor 78 (Olfr78) might play opposite roles in the regulation of blood pressure (Pluznick, 2017) (Pluznick, 2013). Gpr41 was found to localize to the vascular endothelium, and to regulate intrinsic vascular tone. Knocking out Gpr41 would lead to isolated systolic hypertension, a hypertension of "vascular" origin (Natarajan et al., 2016).

On the contrary, localized at the renal afferent arteriole and vascular smooth muscle cells in the peripheral vasculature, Olfr78 might contribute to renin-driven hypertension. Mice showed lower levels of plasma renin, accompanied by lower blood pressure in the absence of Olfr78 (Pluznick et al., 2013). Findings from the clinical literature are also supportive of the concept that microbial SCFAs were involved in the regulation of blood pressure. A pilot study based on 24-h ambulatory blood pressure measurements showed that fecal abundance of SCFAs was significantly different among individuals with different blood pressure, with increases in stool levels of acetate, butyrate, and propionate in individuals with hypertension compared to those with normal blood pressure (Huart et al., 2019). The Healthy Life in an Urban Setting (HELIUS) study was conducted among six different ethnic groups of 4,672 participants. The results revealed that young Dutch participants with lower SBP had significantly lower fecal levels of SCFAs, including acetate and propionate, and their fecal SCFA levels were positively correlated with SBP and DBP (Verhaar et al., 2020).

11.6 Conclusion

In summary, clinical evidence has been accumulated to support the lowering effects of marine n-3 FA on BP, which are more pronounced in hypertensive than normotensive populations. Information on other dietary fatty acids (SFA, linoleic acid, α-linolenic acid) is mostly less robust and therefore their impacts on BP are inconsistent or clinically minor. Nevertheless, it is evident that DASH diet with lower content of SFA and total fat and Mediterranean-style diet with a high ratio of MUFA/SFA are beneficial for the prevention and management of hypertension. Additionally, there are many basic laboratory investigations to explain the biological mechanisms for the n-3 PUFAs' BP-lowering efficacy to some extent, involving the improvements in endothelial functions, anti-inflammatory response, renin-angiotensin system, eicosanoid pathway, and gut-brain axis. Given the published findings, it could be speculated that the different components of dietary fat, rather than the total content of dietary fat, determined the effects on BP. Moreover, the interaction between dietary fat or individual fatty acids and other nutrients on BP should not be ignored. Further prospective epidemiological intervention with different fat subtypes studies should investigate and determine the precise recommendations or guidance of dietary fat in terms of the quality and quantity of each component for the prevention and management of hypertension, which was able to be applied in populations with different dietary patterns and healthy status.

References

Abbasnezhad, A., Falahi, E., Gonzalez, M. J., Kavehi, P., Fouladvand, F., & Choghakhori, R. (2020). Effect of different dietary approaches compared with a regular diet on systolic and diastolic blood pressure in patients with type 2 diabetes: A systematic review and meta-analysis. *Diabetes Research and Clinical Practice*, 163. https://doi.org/10.1016/j.diabres.2020.108108.

AbuMweis, S., Jew, S., Tayyem, R., & Agraib, L. (2018). Eicosapentaenoic acid and docosahexaenoic acid containing supplements modulate risk factors for cardiovascular disease: A meta-analysis of randomised placebo-control human clinical trials. *Journal of Human Nutrition and Dietetics*, 31(1), 67–84. https://doi.org/10.1111/jhn.12493.

Adeloye, D., & Basquill, C. (2014). Estimating the prevalence and awareness rates of hypertension in Africa: A systematic analysis. *PLoS One*, 9(8). https://doi.org/10.1371/journal.pone.0104300.

Alonso, A., Ruiz-Gutierrez, V., & Martínez-González, M. A. (2006). Monounsaturated fatty acids, olive oil and blood pressure: Epidemiological, clinical and experimental evidence. *Public Health Nutrition*, 9(2), 251–257. https://doi.org/10.1079/PHN2005836.

Anchala, R., Kannuri, N. K., Pant, H., Khan, H., Franco, O. H., Di Angelantonio, E., et al. (2014). Hypertension in India: A systematic review and meta-analysis of prevalence, awareness, and control of hypertension. *Journal of Hypertension*, 32(6), 1170–1177. https://doi.org/10.1097/HJH.0000000000000146.

Appel, L. J., Miller, E. R., Seidler, A. J., & Whelton, P. K. (1993). Does supplementation of diet with 'fish oil' reduce blood pressure?: A meta-analysis of controlled clinical trials. *Archives of Internal Medicine*, 153(12), 1429–1438. https://doi.org/10.1001/archinte.1993.00410120017003.

Appel, L. J., Moore, T. J., Obarzanek, E., Vollmer, W. M., Svetkey, L. P., Sacks, F. M., et al. (1997). A clinical trial of the effects of dietary patterns on blood pressure. *New England Journal of Medicine*, 336(16), 1117–1124. https://doi.org/10.1056/NEJM199704173361601.

Biscione, F., Pignalberi, C., Totteri, A., Messina, F., & Altamura, G. (2007). Cardiovascular effects of omega-3 free fatty acids. *Current Vascular Pharmacology*, 5(2), 163–172. https://doi.org/10.2174/157016107780368334.

Cabo, J., Alonso, R., & Mata, P. (2012). Omega-3 fatty acids and blood pressure. *British Journal of Nutrition*, 107(2), S195–S200. https://doi.org/10.1017/S0007114512001584.

Campbell, F., Dickinson, H. O., Critchley, J. A., Ford, G. A., & Bradburn, M. (2013). A systematic review of fish-oil supplements for the prevention and treatment of hypertension. *European Journal of Preventive Cardiology*, 20(1), 107–120. https://doi.org/10.1177/2047487312437056.

Chen, J., Sun, B., & Zhang, D. (2019). Association of dietary n3 and n6 fatty acids intake with hypertension: NHANES 2007–2014. *Nutrients*, 11(6). https://doi.org/10.3390/nu11061232.

Chisaki, K., Okuda, Y., Suzuki, S., Miyauchi, T., Soma, M., Ohkoshi, N., et al. (2003). Eicosapentaenoic acid suppresses basal and insulin-stimulated endothelin-1 production in human endothelial cells. *Hypertension Research*, 26(8), 655–661. https://doi.org/10.1291/hypres.26.655.

Chiu, S., Bergeron, N., Williams, P. T., Bray, G. A., Sutherland, B., & Krauss, R. M. (2016). Comparison of the DASH (dietary approaches to stop hypertension) diet and a higher-fat DASH diet on blood pressure and lipids and lipoproteins: A randomized controlled trial. *American Journal of Clinical Nutrition*, 103(2), 341–347. https://doi.org/10.3945/ajcn.115.123281.

Colussi, G., Catena, C., Novello, M., Bertin, N., & Sechi, L. A. (2017). Impact of omega-3 polyunsaturated fatty acids on vascular function and blood pressure: Relevance for cardiovascular outcomes. *Nutrition, Metabolism and Cardiovascular Diseases*, 27(3), 191–200. https://doi.org/10.1016/j.numecd.2016.07.011.

DuBois, R. N., Abramson, S. B., Crofford, L., Gupta, R. A., Simon, L. S., Van De Putte, L. B. A., et al. (1998). Cyclooxygenase in biology and disease. *FASEB Journal*, 12(12), 1063–1073. https://doi.org/10.1096/fasebj.12.12.1063.

Elena, J., de Any, C. R. M., Dandan, L., Ho, H. V. T., Sonia, B. M., Sievenpiper, J. L., et al. (2019). Effect of high-carbohydrate or high-monounsaturated fatty acid diets on blood pressure: a systematic review and meta-analysis of randomized controlled trials. *Nutrition Reviews*, 19–31. https://doi.org/10.1093/nutrit/nuy040.

Elliott, P., Stamler, J., Nichols, R., Dyer, A. R., Stamler, R., Kesteloot, H., et al. (1996). Intersalt revisited: Further analyses of 24 hour sodium excretion and blood pressure within and across populations. *British Medical Journal*, 312(7041), 1249–1253. https://doi.org/10.1136/bmj.312.7041.1249.

Fields, L. E., Burt, V. L., Cutler, J. A., Hughes, J., Roccella, E. J., & Sorlie, P. (2004). The burden of adult hypertension in the United States 1999 to 2000: A rising tide. *Hypertension*, 44(4), 398–404. https://doi.org/10.1161/01.HYP.0000142248.54761.56.

Filippi, A., Paolini, I., Innocenti, F., Mazzaglia, G., Battaggia, A., & Brignoli, O. (2009). Blood pressure control and drug therapy in patients with diagnosed hypertension: A survey in Italian general practice. *Journal of Human Hypertension*, 23(11), 758–763. https://doi.org/10.1038/jhh.2009.14.

Gao, M., Wang, F., Shen, Y., Zhu, X., Zhang, X., & Sun, X. (2018). Trajectories of mediterranean diet adherence and risk of hypertension in China: Results from the CHNS study, 1997–2011. *Nutrients*, 10(12). https://doi.org/10.3390/nu10122014.

Geldsetzer, P., Manne-Goehler, J., Theilmann, M., Davies, J. I., Awasthi, A., Vollmer, S., et al. (2018). Diabetes and hypertension in India a nationally representative study of 1.3 million adults. *JAMA Internal Medicine*, 178(3), 363–372. https://doi.org/10.1001/jamainternmed.2017.8094.

Geleijnse, J. M., Giltay, E. J., Grobbee, D. E., Donders, A. R. T., & Kok, F. J. (2002). Blood pressure response to fish oil supplementation: Metaregression analysis of randomized trials. *Journal of Hypertension, 20*(8), 1493–1499. https://doi.org/10.1097/00004872-200208000-00010.

Grynberg, A. (2005). Hypertension prevention: From nutrients to (fortified) foods to dietary patterns. Focus on fatty acids. *Journal of Human Hypertension, 19*, S25–S33. https://doi.org/10.1038/sj.jhh.1001957.

Hajjar, I., & Kotchen, T. A. (2003). Trends in prevalence, awareness, treatment, and control of hypertension in the United States, 1988-2000. *Journal of the American Medical Association, 290*(2), 199–206. https://doi.org/10.1001/jama.290.2.199.

Hartweg, J., Farmer, A. J., Holman, R. R., & Neil, H. A. (2007). Meta-analysis of the effects of $n-3$ polyunsaturated fatty acids on haematological and thrombogenic factors in type 2 diabetes. *Diabetologia, 50*(2), 250–258. https://doi.org/10.1007/s00125-006-0486-y.

Hartweg, J., Farmer, A. J., Holman, R. R., & Neil, A. (2009). Potential impact of omega-3 treatment on cardiovascular disease in type 2 diabetes. *Current Opinion in Lipidology, 20*(1), 30–38. https://doi.org/10.1097/MOL.0b013e328321b3be.

Hooper, L., Al-Khudairy, L., Abdelhamid, A. S., Rees, K., Brainard, J. S., Brown, T. J., et al. (2018). Omega-6 fats for the primary and secondary prevention of cardiovascular disease. *Cochrane Database of Systematic Reviews, 2018*(7). https://doi.org/10.1002/14651858.CD011094.pub3.

Hooper, L., Martin, N., Jimoh, O. F., Kirk, C., Foster, E., & Abdelhamid, A. S. (2020). Reduction in saturated fat intake for cardiovascular disease. *Cochrane Database of Systematic Reviews, 2020*(8). https://doi.org/10.1002/14651858.CD011737.pub3.

Hoshi, T., Wissuwa, B., Tian, Y., Tajima, N., Xu, R., Bauer, M., et al. (2013). Omega-3 fatty acids lower blood pressure by directly activating large-conductance $Ca2+$−dependent $K+$ channels. *Proceedings of the National Academy of Sciences of the United States of America, 110*(12), 4816–4821. https://doi.org/10.1073/pnas.1221997110.

Huang, T., Shou, T., Cai, N., Wahlqvist, M. L., & Li, D. (2012). Associations of plasma n3 polyunsaturated fatty acids with blood pressure and cardiovascular risk factors among Chinese. *International Journal of Food Sciences and Nutrition, 63*(6), 667–673. https://doi.org/10.3109/09637486.2011.652076.

Huart, J., Leenders, J., Taminiau, B., Descy, J., Saint-Remy, A., Daube, G., et al. (2019). Gut microbiota and fecal levels of short-chain fatty acids differ upon 24-hour blood pressure levels in men. *Hypertension, 74*(4), 1005–1013. https://doi.org/10.1161/HYPERTENSIONAHA.118.12588.

Hwang, D. (2000). Fatty acids and immune responses—A new perspective in searching for clues to mechanism. *Annual Review of Nutrition, 20*, 431–456. https://doi.org/10.1146/annurev.nutr.20.1.431.

Kannel, W. B., Wolf, P. A., McGee, D. L., McNamara, P., & Castelli, W. P. (1981). Systolic blood pressure, arterial rigidity, and risk of stroke: The Framingham study. *JAMA: The Journal of the American Medical Association, 245*(12), 1225–1229. https://doi.org/10.1001/jama.1981.03310370017013.

Kearney, M., Megan, W., Kristi, R., Paul, M., Whelton, P. K., & Jiang, H. (2005). Global burden of hypertension: Analysis of worldwide data. *The Lancet, 217*–223. https://doi.org/10.1016/s0140-6736(05)17741-1.

Lahoz, C., Alonso, R., Ordovás, J. M., López-Farré, A., De Oya, M., & Mata, P. (1997). Effects of dietary fat saturation on eicosanoid production, platelet aggregation and blood pressure. *European Journal of Clinical Investigation, 27*(9), 780–787. https://doi.org/10.1046/j.1365-2362.1997.1860735.x.

Lee, S. P. S., Dart, A. M., Walker, K. Z., O'Dea, K., Chin-Dusting, J. P. F., & Skilton, M. R. (2012). Effect of altering dietary $n-6:n-3$ PUFA ratio on cardiovascular risk measures in patients treated with statins: A pilot study. *British Journal of Nutrition, 108*(7), 1280–1285. https://doi.org/10.1017/S0007114511006519.

Li, X. C., Zhang, J., & Zhuo, J. L. (2017). The vasoprotective axes of the renin-angiotensin system: Physiological relevance and therapeutic implications in cardiovascular, hypertensive and kidney diseases. *Pharmacological Research, 125*(Pt A), 21–38. https://doi.org/10.1016/j.phrs.2017.06.005.

Li, Z., Chen, J., & Zhang, D. (2019). Association between dietary carotenoid intakes and hypertension in adults: National health and nutrition examination survey 2007-2014. *Journal of Hypertension, 37*(12), 2371–2379. https://doi.org/10.1097/HJH.0000000000002200.

Li, G., Su, H., Zhou, Z., & Yao, W. (2014). Identification of the porcine G protein-coupled receptor 41 and 43 genes and their expression pattern in different tissues and development stages. *PLoS One, 9*(5). https://doi.org/10.1371/journal.pone.0097342.

López, D., Orta, X., Casós, K., Sáiz, M. P., Puig-Parellada, P., Farriol, M., et al. (2004). Upregulation of endothelial nitric oxide synthase in rat aorta after ingestion of fish oil-rich diet. *American Journal of Physiology—Heart and Circulatory Physiology, 287*(2), H567–H572. https://doi.org/10.1152/ajpheart.01145.2003.

Lorente-Cebrián, S., Costa, A. G. V., Navas-Carretero, S., Zabala, M., Martínez, J. A., & Moreno-Aliaga, M. J. (2013). Role of omega-3 fatty acids in obesity, metabolic syndrome, and cardiovascular diseases: A review of the evidence. *Journal of Physiology and Biochemistry, 69*(3), 633–651. https://doi.org/10.1007/s13105-013-0265-4.

Lu, J., Lu, Y., Wang, X., Li, X., Linderman, G. C., Wu, C., et al. (2017). Prevalence, awareness, treatment, and control of hypertension in China: Data from 1.7 million adults in a population-based screening study (China PEACE million persons project). *The Lancet*, 390(10112), 2549–2558. https://doi.org/10.1016/S0140-6736(17)32478-9.

MacDonald, T. M., & Morant, S. V. (2008). Prevalence and treatment of isolated and concurrent hypertension and hypercholesterolaemia in the United Kingdom. *British Journal of Clinical Pharmacology*, 65(5), 775–786. https://doi.org/10.1111/j.1365-2125.2007.03072.x.

Matsumoto, C., Yoruk, A., Wang, L., Gaziano, J. M., & Sesso, H. D. (2019). Fish and omega-3 fatty acid consumption and risk of hypertension. *Journal of Hypertension*, 37(6), 1223–1229. https://doi.org/10.1097/HJH.0000000000002062.

Meydani, S. N., Endres, S., Woods, M. M., Goldin, B. R., Soo, C., Morrill-Labrode, A., et al. (1991). Oral ($n-3$) fatty acid supplementation suppresses cytokine production and lymphocyte proliferation: Comparison between young and older women. *Journal of Nutrition*, 121(4), 547–555. https://doi.org/10.1093/jn/121.4.547.

Miller, P. E., Van Elswyk, M., & Alexander, D. D. (2014). Long-chain Omega-3 fatty acids eicosapentaenoic acid and docosahexaenoic acid and blood pressure: A meta-analysis of randomized controlled trials. *American Journal of Hypertension*, 27(7), 885–896. https://doi.org/10.1093/ajh/hpu024.

Mittal, B. V., & Singh, A. K. (2010). Hypertension in the developing world: Challenges and opportunities. *American Journal of Kidney Diseases*, 55(3), 590–598. https://doi.org/10.1053/j.ajkd.2009.06.044.

Miura, K., Stamler, J., Brown, I. J., Ueshima, H., Nakagawa, H., Sakurai, M., et al. (2013). Relationship of dietary monounsaturated fatty acids to blood pressure: The international study of macro/micronutrients and blood pressure. *Journal of Hypertension*, 31(6), 1144–1150. https://doi.org/10.1097/HJH.0b013e3283604016.

Miyagawa, N., Miura, K., Okuda, N., Kadowaki, T., Takashima, N., Nagasawa, S. Y., et al. (2014). Long-chain $n-3$ polyunsaturated fatty acids intake and cardiovascular disease mortality risk in Japanese: A 24-year follow-up of NIPPON DATA80. *Atherosclerosis*, 232(2), 384–389. https://doi.org/10.1016/j.atherosclerosis.2013.11.073.

Miyajima, T., Tsujino, T., Saito, K., & Yokoyama, M. (2001). Effects of eicosapentaenoic acid on blood pressure, cell membrane fatty acids, and intracellular sodium concentration in essential hypertension. *Hypertension Research*, 24(5), 537–542. https://doi.org/10.1291/hypres.24.537.

Morenga, L. T., & Montez, J. M. (2017). Health effects of saturated and trans-fatty acid intake in children and adolescents: Systematic review and meta-analysis. *PLoS One*, 12(11). https://doi.org/10.1371/journal.pone.0186672.

Mori, T. A., Bao, D. Q., Burke, V., Puddey, I. B., & Beilin, L. J. (1999). Docosahexaenoic acid but not eicosapentaenoic acid lowers ambulatory blood pressure and heart rate in humans. *Hypertension*, 34(2), 253–260. https://doi.org/10.1161/01.HYP.34.2.253.

Morris, M. C., Sacks, F., & Rosner, B. (1993). Does fish oil lower blood pressure? A meta-analysis of controlled trials. *Circulation*, 88(2), 523–533. https://doi.org/10.1161/01.CIR.88.2.523.

Nakamura, H., Hara, A., Tsujiguchi, H., Nguyen, T. T. T., Kambayashi, Y., Miyagi, S., et al. (2018). Relationship between dietary $n-6$ fatty acid intake and hypertension: Effect of glycated hemoglobin levels. *Nutrients*, 10(12). https://doi.org/10.3390/nu10121825.

Nakamura, H., Tsujiguchi, H., Kambayashi, Y., Hara, A., Miyagi, S., Yamada, Y., et al. (2019). Relationship between saturated fatty acid intake and hypertension and oxidative stress. *Nutrition*, 61, 8–15. https://doi.org/10.1016/j.nut.2018.10.020.

Natarajan, N., Hori, D., Flavahan, S., Steppan, J., Flavahan, N. A., Berkowitz, D. E., et al. (2016). Microbial short chain fatty acid metabolites lower blood pressure via endothelial G protein-coupled receptor 41. *Physiological Genomics*, 48(11), 826–834. https://doi.org/10.1152/physiolgenomics.00089.2016.

Nøhr, M. K., Egerod, K. L., Christiansen, S. H., Gille, A., Offermanns, S., Schwartz, T. W., et al. (2015). Expression of the short chain fatty acid receptor GPR41/FFAR3 in autonomic and somatic sensory ganglia. *Neuroscience*, 290, 126–137. https://doi.org/10.1016/j.neuroscience.2015.01.040.

Nyby, M. D., Hori, M. T., Ormsby, B., Gabrielian, A., & Tuck, M. L. (2003). Eicosapentaenoic acid inhibits Ca2+ mobilization and PKC activity in vascular smooth muscle cells. *American Journal of Hypertension*, 16(9 I), 708–714. https://doi.org/10.1016/S0895-7061(03)00980-4.

O'Mahoney, L. L., Matu, J., Price, O. J., Birch, K. M., Ajjan, R. A., Farrar, D., et al. (2018). Omega-3 polyunsaturated fatty acids favourably modulate cardiometabolic biomarkers in type 2 diabetes: A meta-analysis and meta-regression of randomized controlled trials. *Cardiovascular Diabetology*, 17(1). https://doi.org/10.1186/s12933-018-0740-x.

O'Sullivan, T. A., Bremner, A. P., Beilin, L. J., Ambrosini, G. L., Mori, T. A., Huang, R. C., et al. (2012). Polyunsaturated fatty acid intake and blood pressure in adolescents. *Journal of Human Hypertension*, 26(3), 178–187. https://doi.org/10.1038/jhh.2011.7.

Oh, D. Y., Talukdar, S., Bae, E. J., Imamura, T., Morinaga, H., Fan, W. Q., et al. (2010). GPR120 is an omega-3 fatty acid receptor mediating potent anti-inflammatory and insulin-sensitizing effects. *Cell*, 142(5), 687–698. https://doi.org/10.1016/j.cell.2010.07.041.

Oliver, W. J., Cohen, E. I., & Neel, J. V. (1975). Blood pressure, sodium intake, and sodium related hormones in the Yanomamo Indians, a "no salt" culture. *Circulation*, 52(1), 146–151. https://doi.org/10.1161/01.CIR.52.1.146.

Oliw, E. H., & Sprecher, H. W. (1991). Metabolism of polyunsaturated (n−3) fatty acids by monkey seminal vesicles: Isolation and biosynthesis of omega-3 epoxides. *Biochimica et Biophysica Acta (BBA)/Lipids and Lipid Metabolism*, *1086*(3), 287–294. https://doi.org/10.1016/0005-2760(91)90172-E.

Omura, M., Kobayashi, S., Mizukami, Y., Mogami, K., Todoroki-Ikeda, N., Miyake, T., et al. (2001). Eicosapentaenoic acid (EPA) induces Ca2+−independent activation and translocation of endothelial nitric oxide synthase and endothelium-dependent vasorelaxation. *FEBS Letters*, *487*(3), 361–366. https://doi.org/10.1016/S0014-5793(00)02351-6.

Patel, J. V., Tracey, I., Hughes, E. A., & Lip, G. Y. (2010). Omega-3 polyunsaturated acids and cardiovascular disease: Notable ethnic differences or unfulfilled promise? *Journal of Thrombosis and Haemostasis*, *8*(10), 2095–2104. https://doi.org/10.1111/j.1538-7836.2010.03956.x.

Pereira, M., Lunet, N., Azevedo, A., & Barros, H. (2009). Differences in prevalence, awareness, treatment and control of hypertension between developing and developed countries. *Journal of Hypertension*, *27*(5), 963–975. https://doi.org/10.1097/HJH.0b013e3283282f65.

Pluznick, J. L. (2013). A novel SCFA receptor, the microbiota, and blood pressure regulation. *Gut Microbes*, *5*(2). https://doi.org/10.4161/gmic.27492.

Pluznick, J. L. (2017). Microbial short-chain fatty acids and blood pressure regulation. *Current Hypertension Reports*, *19*(4). https://doi.org/10.1007/s11906-017-0722-5.

Pluznick, J. L., Protzko, R. J., Gevorgyan, H., Peterlin, Z., Sipos, A., Han, J., et al. (2013). Olfactory receptor responding to gut microbiota derived signals plays a role in renin secretion and blood pressure regulation. *Proceedings of the National Academy of Sciences of the United States of America*, *110*(11), 4410–4415. https://doi.org/10.1073/pnas.1215927110.

Qian, F., Korat, A. A., Malik, V., & Hu, F. B. (2016). Metabolic effects of monounsaturated fatty acid-enriched diets compared with carbohydrate or polyunsaturated fatty acid-enriched diets in patients with type 2 diabetes: A systematic review and meta-analysis of randomized controlled trials. *Diabetes Care*, *39*(8), 1448–1457. https://doi.org/10.2337/dc16-0513.

Ralston, R. A., Lee, J. H., Truby, H., Palermo, C. E., & Walker, K. Z. (2012). A systematic review and meta-analysis of elevated blood pressure and consumption of dairy foods. *Journal of Human Hypertension*, *26*(1), 3–13. https://doi.org/10.1038/jhh.2011.3.

Ratnayake, W. M. N., & Galli, C. (2009). Fat and fatty acid terminology, methods of analysis and fat digestion and metabolism: A background review paper. *Annals of Nutrition and Metabolism*, *55*(1–3), 8–43. https://doi.org/10.1159/000228994.

Rees, K., Takeda, A., Martin, N., Ellis, L., Wijesekara, D., Vepa, A., et al. (2019). Mediterranean-style diet for the primary and secondary prevention of cardiovascular disease. *Cochrane Database of Systematic Reviews*, *2019*(3). https://doi.org/10.1002/14651858.CD009825.pub3.

Sacks, F. M., Lichtenstein, A. H., Wu, J. H. Y., Appel, L. J., Creager, M. A., Kris-Etherton, P. M., et al. (2017). Dietary fats and cardiovascular disease: A presidential advisory from the American Heart Association. *Circulation*, *136*(3), e1–e23. https://doi.org/10.1161/CIR.0000000000000510.

Saneei, P., Salehi-Abargouei, A., Esmaillzadeh, A., & Azadbakht, L. (2014). Influence of dietary approaches to stop hypertension (DASH) diet on blood pressure: A systematic review and meta-analysis on randomized controlled trials. *Nutrition, Metabolism and Cardiovascular Diseases*, *24*(12), 1253–1261. https://doi.org/10.1016/j.numecd.2014.06.008.

Satoh, A., Arima, H., Ohkubo, T., Nishi, N., Okuda, N., Ae, R., et al. (2017). Associations of socioeconomic status with prevalence, awareness, treatment, and control of hypertension in a general Japanese population: NIPPON DATA2010. *Journal of Hypertension*, *35*(2), 401–408. https://doi.org/10.1097/HJH.0000000000001169.

Schwingshackl, L., Chaimani, A., Schwedhelm, C., Toledo, E., Pünsch, M., Hoffmann, G., et al. (2019). Comparative effects of different dietary approaches on blood pressure in hypertensive and pre-hypertensive patients: A systematic review and network meta-analysis. *Critical Reviews in Food Science and Nutrition*, *59*(16), 2674–2687. https://doi.org/10.1080/10408398.2018.1463967.

Schwingshackl, L., & Hoffmann, G. (2014). Comparison of the long-term effects of high-fat v. low-fat diet consumption on cardiometabolic risk factors in subjects with abnormal glucose metabolism: A systematic review and meta-analysis. *British Journal of Nutrition*, *111*(12), 2047–2058. https://doi.org/10.1017/S0007114514000464.

Schwingshackl, L., Strasser, B., & Hoffmann, G. (2011). Effects of monounsaturated fatty acids on cardiovascular risk factors: A systematic review and meta-analysis. *Annals of Nutrition and Metabolism*, *59*(2–4), 176–186. https://doi.org/10.1159/000334071.

Sekikawa, A., & Hayakawa, T. (2004). Prevalence of hypertension, its awareness and control in adult population in Japan. *Journal of Human Hypertension*, *18*(12), 911–912. https://doi.org/10.1038/sj.jhh.1001765.

Serhan, C. N. (2014). Pro-resolving lipid mediators are leads for resolution physiology. *Nature*, *510*(7503), 92–101. https://doi.org/10.1038/nature13479.

Shah, M., Adams-Huet, B., & Garg, A. (2007). Effect of high-carbohydrate or high-cis-monounsaturated fat diets on blood pressure: A meta-analysis of intervention trials. *American Journal of Clinical Nutrition*, *85*(5), 1251–1256. https://doi.org/10.1093/ajcn/85.5.1251.

Shen, X., Fang, A., He, J., Liu, Z., Guo, M., Gao, R., et al. (2017). Trends in dietary fat and fatty acid intakes and related food sources among Chinese adults: A longitudinal study from the China health and nutrition survey (1997-2011). *Public Health Nutrition*, *20*(16), 2927–2936. https://doi.org/10.1017/S1368980017001781.

Siervo, M., Lara, J., Chowdhury, S., Ashor, A., Oggioni, C., & Mathers, J. C. (2015). Effects of the dietary approach to stop hypertension (DASH) diet on cardiovascular risk factors: A systematic review and meta-analysis. *British Journal of Nutrition*, *113*(1), 1–15. https://doi.org/10.1017/S0007114514003341.

Sukumar, P., Sedo, A., Li, J., Wilson, L. A., O'Regan, D., Lippiat, J. D., et al. (2012). Constitutively active TRPC channels of adipocytes confer a mechanism for sensing dietary fatty acids and regulating adiponectin. *Circulation Research*, *111*(2), 191–200. https://doi.org/10.1161/CIRCRESAHA.112.270751.

Tocci, G., Nati, G., Cricelli, C., Parretti, D., Lapi, F., Ferrucci, A., et al. (2017). Prevalence and control of hypertension in the general practice in Italy: Updated analysis of a large database. *Journal of Human Hypertension*, *31*(4), 258–262. https://doi.org/10.1038/jhh.2016.71.

Ueshima, H., Stamler, J., Elliott, P., Chan, Q., Brown, I. J., Carnethon, M. R., et al. (2007). Food omega-3 fatty acid intake of individuals (total, linolenic acid, long-chain) and their blood pressure: INTERMAP study. *Hypertension*, *50*(2), 313–319. https://doi.org/10.1161/HYPERTENSIONAHA.107.090720.

US Department of Agriculture. (2015). *Scientific report of the 2015 dietary guidelines advisory committee*.

Vasan, R. S., Beiser, A., Seshadri, S., Larson, M. G., Kannel, W. B., D'Agostino, R. B., et al. (2002). Residual lifetime risk for developing hypertension in middle-aged women and men: The Framingham heart study. *Journal of the American Medical Association*, *287*(8), 1003–1010.

Verhaar, B. J. H., Collard, D., Prodan, A., Levels, J. H. M., Zwinderman, A. H., Bäckhed, F., et al. (2020). Associations between gut microbiota, faecal short-chain fatty acids, and blood pressure across ethnic groups: The HELIUS study. *European Heart Journal*, *41*(44), 4259–4267. https://doi.org/10.1093/eurheartj/ehaa704.

Wang, L. (2016). Prevalence and barriers to management of hypertension in Asia: Challenges and opportunities in the Asian century. *Heart Lung and Circulation*, *25*(3), 207–208. https://doi.org/10.1016/j.hlc.2015.12.093.

Wang, Q. Q., Liang, X. H., Wang, L. Y., Lu, X. F., Huang, J., Cao, J., … Gu, D. (2012). Effect of omega-3 fatty acids supplementation on endothelial function: A meta-analysis of randomized controlled trials. *Atherosclerosis*, *221*(2), 536–543. https://doi.org/10.1016/j.atherosclerosis.2012.01.006.

Wang, Z., Chen, Z., Zhang, L., Wang, X., Hao, G., Zhang, Z., et al. (2018). Status of hypertension in China: Results from the China hypertension survey, 2012-2015. *Circulation*, *137*(22), 2344–2356. https://doi.org/10.1161/CIRCULATIONAHA.117.032380.

Watson, H., Mitra, S., Croden, F. C., Taylor, M., Wood, H. M., Perry, S. L., et al. (2018). A randomised trial of the effect of omega-3 polyunsaturated fatty acid supplements on the human intestinal microbiota. *Gut*, *67*(11), 1974–1983. https://doi.org/10.1136/gutjnl-2017-314968.

Wendland, E., Farmer, A., Glasziou, P., & Neil, A. (2006). Effect of α linolenic acid on cardiovascular risk markers: A systematic review. *Heart*, *92*(2), 166–169. https://doi.org/10.1136/hrt.2004.053538.

Whelton, P. K., He, J., & Muntner, P. (2004). Prevalence, awareness, treatment and control of hypertension in North America, North Africa and Asia. *Journal of Human Hypertension*, *18*(8), 545–551. https://doi.org/10.1038/sj.jhh.1001701.

Williams-Bey, Y., Boularan, C., Vural, A., Huang, N. N., Hwang, I. Y., Shan-Shi, C., et al. (2014). Omega-3 free fatty acids suppress macrophage inflammasome activation by inhibiting NF-κB activation and enhancing autophagy. *PLoS One*, *9*(6). https://doi.org/10.1371/journal.pone.0097957.

Wolf-Maier, K., Cooper, R. S., Banegas, J. R., Giampaoli, S., Hense, H. W., Joffres, M., et al. (2003). Hypertension prevalence and blood pressure levels in 6 European countries, Canada, and the United States. *Journal of the American Medical Association*, *289*(18), 2363–2369. https://doi.org/10.1001/jama.289.18.2363.

Wu, S. Y., Mayneris-Perxachs, J., Lovegrove, J. A., Todd, S., & Yaqoob, P. (2014). Fish-oil supplementation alters numbers of circulating endothelial progenitor cells and microparticles independently of eNOS genotype. *American Journal of Clinical Nutrition*, *100*(5), 1232–1243. https://doi.org/10.3945/ajcn.114.088880.

Wyrwoll, C. S., Mark, P. J., Mori, T. A., Puddey, I. B., & Waddell, B. J. (2006). Prevention of programmed hyperleptinemia and hypertension by postnatal dietary ω-3 fatty acids. *Endocrinology*, *147*(1), 599–606. https://doi.org/10.1210/en.2005-0748.

Xanthakis, V., & Vasan, R. S. (2013). Aldosterone and the risk of hypertension. *Current Hypertension Reports*, *15*(2), 102–107. https://doi.org/10.1007/s11906-013-0330-y.

Xin, W., Wei, W., & Li, X. (2012). Effect of fish oil supplementation on fasting vascular endothelial function in humans: A meta-analysis of randomized controlled trials. *PLoS One*, *7*(9). https://doi.org/10.1371/journal.pone.0046028.

Yang, B., Shi, M. Q., Li, Z. H., Yang, J. J., & Li, D. (2016). Fish, long-chain $n-3$ PUFA and incidence of elevated blood pressure: A meta-analysis of prospective cohort studies. *Nutrients*, *8*(1). https://doi.org/10.3390/nu8010058.

Yang, B., Shi, L., Wang, A. M., Shi, M. Q., Li, Z. H., Zhao, F., et al. (2019). Lowering effects of $n-3$ fatty acid supplements on blood pressure by reducing plasma angiotensin II in inner Mongolia hypertensive patients: A double-blind randomized controlled trial. *Journal of Agricultural and Food Chemistry*, *67*(1), 184–192. https://doi.org/10.1021/acs.jafc.8b05463.

Zec, M. M., Schutte, A. E., Ricci, C., Baumgartner, J., Kruger, I. M., & Smuts, C. M. (2019). Long-chain polyunsaturated fatty acids are associated with blood pressure and hypertension over 10-years in black South African adults undergoing nutritional transition. *Foods*, *8*(9), 394–409. https://doi.org/10.3390/foods8090394.

Zeng, F. F., Sun, L. L., Liu, Y. H., Xu, Y., Guan, K., Ling, W. H., et al. (2014). Higher erythrocyte $n-3$ PUFAs are associated with decreased blood pressure in middle-aged and elderly Chinese adults. *Journal of Nutrition*, *144*(8), 1240–1246. https://doi.org/10.3945/jn.114.192286.

Zheng, Z. J., Folsom, A. R., Ma, J., Arnett, D. K., McGovern, P. G., & Eckfeldt, J. H. (1999). Plasma fatty acid composition and 6-year incidence of hypertension in middle-aged adults: The atherosclerosis risk in communities (ARIC) study. *American Journal of Epidemiology*, *150*(5), 492–500. https://doi.org/10.1093/oxfordjournals.aje.a010038.

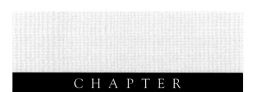

CHAPTER 12

Postprandial lipemia and the relationship to health

Catherine E. Huggins[a], Anthony P. James[b], Maxine P. Bonham[a], Katya M. Clark[b], and Sarah D. Lee[a]

[a]Department of Nutrition, Dietetics and Food, School of Clinical Sciences at Monash Health, Faculty of Medicine Nursing and Health Sciences, Monash University, Clayton, VIC, Australia [b]Nutrition & Dietetics, Curtin School of Population Health, Curtin University, Bentley, WA, Australia

12.1 Introduction

Triglycerides (TG) are the main lipid type in our diet. TG are important for a range of cellular structures and functions including energy production, regulating body temperature, maintaining cell structures, transporting molecules in the circulation, and as physical protection of other organs (in adipose tissue). Under healthy physiological conditions, excess TG are stored in adipocytes until required. When excess TG in the circulation cannot be efficiently stored or metabolized, pathological events arise, including atherogenesis, which can lead to cardiovascular disease (CVD).

Dietary fats are digested by lipases and esterases into free fatty acids, monoglycerides, lysophospholipids, and free cholesterol as they progress through the digestive tract. The products of fat digestion are absorbed into small-intestinal enterocytes where they are mostly reassembled back to TG and packaged into postprandial chylomicron (CM) lipoprotein particles. TG and cholesterol esters make up the core of the CM particle and phospholipids and free cholesterol are present on the surface. Once formed, these TG-rich CM particles are secreted into lacteals and travel via the lymphatic system into the bloodstream. Other TG-rich lipoproteins called very low-density lipoproteins (VLDL) are synthesized in the liver. In the postprandial period, the core of VLDL is TG made from fatty acids (FA) from either de novo lipogenesis (using diet-derived carbohydrate) or from the uptake of circulating lipoprotein remnants associated with FA. During their assembly and once in circulation, CM lipoproteins and VLDL associate with apolipoproteins, which contain hydrophobic and hydrophilic regions, allowing them to interact with both the hydrophobic core and hydrophilic surface of the lipoprotein particle. Apolipoproteins B48 and B100 are structurally important lipoproteins present in CM and VLDL, respectively, and also function as receptor ligands.

Postprandial lipemia is the elevation of TG-rich lipoproteins (TRL), CM, and VLDL in the circulation after a meal. Clearance of TG from the circulation occurs in the postprandial period via two key mechanisms. Firstly, CM TG and VLDL TG are lipolyzed by lipoprotein lipase (LPL) that adheres to the endothelial lining of capillaries. Lipolysis releases FA from the glycerol backbone, which are taken up primarily into adipocytes and reesterified to glycerol and stored as TG. Any TG remaining associated with remnant lipoproteins are removed from the circulation via receptor-mediated uptake by the liver. In the early postprandial period (<4 h after eating), the increase in circulating TG is predominantly due to a greater rate of intestinal CM production, with TG-rich CM particles representing approximately 80% of the increase in plasma TG following a meal (Karpe, Bell, Björkegren, & Hamsten, 1995; Schneeman, Kotite, Todd, & Havel, 1993). Gradually, the concentration of TG-rich VLDL in circulation also increases, initially due to competition with CM for lipolysis by adipose tissue-associated LPL and then later due to increased hepatic de novo lipogenesis (using diet-derived carbohydrate) and increased receptor-mediated uptake of lipoprotein remnant-associated FA for VLDL production and release.

The size of lipoproteins in circulation varies substantially and is affected by TG content. During the postprandial period, as lipolysis progresses, the size of CM and VLDL particles is reduced. Nascent CM particles are generally the largest with a maximal diameter approaching 1000 nm, whereas large VLDL particles are closer to 200 nm in diameter. As lipolysis progresses, the diameter of CM reduces and can reach a size similar to VLDL. In contrast, low-density lipoproteins (LDL) and high-density lipoproteins (HDL) are substantially smaller (20–26 and 6–16 nm, respectively) than CM and VLDL, consisting mostly of apolipoproteins with some cholesterol and/or cholesteryl esters. LDL and HDL have a major role in the transport of cholesterol to and from cells and hence contain much smaller amounts of TG. The rate of TG clearance from circulation is dependent on the rate of lipolysis and receptor-mediated uptake that occurs mainly in the liver. To lower the circulating concentration of TG postprandially, the rate of clearance must exceed the rate of appearance of CM- and VLDL-associated TG in circulation. Impaired postprandial lipid metabolism results in high circulating TG, including in CM and VLDL remnants.

In this chapter, we describe the postprandial dyslipidemia phenotype that is a risk factor for atherogenesis (Section 12.2) and explain potential mechanisms for atherosclerotic plaque formation and endothelial dysfunction (Section 12.3). Postprandial lipemia is affected by a range of modifiable factors that may reduce the risk of dyslipidemia and atherogenesis including the composition of recent meals, habitual dietary fat intake (Section 12.4), and meal timing (Section 12.5). Finally, a brief overview of nonmodifiable factors is considered (Section 12.6) followed by discussion of the relevance of screening for postprandial dyslipidemia (Section 12.7). A graphical summary of the chapter overview is presented in Fig. 12.1.

12.2 Generation of an atherogenic postprandial phenotype

This section provides an overview of how impaired lipolysis and clearance of CM and VLDL lead to the generation of an atherogenic postprandial phenotype. Evidence to implicate TG-rich remnant particles in the development of atherosclerosis (atherogenesis) was first proposed by Zilversmit (1979). As described below, increased competition for lipolysis can result in the generation of cholesterol-enriched proatherogenic CM and VLDL. Postlipolyzed CM

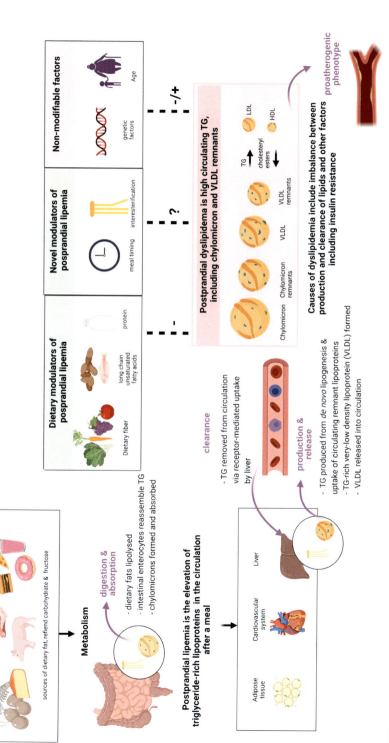

FIG. 12.1 Graphical summary of chapter concepts. When the breakdown of triglyceride (TG) and very low-density lipoprotein (VLDL) is impaired or delayed after a meal, there is an increased production of cholesterol-rich remnants, production of small dense low-density lipoprotein (LDL) particles, and a reduction of high-density lipoprotein (HDL). This is known as a pro-atherogenic phenotype that can lead to fatty streaks in blood vessel walls (Section 12.2). A mechanism for the development of the pro-atherogenic phenotype is discussed (Section 12.3). There are various known and hypothesized modulators of postmeal lipid responses including dietary factors, meal timing, and interesterification of dietary lipids in food processing (Sections 12.4 and 12.5). Nonmodifiable modulators include age and genetic profiles (Section 12.6) created by BioRender.com Dr Catherine Huggins. (n.d.). Monash University. Figure created in BioRender.com.

particles (remnants) may be harmful when they have attained a sufficiently small diameter to penetrate the subendothelial space (Proctor & Mamo, 1998). Once in this space, the small remnants can be engulfed by macrophages, leading to a cascade of events associated with the development of atherosclerosis.

Postprandial dyslipidemia refers to abnormally high or prolonged lipid elevation that suggests impairment in the production, lipolysis, or clearance of lipoproteins and their remnants. When lipolysis is impaired or delayed, the residency time of TRL in the circulation increases, and the opportunity for lipid exchange between the TRL and lipoproteins of lower density (i.e., LDL and HDL) also increases. Such an exchange is mediated by circulating cholesteryl ester transfer protein (CETP) which facilitates the exchange of TG (from the TRL) with cholesteryl esters (from HDL or LDL particles; Barter et al., 2003). This delayed lipolysis of TRL, and subsequent CETP-facilitated lipid transfer results in the production of remnant particles that are partially TG-depleted but are enriched in cholesteryl esters. The amount of cholesterol per particle in these CM and VLDL remnants has been estimated to range from 5- to 20-fold more than that found in LDL particles (Wilhelm & Cooper, 2003). This transfer also results in TG-enriched LDL and HDL particles that are lipolyzed by hepatic lipase resulting in the generation of pro-atherogenic small dense LDL particles and catabolism of the lipid-poor HDL (Barter et al., 2003; Packard, Caslake, & Shepherd, 2000).

Insulin plays an important role in the control of various stages of postprandial lipid metabolism. Under physiological conditions, insulin, which is raised in the postprandial state, suppresses lipolysis in adipose tissue and hepatic production of VLDL. Insulin can also stimulate LDL receptor–related protein 1 (LRP-1) to increase clearance of CM remnants (Laatsch et al., 2009). This action of insulin may be compromised in people who are obese with insulin resistance due to reduced gene expression of LPL (Clemente-Postigo et al., 2011) and LDL receptor (Mamo et al., 2001). Inhibition of these actions of insulin contributes to dyslipidemia and may, in part, mediate increased CVD risk in people who are obese and/or insulin resistant.

In summary, when lipolysis of TG from CM and VLDL is impaired or delayed after a meal, there is an increased production of cholesterol-rich remnants of CM and VLDL, the production of small dense LDL particles, and a reduction of HDL. This is known as a pro-atherogenic phenotype (Fig. 12.2). Potential mechanisms of how this leads to the development of atherogenesis are discussed in the next section (Section 12.3).

12.3 Mechanisms linking postprandial lipids to atherogenesis

Mechanisms that link postprandial lipemia with atherogenesis are complex and interwoven (Alipour, Elte, van Zaanen, Rietveld, & Castro Cabezas, 2008). Initiation of atherogenesis occurs through the infiltration of cholesterol-rich TRL remnants into the subendothelial space of the arterial wall (Fig. 12.2). The TRL remnants include LDL particles, remnants of VLDL, and CM remnants that were not cleared by receptor-mediated processes, for example, in the liver. These circulating remnants can interact with the arterial subendothelium via nonreceptor-mediated processes and accumulate to form fatty streaks. Even though the circulating concentration of CM remnants is relatively low compared to LDL, experimental studies have shown that CM remnant particles are more likely to be retained in the subendothelial space of carotid arteries compared with LDL particles (Nakajima et al., 2011; Proctor, Vine, & Mamo, 2004). The biophysical characteristics of the lipoprotein (size, density, and composition) influence how it anchors and binds with the connective tissue matrix. Differences in apolipoprotein content between LDL and CM remnants may be partly responsible for the difference in their efflux from the subendothelial space. Apolipoprotein (apo) B48, the predominant structural

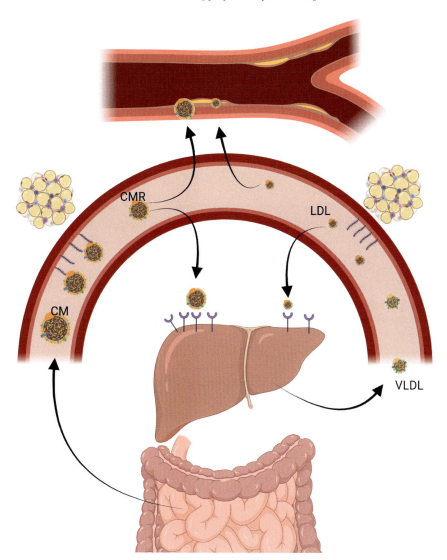

FIG. 12.2 CM and VLDL in circulation. CM are synthesized in small intestine. In blood circulation LPL can lipolyze TG from the core and the fatty acid is taken up into adipocytes. The CM become smaller and relatively cholesterol-rich remnants that can be removed from circulation by LDL receptors, mainly in the liver. VLDL are TG-rich lipoproteins produced in the liver and are similarly acted on by LPL. VLDL remnants are further lipolyzed to become IDL and LDL or cleared from circulation. The CMR and LDL that remain in circulation are dense, cholesterol-rich and risk being part of the atherogenic process, LDL (particularly oxidized LDL) and CMR have the ability to infiltrate the intima of the blood vessels and contribute to atherogenesis. *CM*, chylomicron; *CMR*, chylomicron remnant; *LDL*, low-density lipoprotein; *LIPL*, lipoprotein lipase; *VLDL*, very low-density lipoprotein. *From Katya Clark. (2021). Curtin University. Figure created in BioRender.com.*

apolipoprotein of CM, may exacerbate binding to extracellular proteoglycans compared to apo B100, the predominant apolipoprotein of LDL (Nakajima et al., 2011; Proctor et al., 2004). CM remnant accumulation may explain why impaired postprandial lipid metabolism contributes to arterial cholesterol deposition.

Interactions between lipid metabolism and inflammation contribute to the progression of atherosclerosis. In the postprandial period, monocytes in the blood can develop lipid droplets (Gower et al., 2011). An increase in blood TG is associated with the acute inflammatory response in circulating human monocytes, expression of adhesion molecules, and an inflamed epithelium. Monocytes that infiltrate the arterial tissue are differentiated into macrophages that scavenge more lipid by way of the cholesterol-rich lipoprotein remnants that are trapped in the subendothelial space. The macrophages become lipid-laden foam cells to further contribute to atherosclerotic lesions and CVD susceptibility (Pirillo, Norata, & Catapano, 2014). The propensity of lipoproteins to lead to foam cell formation in human monocyte-derived macrophages is dependent on the lipoprotein type. Experimental studies have found greater accumulation of oxidized LDL compared with LDL that was not oxidized, whereas CM remnants caused extensive lipid accumulation in macrophages irrespective of oxidation status (Batt et al., 2004). CM remnants influence foam cell formation without the need to be oxidized, which is distinct from LDL. In this regard, CM remnants can be considered more atherogenic, as well as being more predisposed to arterial connective tissue matrix retention, which reiterates the contributions of CM lipoprotein remnants in CVD.

Postprandial dyslipidemia is also a causal factor of endothelial dysfunction due to increased oxidative stress resulting from increased availability of lipids in the circulation (Lacroix, Des Rosiers, Tardif, & Nigam, 2012). A high-fat meal can exacerbate postprandial dyslipidemia, depending on the type of fat within the meal (see Section 12.4). High dietary fat intake can promote an inflammatory response by triggering increases in neutrophils, pro-inflammatory cytokines, and the complement system C3 in circulation (Halkes et al., 2001; Pirillo et al., 2014). Furthermore, a high-carbohydrate meal can decrease plasma antioxidant capacity (Lacroix et al., 2012). In situations where excess nutrients exists alongside a low energy demand, for example, metabolic disorders including hyperglycemia or obesity with elevated free fatty acids, cells may generate excessive reactive oxygen species (ROS; Kluge, Fetterman, & Vita, 2013).

In summary, a high affinity of CM remnants for adhering to the artery wall and the contribution of lipoprotein remnants to simulating inflammation and causing endothelial dysfunction highlight postprandial lipemia as a risk factor in CVD. Maintaining an effective mechanism for clearing postprandial lipids from the circulation after a meal is critical for the prevention of a dyslipidemic profile. This also suggests that monitoring nonfasting lipids is important in cardiovascular risk screening, which is discussed further in Section 12.7. There are known and hypothesized modifiers of postprandial lipemia, and these are discussed in Sections 12.4 and 12.5.

12.4 Modulators of postprandial lipemia

The causes of lipid metabolism dysregulation are multifactorial and include primary factors such as age, sex, body mass index, and body composition and secondary factors such as obesity, metabolic syndrome, diabetes, chronic liver or kidney diseases, or medications. Dietary and lifestyle choices may be causal or mediating factors in the development of the secondary factors and therefore contribute to the risk of fasting and nonfasting elevated TG or hypertriglyceridemia. For people who are at risk of hypertriglyceridemia or with established hypertriglyceridemia, making dietary choices that can modulate postprandial responses is important for the protection of cardiometabolic health (as discussed in Section 12.3).

A pioneering study of postprandial metabolism (Berry et al., 2020) identified modifiable lifestyle and environmental factors as the predominant factors affecting postprandial responses. Important exposure factors are now thought to include timing of meals (see Section 12.5), physical activity, sleep, and circadian regulation and their interaction with meal composition and habitual diet (Berry et al., 2020). Several other studies have tested specific foods or nutrients under both acute and/or chronic conditions to examine effects on postprandial TG. A challenge to synthesizing these data is the high heterogeneity between studies with regard to methodological assessment including different populations studied (i.e., healthy or with metabolic impairment), small sample sizes, various measurements of plasma TG (sampling times and calculation of AUC vs. iAUC), differences in the amount and type of dietary fat of the test meal, test meal size, and co-ingestion of nutrients (Lee et al., 2020). This makes it complex to study and to identify dietary factors that may promote a TG-lowering response. This section will largely discuss the role of dietary fat on postprandial TG and also briefly discuss other factors including carbohydrates, proteins, and fiber.

12.4.1 Dietary fats

Short- and medium-chain fatty acids are absorbed directly into the portal system from the intestine and contribute little to the postprandial lipemic response. Long-chain fatty acids are formed into chylomicrons and enter the lymphatic system. An oral fat tolerance test (OFTT) or an acute meal challenge is a common approach used in research to examine the acute postprandial TG response, but this method requires careful consideration to a number of variables. The inconsistency between studies in controlling these different variables leads to an unclear picture of how dietary choices may modulate the postprandial TG response.

It is now accepted that the fat load used in an acute meal challenge has a dose-dependent effect on postprandial lipemia which may, in part, explain the inconsistent findings from acute studies examining the effects of different fat types on lipemic responses. The health status of the participants is also important; if the fasting TG levels are equal to or less than 1 mmol/L (89 mg/dL), there is little effect of different dietary fat types (i.e., saturated, monounsaturated, and polyunsaturated) on the postprandial response. The load or amount of fat used in the OFTT or acute meal challenge will also influence the postprandial TG response, and there appears to be a threshold fat load after which the lipemic response will increase dose-dependently after eating dietary fat, and below this threshold, there is little effect on raising postprandial TG. The fat content of preceding meals will also increase the postprandial lipemic response (Jackson, Denise Robertson, Fielding, Frayn, & Williams, 2002), and there is an interaction between an individual's habitual dietary fat consumption and their response to an OFTT acute meal challenge (Desmarchelier, Borel, Lairon, Maraninchi, & Valéro, 2019). Because of the number of modifiable variables that can influence the lipemic response, experts are calling for a more standardized approach to assessment (Kolovou et al., 2019).

12.4.2 Chain length and degree of saturation of fatty acids affect postprandial lipemia

A review by Desmarchelier et al. (2019) found no clear evidence from acute studies for a hierarchy of lipemia-raising effects based on degree of saturation. Some long-chain saturated fats (SFA) including stearic acid (18:0) and palmitic acid (16:0) have been shown to have a lower lipemic response in healthy adults compared with monounsaturated fats (MUFA) oleic acid (18:1 *cis*-9) and elaidic acid (18:1 *trans*-9). TG containing polyunsaturated fatty acids (PUFA) appear to be absorbed more rapidly than SFA. This may be explained by a slower digestion of saturated fats compared with unsaturated fats, that is, a slower formation of micelles and slower absorption of chylomicrons (Bergeron & Havel, 1995). It may also depend on the experimental conditions, as other studies have shown no difference in the absorption of SFA and PUFA (Demacker, Reijnen, Katan, Stuyt, & Stalenhoef, 1991). Acute experiments using a second meal within the data collection phase may be a useful protocol for assessing the postprandial TG response to different dietary fats. The second meal can stimulate movement of TG present in the enterocyte from the first meal into the circulation. In contrast, Desmarchelier et al. (2019) describe a hierarchal response of postprandial lipemia based on findings from intervention studies (1–4 months) proposing that when diets with similar fat content but different fat types are compared, the postprandial TG is lowest after a PUFA-rich diet, followed by MUFA and then SFA. There is evidence that the class of PUFA (omega-3 (n-3) vs. omega-6 (n-6) PUFA) may also modulate lipemic responses, but these findings have been inconsistent (Demacker et al., 1991; Finnegan et al., 2003).

12.4.3 Postprandial TG-lowering effects of polyunsaturated fatty acids

Consumption of PUFA can have a postprandial TG-lowering effect in comparison to SFA. The early work of Weintraub, Zechner, Brown, Eisenberg, and Breslow (1988) demonstrated that the postprandial response to an acute fat load in people with low fasting TG (less than 100 mg/dL) was affected by the predominant dietary fat type consumed (saturated fat or PUFA) as part of their habitual diet. These experiments showed that the postprandial rise in TG after an acute oral fat load of either SFA or PUFA was lower after 25 days on a PUFA-rich diet, compared with after 25 days on a SFA-rich diet. In contrast, there was no difference in the postprandial TG response to an acute oral load of SFA or PUFA in those following the SFA-rich diet, indicating that the postprandial TG-lowering effects of PUFA are modulated by the habitual dietary fat intake. Subsequently, the study of Bergeron and Havel (1995) also found that a habitual diet plays an important role in the response to an acute meal challenge. It was demonstrated in healthy young participants following an SFA-rich diet that an acute meal challenge rich in PUFA could lower postprandial TG compared with an acute SFA load.

A Cochrane systematic review found high certain evidence for a reduction in fasting TG after consumption of long-chain n-3 PUFA (43,000 participants in 23 trials: mean difference -0.24 mmol/L, 95% CI -0.31 to -0.16; $I^2 = 48$%; Abdelhamid et al., 2020). This TG-lowering effect is not always evident with assessment of the acute response to a meal challenge high in n-3 (Griffo et al., 2014). The rapid gastric emptying associated with n-3 PUFA intake may lead to a greater peak concentration in TG during the postprandial period. Further research is needed to understand the mechanisms of n-3 PUFA in lipid metabolism and association with CVD risk. It could be that TRL remnants are lower after an n-3 PUFA-rich diet compared with an SFA diet, and this may be one mechanism by which n-3 PUFA attenuates the progression of atherosclerosis (Demacker et al., 1991; see Section 12.3). Understanding the physical and chemical interactions between n-3 PUFA and lipoproteins may also help to explain the long-term and acute lipemic responses to n-3 PUFA intake (O'Connell, Mason, Budoff, Navar, & Shearer, 2020).

12.4.4 Fatty acid positioning in triglycerides

Fatty acids are esterified to three stereospecific positions (sn-1, sn-2, and sn-3) on the glycerol backbone of the TG molecule. Both the fatty acid type and stereospecificity affect the physical properties of the fats such as melting point and sensory properties such as mouthfeel. The *sn* positioning (and chain length) of the fatty acids can also determine the metabolic fate of dietary fat during digestion and absorption (Decker, 1996; Small, 1991) with those in positions *sn*-1 and *sn*-3 having different metabolic fates to FA located in the *sn*-2 position.

Fats in the *sn*-1 and *sn*-3 position are preferentially hydrolyzed by pancreatic lipase and LPL resulting in free fatty acids (FFA) and an *sn*-2 monoacylglycerols (Nilsson-Ehle, Egelrud, Belfrage, Olivecrona, & Borgström, 1973; Yang & Kuksis, 1991). The cleaved fatty acids, depending on their chain length, are either reassembled into new TG structures or can form insoluble soaps with calcium and excreted. Those of a shorter length are absorbed directly into the portal system. The FA in position *sn*-2 is absorbed as a monoglyceride and progresses through a more complete absorption and digestion process with slower clearance and, as such, may influence postprandial lipemic responses (Tilakavati & Kalyana, 2007). TG with SFA in *sn*-1 or *sn*-3 positions may produce a lowered postprandial response (Berry, 2009; Mensink et al., 2016; Wang, Wang, & Wang, 2016) compared with SFA present in the *sn*-2 position. A key determinant of the *sn* positioning is the dietary fat source. SFA from vegetable sources is concentrated in the *sn*-1 and *sn*-3 positions, with the unsaturated fats positioned in *sn*-2 (typically oleic and linoleic; Brockerhoff & Yurkowski, 1966; Tilakavati & Kalyana, 2007), whereas SFA from animal sources vary but is often concentrated in *sn*-2 (Berry, 2009; Tilakavati & Kalyana, 2007). This may explain why plant oils, such as palm oil, high in the saturated fatty acid, palmitic acid, do not produce an expected increased lipemic response when compared with, for example, lard (animal source of fat; Berry, 2009).

The position of palmitic acid in palm oil favors *sn*-1 and *sn*-3 unlike for lard where the majority of palmitic acid is concentrated in *sn*-2. Furthermore, stearic-rich fats such as cocoa butter appear to have a neutral effect on cholesterol levels, which is likely a consequence of the position of stearic acid in the outer positions of the TG molecule (Denke, 1994; Kritchevsky, 1994). There are exceptions. Some dairy foods, while typically considered to be high-saturated fat foods, have a proportion of short-chain SFA esterified to positions *sn*-1 and *sn*-3. When compared with equivalent sources of polyunsaturated fatty acids (PUFA) in an acute meal challenge, postprandial TG was observed to be lower (Bonham et al., 2013) after a high-fat dairy meal compared with an equivalent nondairy meal. The higher concentrations of both short- and medium-chain FA present in dairy products in the *sn*-1 and *sn*-3 positions in the TG molecule may have resulted in absorption of these FAs into the portal system rather than incorporation into CM (Jensen, Christensen, & Høy, 1994; Mu & Porsgaard, 2005). The most useful data available to compare the effect of stereospecificity on postprandial lipemia is generated from trials whereby dietary fats are manipulated (interesterified) to change their *sn* positioning. Typically, this involves the manipulation of plant/vegetable fats only. This premise is the background to the industrial transformation/interesterification of fats.

12.4.5 Interesterification (IE)

The repositioning of FA within TG molecules or interesterification (IE) can change specific characteristics of fat such as the melting point and spreadability and is seen as an alternative to hydrogenation. The repositioning of FA in TG molecules can also have implications for absorption, metabolism, and distribution within the body. While commercially, IE offers consumers a more extensive range of products with improved stability and texture, IE relocates palmitic and/or stearic fatty acids into the *sn*-2 position, increasing the potential for saturated fat uptake through chylomicron incorporation, potentially influencing CVD risk. In a recent systematic review, 12 studies (van Rooijen & Mensink, 2020) were identified that have directly compared the effects of higher versus lower proportions of both palmitic ($n=8$) and stearic acid ($n=4$) at the sn-2 position on postprandial metabolism. The majority of the studies compared native fats with IE FA, although the source of fat was not reported for all trials. While IE showed increases in palmitic or stearic FA at the sn-2 position as expected, the consequences of these modifications were mixed with postprandial TG responses, increasing, decreasing, or remaining unchanged for palmitic acid. Of the four studies that investigated stearic acid, three of the four studies reported no change to postprandial TG. The challenge meals varied considerably in the amount of fat provided and duration of follow-up during the postprandial period, making comparisons between studies difficult. However, no adverse consequences were evident from the summarized studies.

While the sn positioning of fats, in theory, provides a hypothesis for observed differences in postprandial TG responses between dietary fat sources, practical comparisons do not exist to explicitly examine these assumptions. While sn positioning should be a consideration in the design of postprandial studies where possible, it is unlikely that the effects of FA positioning can be directly accounted for in postprandial meal studies using existing methods.

12.4.6 Other food components and their effects on postprandial triglycerides (ppTG)

A recent systematic review and meta-analysis synthesized the evidence assessing the effects of different food and nutrients on postprandial lipemia. Although a number of different dietary components have been investigated as modulators of the postprandial TG response, there is a lack of consistent evidence upon which solid conclusions can be formed. A recent meta-analysis (Lee et al., 2020) found there was no significant effect of sugars (including glucose, maltodextrin, and fructose (6 comparisons from 3 trials)) on postprandial TG response. A sensitivity analysis indicated fructose raises postprandial TG, and several other studies which couldn't be included in the meta-analysis have also demonstrated that fructose raises postprandial TG (Jeppesen et al., 1995; Stanhope et al., 2008).

Fiber acts to slow down digestion, and this has been considered a mechanism for lowering postprandial lipemia by forming a water barrier between the intestinal mucosa and the dietary fats. Despite this potential lowering effect, the evidence reviewed in Lee et al. indicated that soluble fiber may lower postprandial TG (Hedges' $g=0.72$; 95% CI: -1.33 to -0.11; $I^2=0.0\%$), but there is insufficient evidence to support a role of insoluble fiber in lowering postprandial TG responses (Lee et al., 2020).

The protein composition of a meal can also influence lipemia. Whey protein appears to have a TG-lowering effect compared with casein (Lee et al., 2020). This difference is likely due to the insulin-stimulating action of whey protein. Insulin increases LPL action and suppresses hormone sensitive lipase (HSL), the latter of which allows the release of fatty acids from adipose tissue (see Section 12.2). Protein also slows down gastric emptying which delays the absorption of dietary fat, thereby lowering the lipemic response to a meal.

There are a range of nutritional compounds or nutraceuticals that have been reported to have positive effects on lowering fasting TG (Cicero et al., 2017). Fewer studies examining postprandial responses to various nutraceuticals are published. A systematic review and meta-analysis of randomized controlled trials (Lee et al., 2020) found that compounds with the most evidence for lowering/raising postprandial TG response include polyphenols of green tea (catechins), calcium, diacylglycerol, and sodium bicarbonate.

In summary, we have described various ways in which dietary factors can modulate the postprandial lipemic response. Some dietary components can suppress the rise in blood lipids while others can exaggerate postprandial lipemia. Dietary patterns that frequently include components that exaggerate the postprandial lipemic response, such as SFA and fructose, increase people's risk of developing dyslipidemia and hence atherogenesis, and those who have obesity and/or insulin resistance are at greater risk (see Section 12.2). There remains to be robust evidence demonstrating that lowering postprandial TG and TRL through diet improves cardiovascular outcomes once dyslipidemia is established, particularly when there is a dearth of studies using alternatives to statins (Marston et al., 2019).

12.5 Meal timing a novel mediator of postprandial triglycerides

Postprandial meal challenges to assess disease risk factors are typically undertaken after an overnight fast when participants are rested. The optimum timing for these meal challenges has been given little consideration. In recent years, there has been considerable interest in the timing of lifestyle behaviors and associations with health outcomes. Physiological processes within our body, such as blood pressure, nutrient metabolism, and body temperature, are governed by endogenous circadian rhythms to ensure they occur at the most appropriate time of the day (Johnston, 2014). Performing behaviors such as eating and sleeping out of synchronization with our body clocks can lead to perturbations in the metabolism of nutrients such as glucose (Leung, Huggins, & Bonham, 2019; Leung, Huggins, Ware, & Bonham, 2020). Long-term implications of unusual meal timings include weight gain and increased risk of diabetes (Wang et al., 2014) in populations such as shift workers (Gao et al., 2020). As such, if we want to understand modulators of postprandial lipemia, postprandial meal challenges should be examined not only when metabolic responses are optimal but also when they are compromised, such as during circadian disruption.

Consuming a meal in the evening, compared with the same meal in the morning, is associated with impaired glucose tolerance and relative insulin resistance (Leung et al., 2020). Lipid metabolism, like the metabolic control of glucose, is also under circadian control in several metabolic organs, including the liver and adipose tissue (Gooley, 2016). Similarly to glucose, there is evidence for diurnal variations in postprandial TG, with higher postprandial lipids observed at night compared to during the day (Sopowski, Hampton, Ribeiro, Morgan, & Arendt, 2001). TRL remnants have also been shown to have a diurnal pattern (Demacker et al., 1991). A recent systematic review summarizing five studies that compared the postprandial TG response to a meal consumed during the day to the same meal consumed found that all studies identified at least one component of the lipemic response (i.e., total concentration or time course kinetics) that differed as a result of meal time (Bonham et al., 2019). The higher TG concentrations at night might reflect increased production of lipoproteins rich in TG (Barter, Carroll, & Nestel, 1971; Schlierf & Dorow, 1973) and/or reduced lipoprotein clearance (Fainaru et al., 1994).

Whereas the reason for this relative lipid intolerance at night is currently unclear, it has been speculated to relate to the aforementioned relative insulin resistance at night (Morgan et al., 1998; Romon et al., 1997). This may cause a reduction in the activity of LPL and a subsequent decrease in the hydrolysis of plasma TG, resulting in higher circulating TG at night (Morgan et al., 1998; also discussed in Section 12.2). With the high population of shift workers who eat throughout the night and an increasing number of people eating for more than 15h a day (Gill & Panda, 2015), we need a greater understanding of how meal timing interacts with the aforementioned dietary modulators of postprandial lipemia.

12.6 Nonmodifiable factors: Evidence of ethnic/genetic influences on postprandial lipemia

In addition to dietary and lifestyle factors that can be modified (Sections 12.4 and 12.5), a number of nonmodifiable factors have been shown to influence postprandial lipid metabolism, including genetic factors, ethnicity, gender, and age. A few genome-wide association studies (GWAS) have been conducted to determine which genetic loci are the biggest contributors to postprandial lipid metabolism as well as to determine the heritability of postprandial lipemia. These studies have found apolipoprotein genes APOA1, APOC3, APOA4, and APOA5 to be involved in the creation of TG-rich lipoproteins as well as ABCA1, CETP, GCKR, HL, IL-6, LPL, PLIN, and TCF7L2 to be involved in the regulation of postprandial lipid metabolism (Perez-Martinez, Lopez-Miranda, Perez-Jimenez, & Ordovas, 2008). As these genes are expressed to varying degrees in different populations, it may help to explain large interindividual variability in postprandial lipid metabolism (Dias, Moughan, Wood, Singh, & Garg, 2017). One recent GWAS conducted in the Netherlands aimed to identify genes that influence postprandial TG independent of fasting TG levels and found the LIPC gene that codes for hepatic lipase to be significant (Ibi et al., 2020).

Ethnicity is another factor that may play a role in postprandial lipid metabolism as some studies have shown that expression of key genes involved in lipid metabolism differ between ethnic groups (Bower, Deshaies, Pfeifer, Tanenberg, & Barakat, 2002; Carr, Brunzell, & Deeb, 2004; Hu, Thomas, & Tomlinson, 2011). For example, African American women have been shown to have lower postprandial TG responses than Caucasian women after consuming identical high-fat meals (Bower et al., 2002). Other studies comparing fasting lipid levels have found distinct lipid profiles between ethnicities irrespective of their glucose status, which suggests an underlying genetic difference in the expression of lipid regulators (Zhang et al., 2010). This is an emerging area of research, and further exploration is warranted to better understand the genetic component of postprandial lipid metabolism.

Sex differences in postprandial lipid metabolism are apparent with males showing slower clearance and high-peak TG concentrations compared to females. These differences are most likely attributed to differences in visceral fat deposition between the genders, as males tend to have more visceral fat than females (Dias et al., 2017; Kolovou et al., 2007). Finally, aging also influences postprandial lipid metabolism with increasing age associated with slower postprandial clearance of TG as well as increased TG responses.

12.7 Assessment of postprandial lipemia is important for CVD risk screening

Traditionally, assessment of the lipid profile for CVD risk is done when the patient is in a fasting (>8h) state. Although it is reasonable to assume that individuals with a dyslipidemic profile in the fasting state would also likely exhibit impaired postprandial metabolism, the converse may not always hold true. Individuals with a normal fasting lipid profile may have impaired postprandial lipid metabolism. As a consequence, there is now increased evidence to advocate for the assessment of lipid profiles in a nonfasting state and to facilitate the detection of impaired postprandial lipid metabolism and hence increased risk for CVD (Bansal et al., 2007; Langsted & Nordestgaard, 2019). In addition, as indicated in Sections 12.2 and 12.3 of this chapter, impaired postprandial lipid metabolism promotes the accumulation of cholesterol-rich CM and VLDL remnants which may attain a size small enough to penetrate the subendothelial space of the arterial wall. The contribution of cholesterol contained in these remnant particles is not captured in the calculation of LDL-cholesterol concentrations but is included in estimations of non-HDL cholesterol or TRL-remnant cholesterol. Indeed, non-HDL cholesterol has been shown to be strongly associated with the risk of CVD and also improvements in its concentration associated with a reduction in CVD events (Varbo & Nordestgaard, 2017).

12.8 Conclusion

There is substantial evidence that elevated postprandial TG, TRL, and TRL remnants are involved in the pathogenesis of atherosclerosis. In this chapter, we described dietary modulators of postprandial lipids and described the gaps in understanding of the effects of dietary modulators on postprandial TG. Novel modulators of postprandial TG were discussed, indicating that there are adverse impacts on postprandial lipid metabolism during the night. Also described was the potential for interesterification of dietary lipids in food processing as a novel approach to modulating postprandial TG. Further research is needed to identify key modulators of postprandial TG which can be tested in clinical trials for benefits on cardiovascular risk reduction. Moreover, studies of the physicochemical effects of dietary fats on lipoproteins may also elucidate mechanisms behind the effects of dietary factors (e.g., n-3 PUFA) on TG. To advance this field of research, a standardized approach to assessment of acute postprandial responses is needed as well as robust intervention studies. Additionally, more systems-level approaches to investigation and new paradigms that extend beyond the reductionist approach would be valuable to understanding the relationship of postprandial lipemia to health.

References

Abdelhamid, A. S., Brown, T. J., Brainard, J. S., Biswas, P., Thorpe, G. C., Moore, H. J., et al. (2020). Omega-3 fatty acids for the primary and secondary prevention of cardiovascular disease. *Cochrane Database of Systematic Reviews, 2020*(3). https://doi.org/10.1002/14651858.CD003177.pub5.

Alipour, A., Elte, J. W. F., van Zaanen, H. C. T., Rietveld, A. P., & Castro Cabezas, M. (2008). Novel aspects of postprandial lipemia in relation to atherosclerosis. *Atherosclerosis. Supplements, 9*(2), 39–44. https://doi.org/10.1016/j.atherosclerosissup.2008.05.007.

Bansal, S., Buring, J. E., Rifai, N., Mora, S., Sacks, F. M., & Ridker, P. M. (2007). Fasting compared with nonfasting triglycerides and risk of cardiovascular events in women. *Journal of the American Medical Association, 298*(3), 309–316. https://doi.org/10.1001/jama.298.3.309.

Barter, P. J., Brewer, H. B., Chapman, M. J., Hennekens, C. H., Rader, D. J., & Tall, A. R. (2003). Cholesteryl ester transfer protein: A novel target for raising HDL and inhibiting atherosclerosis. *Arteriosclerosis, Thrombosis, and Vascular Biology, 23*(2), 160–167. https://doi.org/10.1161/01.ATV.0000054658.91146.64.

Barter, P. J., Carroll, K. F., & Nestel, P. J. (1971). Diurnal fluctuations in triglyceride, free fatty acids, and insulin during sucrose consumption and insulin infusion in man. *The Journal of Clinical Investigation, 50*(3), 583–591. https://doi.org/10.1172/JCI106528.

Batt, K. V., Avella, M., Moore, E. H., Jackson, B., Suckling, K. E., & Botham, K. M. (2004). Differential effects of low-density lipoprotein and chylomicron remnants on lipid accumulation in human macrophages. *Experimental Biology and Medicine (Maywood, N.J.), 229*(6), 528–537.

Bergeron, N., & Havel, R. J. (1995). Influence of diets rich in saturated and omega-6 polyunsaturated fatty acids on the postprandial responses of apolipoproteins B-48, B-100, E, and lipids in triglyceride-rich lipoproteins. *Arteriosclerosis, Thrombosis, and Vascular Biology, 15*(12), 2111–2121. https://doi.org/10.1161/01.ATV.15.12.2111.

Berry, S. E. E. (2009). Triacylglycerol structure and interesterification of palmitic and stearic acid-rich fats: An overview and implications for cardiovascular disease. *Nutrition Research Reviews, 22*(1), 3–17. https://doi.org/10.1017/S0954422409369267.

Berry, S. E., Valdes, A. M., Drew, D. A., Asnicar, F., Mazidi, M., Wolf, J., et al. (2020). Human postprandial responses to food and potential for precision nutrition. *Nature Medicine, 26*(6), 964–973. https://doi.org/10.1038/s41591-020-0934-0.

Bonham, M. P., Kaias, E., Zimberg, I., Leung, G. K. W., Davis, R., Sletten, T. L., et al. (2019). Effect of night time eating on postprandial triglyceride metabolism in healthy adults: A systematic literature review. *Journal of Biological Rhythms, 34*(2), 119–130. https://doi.org/10.1177/0748730418824214.

Bonham, M. P., Linderborg, K. M., Dordevic, A., Larsen, A. E., Nguo, K., Weir, J. M., et al. (2013). Lipidomic profiling of chylomicron triacylglycerols in response to high fat meals. *Lipids, 48*(1), 39–50. https://doi.org/10.1007/s11745-012-3735-5.

Bower, J. F., Deshaies, Y., Pfeifer, M., Tanenberg, R. J., & Barakat, H. A. (2002). Ethnic differences in postprandial triglyceride response to a fatty meal and lipoprotein lipase in lean and obese African American and Caucasian women. *Metabolism, Clinical and Experimental, 51*(2), 211–217. https://doi.org/10.1053/meta.2002.29991.

Brockerhoff, H., & Yurkowski, M. (1966). Stereospecific analyses of several vegetable fats. *Journal of Lipid Research, 7*(1), 62–64.

Carr, M. C., Brunzell, J. D., & Deeb, S. S. (2004). Ethnic differences in hepatic lipase and HDL in Japanese, black, and white Americans: Role of central obesity and LIPC polymorphisms. *Journal of Lipid Research, 45*(3), 466–473.

Cicero, A. F. G., Colletti, A., Bajraktari, G., Descamps, O., Djuric, D. M., Ezhov, M., et al. (2017). Lipid-lowering nutraceuticals in clinical practice: Position paper from an international lipid expert panel. *Nutrition Reviews, 75*(9), 731–767. https://doi.org/10.1093/nutrit/nux047.

Clemente-Postigo, M., Queipo-Ortuño, M. I., Fernandez-Garcia, D., Gomez-Huelgas, R., Tinahones, F. J., & Cardona, F. (2011). Adipose tissue gene expression of factors related to lipid processing in obesity. *PLoS One, 6*(9). https://doi.org/10.1371/journal.pone.0024783, e24783.

Decker, E. A. (1996). The role of stereospecific saturated fatty acid positions on lipid nutrition. *Nutrition Reviews, 54*(4 I), 108–110. https://doi.org/10.1111/j.1753-4887.1996.tb03884.x.

Demacker, P. N. M., Reijnen, I. G. M., Katan, M. B., Stuyt, P. M. J., & Stalenhoef, A. F. H. (1991). Increased removal of remnants of triglyceride-rich lipoproteins on a diet rich in polyunsaturated fatty acids. *European Journal of Clinical Investigation, 21*(2), 197–203. https://doi.org/10.1111/j.1365-2362.1991.tb01809.x.

Denke, M. A. (1994). Effects of cocoa butter on serum lipids in humans: Historical highlights. *The American Journal of Clinical Nutrition*, 1014S–1016S. https://doi.org/10.1093/ajcn/60.6.1014S.

Desmarchelier, C., Borel, P., Lairon, D., Maraninchi, M., & Valéro, R. (2019). Effect of nutrient and micronutrient intake on chylomicron production and postprandial lipemia. *Nutrients, 11*(6). https://doi.org/10.3390/nu11061299.

Dias, C. B., Moughan, P. J., Wood, L. G., Singh, H., & Garg, M. L. (2017). Postprandial lipemia: Factoring in lipemic response for ranking foods for their healthiness. *Lipids in Health and Disease, 16*(1), 178. https://doi.org/10.1186/s12944-017-0568-5.

Fainaru, M., Schafer, Z., Gavish, D., Skurnik, Y., Argov, R., & Kaplan, S. (1994). Diurnal changes in plasma lipoproteins of free-living healthy men consuming a standard diet. *Israel Journal of Medical Sciences, 30*(1), 83–89.

Finnegan, Y. E., Minihane, A. M., Leigh-Firbank, E. C., Kew, S., Meijer, G. W., Muggli, R., et al. (2003). Plant- and marine-derived n-3 polyunsaturated fatty acids have differential effects on fasting and postprandial blood lipid concentrations and on the susceptibility of LDL to oxidative modification in moderately hyperlipidemic subjects. *The American Journal of Clinical Nutrition, 77*(4), 783–795. https://doi.org/10.1093/ajcn/77.4.783.

Gao, Y., Gan, T., Jiang, L., Yu, L., Tang, D., Wang, Y., et al. (2020). Association between shift work and risk of type 2 diabetes mellitus: A systematic review and dose-response meta analysis of observational studies. *Chronobiology International, 37*(1), 29–46. https://doi.org/10.1080/07420528.2019.1683570.

Gill, S., & Panda, S. (2015). A smartphone app reveals erratic diurnal eating patterns in humans that can be modulated for health benefits. *Cell Metabolism, 22*(5), 789–798. https://doi.org/10.1016/j.cmet.2015.09.005.

Gooley, J. J. (2016). Circadian regulation of lipid metabolism. In *Vol. 75. Proceedings of the nutrition society* (pp. 440–450). Cambridge University Press. https://doi.org/10.1017/S0029665116000288. Issue 4.

Gower, R. M., Wu, H., Foster, G. A., Devaraj, S., Jialal, I., Ballantyne, C. M., et al. (2011). CD11c/CD18 expression is upregulated on blood monocytes during hypertriglyceridemia and enhances adhesion to vascular cell adhesion molecule-1. *Arteriosclerosis, Thrombosis, and Vascular Biology, 31*(1), 160–166. https://doi.org/10.1161/ATVBAHA.110.215434.

Griffo, E., Di Marino, L., Patti, L., Bozzetto, L., Annuzzi, G., Cipriano, P., et al. (2014). Test meals rich in marine long-chain n-3 polyunsaturated fatty acids increase postprandial chylomicron response. *Nutrition Research (New York, N.Y.), 34*(8), 661–666. https://doi.org/10.1016/j.nutres.2014.07.005.

Halkes, C. J., van Dijk, H., de Jaegere, P. P., Plokker, H. W., van Der Helm, Y., Erkelens, D. W., et al. (2001). Postprandial increase of complement component 3 in normolipidemic patients with coronary artery disease: Effects of expanded-dose simvastatin. *Arteriosclerosis, Thrombosis, and Vascular Biology, 21*(9), 1526–1530.

Hu, M., Thomas, G. N., & Tomlinson, B. (2011). Lipid disorders in Chinese populations. *Clinical Lipidology, 6*(5),

549–562. https://www.tandfonline.com/doi/abs/10.2217/clp.11.47.

Ibi, D., Noordam, R., Van Klinken, J. B., Li-Gao, R., De Mutsert, R., Trompet, S., et al. (2020). *Genome-wide association study of the postprandial triglyceride response yields common genetic variation in LIPC (hepatic lipase)* (pp. 289–297). Circulation: Genomic and Precision Medicine. https://doi.org/10.1161/CIRCGEN.119.002693.

Jackson, K. G., Denise Robertson, M., Fielding, B. A., Frayn, K. N., & Williams, C. M. (2002). Olive oil increases the number of triacylglycerol-rich chylomicron particles compared with other oils: An effect retained when a second standard meal is fed. *American Journal of Clinical Nutrition*, 76(5), 942–949. https://doi.org/10.1093/ajcn/76.5.942.

Jensen, M. M., Christensen, M. S., & Høy, C. E. (1994). Intestinal absorption of octanoic, decanoic, and linoleic acids: Effect of triglyceride structure. *Annals of Nutrition and Metabolism*, 38(2), 104–116. https://doi.org/10.1159/000177799.

Jeppesen, J., Chen, Y. I., Zhou, M. Y., Schaaf, P., Coulston, A., & Reaven, G. M. (1995). Postprandial triglyceride and retinyl ester responses to oral fat: Effects of fructose. *The American Journal of Clinical Nutrition*, 787–791. https://doi.org/10.1093/ajcn/61.4.787.

Johnston, J. D. (2014). Physiological links between circadian rhythms, metabolism and nutrition. *Experimental Physiology*, 99(9), 1133–1137. https://doi.org/10.1113/expphysiol.2014.078295.

Karpe, F., Bell, M., Björkegren, J., & Hamsten, A. (1995). Quantification of postprandial triglyceride-rich lipoproteins in healthy men by retinyl ester labeling and simultaneous measurement of apolipoproteins B-48 and B-100. *Arteriosclerosis, Thrombosis, and Vascular Biology*, 15(2), 199–207. https://doi.org/10.1161/01.ATV.15.2.199.

Kluge, M. A., Fetterman, J. L., & Vita, J. A. (2013). Mitochondria and endothelial function. *Circulation Research*, 112(8), 1171–1188. https://doi.org/10.1161/CIRCRESAHA.111.300233.

Kolovou, G. D., Anagnostopoulou, K. K., Damaskos, D. S., Mihas, C., Mavrogeni, S., Hatzigeorgiou, G., et al. (2007). Gender influence on postprandial lipemia in heterozygotes for familial hypercholesterolemia. *Annals of Clinical and Laboratory Science*, 37(4), 335–342.

Kolovou, G. D., Watts, G. F., Mikhailidis, D. P., Pérez-Martínez, P., Mora, S., Bilianou, H., et al. (2019). Postprandial hypertriglyceridaemia revisited in the era of non-fasting lipid profiles: Executive summary of a 2019 expert panel statement. *Current Vascular Pharmacology*, 17(5), 538–540. https://doi.org/10.2174/1570161117999190517115432.

Kritchevsky, D. (1994). Stearic acid metabolism and atherogenesis: History. *The American Journal of Clinical Nutrition*, 997S–1001S. https://doi.org/10.1093/ajcn/60.6.997S.

Laatsch, A., Merkel, M., Talmud, P. J., Grewal, T., Beisiegel, U., & Heeren, J. (2009). Insulin stimulates hepatic low density lipoprotein receptor-related protein 1 (LRP1) to increase postprandial lipoprotein clearance. *Atherosclerosis*, 204(1), 105–111. https://doi.org/10.1016/j.atherosclerosis.2008.07.046.

Lacroix, S., Des Rosiers, C., Tardif, J. C., & Nigam, A. (2012). The role of oxidative stress in postprandial endothelial dysfunction. *Nutrition Research Reviews*, 25(2), 288–301. https://doi.org/10.1017/S0954422412000182.

Langsted, A., & Nordestgaard, B. G. (2019). Nonfasting versus fasting lipid profile for cardiovascular risk prediction. *Pathology*, 51(2), 131–141. https://doi.org/10.1016/j.pathol.2018.09.062.

Lee, D. P. S., Low, J. H. M., Chen, J. R., Zimmermann, D., Actis-Goretta, L., & Kim, J. E. (2020). The influence of different foods and food ingredients on acute postprandial triglyceride response: A systematic literature review and Meta-analysis of randomized controlled trials. *Advances in Nutrition*, 11(6), 1529–1543. https://doi.org/10.1093/advances/nmaa074.

Leung, G. K. W., Huggins, C. E., & Bonham, M. P. (2019). Effect of meal timing on postprandial glucose responses to a low glycemic index meal: A crossover trial in healthy volunteers. *Clinical Nutrition*, 38(1), 465–471. https://doi.org/10.1016/j.clnu.2017.11.010.

Leung, G. K. W., Huggins, C. E., Ware, R. S., & Bonham, M. P. (2020). Time of day difference in postprandial glucose and insulin responses: Systematic review and meta-analysis of acute postprandial studies. *Chronobiology International*, 37(3), 311–326. https://doi.org/10.1080/07420528.2019.1683856.

Mamo, J. C., Watts, G. F., Barrett, P. H., Smith, D., James, A. P., & Pal, S. (2001). Postprandial dyslipidemia in men with visceral obesity: An effect of reduced LDL receptor expression? *American Journal of Physiology. Endocrinology and Metabolism*, 281(3), E626–E632.

Marston, N. A., Giugliano, R. P., Im, K. A., Silverman, M. G., O'Donoghue, M. L., Wiviott, S. D., et al. (2019). Association between triglyceride lowering and reduction of cardiovascular risk across multiple lipid-lowering therapeutic classes. *Circulation*, 140(16), 1308–1317. https://doi.org/10.1161/CIRCULATIONAHA.119.041998.

Mensink, R. P., Sanders, T. A., Baer, D. J., Hayes, K. C., Howles, P. N., & Marangoni, A. (2016). The increasing use of interesterified lipids in the food supply and their effects on health parameters. *Advances in Nutrition*, 7(4), 719–729. https://doi.org/10.3945/an.115.009662.

Morgan, L., Arendt, J., Owens, D., Folkard, S., Hampton, S., Deacon, S., et al. (1998). Effects of the endogenous clock and sleep time on melatonin, insulin, glucose and lipid metabolism. *Journal of Endocrinology*, 157(3), 443–451. https://doi.org/10.1677/joe.0.1570443.

Mu, H., & Porsgaard, T. (2005). The metabolism of structured triacylglycerols. *Progress in Lipid Research*, 44(6), 430–448. https://doi.org/10.1016/j.plipres.2005.09.002.

Nakajima, K., Nakano, T., Tokita, Y., Nagamine, T., Inazu, A., Kobayashi, J., et al. (2011). Postprandial lipoprotein metabolism: VLDL vs chylomicrons. *Clinica Chimica Acta*, 412(15–16), 1306–1318. https://doi.org/10.1016/j.cca.2011.04.018.

Nilsson-Ehle, P., Egelrud, T., Belfrage, P., Olivecrona, T., & Borgström, B. (1973). Positional specificity of purified milk lipoprotein lipase. *Journal of Biological Chemistry*, 248(19), 6734–6737.

O'Connell, T. D., Mason, R. P., Budoff, M. J., Navar, A. M., & Shearer, G. C. (2020). Mechanistic insights into cardiovascular protection for omega-3 fatty acids and their bioactive lipid metabolites. *European Heart Journal Supplements*, J3–J20. https://doi.org/10.1093/eurheartj/suaa115.

Packard, C., Caslake, M., & Shepherd, J. (2000). The role of small, dense low density lipoprotein (LDL): A new look. *International Journal of Cardiology*, 74.

Perez-Martinez, P., Lopez-Miranda, J., Perez-Jimenez, F., & Ordovas, J. M. (2008). Influence of genetic factors in the modulation of postprandial lipemia. *Atherosclerosis Supplements*, 9(2), 49–55. https://doi.org/10.1016/j.atherosclerosissup.2008.05.005.

Pirillo, A., Norata, G. D., & Catapano, A. L. (2014). Postprandial lipemia as a cardiometabolic risk factor. *Current Medical Research and Opinion*, 30(8), 1489–1503. https://doi.org/10.1185/03007995.2014.909394.

Proctor, S. D., & Mamo, J. C. (1998). Retention of fluorescent-labelled chylomicron remnants within the intima of the arterial wall—Evidence that plaque cholesterol may be derived from post-prandial lipoproteins. *European Journal of Clinical Investigation*, 28(6), 497–503.

Proctor, S. D., Vine, D. F., & Mamo, J. C. L. (2004). Arterial permeability and efflux of apolipoprotein B-containing lipoproteins assessed by in situ perfusion and three-dimensional quantitative confocal microscopy. *Arteriosclerosis, Thrombosis, and Vascular Biology*, 24(11), 2162–2167. https://doi.org/10.1161/01.ATV.0000143859.75035.5a.

Romon, M., Le Fur, C., Lebel, P., Edmé, J. L., Fruchart, J. C., & Dallongeville, J. (1997). Circadian variation of postprandial lipemia. *The American Journal of Clinical Nutrition*, 934–940. https://doi.org/10.1093/ajcn/65.4.934.

van Rooijen, M. A., & Mensink, R. P. (2020). Palmitic acid versus stearic acid: Effects of interesterification and intakes on cardiometabolic risk markers-a systematic review. *Nutrients*, 12(3). https://doi.org/10.3390/nu12030615.

Schlierf, G., & Dorow, E. (1973). Diurnal patterns of triglycerides, free fatty acids, blood sugar, and insulin during carbohydrate-induction in man and their modification by nocturnal suppression of lipolysis. *The Journal of Clinical Investigation*, 52(3), 732–740. https://doi.org/10.1172/JCI107235.

Schneeman, B. O., Kotite, L., Todd, K. M., & Havel, R. J. (1993). Relationships between the responses of triglyceride-rich lipoproteins in blood plasma containing apolipoproteins B-48 and B-100 to a fat-containing meal in normolipidemic humans. *Proceedings of the National Academy of Sciences*, 2069–2073. https://doi.org/10.1073/pnas.90.5.2069.

Small, D. M. (1991). The effects of glyceride structure on absorption and metabolism. *Annual Review of Nutrition*, 11, 413–434. https://doi.org/10.1146/annurev.nu.11.070191.002213.

Sopowski, M. J., Hampton, S. M., Ribeiro, D. C. O., Morgan, L., & Arendt, J. (2001). Postprandial triacylglycerol responses in simulated night and day shift: Gender differences. *Journal of Biological Rhythms*, 16(3), 272–276. https://doi.org/10.1177/074873001129001881.

Stanhope, K. L., Griffen, S. C., Bair, B. R., Swarbrick, M. M., Keim, N. L., & Havel, P. J. (2008). Twenty-four-hour endocrine and metabolic profiles following consumption of high-fructose corn syrup-, sucrose-, fructose-, and glucose-sweetened beverages with meals. *American Journal of Clinical Nutrition*, 87(5), 1194–1203. https://doi.org/10.1093/ajcn/87.5.1194.

Tilakavati, K., & Kalyana, S. (2007). Effects of stereospecific positioning of fatty acids in triacylglycerol structures in native and randomized fats: A review of their nutritional implications. *Nutrition and Metabolism*, 16. https://doi.org/10.1186/1743-7075-4-16.

Varbo, A., & Nordestgaard, B. G. (2017). Remnant lipoproteins. *Current Opinion in Lipidology*, 28(4), 300–307. https://doi.org/10.1097/MOL.0000000000000429.

Wang, J. B., Patterson, R. E., Ang, A., Emond, J. A., Shetty, N., & Arab, L. (2014). Timing of energy intake during the day is associated with the risk of obesity in adults. *Journal of Human Nutrition and Dietetics*, 27(2), 255–262. https://doi.org/10.1111/jhn.12141.

Wang, T., Wang, X., & Wang, X. (2016). Effects of lipid structure changed by interesterification on melting property and Lipemia. *Lipids*, 51(10), 1115–1126. https://doi.org/10.1007/s11745-016-4184-3.

Weintraub, M. S., Zechner, R., Brown, A., Eisenberg, S., & Breslow, J. L. (1988). Dietary polyunsaturated fats of the W-6 and W-3 series reduce postprandial lipoprotein levels. Chronic and acute effects of fat saturation on postprandial lipoprotein metabolism. *Journal of Clinical Investigation*, 82(6), 1884–1893. https://doi.org/10.1172/JCI113806.

Wilhelm, M. G., & Cooper, A. D. (2003). Induction of atherosclerosis by human chylomicron remnants: A hypothesis. *Journal of Atherosclerosis and Thrombosis, 10*(3), 132–139.

Yang, L. Y., & Kuksis, A. (1991). Apparent convergence (at 2-monoacylglycerol level) of phosphatidic acid and 2-monoacylglycerol pathways of synthesis of chylomicron triacylglycerols. *Journal of Lipid Research, 32*(7), 1173–1186.

Zhang, L., Qiao, Q., Tuomilehto, J., Janus, E. D., Lam, T. H., Ramachandran, A., et al. (2010). Distinct ethnic differences in lipid profiles across glucose categories. *The Journal of Clinical Endocrinology and Metabolism, 95*(4), 1793–1801. https://doi.org/10.1210/jc.2009-2348.

Zilversmit, D. B. (1979). Atherogenesis: A postprandial phenomenon. *Circulation, 60*(3), 473–485. https://doi.org/10.1161/01.CIR.60.3.473.

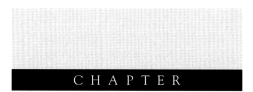

CHAPTER

13

The metabolites derived from lipids and their effects on human health

Li-Li Xiu[a], Ling-Shen Hung[b], Ling Wang[c], Jian-Ying Huang[a], and Xiang-Yang Wang[a]

[a]Department of Food Science and Technology, School of Food Science and Biotechnology, Zhejiang Gongshang University, Hangzhou, China [b]Department of Food Science, College of Chemistry and Food Science, Yulin Normal University, Yulin, Guangxi, China [c]Department of Food Micrology, College of Food Science and Technology, Huazhong Agricultural University, Wuhan, Hubei, China

13.1 Introduction

Lipids are essential for life. The reactions that produce, consume, and regenerate lipids are called lipid metabolism, which includes the biosynthesis and degradation of lipids. However, it is also the least understood compared with proteins, polynucleotides, and sugars (German, 2011). The body breaks down lipids in digestion, some for immediate energy needs and some for storage. In recent years, many more functions associated with lipid and lipid metabolites have been discovered. They play many key biological functions in energy storage and supply, providing body insulation and protection, cell and tissue structure, and signaling messengers. Lipid metabolites participate in the regulation of cellular processes including cell proliferation, growth, differentiation, and apoptosis. Lipid metabolism is associated with carbohydrate and protein metabolism and is regulated by genetic, gut microbiota, or environmental factors. Lipid metabolism generates many biological intermediates which are produced by the activation of multiple signaling pathways and can also regulate multiple signaling pathways, which raises a growing interest in potential biomarkers in many clinical conditions. Lipid metabolism is altered to an unhealthy status, or it could be disease status changing lipid metabolism. Lipid metabolism disorder (LMD) or dyslipidemia is the condition of metabolic syndrome and the pathogenesis of cardiovascular diseases (CVDs), fatty liver, and type 2 diabetes, among others. The International Diabetes Federation has reported that approximately 25% of global adults have LMDs (Cornier et al., 2008). LMDs are recognized to induce and modulate a wide range of chronic diseases. In clinics, lipid status is estimated based on serum concentrations of total cholesterol (TC), high-density lipoprotein (HDL), low-density lipoprotein (LDL), and triacylglycerols (TAGs), which induces abnormally high levels of the blood and liver index including triglyceride (TG), total cholesterol (TC), low-density lipoprotein cholesterol (LDL-C), and low levels of high-density lipoprotein cholesterol (HDL-C), while only limited information can be obtained from the analysis of structure and function of some specific lipid species. There are two sources of lipids for human metabolism, exogenously derived (dietary) lipids and endogenously synthesized lipids. In humans, lipids are obtained from food or synthesized by the liver. The liver is the site of most lipid transformations. Lipids are transported from the gut to the liver by lipoproteins. The chemical process in lipid metabolism includes lipolysis, beta-oxidation, lipid peroxidation, and so on.

13.1.1 Lipolysis

Lipolysis is the metabolic pathway through which one TAG molecule is hydrolyzed into three free fatty acids and one glycerol by lipases. Lipolysis takes place in the cytoplasm. Several hormones are involved in lipolysis, including growth hormone, brain natriuretic peptide, and cortisol glucagon (Nielsen, Jørgensen, Møller, & Lund, 2014). Major regulators of human lipolysis are catecholamines, natriuretic peptides, and insulin (Jocken & Blaak, 2008; Koppo et al., 2010). The resulting free fatty acids are oxidized by β-oxidation into acetyl CoA or other fatty acid metabolism pathways, while the glycerol released from triglycerides directly enters the glycolysis pathway.

13.1.2 β-Oxidation

β-Oxidation is a catabolic process involving multiple steps by which fatty acid molecules are broken down to produce energy. It is named as β-oxidation because the β carbon in the fatty acid undergoes oxidation to a carbonyl group. Fatty acyl CoA molecules combine with carnitine to create a fatty acylcarnitine molecule, which helps to transport the fatty acid across the mitochondrial membrane. The fatty acylcarnitine molecule is converted back into fatty acyl CoA and then into acetyl CoA in the mitochondrial matrix. The newly formed acetyl CoA enters the Krebs cycle and is used to produce energy.

13.1.3 Lipogenesis

Lipogenesis is the metabolic process where acetyl-CoA is converted to fatty acid and subsequent TAGs. TAGs and other lipids from lipogenesis are stored in adipose tissue until they are needed. Lipogenesis is mainly regulated by nutrient intake, individual endogenous status and environmental factors. The hormones that regulate lipogenesis include insulin, leptin, and growth hormones. Lipogenesis can be regulated by diet. Polyunsaturated fatty acids decrease lipogenesis by suppressing fatty acid synthase and stearoyl-CoA desaturase gene expression in the liver (Jump, Clarke, Thelen, & Liimatta, 1994). Lifestyle is another important environmental factor modifying lipid parameters. Smoking changes lipid profile, which is thought to contribute to smoking-related diseases such as CVD (Attard et al., 2017), but smoking cessation can renormalize plasma lipid profiles. The rate of lipogenesis is highly induced in cancer cells. On the other hand, inhibition of fatty acid synthase expression decreases tumor growth and induces apoptosis of cancer cells (Kuhajda, 2000).

13.1.4 Ketogenesis

Ketogenesis is a metabolic pathway that produces ketone bodies including acetone, acetoacetate, and beta-hydroxybutyrate molecules by breaking down fatty acids or ketogenic amino acids. The body continually produces small amounts of ketone bodies for health and the number in the blood increases when fasting. If excessive acetyl CoA is produced from the oxidation of fatty acids and the TCA cycle is overloaded, acetyl CoA generates ketone bodies to supply an alternative form of energy for certain organs, particularly the brain, heart, and skeletal muscle under unavailability of blood glucose circumstances. Ketone bodies are formed predominantly from fatty acids but also ketogenic amino acids such as leucine and lysine. Ketolytic enzymes include mitochondrial acetoacetyl-CoA thiolase. Ketogenesis is regulated in multiple stages. Hormones such as glucagon, cortisol, thyroid hormones, and catecholamines are involved in the ketogenesis process (Wolfrum, Asilmaz, Luca, Friedman, & Stoffel, 2004). Glucagon is the main catabolic hormone that activates hormone-sensitive lipase and inhibits acetyl-CoA carboxylase, therefore stimulating ketone body production. In contrast, insulin inhibits hormone-sensitive lipase and 3-hydroxy-3-methylglutaryl (HMG) CoA lyase, further inhibiting ketone body production. In addition to its effects on cellular energy supply, ketone bodies act as vital metabolic and signaling mediators when carbohydrates are abundant (Puchalska & Crawford, 2017). The ketone body β-hydroxybutyrate is beneficial in human neurodegenerative disease as signaling metabolites (Newman & Verdin, 2014).

13.1.5 Ketolysis

Ketolysis is the opposite process to ketogenesis, which involves a set of reactions that aim to regain energy via oxidation of ketone bodies. When glucose is insufficient, ketone bodies can be oxidized to produce acetyl CoA in the mitochondria of extrahepatic tissues to be used in the tricarboxylic acid cycle to generate energy.

13.1.6 Lipid peroxidation

Lipid peroxidation is a complex free radical-related process that is generated naturally in biological systems with or without enzymatic control. The products of lipid peroxidation are known as lipid peroxides. In this process, free radicals attack an allylic carbon of lipids to form a carbon-centered radical, which reacts with oxygen to form peroxyl radicals. The lipid peroxidation process has three well-described phases that form a free radical chain reaction, including initiation, propagation, and termination. After the production of a fatty acid radical in the initiation phase, the unstable fatty acid radical quickly reacts with molecular oxygen in the propagation step to form a peroxyl-fatty acid radical. This unstable peroxyl-fatty acid radical further reacts with a free fatty acid to produce hydrogen peroxide or cyclic peroxide and another fatty acid radical. The chain reaction continues until a nonradical species is formed by the combination of two free radicals in the termination step. Lipid peroxidation most often affects polyunsaturated fatty acids (PUFAs) such as linoleic acid and arachidonic acid. The composition, structure, and normal function of cellular membranes were altered because peroxidation of membrane lipids alters the physical properties of lipid bilayers including membrane fluidity, membrane permeability, and lipid interactions. Some end products of lipid peroxidation are not stable and they suffer from further chemical reactions with biofunctional protein or DNA that result in some products of lipid peroxides exhibiting additional toxicity. The aldehydes, one of the degradation products of lipid peroxides, are toxic to cells because they react with proteins or DNA. Oxidative stress, proinflammatory, and free radical-mediated injury are the major causes of the pathophysiology of disease (Ramana, Srivastava, & Singhal, 2019).

Oxylipins are a group of lipid oxidation metabolites generated by the oxidation of polyunsaturated fatty acids involved in the processes of inflammation and immunity. The oxylipins from n-6 PUFA mainly induce inflammation, but oxylipins from n-3 PUFA are effective in inflammation resolving actions although there are notable exceptions. Oxylipins can be generated in a controlled manner by cyclooxygenases (COXs), lipoxygenases (LOXs), and cytochrome p450s (CYPs), or non-enzymatic processes in the human body. COXs synthesize lipid endoperoxides, LOXs synthesize lipid hydroperoxides and CYPs synthesize EETs.

Balancing redox reactions is necessary for life. Overproduction of lipid peroxides in the organism results from the accumulation of oxidants which can oxidize biomolecules, including DNA, proteins, and lipids. There are a variety of pathways for reducing lipid peroxides in biological systems. The glutathione peroxidase (GPx) enzymes are key regulators of lipid peroxidation to reduce lipid peroxides. There are eight different isoforms of GPxs in humans. The GPx4 enzyme is the primary reductant of lipid peroxides which converts lipid hydroperoxides to lipid alcohols. Inhibition of GPx4 results in the accumulation of lipid peroxides and cell death. The most common strategy for reducing lipid peroxides is to inhibit the enzymes which are involved in lipid peroxidation. Vitamin E serves as a radical scavenging agent to reduce lipid peroxides, which donates a single electron to the peroxyl radical, terminating the lipid peroxidation. Plant poly phenols, such as tannic acid, also have the function of radical scavenging.

13.2 The gut microbiota and lipid metabolism

There are at least 1000 distinct species of bacteria in the human intestinal track with a number of over 100 trillion organisms (Bäckhed, Ley, Sonnenburg, Peterson, & Gordon, 2005). Gut microbiota consumes, stores, and redistributes energy. It mediates physiologically chemical transformations and plays an important role in maintaining metabolic homeostasis. Host immune and inflammatory responses were influenced by the composition and products of the gut microbiota (Maslowski & MacKay, 2011). In addition, the production of these metabolites by microbes contributes to the host metabolic phenotype. Evidence is now accumulating to indicate that gut microbiota composition may play an important role in the development of diseases associated with altered metabolism. Gut bacterial composition dysbiosis has been associated with the pathogenesis of many diseases, including obesity, CVD, cancer, mental disease, among others. The intestinal microbiota is derived in part from the mother and is modified by factors such as diet, host genetics and other environmental factors. The function and composition of the gut microbiota is affected by diet properties, which are considered as one of the main drivers in shaping the gut microbiota. Lipids as important diet components and as substrates for bacterial metabolic processes involved in shaping the gut microbiota.

13.2.1 Dietary lipids affect the phylogenetic diversity of the gut microbiota

Lipids play an important role in shaping the composition and further for the function of the gut microbiota. Dietary lipids can dramatically alter the gut microbiome. The lower-fat diet increased α-diversity, increased abundance of *Blautia*, *Faecalibacterium*, decreased the p-cresol and indole levels which are associated with host metabolic disorders and the higher-fat diet increased *Alistipes*, *Bacteroides*, and decreased *Faecalibacterium* in a 6-month randomized controlled-feeding human study (Wan et al., 2019). Carlotta De Filippo et al. compared the fecal microbiota from two groups of children with different diets. One group was from Europe and consumed a typical modern western diet, high in fat content, and one group was from a rural African village of Burkina Faso on a rural diet, high in fiber content. Burkina Faso children with a unique abundance of bacteria from the genus Prevotella and Xylanibacter, which can hydrolyze cellulose and xylan, are completely lacking in the EU children. Significantly more short-chain fatty acids were found in Burkina Faso than in European children (De Filippo et al., 2010). Animal studies also found that high dietary fat intake can cause gut microbiota dysbiosis. Switching from a low-fat, plant-rich diet to a high-fat, high-sugar diet shifted the structure of the microbiota, altered microbiome gene expression, and changed the representation of metabolic pathways within a single day in a humanized study (Turnbaugh et al., 2009).

Lipids with different fatty acid profiles may contribute to different gut microbiota composition. Fish oil rich in n-3 PUFA increases the diversity of the gut microbiota. In contrast, lard enriched in saturated fatty acid decreases it. The lard diet promotes a shift in gut microbiota composition and function. *Actinobacteria, lactic acid bacteria, Verrucomicrobia, Alphaproteobacteria,* and *Deltaproteobacteria* were increased in n-3 PUFA-fed mice, while *Bacteroides, Turicibacter,* and *Bilophila* were increased in lard-fed mice (Baptista, Sun, Carter, & Buford, 2020). *Akkermansia* and Lactobacillus were increased in the cecum contents of mice fed fish oil compared to lard for 11 weeks (Baptista et al., 2020). Mice fed lard increased toll-like receptor activation and white adipose tissue inflammation and reduced insulin sensitivity compared with mice fed fish oil. The phenotypic differences between the dietary groups can be partly attributed to differences in microbiota composition (Caesar, Tremaroli, Kovatcheva-Datchary, Cani, & Bäckhed, 2015). *Bilophila wadsworthia* is a gram-negative sulfite-reducing, bile-resistant asaccharolytic bacillus. *B. wadsworthia* aggravates high fat diet induced inflammation, intestinal barrier dysfunction, and bile acid dysmetabolism, leading to higher glucose dysmetabolism and hepatic steatosis (Natividad et al., 2018). The antibacterial action of fatty acids is another reason for changes in gut microbiota. The fatty acid antibacterial characteristics are determined by carbon chain length, saturation, and double bond position, among others. Long-chain unsaturated fatty acids, such as linoleic acid, show antibacterial activity (Zheng et al., 2005).

13.2.2 The gut microbiota modulates lipid metabolism

It is well established that the gut microbiota plays a role in regulating host lipid metabolism through direct and indirect biological mechanisms. The gut microbiota can perform their own lipid metabolic processes which can produce metabolites that function as biologically active substances impacting the health of the host. Dietary probiotics interfere with the gut microbiota and exert beneficial health effects on humans. Some metabolites of probiotics positively affect host physiology. After being administered with lactobacilli suspension (10^8 CFU) for 8 weeks, the serum blood lipid levels were significantly improved, and the liver lipid accumulation was significantly inhibited (Li et al., 2020).

The gut microbiota affects host lipid metabolism through interaction with the diet. A human gram-positive intestinal bacteria, *Roseburia* species, metabolized linoleic acid (*cis*-9, *cis*-12-18:2) into a 10-hydroxy-18:1 fatty acid which is a precursor of the conjugated linoleic acid (*cis*-9,-*trans*-11-18:2, CLA) (Devillard, McIntosh, Duncan, & Wallace, 2007). Other gut bacteria, including *Lactobacillus, Butyrivibrio,* and *Megasphaera*, can also produce conjugated linoleic acid. Arabinoxylans supplementation as a prebiotic increased conjugated linoleic acid concentration in the cecal tissue by increasing Roseburia spp. abundance (Druart et al., 2013). The gut microbiota can regulate lipid metabolism by regulating bile-acid metabolism. Bile acids synthesized in the human liver from cholesterol are important for ensuring dietary lipids are soluble and absorbable. The gut microbiota deconjugate bile acids and further metabolize these bile acids into secondary bile acids, which increases the bile acid diversity.

13.2.3 Short chain fatty acids produced by the gut microbiota and their impacts on human lipid metabolism

The gut microbiota can metabolize complex carbohydrates through their own pathways which are different from humans'. Short chain fatty acids (SCFAs), including formate, acetate, propionate, and butyrate are the primary end metabolic products of human nondigestible carbohydrates through the gut microbiota. Increased circulating SCFAs are associated with reduced adipocyte lipolysis and adipogenesis.

13.3 Effects of lipid metabolites on CVDs

CVDs are a group of disorders that affect the heart or blood vessels including coronary heart disease, heart failure, hypertension, cerebral vascular disease, and other conditions. It is characterized by lipid and cholesterol accumulation and the development of fibrotic plaques within the walls of large and medium arteries. CVD is the leading cause of mortality and morbidity globally, representing 31% of all global deaths in 2015 (Ruan et al., 2018). Globally, 1.39 billion persons have hypertension, which is one of the most important risk factors for CVD (Bloch, 2016). The other risk factors for CVDs include tobacco, an unhealthy diet, a sedentary lifestyle, and harmful use of alcohol. Most CVDs could be prevented if a precise method has been established for early detection. Lipid metabolites have received more attention in CVD pathology. Since Gofman et al. found that the risk of myocardial infarction is associated with increased levels of LDL-C in 1954, the relationship between LDL-C levels and CVDs is well described (Goldstein & Brown, 2015). LDL-C has been used as a primary target of lipid-lowering therapy for many years. But CVDs are recognized as a group of multifactorial disorders, some individuals with normal levels of LDL-C still develop CVD, which means that LDL-C alone as a risk marker is not sufficient to identify patients at high risk (Sachdeva et al., 2009). Specific lipid or lipid metabolites are necessary for CVD prediction and identification.

13.3.1 Association between ceramides and CVDs

Ceramides have functions in LDL-C aggregation (Perman et al., 2011). Ceramides have been put forward as predictors of mortality in patients with CVDs, such as coronary artery disease, stroke, and heart failure (Havulinna et al., 2016; Laaksonen et al., 2016). Increased plasma concentrations of four ceramides, d18:1/16:0, d18:1/18:0, d18:1/24:0, and d18:1/24:1, were found independently associated with serious adverse cardiovascular events in CVD patients. The higher levels of plasma ceramides are associated with coronary artery stenosis in coronary artery disease patients. Higher levels of plasma ceramide (d18:1/20:0), ceramide (d18:1/22:0) and ceramide (d18:1/24:0) were significantly associated with the presence of coronary artery stenosis (Mantovani et al., 2020).

13.3.2 Association between eicosanoids and CVDs

Epoxyeicosatrienoic acids (EETs) are metabolites of arachidonic acid via cytochrome P450 (CYP) epoxylgenases. There are four regioisomers of EETs, which are denoted as 5,6-EET, 8,9-EET, 11,12-EET, and 14,15-EET. EETs have beneficial effects on vasodilation. Studies found that the elevation of EETs had protective effects in various cardiovascular diseases, including hypertension, myocardial infarction, and heart failure (Lai & Chen, 2021). Inhibiting the hydrolase of EETs has been considered as a therapeutic target for CVD disease (Imig & Hammock, 2009; Ni, Chen, Chen, & Yang, 2011). Thromboxane is also a member of eicosanoids, which are metabolites of arachidonic acid catalyzed by COXs and CYPs. The major known active thromboxane is thromboxane A_2. Thromboxane A_2 is a constrictor of smooth muscle and a potent hypertensive agent. Prostacyclin is the precursor of thromboxane A_2, but it is an effective vasodilator. Thromboxane A_2 is in homeostatic balance with prostacyclin in the circulatory system to keep normal function. Aspirin, a COX1 inhibitor, decreases atherothrombotic associated mortality and these potent effects of aspirin have shown the utility of its ability to inhibit the production of Thromboxane A2 to decrease CVD mortality (Zordoky & El-Kadi, 2010).

13.4 Metabolites derived from lipids that correlate with cancer incidence

Cancers are a large family of diseases that involve abnormal cell growth with the potential to invade or spread to other parts of the body. Lipid metabolites take part in the pathology of cancer. Lipid metabolism in cancer cells is regulated by the oncogenic signaling pathways and is important for the initiation and progression of tumors (Menendez & Lupu, 2007). Some lipid metabolites may induce cancer incidence.

13.4.1 The effects of fatty acid and its metabolites on cancer incidence and progress

Cancer cells can connect their metabolism to sustain the production needed for cell survival, growth, and division. Lipid metabolites play an important role in these chemical processes as substrates or signal mediators. Cancer cells mainly use de novo synthesized lipids. Continuous de novo lipogenesis provides cancer cells with membrane building blocks, signaling lipid molecules as well as energy supply to support cell proliferation. Lipids from diet also play an important role in the incidence and progress of cancer. Lipid can be consumed through β-oxidation to provide key substitute energy for cancer cell survival in a glucose-limited situation. Epidemiologic studies show that people with a predominantly low-fat diet had a much lower prostate cancer, breast cancer incidence, recurrence, or mortality of cancer (Lee, Demissie, Lu, & Rhoads, 2007; Xing, Xu, & Shen, 2014). Dietary intake of SFAs correlated positively with cancer. An increase in the incidence of cancer in eastern populations may result from a change in dietary preferences in favor of an SFA-rich Western style diet (Arnold et al., 2017). SFA increases cancer partly due to SFAs changing the lipid metabolism. Some known mechanisms of SFAs inducing cancer include the activation or upregulation of factors involved in carcinogenesis, including nuclear factor κB and toll-like receptors (Huang et al., 2012). SFAs and polyunsaturated fatty acids affect lipid metabolism and contribute to cancer. Inflammation is one of the hallmarks of cancer. SFA increases the products from COX2, which are considered as proinflammatory chemicals. n-3 PUFAs and their metabolites are known to exhibit antiinflammatory properties. In contrast, most n-6 PUFAs show proinflammatory properties. The eicosapentaenoic acid (EPA, C20:5n-3) proportion in the plasma and red blood cells of the total phospholipid fractions was significantly lower in patients with cancer than in the controls (Okuno et al., 2013). The balance between n-3 and n-6 PUAFs plays a role in cancer. The ratio of n-6/n-3 PUFAs in cancerous tissue was significantly higher than in normal tissue (Bagga, Anders, Wang, & Glaspy, 2002). Increased n-6/n-3 PUFA ratio in diet has been found as

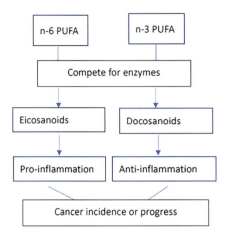

FIG. 13.1 Effects of metabolites from n-3 and n-6 fatty acids on cancer.

an important risk factor of cancer, such as aggressive prostate cancer (Williams et al., 2011), breast cancer (Yang, Ren, Fu, Gao, & Li, 2014), and invasive lung cancer (Xia, Wang, & Kang, 2005). Both n-3 and n-6 PUFAs are precursors of signaling molecules with opposing effects. Arachidonic acid (ARA, 20:4n-6), as the predominant n-6 fatty acid in the human body, is converted to prostaglandins (PGs), leukotrienes, and other eicosanoid products. These products are important regulators of cellular functions with inflammatory and carcinogenic effects. Eicosanoids from ARA, including prostaglandin E_2 (PGE_2), 5-hydroxyeicosatetraenoic acid (5-HETE), and 12-HETE have been found to stimulate the proliferation of cancer cells and promote tumor development (Chang et al., 2019). 12S-HETE was shown to promote the invasiveness of colorectal adenocarcinoma cells (Stadler et al., 2017). Increased production of leukotriene B_4 (LTB_4), 5-HETE, and 12-HETE have also been found in the mucosa of colon cancer patients and the saliva of oral cancer patients (Metzger, Angres, Maier, & Lehmann, 1995; Nielsen et al., 2005). Some EETs induce cancer cellular proliferation, migration, and angiogenesis. Inflammations may increase the cancer development, progression, and metastasis (Mantovani, Allavena, Sica, & Balkwill, 2008). The n-3 PUFA EPA and DHA have antiinflammatory properties where they compete with arachidonic acid for the enzymes (Serhan, 2014). This competition results in a changed pattern between eicosanoids and docosanoids. Resolvins and marisons derived from EPA and DHA have been recognized as specialized pro-resoling mediators that suppress tumor growth and enhance cancer therapy (Sulciner et al., 2018) (Fig. 13.1).

13.4.2 The lipogenic enzymes implicated in the development of cancer

Lipogenesis is increased in cancer cells (Swinnen, Brusselmans, & Verhoeven, 2006). Enzymes that are involved in lipid biogenesis play a pivotal role in cancer progression. This lipogenesis in tumor cells is reflected by the significantly increased activity and expression of lipogenic enzymes. Markedly increased ATP citrate lyase (ACLY) expression and activity have been reported in cancer cells, including colorectal cancer, breast cancer, nonsmall cell lung cancer, and hepatocellular carcinoma. An increased de novo synthesis of fatty acid is a hallmark of the transformed phenotype of cancer, which is observed in many cancer types. Various tumors and their precursor lesions undergo exacerbated endogenous fatty acid biosynthesis. Cancer cells can use the excess pyruvate from glycolytic metabolism for de novo fatty acid synthesis, which is necessary to maintain a constant supply of lipids and lipid precursors to membrane production in highly proliferating cancer cells (Costello & Franklin, 2006). The predominant product of endogenously synthesized fatty acids by fatty acid synthase (FASN) is palmitate, a 16-carbon saturated fatty acid (Asturias et al., 2005). The activity of elongation of very long-chain fatty acid enzymes (ELOVLs) determines the rate of fatty acid elongation. Seven distinct ELOVLs subtypes are reported in mammals. ELOVLs are responsible for the addition of two carbon units to the fatty acid chain and catalyze specifically for different chain lengths of saturated or unsaturated fatty acids. The activity of ELOVLs is cancer type-specific. For example, ELOVL2 is involved in breast cancer (González-Bengtsson, Asadi, Gao, Dahlman-Wright, & Jacobsson, 2016), ELOVL1 and ELOVL6 in triple negative breast cancer (Yamashita et al., 2017) and ELVOL7 in prostate cancer (Tamura et al., 2009). The expression level of ELOVL1 is increased in colorectal cancer tissues (Hama et al., 2021). Some studies demonstrated that colorectal cancer was associated with a significant increase in serum levels of very long chain saturated fatty acids, such as 24:0, 25:0, 26:0, 28:0 and 30:0 (Kondo et al., 2011). Cancerous tissue contained more 22:0, 24:0, and 26:0 carbon SFAs than healthy controls or normal colonic tissue (Mika et al., 2017).

13.4.3 The effects of lipid peroxidation metabolites on cancer development

Oxidative stress can induce carcinogenesis. The end products of reactive oxygen species-mediated lipid breakdown are 4-hydroxynonenal (HNE) and malondialdehyde (MDA), both found at elevated concentrations in colorectal cancer tissues (Zhong & Yin, 2015). MDA and 4-HNE are established mutagenic in human cells (Niedernhofer, Daniels, Rouzer, Greene, & Marnett, 2003).

13.5 Metabolites derived from lipids that correlated with neurodegenerative disease

Neurodegenerative diseases are characterized by the slow progressive degeneration of the structure and function of the central nervous system or peripheral nervous system, which leads to deficits in specific brain functions (Heemels, 2016). There is no cure for these neurodegenerative diseases currently. Lipid and lipid metabolites play a pivotal role in the normal physiological function of the neurons and structural development of the brain. Lipids constitute 50% of the brain's dry weight (Bruce, Zsombok, & Eckel, 2017). The fatty acid composition of the brain is mainly long-chain polyunsaturated fatty acids, particularly arachidonic acid (ARA, 20:4n-6), EPA and docosahexaenoic acid (DHA, C22:6n-3). These lipids and their metabolites affect the overall normal physiology of the brain. The high content of oxygen in the brain causes the polyunsaturated fat to easily peroxidate. The brain consumes a large volume of oxygen and generates a high quantity of lipid peroxides. Lipid peroxidation and its degeneration products are particularly important in degenerative diseases of the brain and the central nervous system. The lipid peroxidation and degradation products have been shown to induce apoptosis in neurons. There were elevated levels of lipid peroxidation products in diseased regions of the brain obtained postmortem from patients with neurodegenerative disease. One of the characteristics of neurodegenerative diseases is the accumulation of protein aggregates (Forman, Trojanowski, & Lee, 2004). The amyloid-beta peptide plays an important role in the pathology of Alzheimer's type neurodegenerative disease. 4-HNE can crosslink amyloid β peptides to each other, covalently modifying amyloid β peptide via 1,4-conjugate addition and triggering its aggregation and accelerating the formation of protofibrils. Both 4-HNE and acrolein are neurotoxic for hippocampal cultured cells. The growing body of evidence for the involvement of lipid peroxidation and general oxidative stress as a driving force of neurodegenerative disease has generated much interest in using antioxidants as therapeutics. Techniques to prevent oxidative stress accompanied by neurodegeneration have the potential to offer new therapeutic options for neurodegenerative diseases.

13.6 Conclusions

Lipid metabolites and the relevant enzymes play important roles in cardiovascular disease, cancer, and neurodegenerative disease. Inflammation is a common feature of these pathologies. As one hallmark of inflammation, the peroxidation metabolites from AA, such as eicosanoids, have a pivotal effect on disease pathology, but docosanoids from DHA and EPA as specialized pro-resolving mediators play protective effects.

References

Arnold, M., Sierra, M. S., Laversanne, M., Soerjomataram, I., Jemal, A., & Bray, F. (2017). Global patterns and trends in colorectal cancer incidence and mortality. *Gut, 66*(4), 683–691. https://doi.org/10.1136/gutjnl-2015-310912.

Asturias, F. J., Chadick, J. Z., Cheung, I. K., Stark, H., Witkowski, A., Joshi, A. K., et al. (2005). Structure and molecular organization of mammalian fatty acid synthase. *Nature Structural and Molecular Biology, 12*(3), 225–232. https://doi.org/10.1038/nsmb899.

Attard, R., Dingli, P., Doggen, C. J. M., Cassar, K., Farrugia, R., & Wettinger, S. B. (2017). The impact of passive and active smoking on inflammation, lipid profile and the risk of myocardial infarction. *Open Heart, 4*(2). https://doi.org/10.1136/openhrt-2017-000620.

Bäckhed, F., Ley, R. E., Sonnenburg, J. L., Peterson, D. A., & Gordon, J. I. (2005). Host-bacterial mutualism in the human intestine. *Science, 307*(5717), 1915–1920. https://doi.org/10.1126/science.1104816.

Bagga, D., Anders, K. H., Wang, H. J., & Glaspy, J. A. (2002). Long-chain n-3-to-n-6 polyunsaturated fatty acid ratios in breast adipose tissue from women with and without breast cancer. *Nutrition and Cancer, 42*(2), 180–185. https://doi.org/10.1207/S15327914NC422_5.

Baptista, L. C., Sun, Y., Carter, C. S., & Buford, T. W. (2020). Crosstalk between the gut microbiome and bioactive lipids: Therapeutic targets in cognitive frailty. *Frontiers in Nutrition, 7*. https://doi.org/10.3389/fnut.2020.00017.

Bloch, M. J. (2016). Worldwide prevalence of hypertension exceeds 1.3 billion. *Journal of the American Society of Hypertension, 10*(10), 753–754. https://doi.org/10.1016/j.jash.2016.08.006.

Bruce, K. D., Zsombok, A., & Eckel, R. H. (2017). Lipid processing in the brain: A key regulator of systemic metabolism. *Frontiers in Endocrinology, 8*, 60. https://doi.org/10.3389/fendo.2017.00060.

Caesar, R., Tremaroli, V., Kovatcheva-Datchary, P., Cani, P. D., & Bäckhed, F. (2015). Crosstalk between gut microbiota and dietary lipids aggravates WAT inflammation through TLR signaling. *Cell Metabolism, 22*(4), 658–668. https://doi.org/10.1016/j.cmet.2015.07.026.

Chang, J., Tang, N., Fang, Q., Zhu, K., Liu, L., Xiong, X., et al. (2019). Inhibition of COX-2 and 5-LOX regulates the progression of colorectal cancer by promoting PTEN and suppressing PI3K/AKT pathway. *Biochemical and Biophysical Research Communications, 517*(1), 1–7. https://doi.org/10.1016/j.bbrc.2018.01.061.

Cornier, M. A., Dabelea, D., Hernandez, T. L., Lindstrom, R. C., Steig, A. J., Stob, N. R., et al. (2008). The metabolic syndrome. *Endocrine Reviews, 29*(7), 777–822. https://doi.org/10.1210/er.2008-0024.

Costello, L. C., & Franklin, R. B. (2006). Tumor cell metabolism: The marriage of molecular genetics and proteomics with cellular intermediary metabolism; proceed with caution! *Molecular Cancer, 5*(59). https://doi.org/10.1186/1476-4598-5-59.

De Filippo, C., Cavalieri, D., Di Paola, M., Ramazzotti, M., Poullet, J. B., Massart, S., et al. (2010). Impact of diet in shaping gut microbiota revealed by a comparative study in children from Europe and rural Africa. *Proceedings of the National Academy of Sciences of the United States of America, 107*(33), 14691–14696. https://doi.org/10.1073/pnas.1005963107.

Devillard, E., McIntosh, F. M., Duncan, S. H., & Wallace, R. J. (2007). Metabolism of linoleic acid by human gut bacteria: Different routes for biosynthesis of conjugated linoleic acid. *Journal of Bacteriology, 189*(6), 2566–2570. https://doi.org/10.1128/JB.01359-06.

Druart, C., Neyrinck, A. M., Dewulf, E. M., De Backer, F. C., Possemiers, S., Van De Wiele, T., et al. (2013). Implication of fermentable carbohydrates targeting the gut microbiota on conjugated linoleic acid production in high-fat-fed mice. *British Journal of Nutrition, 110*(6), 998–1011. https://doi.org/10.1017/S0007114513000123.

Forman, M. S., Trojanowski, J. Q., & Lee, V. M. Y. (2004). Neurodegenerative diseases: A decade of discoveries paves the way for therapeutic breakthroughs. *Nature Medicine*, 10(10), 1055–1063. https://doi.org/10.1038/nm1113.

German, J. B. (2011). Dietary lipids from an evolutionary perspective: Sources, structures and functions. *Maternal & Child Nutrition*, 7(2), 2–16. https://doi.org/10.1111/j.1740-8709.2011.00300.x.

Goldstein, J. L., & Brown, M. S. (2015). A century of cholesterol and coronaries: From plaques to genes to statins. *Cell*, 161(1), 161–172. https://doi.org/10.1016/j.cell.2015.01.036.

González-Bengtsson, A., Asadi, A., Gao, H., Dahlman-Wright, K., & Jacobsson, A. (2016). Estrogen enhances the expression of the polyunsaturated fatty acid elongase Elovl 2 via ERα in breast cancer cells. *PLoS One*, 11(10). https://doi.org/10.1371/journal.pone.0164241.

Hama, K., Fujiwara, Y., Hayama, T., Ozawa, T., Nozawa, K., Matsuda, K., et al. (2021). Very long-chain fatty acids are accumulated in triacylglycerol and nonesterified forms in colorectal cancer tissues. *Scientific Reports*, 2021(11). https://doi.org/10.1038/s41598-021-85603-w.

Havulinna, A. S., Sysi-Aho, M., Hilvo, M., Kauhanen, D., Hurme, R., Ekroos, K., et al. (2016). Circulating ceramides predict cardiovascular outcomes in the population-based FINRISK 2002 cohort. *Arteriosclerosis, Thrombosis, and Vascular Biology*, 36(12), 2424–2430. https://doi.org/10.1161/ATVBAHA.116.307497.

Heemels, M. T. (2016). Neurodegenerative diseases. *Nature*, 539(7628), 179. https://doi.org/10.1038/539179a.

Huang, S., Rutkowsky, J. M., Snodgrass, R. G., Ono-Moore, K. D., Schneider, D. A., Newman, J. W., et al. (2012). Saturated fatty acids activate TLR-mediated proinflammatory signaling pathways. *Journal of Lipid Research*, 53(9), 2002–2013. https://doi.org/10.1194/jlr.D029546.

Imig, J. D., & Hammock, B. D. (2009). Soluble epoxide hydrolase as a therapeutic target for cardiovascular diseases. *Nature Reviews Drug Discovery*, 8(10), 794–805. https://doi.org/10.1038/nrd2875.

Jocken, J. W. E., & Blaak, E. E. (2008). Catecholamine-induced lipolysis in adipose tissue and skeletal muscle in obesity. *Physiology and Behavior*, 94(2), 219–230. https://doi.org/10.1016/j.physbeh.2008.01.002.

Jump, D. B., Clarke, S. D., Thelen, A., & Liimatta, M. (1994). Coordinate regulation of glycolytic and lipogenic gene expression by polyunsaturated fatty acids. *Journal of Lipid Research*, 35(6), 1076–1084.

Kondo, Y., Nishiumi, S., Shinohara, M., Hatano, N., Ikeda, A., Yoshie, T., et al. (2011). Serum fatty acid profiling of colorectal cancer by gas chromatography/mass spectrometry. *Biomarkers in Medicine*, 5(4), 451–460. https://doi.org/10.2217/bmm.11.41.

Koppo, K., Larrouy, D., Marques, M. A., Berlan, M., Bajzova, M., Polak, J., et al. (2010). Lipid mobilization in subcutaneous adipose tissue during exercise in lean and obese humans. Roles of insulin and natriuretic peptides. *American Journal of Physiology. Endocrinology and Metabolism*, 299(2), E258–E265. https://doi.org/10.1152/ajpendo.00767.2009.

Kuhajda, F. P. (2000). Fatty-acid synthase and human cancer: New perspectives on its role in tumor biology. *Nutrition*, 16(3), 202–208. https://doi.org/10.1016/S0899-9007(99)00266-X.

Laaksonen, R., Ekroos, K., Sysi-Aho, M., Hilvo, M., Vihervaara, T., Kauhanen, D., et al. (2016). Plasma ceramides predict cardiovascular death in patients with stable coronary artery disease and acute coronary syndromes beyond LDL-cholesterol. *European Heart Journal*, 37(25), 1967–1976. https://doi.org/10.1093/eurheartj/ehw148.

Lai, J., & Chen, C. (2021). The role of epoxyeicosatrienoic acids in cardiac remodeling. *Frontiers in Physiology*, 12. https://doi.org/10.3389/fphys.2021.642470.

Lee, J., Demissie, K., Lu, S. E., & Rhoads, G. G. (2007). Cancer incidence among Korean-American immigrants in the United States and native Koreans in South Korea. *Cancer Control*, 14(1), 78–85. https://doi.org/10.1177/107327480701400111.

Li, H., Liu, F., Lu, J., Shi, J., Guan, J., Yan, F., et al. (2020). Probiotic mixture of Lactobacillus plantarum strains improves lipid metabolism and gut microbiota structure in high fat diet-fed mice. *Frontiers in Microbiology*, 11. https://doi.org/10.3389/fmicb.2020.00512.

Mantovani, A., Allavena, P., Sica, A., & Balkwill, F. (2008). Cancer-related inflammation. *Nature*, 454(7203), 436–444. https://doi.org/10.1038/nature07205.

Mantovani, A., Bonapace, S., Lunardi, G., Canali, G., Dugo, C., Vinco, G., et al. (2020). Associations between specific plasma ceramides and severity of coronary-artery stenosis assessed by coronary angiography. *Diabetes & Metabolism*, 46(2), 150–157. https://doi.org/10.1016/j.diabet.2019.07.006.

Maslowski, K. M., & MacKay, C. R. (2011). Diet, gut microbiota and immune responses. *Nature Immunology*, 12(1), 5–9. https://doi.org/10.1038/ni0111-5.

Menendez, J. A., & Lupu, R. (2007). Fatty acid synthase and the lipogenic phenotype in cancer pathogenesis. *Nature Reviews Cancer*, 7(10), 763–777. https://doi.org/10.1038/nrc2222.

Metzger, K., Angres, G., Maier, H., & Lehmann, W. D. (1995). Lipoxygenase products in human saliva: Patients with oral cancer compared to controls. *Free Radical Biology and Medicine*, 18(2), 185–194. https://doi.org/10.1016/0891-5849(94)00108-V.

Mika, A., Kobiela, J., Czumaj, A., Chmielewski, M., Stepnowski, P., & Sledzinski, T. (2017). Hyper-elongation in colorectal Cancer tissue-cerotic acid is a potential novel serum metabolic marker of colorectal malignancies. *Cellular Physiology and Biochemistry*, 41(2), 722–730. https://doi.org/10.1159/000458431.

Natividad, J. M., Lamas, B., Pham, H. P., Michel, M. L., Rainteau, D., Bridonneau, C., et al. (2018). Bilophila wadsworthia aggravates high fat diet induced metabolic dysfunctions in mice. *Nature Communications, 2018*(1). https://doi.org/10.1038/s41467-018-05249-7.

Newman, J. C., & Verdin, E. (2014). Ketone bodies as signaling metabolites. *Trends in Endocrinology and Metabolism, 25*(1), 42–52. https://doi.org/10.1016/j.tem.2013.09.002.

Ni, G. H., Chen, J. F., Chen, X. P., & Yang, T. L. (2011). Soluble epoxide hydrolase: A promising therapeutic target for cardiovascular diseases. *Pharmazie, 66*(3), 153–157. https://doi.org/10.1692/ph.2011.0709.

Niedernhofer, L. J., Daniels, J. S., Rouzer, C. A., Greene, R. E., & Marnett, L. J. (2003). Malondialdehyde, a product of lipid peroxidation, is mutagenic in human cells. *Journal of Biological Chemistry, 278*(33), 31426–31433. https://doi.org/10.1074/jbc.M212549200.

Nielsen, C. K., Campbell, J. I. A., Öhd, J. F., Mörgelin, M., Riesbeck, K., Landberg, G., et al. (2005). A novel localization of the G-protein-coupled CysLT1 receptor in the nucleus of colorectal adenocarcinoma cells. *Cancer Research, 65*(3), 732–742.

Nielsen, J., Jørgensen, J. O. L., Møller, N., & Lund, S. (2014). Dissecting adipose tissue lipolysis: Molecular regulation and implications for metabolic disease. *Journal of Molecular Endocrinology, 52*(3), R199–R222. https://doi.org/10.1530/JME-13-0277.

Okuno, M., Hamazaki, K., Ogura, T., Kitade, H., Matsuura, T., Yoshida, R., et al. (2013). Abnormalities in fatty acids in plasma, erythrocytes and adipose tissue in japanese patients with colorectal cancer. *In Vivo, 27*(2), 203–210. http://iv.iiarjournals.org/content/27/2/203.full.pdf+html.

Perman, J. C., Boström, P., Lindbom, M., Lidberg, U., StÅhlman, M., Hägg, D., et al. (2011). The VLDL receptor promotes lipotoxicity and increases mortality in mice following an acute myocardial infarction. *Journal of Clinical Investigation, 121*(7), 2625–2640. https://doi.org/10.1172/JCI43068.

Puchalska, P., & Crawford, P. A. (2017). Multi-dimensional roles of ketone bodies in fuel metabolism, signaling, and therapeutics. *Cell Metabolism, 25*(2), 262–284. https://doi.org/10.1016/j.cmet.2016.12.022.

Ramana, K. V., Srivastava, S., & Singhal, S. S. (2019). Lipid peroxidation products in human health and disease 2019. *Oxidative Medicine and Cellular Longevity, 2019*. https://doi.org/10.1155/2019/7147235.

Ruan, Y., Guo, Y., Zheng, Y., Huang, Z., Sun, S., Kowal, P., et al. (2018). Cardiovascular disease (CVD) and associated risk factors among older adults in six low-and middle-income countries: Results from SAGE wave 1. *BMC Public Health, 18*(1). https://doi.org/10.1186/s12889-018-5653-9.

Sachdeva, A., Cannon, C. P., Deedwania, P. C., LaBresh, K. A., Smith, S. C., Dai, D., et al. (2009). Lipid levels-in patients hospitalized with coronary artery disease: An analysis of 136,905 hospitalizations in get with the guidelines. *American Heart Journal, 157*(1), 111–117. https://doi.org/10.1016/j.ahj.2008.08.010.

Serhan, C. N. (2014). Pro-resolving lipid mediators are leads for resolution physiology. *Nature, 510*(7503), 92–101. https://doi.org/10.1038/nature13479.

Stadler, S., Nguyen, C. H., Schachner, H., Milovanovic, D., Holzner, S., Brenner, S., et al. (2017). Colon cancer cell derived 12(S) HETE induces the retraction of cancer-associated fibroblast via MLC2, RHO/ROCK and Ca2+ signalling. *Cellular and Molecular Life Sciences, 74*(10), 1907–1921. https://doi.org/10.1007/s00018-016-2441-5.

Sulciner, M. L., Serhan, C. N., Gilligan, M. M., Mudge, D. K., Chang, J., Gartung, A., et al. (2018). Resolvins suppress tumor growth and enhance cancer therapy. *Journal of Experimental Medicine, 215*(1), 115–140. https://doi.org/10.1084/jem.20170681.

Swinnen, J. V., Brusselmans, K., & Verhoeven, G. (2006). Increased lipogenesis in cancer cells: New players, novel targets. *Current Opinion in Clinical Nutrition and Metabolic Care, 9*(4), 358–365. https://doi.org/10.1097/01.mco.0000232894.28674.30.

Tamura, K., Makino, A., Hullin-Matsuda, F., Kobayashi, T., Furihata, M., Chung, S., et al. (2009). Novel lipogenic enzyme ELOVL7 is involved in prostate cancer growth through saturated long-chain fatty acid metabolism. *Cancer Research, 69*(20), 8133–8140. https://doi.org/10.1158/0008-5472.CAN-09-0775.

Turnbaugh, P. J., Ridaura, V. K., Faith, J. J., Rey, F. E., Knight, R., & Gordon, J. I. (2009). The effect of diet on the human gut microbiome: A metagenomic analysis in humanized gnotobiotic mice. *Science Translational Medicine, 1*(6). https://doi.org/10.1126/scitranslmed.3000322.

Wan, Y., Wang, F. L., Yuan, J. H., Li, J., Jiang, D. D., Zhang, J. J., et al. (2019). Effects of dietary fat on gut microbiota and faecal metabolites, and their relationship with cardiometabolic risk factors: A 6-month randomised controlled-feeding trial. *Gut, 2019*(8). https://doi.org/10.1136/gutjnl-2018-317609.

Williams, C. D., Whitley, B. M., Hoyo, C., Grant, D. J., Iraggi, J. D., Newman, K. A., et al. (2011). A high ratio of dietary n-6/n-3 polyunsaturated fatty acids is associated with increased risk of prostate cancer. *Nutrition Research, 31*(1), 1–8. https://doi.org/10.1016/j.nutres.2011.01.002.

Wolfrum, C., Asilmaz, E., Luca, E., Friedman, J. M., & Stoffel, M. (2004). Foxa2 regulates lipid metabolism and ketogenesis in the liver during fasting and in diabetes. *Nature, 432*(7020), 1027–1032. https://doi.org/10.1038/nature03047.

Xia, S. H., Wang, J., & Kang, J. X. (2005). Decreased n-6/n-3 fatty acid ratio reduces the invasive potential of human lung cancer cells by downregulation of cell adhesion/invasion-related genes. *Carcinogenesis*, 26(4), 779–784. https://doi.org/10.1093/carcin/bgi019.

Xing, M. Y., Xu, S. Z., & Shen, P. (2014). Effect of low-fat diet on breast cancer survival: A meta-analysis. *Asian Pacific Journal of Cancer Prevention*, 15(3), 1141–1144. https://doi.org/10.7314/APJCP.2014.15.3.1141.

Yamashita, Y., Nishiumi, S., Kono, S., Takao, S., Azuma, T., & Yoshida, M. (2017). Differences in elongation of very long chain fatty acids and fatty acid metabolism between triple-negative and hormone receptor-positive breast cancer. *BMC Cancer*, 17(1). https://doi.org/10.1186/s12885-017-3554-4.

Yang, B., Ren, X. L., Fu, Y. Q., Gao, J. L., & Li, D. (2014). Ratio of n-3/n-6 PUFAs and risk of breast cancer: A meta-analysis of 274135 adult females from 11 independent prospective studies. *BMC Cancer*, 14(1). https://doi.org/10.1186/1471-2407-14-105.

Zheng, C. J., Yoo, J. S., Lee, T. G., Cho, H. Y., Kim, Y. H., & Kim, W. G. (2005). Fatty acid synthesis is a target for antibacterial activity of unsaturated fatty acids. *FEBS Letters*, 579(23), 5157–5162. https://doi.org/10.1016/j.febslet.2005.08.028.

Zhong, H., & Yin, H. (2015). Role of lipid peroxidation derived 4-hydroxynonenal (4-HNE) in cancer: Focusing on mitochondria. *Redox Biology*, 4, 193–199. https://doi.org/10.1016/j.redox.2014.12.011.

Zordoky, B. N. M., & El-Kadi, A. O. S. (2010). Effect of cytochrome P450 polymorphism on arachidonic acid metabolism and their impact on cardiovascular diseases. *Pharmacology and Therapeutics*, 125(3), 446–463. https://doi.org/10.1016/j.pharmthera.2009.12.002.

CHAPTER 14

Marine n-3 polyunsaturated fatty acids and inflammatory diseases

Yuanqing Fu

Laboratory of Precision Nutrition and Computational Medicine, School of Life Sciences, Westlake University, Hangzhou, China

14.1 Marine n-3 polyunsaturated fatty acids and inflammatory processes

Omega-3 (or n-3) fatty acids is a family of polyunsaturated fatty acids that have the last double bond between carbon numbers 3 and 4 in the hydrocarbon chain. Long chain n-3 fatty acids include docosahexaenoic acid (DHA; 22:6n-3), docosapentaenoic acid (DPA; 22:5n-3) and eicosapentaenoic acid (EPA; 20:5n-3), which are found rich in oily fish, and so these long chain n-3 PUFAs are collectively referred to as marine n-3 fatty acids. Marine n-3 PUFAs are generally regarded as safe at a dose up to 3 g/day, stated by the US Food and Drug Administration (FDA) since 2018. In addition, fish consumption is recommended in the 2015–2020 Dietary Guidelines for Americans by the American Heart Association (Rimm et al., 2018). However, caution should be taken when suggesting the use of n-3 PUFAs supplementation for preventing cardiovascular diseases or reducing major adverse cardiovascular events, as several high-quality systematic reviews, pool analysis, and recent randomized controlled trials (RCTs) yielded inconsistent results (Aung et al., 2018; Del Gobbo et al., 2016; Nicholls et al., 2020; Rizos, Ntzani, Bika, Kostapanos, & Elisaf, 2012).

Inflammation is an important part of the normal host defense mechanism against infection or injury. As a response to the pathogens, the host initiates the inflammatory processes that are involved with interactions between many cell types and the production of a series of mediators. The mediators include lipid-derived prostaglandins (PGs), thromboxane (TXs), leukotrienes (LTs), endocannabinoids, platelet-activating factors, cytokines and chemokines (Calder, 2015). On the one hand, the inflammatory response is hostile to pathogens, but on the other hand, the uncontrolled inflammation causes damage to host tissues. Nevertheless, the inflammatory response is normally self-limiting and well regulated, since the activation of negative feedback mechanisms, including secretion of antiinflammatory cytokines and resolving lipid mediators, inhibiting the pro-inflammatory signaling and activation of regulatory cells. However, in some cases, abnormal regulation of the inflammation process may occur, and thus lead to excessive or chronic inflammation which is harmful to the host (Bäck, Yurdagul, Tabas, Öörni, & Kovanen, 2019; Kidane et al., 2014; Urman, Taklalsingh, Sorrento, & McFarlane, 2018). Chronic inflammation has been widely considered to play an important role in the progression of several chronic diseases, including atherosclerosis, inflammatory bowel diseases, rheumatoid arthritis, cancer and neurodegenerative syndromes (Chamani et al., 2020; Fiala & Veerhuis, 2010; Greten & Grivennikov, 2019; Marchio et al., 2019; Wolf & Ley, 2019).

One of the most important links between n-3 PUFAs and inflammation is eicosanoids, which play a key role in mediating and regulating the inflammation (Calder, 2006). Arachidonic acid (20:4n-6) is the major substrate for eicosanoid synthesis. The products of the eicosanoid pathway, including PGs, TXs, and LTs, are produced from arachidonic acid through the action of cyclooxygenases (COX) and lipoxygenase (LOX). These AA-derived eicosanoids exert significant influence on the inflammatory response. PGs are involved in the classic signs of inflammation, such as vascular permeability, tissue regeneration, fibrosis, pain perception, and leukocyte migration into inflammatory tissues (Sano et al., 1992). Thromboxane A2 is formed by platelets, macrophages, and polymorphonuclear leukocytes (PMNs) and can promote aggregation of platelets as well as adhesiveness of PMNs (Verstraete, 1983). LTs also play as pro-inflammatory mediators which increase COX-2 expression and enhance local blood flow through stimulating neutrophil secretion (Henderson, 1994). Marine n-3 PUFAs were reported to reduce the amount of AA in immune cells and thus to reduce AA derivatives (Rees et al., 2006). To assess the effect of marine n-3 PUFAs on AA-derived major eicosanoids, a systematic review and meta-analysis of 18 RCTs involving 826 subjects found that the supplementation of marine n-3 PUFA significantly decreased concentrations of circulating thromboxane B_2 (TXB_2) in subjects with high risk of cardiovascular diseases and leukotriene B_4 (LTB_4) in neutrophils among patients with chronic inflammatory diseases (Jiang et al., 2016). Regarding the mechanisms, marine n-3 PUFA, especially EPA, can competitively inhibit the synthesis of AA-derived eicosanoids, through acting as a substrate catalyzed by 5-LOX enzymes and COX enzymes. The EPA-derived eicosanoids, including leukotriene B_5 (LTB_5) and leukotriene E_5 (LTE_5), possess less potent pro-inflammatory activity in comparison with AA-derived eicosanoids (Goldman, Pickett, & Goetzl, 1983). Additionally, n-3 PUFAs can also exhibit antiinflammatory activity by indirectly altering the expression of inflammatory genes through effects on transcription factor genes (Lo, Chiu, Fu, Lo, & Helton, 1999; Novak, Babcock, Jho, Helton, & Espat, 2003). In animal models, marine n-3 PUFAs supplementation is associated with a lower production of TNF-α, IL-1β and IL-6, while an increased level of IL-10 after the challenge of endotoxin injection (Billiar et al., 1988; Sadeghi, Wallace, & Calder, 1999). Furthermore, marine n-3 PUFAs also generate a series of antiinflammatory mediators, termed specialized pro-resolving mediators, including resolvins, protectins, and maresins (Bannenberg & Serhan, 2010; Serhan & Levy, 2018). The metabolism of EPA can lead to the formation of resolvin E series, the metabolism of DPA can lead to the biosynthesis of protectin D family members (e.g., PD1 and PD2) and the metabolism of DHA can lead to the formation of resolvin D series, maresins and protectins, which were believed possessing higher inflammation-resolving ability than the competitive inhibition on the generation of AA-derived eicosanoids (Arita et al., 2007; Chiurchiù et al., 2016; Hudert et al., 2006). The overview of metabolism pathways and antiinflammatory actions of marine n-3 PUFA is summarized in Fig. 14.1. Numerous studies have shown that increased intake of marine n-3 PUFA is beneficial for the balance of inflammatory factors and therefore has a

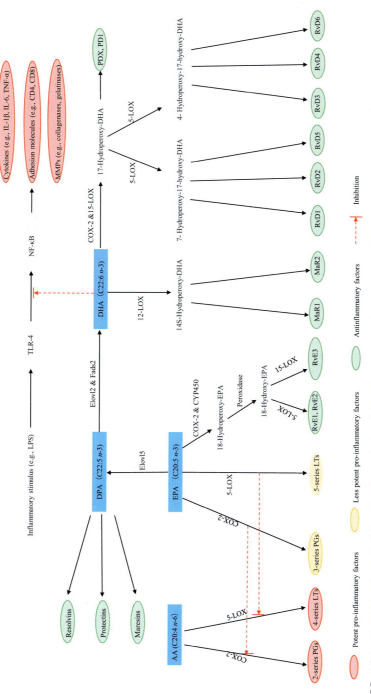

FIG. 14.1 Overview of metabolism pathways and antiinflammatory actions of marine n-3 PUFAs.

protective effect on inflammatory diseases, including rheumatoid arthritis, inflammatory bowel disease and Alzheimer's disease although definite conclusions are yet to be drawn. A summary of existing evidence from meta-analysis of RCTs or observational studies on marine n-3 PUFAs and typical inflammatory diseases is in Table 14.1.

14.2 Marine n-3 polyunsaturated fatty acids and inflammatory diseases

14.2.1 Rheumatoid arthritis

Rheumatoid arthritis (RA) is a chronic systemic autoimmune disorder characterized by inflammation of joints with severe pain, swelling, and irreversible destruction of cartilage and bone (Choy & Panayi, 2001; Smolen, Daniel, & McInnes, 2016). COX-1 and COX-2 expressions are increased in the synovium of RA patients, and the levels of pro-inflammatory eicosanoid products, cytokines and chemokines are relatively high in the synovial fluid of patients with RA (Mateen, Zafar, Moin, Khan, & Zubair, 2016; Sano et al., 1992). The conventional therapeutic options employed in the management of RA are corticosteroids, immunosuppressive drugs and nonsteroidal antiinflammatory drugs (NSAIDs). Notably, one of the mechanisms underlying the efficacy of the most commonly used NSAIDs is the inhibition on the COX metabolism of AA, indicating marine n-3 PUFAs may have great potential for treating RA (Calder, 2015).

Studies based on animal models of arthritis consistently report promising efficacy of marine n-3 PUFAs in relieving the severity of arthritis and improving joint pathology (Ierna, Kerr, Scales, Berge, & Griinari, 2010; Volker, FitzGerald, & Garg, 2000). The reported effects of marine n-3 PUFAs were mainly obtained through the reduction of pro-inflammatory cytokines and metalloproteinases production and the decrease of leukocytes migration (Navarini, Afeltra, Gallo Afflitto, & Margiotta, 2017). One of the latest animal studies investigated whether n-3 PUFAs attenuate arthritis in a collagen antibody-induced arthritis model using fat-1 transgenic mice (Kim et al., 2018). The fat-1 gene encodes an n-3 fatty acid desaturase that converts n-6 to n-3 fatty acids, leading to abundant n-3 fatty acids without the need for a dietary n-3 supply. The results showed that clinical arthritis score was attenuated, ankle thickness was decreased, and the inflammatory cell infiltration was reduced in fat-1 mice compared to wild type (WT) mice. The expression levels of IL-17 and related cytokines including IL-6 and IL-23 decreased in the spleen and ankle joint tissue of fat-1 mice. Furthermore, Treg cell differentiation was also found relatively high in fat-1 mice. Overall, data from animal models provided consistent evidence indicating marine n-3 PUFAs could be beneficial for treating arthritis although the level of animal study derived evidence is low.

Prospective cohort studies also support a protective effect of marine n-3 PUFA against the development of RA. In a large cohort study involving 57,053 Danish participants, after an average follow-up of 5.3 years, per 30 g increment in fat fish intake was associated with 49% reduced risk of RA (Pedersen et al., 2005). Another cohort study including 32,232 women from Sweden, identified 205 RA cases during a mean follow-up of 7.5 years (Di Giuseppe et al., 2014). An intake of more than 0.21 g n-3 PUFAs per day was associated with a 35% lower risk of RA, compared to lower intake. Furthermore, long-term dietary n-3 PUFA intake consistently higher than 0.21 g/day was associated with a 52% reduced risk of RA (Di Giuseppe et al., 2014).

In the past decades, numerous clinical studies explored the effects of marine n-3 PUFAs on RA. An RCT of marine n-3 PUFAs enriched lipid extract performed in 50 RA patients reported improvements in several clinical outcomes including reduced tender joint counts (TJC) and swollen joint counts (SJC), and duration of morning stiffness (Fu et al., 2015). In consistent with

TABLE 14.1 Key meta-analysis of RCTs or observational studies on marine n-3 PUFAs and inflammatory diseases.

Disease	Study design	Participants	Intervention/exposure	Dosage	Outcome	Intervention/follow-up duration	Main findings	References
Rheumatoid arthritis (RA)	Meta-analysis of RCTs ($n=20$)	Patients with RA ($n=1288$)	n-3 PUFAs	EPA+DHA: 0.3–5.4 g/day	RA disease activity, inflammation, and CVD risk	12–72 weeks	Oral supplementation with n-3 PUFAs (e.g., EPA, DHA) resulted in significant amelioration of disease severity markers, including EMS, number of tender joints, erythrocyte sedimentation rate (ESR), pain scale, and LTB4.	Gioxari, Kaliora, Marantidou, and Panagiotakos (2018)
	Meta-analysis of RCTs ($n=42$)	Arthritis patients (including RA, Osteoarthritis, and other/mixed types of arthritis; $n=2751$)	n-3 PUFAs	EPA: 0.013–4.05 g/day; DHA: 0.01–2.70 g/day	Arthritis pain	2 weeks–18 months	A significant effect was found in patients with rheumatoid arthritis (22 trials) and other or mixed diagnoses (3 trials), but not in osteoarthritis patients (5 trials). The evidence for using marine oil to alleviate pain in arthritis patients was overall of low quality, but of moderate quality in rheumatoid arthritis patients.	Senftleber et al. (2017)
	Meta-analysis of observational studies ($n=7$)	174,701 participants and 3346 cases of RA	Fish consumption	NA	Risk of rheumatoid arthritis	7–8 years (for prospective studies)	For each one serving per week increment in fish consumption, the relative risk of RA was 0.96 (95% confidence interval (CI) 0.91 to 1.01), which showed a nonstatistically significant inverse association between fish consumption and RA.	Di Giuseppe, Wallin, Bottai, Askling, and Wolk (2014)

Continued

TABLE 14.1 Key meta-analysis of RCTs or observational studies on marine n-3 PUFAs and inflammatory diseases—cont'd

Disease	Study design	Participants	Intervention/exposure	Dosage	Outcome	Intervention/follow-up duration	Main findings	References
	Meta-analysis of RCTs ($n=10$)	Patients with RA ($n=370$)	n-3 PUFAs	2.9–9.6 g/day	TJC, number of swollen joints, patient global assessment of disease-associated pain, physician global assessment of disease activity, pain, morning stiffness, physical function, ESR, C-reactive protein and nonselective nonsteroidal antiinflammatory drug (NSAID) consumption	12 weeks–15 months	No significant improvement was observed in the n-3 PUFA group as compared with controls for any clinical outcomes except reduced NSAID consumption. The use of n-3 PUFAs at dosages >2.7 g/day for >3 months reduces NSAID consumption by RA patients.	Lee, Bae, and Song (2012)
	Meta-analysis of RCTs ($n=17$)	Patients with RA or joint pain secondary to inflammatory bowel disease and dysmenorrhea ($n=823$)	n-3 PUFAs	1.7–9.6 g/day	Patient assessed pain, physician assessed pain, duration of morning stiffness, number of painful and/or tender joints, Ritchie articular index, and NSAID consumption	1–15 months	Supplementation with omega-3 PUFAs for 3–4 months significantly reduces patient reported joint pain intensity, minutes of morning stiffness, number of painful and/or tender joints, and NSAID consumption. n-3 PUFAs are an attractive adjunctive treatment for joint pain associated with rheumatoid arthritis, inflammatory bowel disease, and dysmenorrhea.	Goldberg and Katz (2007)
Inflammatory bowel disease (IBD)	Meta-analysis of RCTs ($n=83$, with 13 specifically recruiting participants with IBD)	Adult participants with or without a diagnosis of IBD ($n=41{,}751$)	n-3 PUFAs; n-6 PUFAs	EPA: 0.54–3.99 g/day; DHA: 0.36–1.72 g/day	Rates of induced IBD relapse (or remission), IBD severity or worsening and inflammatory markers (e.g., CRP, ESR and IL-6)	6 months–4.9 years	Increasing n-3 PUFAs intakes may reduce risk of IBD relapse and IBD worsening, and reduce EST, but may increase IBD diagnosis risk. Supplementation with PUFAs has little or no effect on prevention or treatment of IBD and provides little support for modification of long-term inflammatory status.	Ajabnoor, Thorpe, Abdelhamid, and Hooper (2020)

Disease	Study type	Population	Intervention	Dose	Outcome measures	Duration	Main findings	Reference
Inflammatory bowel disease (IBD)	Meta-analysis of cohort studies ($n=10$)	General populations ($n=282{,}610$) including 2002 cases of IBD.	n-3 PUFAs, fish consumption	NA	Risk of IBD	10.4–26 years (for prospective follow-up studies)	There was no relationship between total dietary n-3 PUFAs intake and IBD ($p=0.41$). A significant inverse association was observed between dietary long-chain n-3 PUFAs and the risk of ulcerative colitis ($p=0.03$).	Mozaffari, Daneshzad, Larijani, Bellissimo, and Azadbakht (2020)
Inflammatory bowel disease (IBD)	Meta-analysis of RCTs ($n=9$)	IBD patients ($n=1039$ for CD; $n=138$ for UC) in remission	n-3 PUFAs	EPA: 1.2–3.3 g/day; DHA: 0.6–2.1 g/day	Relapse rate	1–2 years	There was a statistically significant benefit for n-3 in CD. A sensitivity analysis excluding a small pediatric study resulted in the pooled RR being no longer statistically significant. For UC, there was no difference in the relapse rate between the n-3 and control groups. The existing data do not support routine treatment with n-3 fatty acids for maintaining remission in IBD.	Turner, Shah, Steinhart, Zlotkin, and Griffiths (2011)
Inflammatory bowel disease (IBD)	Meta-analysis of RCTs ($n=13$)	IBD patients ($n=741$)	n-3 PUFAs	NR	Clinical sigmoidoscopic/histologic scores; rates of induced remission or relapse; or requirements for steroids and other immunosuppressive agents	3–24 months	n-3 Fatty acids reduce corticosteroid requirements, although statistical significance was shown in only 1 of the studies. The available data are insufficient to draw conclusions about the effects of n-3 fatty acids on clinical, endoscopic, or histologic scores or remission or relapse rates.	MacLean et al. (2005)
Alzheimer's disease (AD)	Meta-analysis of RCTs ($n=6$)	Patients diagnosed with AD ($n=758$)	n-3 PUFAs	EPA: 0.60–1.0 g/day; DHA: 0.625–2.0 g/day	Cognitive function (e.g., memory, praxis, or language skills)	3–18 months	There is no consistent evidence to support the effectiveness of n-3 supplementation in improving cognitive function in AD patients in the short and medium term.	Araya-Quintanilla et al. (2020)

Continued

TABLE 14.1 Key meta-analysis of RCTs or observational studies on marine n-3 PUFAs and inflammatory diseases—cont'd

Disease	Study design	Participants	Intervention/exposure	Dosage	Outcome	Intervention/follow-up duration	Main findings	References
Alzheimer's disease (AD)	Meta-analysis of prospective cohort studies (n=21)	General populations (n=181,580) with 4438 cases	n-3 PUFAs, PUFAs, fish consumption	NA	Risk estimates for mild cognitive impairment, cognitive decline, dementia, AD or Parkinson's disease	3–21 years	Higher consumption of fish and marine derived DHA may be associated with lower risks of dementia and AD. However, total n-3 PUFAs are not inversely associated with all investigated cognitive risks. Overall, fishery products are recommended as dietary sources and are associated with lower risks of cognitive impairment. Marine-derived DHA was associated with lower risks of dementia and AD but without a linear dose-response relation.	Zhang et al. (2016)
Alzheimer's disease (AD)	Meta-analysis of prospective cohort studies (n=6)	General populations or people at high risk of dementia or AD (n=22,402)	n-3 PUFAs, fish consumption	NA	Incidence of dementia or AD	Mean: 2.1–9.6 years	Long-chain n-3 PUFAs intake didn't reduce the risk of dementia or Alzheimer's disease. A higher intake of fish was associated with a 36% lower risk of AD, and an increment of 100g per week of fish intake was associated with an 11% lower risk of AD.	Wu et al. (2015)
Alzheimer's disease (AD)	Meta-analysis of RCTs (n=10)	Cognitively normal elderly adults (healthy), elderly adults with memory complaints and objective cognitive decline (CIND), and patients with dementia or AD (totally n=2507)	n-3 PUFAs	EPA:0.02–1.67g/day; DHA: 0.06–1.55g/day	Cognitive performance	12.8–108 weeks	n-3 Fatty acid treatment was associated with a small, but significant, benefit for immediate recall and attention and processing speed in subjects with CIND but not in healthy subjects or those with AD.	Mazereeuw, Lanctôt, Chau, Swardfager, and Herrmann (2012)

this study, other RCT studies of fish oil in RA patients also reported improvements in clinical outcomes such as reduced duration of morning stiffness, reduced joint pain and reduced time to fatigue (Rajaei et al., 2015). A more recent RCT examined the antiinflammatory effects of high-dose n-3 PUFA alone or in combination with gamma linolenic acid in 60 patients with active RA (Veselinovic et al., 2017). The disease activity score 28 (DAS28; a disease activity score calculated based on assessments of tenderness and/or swelling of 28 joints), the number of tender joints and visual analog scale score decreased significantly in both the supplemented groups after 12 weeks of supplementation, but not in the control group. Notably, the dose of marine n-3 PUFAs used in the trials was relatively high (Veselinovic et al., 2017). A meta-analysis of 17 RCTs assessing the pain-relieving effects of n-3 PUFAs in patients with RA or joint pain also confirmed the abovementioned evidence about the capacity of adequate doses of marine n-3 PUFAs to improve clinically typical outcomes (Goldberg & Katz, 2007). This study found that fish oil reduced patient-assessed joint pain, duration of morning stiffness, and number of tender joints. Another meta-analysis of 10 RCTs investigating the effects of n-3 PUFAs at doses ≥ 2.7 g/day for a minimum of 3 months on clinical outcomes among RA patients suggested that the improvement in TJC, SJC, and physical function did not reach statistical significance, but NSAID consumption could be reduced (Lee et al., 2012). The beneficial properties of n-3 PUFAs on RA disease activity were also confirmed by another meta-analysis involving 20 RCTs and 1288 RA patients, which found oral supplementation with n-3 PUFAs resulted in significant amelioration of disease severity markers, including early morning stiffness, TJC, erythrocyte sedimentation rate, pain scale, and leukotriene B4 (Gioxari et al., 2018). Overall, there are relatively strong evidence to suggest that the high doses of marine n-3 PUFAs exhibit clinical benefits for RA patients.

14.2.2 Inflammatory bowel disease

Ulcerative colitis (UC) and Crohn's disease (CD) are collectively called inflammatory bowel disease (IBD), which affects the gastrointestinal mucosa and possesses a lifelong burden of disease for the patients (Baumgart & Sandborn, 2007; Wang, Fu, Cai, Sinclair, & Li, 2016). Regarding the inflammation process or immune cell response profile, CD is characterized by a Th1 pattern of cytokine formation with upregulated expression of TNF-α, interferon-γ, IL-1β, and IL-6, while UC has a modified Th2 profile in which IL-5 expression was increased (Calder, 2015). In addition, AA-derived eicosanoids such as PGE_2, PGD_2, TXB_2, and LTB_4 were involved in IBD development, and these mediators were increased in the intestinal mucosa of IBD mice model (Hirata et al., 2001; Nieto, Torres, Ŕos, & Gil, 2002). The first evidence of the importance of dietary intake of n-3 polyunsaturated fatty acids for IBD was derived from epidemiologic observations of the low incidence of IBD in Eskimos, whose diet is particularly rich in marine n-3 PUFAs (Belluzzi et al., 2000). Thereafter, marine n-3 PUFAs have been thoroughly examined in this condition, and most of these studies demonstrated that the reduction in the amount of AA-derived eicosanoids including PGE_2, LTB_4, TXB_2, and LTC_4 in the colonic mucosa might underlie the protective effects of marine n-3 PUFAs on relieving the disease severity (Barbalho, Goulart, Quesada, Bechara, & De Carvalho, 2016; Charpentier et al., 2018). Besides, the lower level of Th17 cell number in lymphoid tissues in fat-1 mice with colitis suggested the potential effects of marine n-3 PUFAs on Th17 lymphocytes (Monk et al., 2012). Another study also investigated the colitis model in fat-1 mice and found that NF-kB activation was lower in fat-1 mice and the specialized pro-resolving mediators including resolvin E1, resolvin D3, and protectin D1 were present in the colonic tissue from fat-1 mice (Hudert et al., 2006). These specialized pro-resolving mediators may become important tools for understanding and treatment of IBDs (Abdolmaleki et al., 2020; Schwanke, Marcon, Bento, & Calixto, 2016). The antiinflammatory effects of the resolvins were further examined in an animal study, in which administration of resolvin E1 to mice with chemically induced colitis could decrease the infiltration of granulocytes into colonic tissue and the expression of a number of pro-inflammatory genes, such as TNF and COX-2 (Arita et al., 2005).

Even though animal studies consistently reported that marine n-3 fatty acids decreased the disease severity of chemically induced colitis in accompany with reduction of the AA-derived eicosanoids, the evidence from RCTs is not that consistent. Colonic mucosa of patients with active UC is characterized by a significant increase in the availability of AA, while decreased levels of n-3 PUFAs (Kohli & Levy, 2009; Scaioli, Liverani, & Belluzzi, 2017). More importantly, supplemental intake of fish oil could lead to the incorporation of EPA and DHA into gut mucosal tissue of patients with IBD (Hillier, Jewell, Dorrell, & Smith, 1991). The investigation into the effects of dietary n-3 PUFAs on the erythrocyte membrane fatty acids composition of IBD patients also found significantly increased erythrocyte membrane n-3/n-6 ratio, especially among those in the remission group (Uchiyama et al., 2010). Based on a one-year, double-blind, placebo-controlled study among patients with CD, a significant difference in the proportion of patients who remained in remission at 12 months of intervention was observed between groups (59% in the fish oil group, 26% in the placebo group) (Belluzzi et al., 1996). Another double-blind, placebo-controlled trial showed that fish oil supplementation (4.2 g/day) could yield clinical improvement among patients with UC (Aslan & Triadafilopoulos, 1992). These findings suggested that n-3 PUFAs might be a potential adjuvant therapy for improving the clinical activity of IBD patients. However, there are also studies reporting that limited clinical benefits for IBD patients were generated from the marine n-3 PUFAs supplementation. In the Epanova Program in Crohn's Study (EPIC-1) and EPIC-2 which included 760 patients with CD, no significant difference in the rate of relapse at 1 year was observed among patients who received n-3 PUFAs or placebo (Feagan et al., 2008). Another RCT found that the supplementation of EPA and DHA (2.7 g/day) and antioxidants for 24 weeks exhibited no effects on disease activity in 61 patients with CD (Trebble et al., 2005). In an RCT involving 87 UC patients who kept their own standard drug therapy, fish oil (4.5 g EPA daily) and olive oil placebo were randomly assigned to two groups for 1 year. The authors found that treatment with fish oil resulted in measurable, but only limited, clinical benefit (Hawthorne et al., 1992). For patients in remission at trial entry or during the trial, there was no significant difference in the rate of relapse (Hawthorne et al., 1992). The relapse prevention effects of dietary n-3 fatty acids (5.1 g/day) were further examined in a double-blind, placebo-controlled trial of 64 patients with UC in remission, and the cumulative relapse rate at 2 years was similar for both groups (Loeschke et al., 1996). Moreover, there was also no consistent difference in clinical, macroscopic and histologic disease activity between groups. A systematical review and meta-analysis of n-3 PUFAs for maintenance of remission in IBD included 9 RCTs and summarized the efficacy and safety of fish oil in CD and UC patients (Turner et al., 2011). Although a significant benefit for n-3 PUFA in CD was observed with a 23% reduced risk for relapse, sensitivity analysis found the pooled RR no longer statistically significant after excluding a small pediatric study (Turner et al., 2011). Notably, two well-performed studies with a large sample size, among the included studies, reported no benefit from n-3 PUFAs. For UC, no difference in the relapse rate between the n-3 PUFAs and control groups was observed, and the pooled analysis showed a higher rate of adverse events in the n-3 PUFAs treatment group (Turner et al., 2011). A recently published comprehensive meta-analysis of RCTs investigating long-term effects of n-3, n-6 and total PUFAs on IBD and inflammatory markers found low-quality evidence supporting protective effects of n-3 PUFAs on IBD relapse and worsening (Ajabnoor et al., 2020). Therefore, the existing data are insufficient to suggest n-3 PUFA supplementation for patients with CD or UC.

Several large sample-size prospective cohort studies supported that higher intake of dietary DHA was associated with a lower risk of UC, which suggested the potential of preventative effect of marine n-3 PUFAs supplementation on the development of IBD (Hart et al., 2009; John et al., 2010). However, a recent meta-analysis of observational studies involving 282,610 participants found that there were no relationships between total dietary n-3 PUFAs intake and IBD although a significant inverse association was observed between dietary long-chain n-3 PUFAs and the risk of ulcerative colitis (Mozaffari et al., 2020). These results highlight that the potential biases, including the sample size, the mode of consumption and the type of formulation used, may be introduced into these cohort studies. Therefore, although many studies have shown the potential preventative and therapeutic role of marine n-3 PUFAs in IBD development, further well-designed studies are still needed to clarify the necessary doses and optimal way of delivery that could be beneficial for IBD prevention and treatment, before suggesting the use of n-3 PUFAs in clinical settings.

14.2.3 Alzheimer's disease

The chronic low-grade inflammation in the brain is also observed in neurodegenerative diseases, including Alzheimer's disease (AD). AD, characterized by impairments of memory, language, and other cognitive functions, has been the most common neurodegenerative disorder (Alzheimer's Association, 2016). The numbers of people living with dementia are expected to be 65.7 million in 2030 and 115.4 million in 2050 (Prince et al., 2013). Although symptomatic improvements could be achieved, AD is yet an incurable disease with most currently approved drugs for AD not addressing the progressive neurodegeneration (Oboudiyat, Glazer, Seifan, Greer, & Isaacson, 2013). As neuroinflammation plays a key role in the advancement of this disorder, limiting neuroinflammation through antiinflammatory agents such as n-3 PUFAs has been suggested as an important strategy for preventing and treating AD.

The neuroinflammation is characterized by increased microglia and astrocyte activation, which partly mediated the effects of amyloid-beta peptide on neuronal death and synaptic impairment (Sawikr et al., 2017). Glial activation can induce the production of pro-inflammatory cytokines and reactive oxygen species, which lead to a chronic inflammatory process (Sawikr et al., 2017). In vitro experiments in immortalized BV-2 microglial cells showed that n-3 PUFAs administration decreased the expression of pro-inflammatory factors including IL-1β, TNF-α, and COX-2 (Lu, Tsao, Leung, & Su, 2010; Moon et al., 2007). Moreover, the cell-surface expression of the CD14 and Toll-like receptor 4 receptors was also downregulated by the EPA or DHA administration (De Smedt-Peyrusse et al., 2008). EPA could also downregulate the expression of proinflammatory cytokines (e.g., IL-1β and IL-6) and upregulate the expression of antiinflammatory cytokines in glioma cells and rat hippocampus (Kavanagh, Lonergan, & Lynch, 2004; Kawashima, Harada, Imada, Yano, & Mizuguchi, 2008; Lonergan, Martin, Horrobin, & Lynch, 2004). These studies provide the mechanistic clues supporting further study on the relationship between n-3 PUFAs and neurodegenerative disorders.

Based on a prospective study involving 815 participants conducted from 1993 through

2000, investigators found that consuming fish once per week or more could reduce the risk of developing AD by 60%, compared with those who rarely or never ate fish (Morris et al., 2003). In addition, both the total intake of n-3 PUFAs and individual DHA intake were associated with reduced risk of AD, but the protective association of EPA with AD was not observed (Morris et al., 2003). A long-term prospective study involving more than 5000 participants aged ≥55 years was conducted between 1990 and 2004, and 465 participants developed dementia with 365 AD cases. In this study, the dietary intakes of n-3 PUFAs were not associated with dementia risk or AD risk (Devore et al., 2009). As inconsistent findings regarding the associations between n-3 PUFAs intakes and AD risk were reported, a systematic review and meta-analysis of 21 studies involving 181,580 participants and 4438 cases was conducted and demonstrated that a 1-serving/week increment of dietary fish was associated with 5% lower risk of dementia and 7% reduced risk of AD (Zhang et al., 2016). Neuroprotective effects on AD were also observed for individual DHA intake, with a per 0.1 g/day increment of DHA intake associated with a 37% lower risk of AD (Zhang et al., 2016). Additionally, many epidemiological studies also report high n-3 PUFAs in the blood are associated with protection against cognitive decline. In the Atherosclerosis Risk in Communities Study including more than 2000 subjects, the risk of global cognitive decline increased with elevated circulating saturated fatty acids and n-6 fatty acids, while circulating n-3 unsaturated fatty acids reduced the risk of cognitive decline (Beydoun, Kaufman, Satia, Rosamond, & Folsom, 2007). A recent study investigated the association of a plasma n-3 PUFA index (the sum of circulating EPA and DHA concentrations) with several dementia-related outcomes in a large cohort of older adults over a 17-year follow-up. Higher levels of plasma EPA and DHA were associated with a lower risk of dementia, with a hazard ratio of 0.87 for 1 standard deviation, and protective effects on global cognition, memory, and medical temporal lobe volume were also observed for combined plasma EPA and DHA (Thomas et al., 2020).

Although most meta-analysis of observational studies suggested that DHA and their food sources were associated with lower risk of AD and AD related outcomes, interventional studies with n-3 PUFAs did not yield conclusive results. In a study on participants with subjective memory complaints, supplementation of combined EPA, DHA, and phosphatidylserine for 6 weeks exerted improvements in cognitive functions (Richter, Herzog, Cohen, & Steinhart, 2010). Another randomized, double-blind study reported that 1.8 g/day n-3 PUFA supplementation for 24 weeks improved the cognitive function only among patients with mild cognitive impairment but not among patients with AD (Chiu et al., 2008). Moreover, the Omega AD study also observed similar results, which indicated that the supplementation of DHA and EPA for 6 months exhibited clinical benefits for patients with mild AD but not for severe AD patients (Freund-Levi et al., 2006). A systematic review included seven intervention studies to assess the impact of supplementation or dietary intake of n-3 PUFAs on cognitive function in humans with AD, and most of the included studies did not find statistically significant results for n-3 fatty acid supplementation compared to placebo (Canhada, Castro, Perry, & Luft, 2018). A 2020 meta-analysis of six RCTs concluded that there was no consistent evidence to support the effectiveness of n-3 PUFAs supplementation in improving cognitive function in AD patients in the short and medium term (Araya-Quintanilla et al., 2020). Discrepancies between studies may be due in part to the AD-associated genotype (e.g., APOE ε4) and the DHA or EPA status at baseline, and it is also not clear whether supplementation for long durations or at specific ages may be more protective and whether age-related changes in the metabolism in n-3 PUFAs may be involved in the inconsistent results (Dacks, Shineman, & Fillit, 2013). In summary, the existing evidence is still insufficient to recommend the use of n-3 PUFAs for improving cognitive function in AD patients, and more robust evidence is warranted.

14.3 What are the gaps in evidence that need attention?

Although the relationship between n-3 marine PUFAs and the inflammation process has been well elucidated, especially regarding the eicosanoid pathway and specialized pro-resolving lipid mediators, the protective or therapeutic effects of the n-3 marine PUFAs on inflammatory diseases are less consistent. The gap still exists between preclinical studies and the translation of the n-3 marine PUFAs in clinical settings. In summary, the current evidence is relatively strong as to supporting the clinical benefits of marine n-3 PUFAs supplementation for RA, but not robust enough to suggest the therapeutic effects of n-3 PUFAs on IBD or AD. Additionally, most of the previous studies applied the mixed EPA and DHA or fish oil as interventional supplements, but the effects of individual n-3 PUFAs might be different from each other. The investigation on potential protective effects of individual n-3 PUFAs, especially DPA, on inflammatory diseases has received relatively less attention, and further research aiming to clarify the unique functionality of the individual marine n-3 PUFAs is warranted.

References

Abdolmaleki, F., Kovanen, P. T., Mardani, R., Gheibi-hayat, S. M., Bo, S., & Sahebkar, A. (2020). Resolvins: Emerging players in autoimmune and inflammatory diseases. *Clinical Reviews in Allergy and Immunology*, 58(1), 82–91. https://doi.org/10.1007/s12016-019-08754-9.

Ajabnoor, S. M., Thorpe, G., Abdelhamid, A., & Hooper, L. (2020). Long-term effects of increasing omega-3, omega-6 and total polyunsaturated fats on inflammatory bowel disease and markers of inflammation: A systematic review and meta-analysis of randomized controlled trials. *European Journal of Nutrition*. https://doi.org/10.1007/s00394-020-02413-y.

Alzheimer's Association. (2016). 2016 Alzheimer's disease facts and figures. *Alzheimer's & Dementia*, 459–509. https://doi.org/10.1016/j.jalz.2016.03.001.

Araya-Quintanilla, F., Gutiérrez-Espinoza, H., Sánchez-Montoya, U., Muñoz-Yañez, M. J., Baeza-Vergara, A., Petersen-Yanjarí, M., et al. (2020). Efectividad de la suplementación de ácidos grasos omega-3 en pacientes con enfermedad de Alzheimer: revisión sistemática con metaanálisis. *Neurología*, 105–114. https://doi.org/10.1016/j.nrl.2017.07.009.

Arita, M., Ohira, T., Sun, Y. P., Elangovan, S., Chiang, N., & Serhan, C. N. (2007). Resolvin E1 selectively interacts with leukotriene B4 receptor BLT1 and ChemR23 to regulate inflammation. *Journal of Immunology*, 178(6), 3912–3917. https://doi.org/10.4049/jimmunol.178.6.3912.

Arita, M., Yoshida, M., Hong, S., Tjonahen, E., Glickman, J. N., Petasis, N. A., et al. (2005). Resolvin E1, an endogenous lipid mediator derived from omega-3 eicosapentaenoic acid, protects against 2,4,6-trinitrobenzene sulfonic acid-induced colitis. *Proceedings of the National Academy of Sciences of the United States of America*, 102(21), 7671–7676. https://doi.org/10.1073/pnas.0409271102.

Aslan, A., & Triadafilopoulos, G. (1992). Fish oil fatty acid supplementation in active ulcerative colitis: A double-blind, placebo-controlled, crossover study. *The American Journal of Gastroenterology*, 87(4), 432–437. https://doi.org/10.1111/j.1572-0241.1992.tb02850.x.

Aung, T., Halsey, J., Kromhout, D., Gerstein, H. C., Marchioli, R., Tavazzi, L., et al. (2018). Associations of omega-3 fatty acid supplement use with cardiovascular disease risks meta-analysis of 10 trials involving 77 917 individuals. *JAMA Cardiology*, 3(3), 225–234. https://doi.org/10.1001/jamacardio.2017.5205.

Bäck, M., Yurdagul, A., Tabas, I., Öörni, K., & Kovanen, P. T. (2019). Inflammation and its resolution in atherosclerosis: Mediators and therapeutic opportunities. *Nature Reviews Cardiology*, 16(7), 389–406. https://doi.org/10.1038/s41569-019-0169-2.

Bannenberg, G., & Serhan, C. N. (2010). Specialized pro-resolving lipid mediators in the inflammatory response: An update. *Biochimica et Biophysica Acta-Molecular and Cell Biology of Lipids*, 1801(12), 1260–1273. https://doi.org/10.1016/j.bbalip.2010.08.002.

Barbalho, S. M., Goulart, R. D. A., Quesada, K., Bechara, M. D., & De Carvalho, A. D. C. A. (2016). Inflammatory bowel disease: Can omega-3 fatty acids really help? *Annals of Gastroenterology*, 29(1), 37–43. http://www.annalsgastro.gr/index.php/annalsgastro/article/download/2366/1662.

Baumgart, D. C., & Sandborn, W. J. (2007). Inflammatory bowel disease: Clinical aspects and established and evolving therapies. *Lancet*, 369(9573), 1641–1657. https://doi.org/10.1016/S0140-6736(07)60751-X.

Belluzzi, A., Boschi, S., Brignola, C., Munarini, A., Cariani, G., & Miglio, F. (2000). Polyunsaturated fatty acids and inflammatory bowel disease. *American Journal of Clinical Nutrition*, 71(1). https://doi.org/10.1093/ajcn/71.1.339s. American Society for Nutrition.

Belluzzi, A., Brignola, C., Campieri, M., Pera, A., Boschi, S., & Miglioli, M. (1996). Effect of an enteric-coated fish-oil preparation on relapses in Crohn's disease. *New England Journal of Medicine*, 334(24), 1557–1560. https://doi.org/10.1056/NEJM199606133342401.

Beydoun, M. A., Kaufman, J. S., Satia, J. A., Rosamond, W., & Folsom, A. R. (2007). Plasma n-3 fatty acids and the risk of cognitive decline in older adults: The atherosclerosis risk in communities study. *American Journal of Clinical Nutrition*, 85(4), 1103–1111. https://doi.org/10.1093/ajcn/85.4.1103.

Billiar, T. R., Bankey, P. E., Svingen, B. A., Curran, R. D., West, M. A., Holman, R. T., et al. (1988). Fatty acid intake and Kupffer cell function: Fish oil alters eicosanoid and monokine production to endotoxin stimulation. *Surgery*, 104(2), 343–349.

Calder, P. C. (2006). n-3 Polyunsaturated fatty acids, inflammation, and inflammatory diseases. *American Journal of Clinical Nutrition*, 83(6 Suppl), 1505S-19S.

Calder, P. C. (2015). Marine omega-3 fatty acids and inflammatory processes: Effects, mechanisms and clinical relevance. *Biochimica et Biophysica Acta*, 1851(4), 469–484. https://doi.org/10.1016/j.bbalip.2014.08.010.

Canhada, S., Castro, K., Perry, I. S., & Luft, V. C. (2018). Omega-3 fatty acids' supplementation in Alzheimer's disease: A systematic review. *Nutritional Neuroscience*, 21(8), 529–538. https://doi.org/10.1080/1028415X.2017.1321813.

Chamani, S., Bianconi, V., Tasbandi, A., Pirro, M., Barreto, G. E., Jamialahmadi, T., et al. (2020). Resolution of inflammation in neurodegenerative diseases: The role of Resolvins. *Mediators of Inflammation*, 2020. https://doi.org/10.1155/2020/3267172.

Charpentier, C., Chan, R., Salameh, E., Mbodji, K., Ueno, A., Coëffier, M., et al. (2018). Dietary n-3 PUFA may attenuate experimental colitis. *Mediators of Inflammation*, 2018. https://doi.org/10.1155/2018/8430614.

Chiu, C. C., Su, K. P., Cheng, T. C., Liu, H. C., Chang, C. J., Dewey, M. E., et al. (2008). The effects of omega-3 fatty acids monotherapy in Alzheimer's disease and mild cognitive impairment: A preliminary randomized double-blind placebo-controlled study. *Progress in Neuro-Psychopharmacology and Biological Psychiatry*, 32(6), 1538–1544. https://doi.org/10.1016/j.pnpbp.2008.05.015.

Chiurchiù, V., Leuti, A., Dalli, J., Jacobsson, A., Battistini, L., MaCcarrone, M., et al. (2016). Proresolving lipid mediators resolvin D1, resolvin D2, and maresin 1 are critical in modulating T cell responses. *Science Translational Medicine*, 8(353). https://doi.org/10.1126/scitranslmed.aaf7483.

Choy, E. H. S., & Panayi, G. S. (2001). Cytokine pathways and joint inflamation in rheumatoid arthritis. *New England Journal of Medicine*, 344(12), 907–916. https://doi.org/10.1056/NEJM200103223441207.

Dacks, P. A., Shineman, D. W., & Fillit, H. M. (2013). Current evidence for the clinical use of long-chain polyunsaturated N-3 fatty acids to prevent age-related cognitive decline and Alzheimer's disease. *The Journal of Nutrition, Health & Aging*, 17(3), 240–251. https://doi.org/10.1007/s12603-012-0431-3.

De Smedt-Peyrusse, V., Sargueil, F., Moranis, A., Harizi, H., Mongrand, S., & Layé, S. (2008). Docosahexaenoic acid prevents lipopolysaccharide-induced cytokine production in microglial cells by inhibiting lipopolysaccharide receptor presentation but not its membrane subdomain localization. *Journal of Neurochemistry*, 105(2), 296–307. https://doi.org/10.1111/j.1471-4159.2007.05129.x.

Del Gobbo, L. C., Imamura, F., Aslibekyan, S., Marklund, M., Virtanen, J. K., Wennberg, M., et al. (2016). ω-3 Polyunsaturated fatty acid biomarkers and coronary heart disease: Pooling project of 19 cohort studies. *JAMA Internal Medicine*, 176(8), 1155–1166. https://doi.org/10.1001/jamainternmed.2016.2925.

Devore, E. E., Grodstein, F., Van Rooij, F. J. A., Hofman, A., Rosner, B., Stampfer, M. J., et al. (2009). Dietary intake of fish and omega-3 fatty acids in relation to long-term dementia risk. *American Journal of Clinical Nutrition*, 90(1), 170–176. https://doi.org/10.3945/ajcn.2008.27037.

Di Giuseppe, D., Wallin, A., Bottai, M., Askling, J., & Wolk, A. (2014). Long-term intake of dietary long-chain n-3 polyunsaturated fatty acids and risk of rheumatoid arthritis: A prospective cohort study of women. *Annals of the Rheumatic Diseases*, 73(11), 1949–1953. https://doi.org/10.1136/annrheumdis-2013-203338.

Feagan, B. G., Sandborn, W. J., Mittmann, U., Bar-Meir, S., D'Haens, G., Bradette, M., et al. (2008). Omega-3 free fatty acids for the maintenance of remission in crohn disease: The EPIC randomized controlled trials. *JAMA : The Journal of the American Medical Association*, 299(14), 1690–1697. https://doi.org/10.1001/jama.299.14.1690.

Fiala, M., & Veerhuis, R. (2010). Biomarkers of inflammation and amyloid-β phagocytosis in patients at risk of Alzheimer disease. *Experimental Gerontology*, 45(1), 57–63. https://doi.org/10.1016/j.exger.2009.08.003.

Freund-Levi, Y., Eriksdotter-Jönhagen, M., Cederholm, T., Basun, H., Faxén-Irving, G., Garlind, A., et al. (2006). ω-3 Fatty acid treatment in 174 patients with mild to moderate Alzheimer disease: OmegAD study—A randomized double-blind trial. *Archives of Neurology, 63*(10), 1402–1408. https://doi.org/10.1001/archneur.63.10.1402.

Fu, Y., Li, G., Zhang, X., Xing, G., Hu, X., Yang, L., et al. (2015). Lipid extract from hard-shelled mussel (mytilus coruscus) improves clinical conditions of patients with rheumatoid arthritis: A randomized controlled trial. *Nutrients, 7*(1), 625–645. https://doi.org/10.3390/nu7010625.

Gioxari, A., Kaliora, A. C., Marantidou, F., & Panagiotakos, D. P. (2018). Intake of ω-3 polyunsaturated fatty acids in patients with rheumatoid arthritis: A systematic review and meta-analysis. *Nutrition, 114-124*. https://doi.org/10.1016/j.nut.2017.06.023, e4.

Goldberg, R. J., & Katz, J. (2007). A meta-analysis of the analgesic effects of omega-3 polyunsaturated fatty acid supplementation for inflammatory joint pain. *Pain, 129*(1–2), 210–223. https://doi.org/10.1016/j.pain.2007.01.020.

Goldman, D. W., Pickett, W. C., & Goetzl, E. J. (1983). Human neutrophil chemotactic and degranulating activities of leukotriene B5 (LTB5) derived from eicosapentaenoic acid. *Biochemical and Biophysical Research Communications, 117*(1), 282–288. https://doi.org/10.1016/0006-291X(83)91572-3.

Greten, F. R., & Grivennikov, S. I. (2019). Inflammation and Cancer: Triggers, mechanisms, and consequences. *Immunity, 51*(1), 27–41. https://doi.org/10.1016/j.immuni.2019.06.025.

Hart, A., Tjonneland, A., Olsen, A., Overvad, K., Bergmann, M. M., Boeing, H., et al. (2009). Linoleic acid, a dietary n-6 polyunsaturated fatty acid, and the aetiology of ulcerative colitis: A nested case-control study within a European prospective cohort study. *Gut, 58*(12), 1606–1611. https://doi.org/10.1136/gut.2008.169078.

Hawthorne, A. B., Daneshmend, T. K., Hawkey, C. J., Belluzzi, A., Everitt, S. J., Holmes, G. K. T., et al. (1992). Treatment of ulcerative colitis with fish oil supplementation: A prospective 12 month randomised controlled trial. *Gut, 33*(7), 922–928. https://doi.org/10.1136/gut.33.7.922.

Henderson, W. R. (1994). The role of leukotrienes in inflammation. *Annals of Internal Medicine, 121*(9), 684–697. https://doi.org/10.7326/0003-4819-121-9-199411010-00010.

Hillier, K., Jewell, R., Dorrell, L., & Smith, C. L. (1991). Incorporation of fatty acids from fish oil and olive oil into colonic mucosal lipids and effects upon eicosanoid synthesis in inflammatory bowel disease. *Gut, 32*(10), 1151–1155. https://doi.org/10.1136/gut.32.10.1151.

Hirata, I., Murano, M., Nitta, M., Sasaki, S. I., Toshina, K., Maemura, K., et al. (2001). Estimation of mucosal inflammatory mediators in rat DSS-induced colitis: Possible role of PGE2 in protection against mucosal damage. *Digestion, 63*(1), 73–80. https://doi.org/10.1159/000051915.

Hudert, C. A., Weylandt, K. H., Lu, Y., Wang, J., Hong, S., Dignass, A., et al. (2006). Transgenic mice rich in endogenous omega-3 fatty acids are protected from colitis. *Proceedings of the National Academy of Sciences of the United States of America, 103*(30), 11276–11281. https://doi.org/10.1073/pnas.0601280103.

Ierna, M., Kerr, A., Scales, H., Berge, K., & Griinari, M. (2010). Supplementation of diet with krill oil protects against experimental rheumatoid arthritis. *BMC Musculoskeletal Disorders, 11*. https://doi.org/10.1186/1471-2474-11-136.

Jiang, J., Li, K., Wang, F., Yang, B., Fu, Y., Zheng, J., et al. (2016). Effect of marine-derived n-3 polyunsaturated fatty acids on major eicosanoids: A systematic review and meta-analysis from 18 randomized controlled trials. *PLoS One, 11*(1). https://doi.org/10.1371/journal.pone.0147351.

John, S., Luben, R., Shrestha, S. S., Welch, A., Khaw, K. T., & Hart, A. R. (2010). Dietary n-3 polyunsaturated fatty acids and the aetiology of ulcerative colitis: A UK prospective cohort study. *European Journal of Gastroenterology and Hepatology, 22*(5), 602–606. https://doi.org/10.1097/MEG.0b013e3283352d05.

Kavanagh, T., Lonergan, P. E., & Lynch, M. A. (2004). Eicosapentaenoic acid and gamma-linolenic acid increase hippocampal concentrations of IL-4 and IL-10 and abrogate lipopolysaccharide-induced inhibition of long-term potentiation. *Prostaglandins, Leukotrienes, and Essential Fatty Acids, 70*(4), 391–397. Churchill Livingstone https://doi.org/10.1016/j.plefa.2003.12.014.

Kawashima, A., Harada, T., Imada, K., Yano, T., & Mizuguchi, K. (2008). Eicosapentaenoic acid inhibits interleukin-6 production in interleukin-1β-stimulated C6 glioma cells through peroxisome proliferator-activated receptor-gamma. *Prostaglandins, Leukotrienes, and Essential Fatty Acids, 79*(1–2), 59–65. https://doi.org/10.1016/j.plefa.2008.07.002.

Kidane, D., Chae, W. J., Czochor, J., Eckert, K. A., Glazer, P. M., Bothwell, A. L. M., et al. (2014). Interplay between DNA repair and inflammation, and the link to cancer. *Critical Reviews in Biochemistry and Molecular Biology, 49*(2), 116–139. https://doi.org/10.3109/10409238.2013.875514.

Kim, J. Y., Lim, K., Kim, K. H., Kim, J. H., Choi, J. S., & Shim, S. C. (2018). n-3 Polyunsaturated fatty acids restore Th17 and Treg balance in collagen antibody-induced arthritis. *PLoS One, 13*(3). https://doi.org/10.1371/journal.pone.0194331.

Kohli, P., & Levy, B. D. (2009). Resolvins and protectins: Mediating solutions to inflammation. *British Journal of Pharmacology, 158*(4), 960–971. https://doi.org/10.1111/j.1476-5381.2009.00290.x.

Lee, Y. H., Bae, S. C., & Song, G. G. (2012). Omega-3 polyunsaturated fatty acids and the treatment of rheumatoid arthritis: A meta-analysis. *Archives of Medical Research, 43*(5), 356–362. https://doi.org/10.1016/j.arcmed.2012.06.011.

Lo, C. J., Chiu, K. C., Fu, M., Lo, R., & Helton, S. (1999). Fish oil decreases macrophage tumor necrosis factor gene transcription by altering the NFκB activity. *Journal of Surgical Research, 82*(2), 216–221. https://doi.org/10.1006/jsre.1998.5524.

Loeschke, K., Ueberschaer, B., Pietsch, A., Gruber, E., Ewe, K., Wiebecke, B., et al. (1996). n 3 Fatty acids only delay early relapse of ulcerative colitis in remission. *Digestive Diseases and Sciences, 41*(10), 2087–2094. https://doi.org/10.1007/BF02093614.

Lonergan, P. E., Martin, D. S. D., Horrobin, D. F., & Lynch, M. A. (2004). Neuroprotective actions of eicosapentaenoic acid on lipopolysaccharide- induced dysfunction in rat hippocampus. *Journal of Neurochemistry, 91*(1), 20–29. https://doi.org/10.1111/j.1471-4159.2004.02689.x.

Lu, D. Y., Tsao, Y. Y., Leung, Y. M., & Su, K. P. (2010). Docosahexaenoic acid suppresses neuroinflammatory responses and induces heme oxygenase-1 expression in BV-2 microglia: Implications of antidepressant effects for omega-3 fatty acids. *Neuropsychopharmacology, 35*(11), 2238–2248. https://doi.org/10.1038/npp.2010.98.

MacLean, C. H., Mojica, W. A., Newberry, S. J., Pencharz, J., Garland, R. H., & Tu, W. (2005). Systematic review of the effects of n-3 fatty acids in inflammatory bowel disease. *American Journal of Clinical Nutrition, 82*(3), 611–619. https://doi.org/10.1093/ajcn.82.3.611.

Marchio, P., Guerra-Ojeda, S., Vila, J. M., Aldasoro, M., Victor, V. M., & Mauricio, M. D. (2019). Targeting early atherosclerosis: A focus on oxidative stress and inflammation. *Oxidative Medicine and Cellular Longevity, 2019*. https://doi.org/10.1155/2019/8563845.

Mateen, S., Zafar, A., Moin, S., Khan, A. Q., & Zubair, S. (2016). Understanding the role of cytokines in the pathogenesis of rheumatoid arthritis. *Clinica Chimica Acta, 455*, 161–171. https://doi.org/10.1016/j.cca.2016.02.010.

Mazereeuw, G., Lanctôt, K. L., Chau, S. A., Swardfager, W., & Herrmann, N. (2012). Effects of ω-3 fatty acids on cognitive performance: A meta-analysis. *Neurobiology of Aging, 33*(7), 1482.e17–1482.e29. https://doi.org/10.1016/j.neurobiolaging.2011.12.014.

Monk, J. M., Jia, Q., Callaway, E., Weeks, B., Alaniz, R. C., Mcmurray, D. N., et al. (2012). Th17 cell accumulation is decreased during chronic experimental colitis by (n-3) PUFA in fat-1 mice. *Journal of Nutrition, 142*(1), 117–124. https://doi.org/10.3945/jn.111.147058.

Moon, D. O., Kim, K. C., Jin, C. Y., Han, M. H., Park, C., Lee, K. J., et al. (2007). Inhibitory effects of eicosapentaenoic acid on lipopolysaccharide-induced activation in BV2 microglia. *International Immunopharmacology, 7*(2), 222–229. https://doi.org/10.1016/j.intimp.2006.10.001.

Morris, M. C., Evans, D. A., Bienias, J. L., Tangney, C. C., Bennett, D. A., Wilson, R. S., et al. (2003). Consumption of fish and n-3 fatty acids and risk of incident Alzheimer disease. *Archives of Neurology, 60*(7), 940–946. https://doi.org/10.1001/archneur.60.7.940.

Mozaffari, H., Daneshzad, E., Larijani, B., Bellissimo, N., & Azadbakht, L. (2020). Dietary intake of fish, n-3 polyunsaturated fatty acids, and risk of inflammatory bowel disease: A systematic review and meta-analysis of observational studies. *European Journal of Nutrition, 59*(1). https://doi.org/10.1007/s00394-019-01901-0.

Navarini, L., Afeltra, A., Gallo Afflitto, G., & Margiotta, D. P. E. (2017). Polyunsaturated fatty acids: Any role in rheumatoid arthritis? *Lipids in Health and Disease, 16*(1). https://doi.org/10.1186/s12944-017-0586-3.

Nicholls, S. J., Lincoff, A. M., Garcia, M., Bash, D., Ballantyne, C. M., Barter, P. J., et al. (2020). Effect of high-dose Omega-3 fatty acids vs corn oil on major adverse cardiovascular events in patients at high cardiovascular risk: The STRENGTH randomized clinical trial. *JAMA: The Journal of the American Medical Association, 324*(22), 2268–2280. https://doi.org/10.1001/jama.2020.22258.

Nieto, N., Torres, M. I., Ríos, A., & Gil, A. (2002). Dietary polyunsaturated fatty acids improve histological and biochemical alterations in rats with experimental ulcerative colitis. *Journal of Nutrition, 132*(1), 11–19. https://doi.org/10.1093/jn/132.1.11.

Novak, T. E., Babcock, T. A., Jho, D. H., Helton, W. S., & Espat, N. J. (2003). NF-κB inhibition by ω-3 fatty acids modulates LPS-stimulated macrophage TNF-α-transcription. *American Journal of Physiology - Lung Cellular and Molecular Physiology, 284*(1), L84–L89. https://doi.org/10.1152/ajplung.00077.2002.

Oboudiyat, C., Glazer, H., Seifan, A., Greer, C., & Isaacson, R. S. (2013). Alzheimer's disease. *Seminars in Neurology, 33*(4), 313–329. https://doi.org/10.1055/s-0033-1359319.

Pedersen, M., Stripp, C., Klarlund, M., Olsen, S. F., Tjønneland, A. M., & Frisch, M. (2005). Diet and risk of rheumatoid arthritis in a prospective cohort. *Journal of Rheumatology, 32*(7), 1249–1252.

Prince, M., Bryce, R., Albanese, E., Wimo, A., Ribeiro, W., & Ferri, C. P. (2013). The global prevalence of dementia: A systematic review and metaanalysis. *Alzheimer's & Dementia, 9*(1), 63–75.e2. https://doi.org/10.1016/j.jalz.2012.11.007.

Rajaei, E., Mowla, K., Ghorbani, A., Bahadoram, S., Bahadoram, M., & Dargahi-Malamir, M. (2015). The effect of Omega-3 fatty acids in patients with active rheumatoid arthritis receiving DMARDs therapy: Double-blind randomized controlled trial. *Global Journal of Health Science, 8*(7), 18–25. https://doi.org/10.5539/gjhs.v8n7p18.

Rees, D., Miles, E. A., Banerjee, T., Wells, S. J., Roynette, C. E., Wahle, K. W. J., et al. (2006). Dose-related effects of eicosapentaenoic acid on innate immune function in healthy humans: A comparison of young and older men. *American Journal of Clinical Nutrition, 83*(2), 331–342. https://doi.org/10.1093/ajcn/83.2.331.

Richter, Y., Herzog, Y., Cohen, T., & Steinhart, Y. (2010). The effect of phosphatidylserine-containing omega-3 fatty acids on memory abilities in subjects with subjective memory complaints: A pilot study. *Clinical Interventions in Aging, 5*, 313–316. https://doi.org/10.2147/cia.s13432.

Rimm, E. B., Appel, L. J., Chiuve, S. E., Djoussé, L., Engler, M. B., Kris-Etherton, P. M., et al. (2018). Seafood long-chain n-3 polyunsaturated fatty acids and cardiovascular disease: A science advisory from the American Heart Association. *Circulation, 138*(1), e35–e47. https://doi.org/10.1161/CIR.0000000000000574.

Rizos, E. C., Ntzani, E. E., Bika, E., Kostapanos, M. S., & Elisaf, M. S. (2012). Association between omega-3 fatty acid supplementation and risk of major cardiovascular disease events: A systematic review and meta-analysis. *JAMA : The Journal of the American Medical Association, 308*(10), 1024–1033. https://doi.org/10.1001/2012.jama.11374.

Sadeghi, S., Wallace, F. A., & Calder, P. C. (1999). Dietary lipids modify the cytokine response to bacterial lipopolysaccharide in mice. *Immunology, 96*(3), 404–410. https://doi.org/10.1046/j.1365-2567.1999.00701.x.

Sano, H., Hla, T., Maier, J. A. M., Crofford, L. J., Case, J. P., Maciag, T., et al. (1992). In vivo cyclooxygenase expression in synovial tissues of patients with rheumatoid arthritis and osteoarthritis and rats with adjuvant and streptococcal cell wall arthritis. *Journal of Clinical Investigation, 89*(1), 97–108. https://doi.org/10.1172/JCI115591.

Sawikr, Y., Yarla, N. S., Peluso, I., Kamal, M. A., Aliev, G., & Bishayee, A. (2017). Neuroinflammation in Alzheimer's disease: The preventive and therapeutic potential of polyphenolic nutraceuticals. *Advances in Protein Chemistry and Structural Biology, 108*, 33–57. Academic Press Inc https://doi.org/10.1016/bs.apcsb.2017.02.001.

Scaioli, E., Liverani, E., & Belluzzi, A. (2017). The imbalance between N-6/N-3 polyunsaturated fatty acids and inflammatory bowel disease: A comprehensive review and future therapeutic perspectives. *International Journal of Molecular Sciences, 18*(12). https://doi.org/10.3390/ijms18122619.

Schwanke, R. C., Marcon, R., Bento, A. F., & Calixto, J. B. (2016). EPA- and DHA-derived resolvins' actions in inflammatory bowel disease. *European Journal of Pharmacology, 785*, 156–164. https://doi.org/10.1016/j.ejphar.2015.08.050.

Senftleber, N. K., Nielsen, S. M., Andersen, J. R., Bliddal, H., Tarp, S., & Lauritzen, L. (2017). Marine oil supplements for arthritis pain: A systematic review and meta-analysis of randomized trials. *Nutrients, 9*(1). https://doi.org/10.3390/nu9010042.

Serhan, C. N., & Levy, B. D. (2018). Resolvins in inflammation: Emergence of the pro-resolving superfamily of mediators. *Journal of Clinical Investigation, 128*(7), 2657–2669. https://doi.org/10.1172/JCI97943.

Smolen, J. S., Daniel, A., & Mclnnes, B. I. (2016). Rheumatoid arthritis. *The Lancet*, 2023–2038. https://doi.org/10.1016/s0140-6736(16)30173-8.

Thomas, A., Baillet, M., Proust-Lima, C., Féart, C., Foubert-Samier, A., Helmer, C., et al. (2020). Blood polyunsaturated omega-3 fatty acids, brain atrophy, cognitive decline, and dementia risk. *Alzheimer's & Dementia*. https://doi.org/10.1002/alz.12195.

Trebble, T. M., Stroud, M. A., Wootton, S. A., Calder, P. C., Fine, D. R., Mullee, M. A., et al. (2005). High-dose fish oil and antioxidants in Crohn's disease and the response of bone turnover: A randomised controlled trial. *British Journal of Nutrition, 94*(2), 253–261. https://doi.org/10.1079/BJN20051466.

Turner, D., Shah, P. S., Steinhart, A. H., Zlotkin, S., & Griffiths, A. M. (2011). Maintenance of remission in inflammatory bowel disease using omega-3 fatty acids (fish oil): A systematic review and meta-analyses. *Inflammatory Bowel Diseases, 17*(1), 336–345. https://doi.org/10.1002/ibd.21374.

Uchiyama, K., Nakamura, M., Odahara, S., Koido, S., Katahira, K., Shiraishi, H., et al. (2010). N-3 polyunsaturated fatty acid diet therapy for patients with inflammatory bowel disease. *Inflammatory Bowel Diseases, 16*(10), 1696–1707. https://doi.org/10.1002/ibd.21251.

Urman, A., Taklalsingh, N., Sorrento, C., & McFarlane, I. M. (2018). Inflammation beyond the joints: Rheumatoid arthritis and cardiovascular disease. *SciFed Journal of Cardiology, 2*(3).

Verstraete, M. (1983). Introduction: Thromboxane in biological systems and the possible impact of its inhibition. *British Journal of Clinical Pharmacology*, 7S–11S. https://doi.org/10.1111/j.1365-2125.1983.tb02100.x.

Veselinovic, M., Vasiljevic, D., Vucic, V., Arsic, A., Petrovic, S., Tomic-Lucic, A., et al. (2017). Clinical benefits of n-3 PUFA and -linolenic acid in patients with rheumatoid arthritis. *Nutrients, 9*(4). https://doi.org/10.3390/nu9040325.

Volker, D. H., FitzGerald, P. E. B., & Garg, M. L. (2000). The eicosapentaenoic to docosahexaenoic acid ratio of diets affects the pathogenesis of arthritis in Lew/SSN rats. *Journal of Nutrition, 130*(3), 559–565. https://doi.org/10.1093/jn/130.3.559.

Wang, F., Fu, Y., Cai, W., Sinclair, A. J., & Li, D. (2016). Anti-inflammatory activity and mechanisms of a lipid extract from hard-shelled mussel (*Mytilus coruscus*) in mice with dextran sulphate sodium-induced colitis. *Journal of Functional Foods, 23*, 389–399. https://doi.org/10.1016/j.jff.2016.03.002.

Wolf, D., & Ley, K. (2019). Immunity and inflammation in atherosclerosis. *Circulation Research*, *124*(2), 315–327. https://doi.org/10.1161/CIRCRESAHA.118.313591.

Wu, S., Ding, Y., Wu, F., Li, R., Hou, J., & Mao, P. (2015). Omega-3 fatty acids intake and risks of dementia and Alzheimer's disease: A meta-analysis. *Neuroscience & Biobehavioral Reviews*, *48*, 1–9. https://doi.org/10.1016/j.neubiorev.2014.11.008.

Zhang, Y., Chen, J., Qiu, J., Li, Y., Wang, J., & Jiao, J. (2016). Intakes of fish and polyunsaturated fatty acids and mild-to-severe cognitive impairment risks: A dose-response meta-analysis of 21 cohort studies. *American Journal of Clinical Nutrition*, *103*(2), 330–340. https://doi.org/10.3945/ajcn.115.124081.

CHAPTER 15

Lipids and birth defects

Kelei Li[a,b] and Yan Shi[a,b]

[a]Institute of Nutrition and Health, Qingdao University, Qingdao, China [b]Department of Nutrition and Food Hygiene, School of Public Health, Qingdao University, Qingdao, China

15.1 Introduction

Birth defects are congenital structural or genetic conditions that cause significant health and developmental complications, and the prevalence is about 3%–5% in all births (Mai et al., 2019). The common types include birth defects of the central nervous system (such as neural tube defects), birth defects of the eye (such as anophthalmia/microphthalmia), cardiovascular birth defects (such as atrioventricular septal defect, coarctation of the aorta), orofacial birth defects (such as cleft lip, cleft palate), gastrointestinal birth defects (such as esophageal atresia, tracheoesophageal fistula), musculoskeletal birth defects (such as clubfoot, gastroschisis), chromosomal birth defects (such as trisomy 13, trisomy 18, trisomy 21), and so on (Mai et al., 2019).

Genetic and environmental factors and their interaction all play an important role in the development of birth defects. Candidate gene studies and genome-wide association studies (GWASs) have identified many single nuclear polymorphisms (SNPs) in genes involved in the Wnt signaling pathway, BMP signaling pathway, Hedgehog signaling pathway, folate-homocysteine pathway, oxidative stress pathway, and so on (Hobbs et al., 2014). In addition, epigenetic alteration is also involved in many birth defects, such as Prader-Willi syndrome, Angelman syndrome, Beckwith-Wiedemann syndrome, and Russell-Silver syndrome (Hobbs et al., 2014). Major environmental risk factors include smoking, alcohol consumption, illicit drug use, obesity, diabetes mellitus, phenylketonuria, multiple gestations, advanced maternal/paternal age, folic acid deficiency, and medication exposure (such as folic acid antagonists, antiepileptics) (Harris et al., 2017).

Lipids are important structural components of the human body. They play a crucial role in embryo growth and development via modulating metabolism, oxidative stress, cell signaling, and gene expression (McKeegan & Sturmey, 2011; Niringiyumukiza, Cai, & Xiang, 2018). In recent years, disturbance of lipid metabolism has been shown to be one important cause of birth defects, and relevant evidence will be discussed in this chapter.

15.2 Evidence relating lipids to birth defects risk in human studies

The National Birth Defects Prevention Study (NBDPS), a population-based case–control study, provided evidence for the relationship between dietary lipids intake and several birth defects: per 10g increase in periconceptional total fat intake was associated with a 10% decrease in the risk of offspring double-inlet ventricle congenital heart disease (number of cases/controls: 200/11,063) (Paige et al., 2019); higher periconceptional total fat intake was associated with lower risk of offspring pulmonary valve stenosis and higher risk of aorta coarctation in combination with ventricular septal defect (number of cases/controls: 11,393/11,029) (Collins et al., 2020); the middle tertile of periconceptional cholesterol intake was associated with lower risk of gastroschisis, compared with the lowest tertile of cholesterol intake (number of cases/controls: 304/3313) (Siega-Riz, Olshan, Werler, & Moore, 2006). Another case–control study (number of cases/controls: 276/324) showed that a mother of a child with outflow tract defects tended to have a higher dietary intake of saturated fat and a lower dietary intake of riboflavin and nicotinamide (two co-enzymes in lipid metabolism) than controls, and a lower dietary intake of monounsaturated fat was associated with a lower risk of outflow tract defects (Smedts et al., 2008).

Fatty acids and eicosanoid composition are also involved in the development of birth defects. Our previous case–control study found that the proportions of several polyunsaturated fatty acids (PUFAs), such as C18:2n-6, C18:3n-6, C20:3n-6, C18:3n-3, C20:3n-3, C20:5n-3, and C22:5n-3, were significantly lower in the placenta of cases with neural tube defects than in controls, and all of these PUFAs were negatively associated with the risk of neural tube defects (Li et al., 2017). In addition, we also found that the ratios of C20:4n-6/C20:5n-3 and thromboxane B_2 (TXB_2)/6-keto-prostaglandin $F_{1\alpha}$ (6-keto-$PGF_{1\alpha}$) were significantly higher in the placenta of subjects with neural tube defects than in controls, and higher ratios of placental C20:4n-6/C20:5n-3 and TXB_2/6-keto-$PGF_{1\alpha}$ were associated with a higher risk of neural tube defects (number of cases/controls: 77/142) (Li et al., 2017). Another case–control study indicated that maternal serum level of total fatty acids and unsaturated fatty acids, and the ratio of C18:1n-9/C18:0 were lower, but the ratio of C16:0/C18:2n-6 was higher in the gastroschisis group than in the control group (number of cases/controls: 57/114) (Centofanti et al., 2018). The ratio of unsaturated/saturated fatty acids and long-chain/medium-chain fatty acids in myelin in patients with genetic phenylketonuria ($n=4$) was lower than in nonphenylketonuria subjects ($n=4$) (Johnson, McKean, & Shah, 1977). The content of very-long-chain fatty acids (VLFAs, number of carbons ≥ 24), such as C26:1 and C26:0, in fibroblasts of subjects with genetic peroxisomal diseases is higher than that in healthy controls (Molzer et al., 1986).

Inositol, also called 1,2,3,4,5,6-hexahydroxycyclohexane, can be incorporated as the polar head-group of membrane lipids based on phosphatidylinositol (Greene, Leung, & Copp, 2017). Observational studies showed contradictory results about inositol and neural tube defects: both nonsignificant and negative associations were observed between maternal inositol levels (dietary intake or blood level) and the risk of neural tube defects (Groenen et al., 2003; Shaw, Carmichael, Yang, & Schaffer, 2005). Results from a nutrigenetic study demonstrated that mutation of the ITPK1 gene was associated with a lower maternal plasma inositol hexakisphosphate (IP6) level, a lower expression of ITPK1, and a higher risk of neural tube defects, supporting the beneficial effect of inositol on birth defects (Guan et al., 2014). An intervention study in humans indicated that a couple with a history of two consecutive pregnancies of folate-resistant neural tube defects gave birth to a healthy baby after supplementation of 500 mg/d inositol and 2.5 mg/d folic acid together starting from 3 months before conception until 60 days of pregnancy (Cavalli & Copp, 2002). A similar prevention effect of inositol supplementation for women with a history of neural tube defects during pregnancy was observed in other two intervention studies (Cavalli, Tedoldi, & Riboli, 2008; Cavalli, Tonni, Grosso, & Poggiani, 2011).

15.3 Evidence relating lipids to birth defects in animal studies

C20:4n-6 can decrease the rate of malformation (neural tube defects, cleft palate, and micrognathia) induced by hyperglycemia in mouse embryo culture study and rat in vivo study, indicating C20:4n-6 deficiency is involved in hyperglycemia-induced teratogenesis (Goldman et al., 1985). A study in rats indicated that safflower oil, which is rich in C18:2n-6, significantly reduced the malformation rate in offspring of diabetic rats (Reece et al., 1996). We previously used sodium valproate (VPA) to build a mouse model of neural tube defects to evaluate the effect of different PUFA supplementations during pregnancy on neural tube defects (Li et al., 2018). Sodium valproate is an antiepileptic drug, which can disturb folate-homocysteine metabolism and lead to the occurrence of exencephaly (Li et al., 2018). The results indicated that compared with monounsaturated fatty acids in olive oil, PUFAs from flaxseed oil (mainly C18:3n-3), fish oil (mainly n-3 long-chain PUFA: C20:5n-3, C22:6n-3, and C22:5n-3), and corn oil (mainly C18:2n-6) all effectively reduced the incidence of neural tube defects induced by VPA, and n-3 long-chain PUFAs from fish oil had the best prevention effect (Li et al., 2018).

Inositol deficiency has been shown to cause cranial neural tube defects in mice (Cockroft, 1979; Cockroft, Brook, & Copp, 1992). Lack of PIP5KIγ (an enzyme that catalyzes the synthesis of PIP2 by phosphorylating phosphatidylinositol 4 phosphate) can lead to neural tube defects in mice embryos, demonstrating the important role of inositol metabolism in the process of neural tube normal closure (Wang, Lian, Golden, Morrisey, & Abrams, 2007). However, inositol supplementation shows different effects in different mouse models of neural tube defects. Inositol supplementation can effectively prevent the occurrence of neural tube defects in curly tail mice (a model of folate-resistant neural tube defects), in mice exposed to hyperglycemia, and in *splotch mice* that carry an intragenic deletion in the Pax3 gene (a model of neural tube defects that can be prevented by folic acid), but this prevention effect disappears in Grhl3-null mice (which has now been recognized as a model of folate- and inositol-resistant neural tube defects), Bent tail mice, and Mekk4 knock-out mice (Greene et al., 2017).

15.4 The possible mechanism for the relationship between lipids and birth defects

Folate, also called vitamin B_9, has long been known as a nutrient effectively protecting against birth defects (especially neural tube defects), and its most important role is involved in homocysteine metabolism, one-carbon metabolism, and DNA synthesis (Li, Wahlqvist, & Li, 2016). The teratogenicity of homocysteine has been demonstrated in both human and animal studies (Rosenquist, Ratashak, & Selhub, 1996; Yang, Li, Wan, & Du, 2017). Our previous randomized controlled trial (RCT) indicated that n-3 long-chain PUFAs and vitamin B_{12} could synergistically lower plasma homocysteine levels (Huang, Li, Asimi, Chen, & Li, 2015). A study in rats demonstrated that PUFA supplementation could lower plasma homocysteine levels via regulating the mRNA expression of key enzymes involved in folate-homocysteine metabolisms, such as methylenetetrahydrofolate reductase

(MTHFR), methionine adenosyltransferase (MAT), cystathionine-β-synthase (CBS), phosphatidylethanolamine N-methyltransferase (PEMT), glycine N-methyltransferase (GNMT), 5-methyltetrahydrofolate-homocysteine methyltransferase reductase (MTRR), and betaine aldehyde dehydrogenase (BAD) (Huang, Hu, Khan, Yang, & Li, 2013). This modulating effect on gene expression was also observed in an ex vivo study (Huang, Wahlqvist, & Li, 2012). In addition, PUFAs, especially n-3 long-chain PUFAs, could upregulate the activity of MAT (Huang, Wahlqvist, & Li, 2010). Our previous study indicated that VPA injection for pregnant mice could lead to embryo neural tube defects, accompanied by the inhibited expression of several enzymes involved in folate-homocysteine metabolism (such as guanidinoacetate N-methyltransferase (GAMT), CBS, dihydrofolate reductase (DHFR), MTRR, and cystathionine-γ-lyase (CSE)) in the liver, increased expression of these enzymes and homocysteine level in embryos. However, PUFA supplementation could prevent neural tube defects and alleviate this disturbance of folate-homocysteine metabolism in both embryos and the liver of pregnant mice (Li et al., 2018). The evidence above demonstrates that PUFAs may prevent birth defects via modulating folate-homocysteine metabolism.

Moreover, eicosanoid metabolism may be another mechanism behind the association between lipids and birth defects. C20:5n-3 and C20:4n-6 are two precursors for eicosanoid synthesis under the catalyzation of cyclooxygenase (COX) and lipoxygenase (LOX). Under the catalyzation of COX and LOX, C20:4n-6 can be metabolized to 2-series prostaglandin (PG, such as PGI_2), 2-series thromboxane (TX, such as TXA_2), and 4-series leukotriene (LT, such as LTB_4), while C20:5n-3 can be metabolized to 3-series PG, 3-series TX, and 5-series LT (Calder, 2003). As mentioned before, a high ratio of TXB_2/6-keto-PGF_{1a} (stable metabolites of TXA_2 and PGI_2) is a risk factor for neural tube defects, and this ratio is also positively correlated with the ratio of C20:4n-6/C20:5n-3 (Li et al., 2017). PGI_2 is a potent vasodilator, but TXA_2 is a vasoconstrictor (Moncada & Higgs, 1988). They play a reverse role in regulating vascular tone. A human placenta perfusion study ex vivo found that inhibitors of COX could reduce placenta transfer by reducing the production of 6-keto-PGF_{1a}, but this effect can be reversed by perfusion of the PGI_2 analog (Kuhn & Stuart, 1987). The role of PG and TX in placenta transfer has also been demonstrated in several other studies (Shellhaas, Coffman, Dargie, Killam, & Helen, 1997; Tuvemo, 1980). Based on this evidence, we hypothesized that a high ratio of C20:4n-6/C20:5n-3 leads to a high ratio of TXA_2/PGI_2 in the placenta, and this abnormal eicosanoid metabolism leads to vascular constriction and reduced blood flow and thus hinders the placenta transfer of oxygen and nutrients from mother to fetus and finally causes the occurrence of neural tube defects (Li et al., 2017).

The mechanism for the prevention effect of inositol against birth defects includes its regulation of protein kinase C (PKC) and C20:4n-6 metabolism. The rat study found that inositol can prevent folate-resistant neural tube defects via stimulating PKC activity (Greene & Copp, 1997). In humans, phosphatidylinositol can be phosphorylated into PI(4)P and then PI(4,5)P2 under the catalyzation of PI4K and PIP5K, respectively (Greene et al., 2017). PI(4,5)P2 can be hydrolyzed into diacylglycerol and I(1,4,5)P3 (Greene et al., 2017). I(1,4,5)P3 can mobilize intracellular Ca^{2+} from the endoplasmic reticulum and thus recover PKC from its soluble fraction (inactive form) and translocate it to membranes as an active form, while DG can increase the affinity of PKC for Ca^{2+} (Berridge, 1984; Nishizuka, 1986). The prevention effect of inositol against neural tube defects induced by high glucose exposure of cultured mouse embryos can be reversed by indomethacin, an inhibitor of eicosanoid synthesis from C20:4n-6 (Baker, Piddington, Goldman, Egler, & Moehring, 1990). However, adding eicosanoids derived from C20:4n-6 to the culture medium

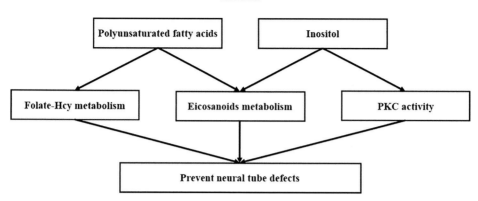

FIG. 15.1 Summary of the relationship between lipids and birth defects.

can also protect against glucose-induced neural tube defects (Baker et al., 1990).

The prevention effect of lipids on neural tube defects is summarized in Fig. 15.1.

15.5 Conclusion

Abnormal lipid metabolism is an important reason for birth defects, and the possible mechanism includes its effect on folate-homocysteine metabolism, eicosanoid metabolism, and inositol metabolism. Increased dietary intake of PUFAs and inositol is recommended.

References

Baker, L., Piddington, R., Goldman, A., Egler, J., & Moehring, J. (1990). Myo-inositol and prostaglandins reverse the glucose inhibition of neural tube fusion in cultured mouse embryos. *Diabetologia, 33*(10), 593–596. https://doi.org/10.1007/BF00400202.

Berridge, M. J. (1984). Inositol trisphosphate and diacylglycerol as second messengers. *The Biochemical Journal, 220*(2), 345–360. https://doi.org/10.1042/bj2200345.

Calder, P. C. (2003). Long-chain n-3 fatty acids and inflammation: Potential application in surgical and trauma patients. *Brazilian Journal of Medical and Biological Research, 36*(4), 433–446. https://doi.org/10.1590/S0100-879X2003000400004.

Cavalli, P., & Copp, A. J. (2002). Inositol and folate resistant neural tube defects. *Journal of Medical Genetics, 39*(2), E5. https://doi.org/10.1136/jmg.39.2.e5.

Cavalli, P., Tedoldi, S., & Riboli, B. (2008). Inositol supplementation in pregnancies at risk of apparently folate-resistant NTDs. *Birth Defects Research Part A-Clinical and Molecular Teratology, 82*(7), 540–542. https://doi.org/10.1002/bdra.20454.

Cavalli, P., Tonni, G., Grosso, E., & Poggiani, C. (2011). Effects of inositol supplementation in a cohort of mothers at risk of producing an NTD pregnancy. *Birth Defects Research Part A - Clinical and Molecular Teratology, 91*(11), 962–965. https://doi.org/10.1002/bdra.22853.

Centofanti, S. F., Francisco, R. P. V., Phillippi, S. T., Castro, I. A., Hoshida, M. S., Curi, R., et al. (2018). Low serum fatty acid levels in pregnancies with fetal gastroschisis: A prospective study. *American Journal of Medical Genetics, Part A, 176*(4), 915–924. https://doi.org/10.1002/ajmg.a.38638.

Cockroft, D. L. (1979). Nutrient requirements of rat embryos undergoing organogenesis in vitro. *Journal of Reproduction and Fertility, 57*(2), 505–510. https://doi.org/10.1530/jrf.0.0570505.

Cockroft, D. L., Brook, F. A., & Copp, A. J. (1992). Inositol deficiency increases the susceptibility to neural tube defects of genetically predisposed (curly tail) mouse embryos in vitro. *Teratology, 45*(2), 223–232. https://doi.org/10.1002/tera.1420450216.

Collins, R. T., Yang, W., Carmichael, S. L., Bolin, E. H., Nembhard, W. N., & Shaw, G. M. (2020). Maternal dietary fat intake and the risk of congenital heart defects in offspring. *Pediatric Research, 88*(5), 804–809. https://doi.org/10.1038/s41390-020-0813-x.

Goldman, A. S., Baker, L., Piddington, R., Marx, B., Herold, R., & Egler, J. (1985). Hyperglycemia-induced teratogenesis is mediated by a functional deficiency of arachidonic acid. *Proceedings of the National Academy of Sciences of the United States of America, 82*(23), 8227–8231. https://doi.org/10.1073/pnas.82.23.8227.

Greene, N. D. E., & Copp, A. J. (1997). Inositol prevents folate-resistant neural tube defects in the mouse. *Nature Medicine, 3*(1), 60–66. https://doi.org/10.1038/nm0197-60.

Greene, N. D. E., Leung, K. Y., & Copp, A. J. (2017). Inositol, neural tube closure and the prevention of neural tube defects. *Birth Defects Research, 109*(2), 68–80. https://doi.org/10.1002/bdra.23533.

Groenen, P. M., Peer, P. G., Wevers, R. A., Swinkels, D. W., Frankc, B., Mariman, E. C., et al. (2003). Maternal myo-inositol, glucose, and zinc status is associated with the risk of offspring with spina bifida. *American Journal of Obstetrics and Gynecology, 189*(6), 1713–1719. https://doi.org/10.1016/S0002-9378(03)00807-X.

Guan, Z., Wang, J., Guo, J., Wang, F., Wang, X., Li, G., et al. (2014). The maternal ITPK1 gene polymorphism is associated with neural tube defects in a high-risk Chinese population. *PLoS One, 9*(1). https://doi.org/10.1371/journal.pone.0086145.

Harris, B. S., Bishop, K. C., Kemeny, H. R., Walker, J. S., Rhee, E., & Kuller, J. A. (2017). Risk factors for birth defects. *Obstetrical and Gynecological Survey, 72*(2), 123–135. https://doi.org/10.1097/OGX.0000000000000405.

Hobbs, C. A., Chowdhury, S., Cleves, M. A., Erickson, S., MacLeod, S. L., Shaw, G. M. S., et al. (2014). Genetic epidemiology and nonsyndromic structural birth defects from candidate genes to epigenetics. *JAMA Pediatrics, 168*(4), 371–377. https://doi.org/10.1001/jamapediatrics.2013.4858.

Huang, T., Hu, X., Khan, N., Yang, J., & Li, D. (2013). Effect of polyunsaturated fatty acids on homocysteine metabolism through regulating the gene expressions involved in methionine metabolism. *The Scientific World Journal, 2013.* https://doi.org/10.1155/2013/931626.

Huang, T., Li, K., Asimi, S., Chen, Q., & Li, D. (2015). Effect of vitamin B-12 and n-3 polyunsaturated fatty acids on plasma homocysteine, ferritin, C-reactive protein, and other cardiovascular risk factors: A randomized controlled trial. *Asia Pacific Journal of Clinical Nutrition, 24*(3), 403–411. https://doi.org/10.6133/apjcn.2015.24.3.19.

Huang, T., Wahlqvist, M. L., & Li, D. (2010). Docosahexaenoic acid decreases plasma homocysteine via regulating enzyme activity and mRNA expression involved in methionine metabolism. *Nutrition, 26*(1), 112–119. https://doi.org/10.1016/j.nut.2009.05.015.

Huang, T., Wahlqvist, M. L., & Li, D. (2012). Effect of n-3 polyunsaturated fatty acid on gene expression of the critical enzymes involved in homocysteine metabolism. *Nutrition Journal, 11*(1). https://doi.org/10.1186/1475-2891-11-6.

Johnson, R. C., McKean, C. M., & Shah, S. N. (1977). Fatty acid composition of lipids in cerebral myelin and synaptosomes in phenylketonuria and down syndrome. *Archives of Neurology, 34*(5), 288–294. https://doi.org/10.1001/archneur.1977.00500170042008.

Kuhn, D. C., & Stuart, M. J. (1987). Cyclooxygenase inhibition reduces placental transfer: Reversal by carbacyclin. *American Journal of Obstetrics and Gynecology, 157*(1), 194–198. https://doi.org/10.1016/S0002-9378(87)80379-4.

Li, K., Li, J., Gu, J., Guo, X., Gao, T., & Li, D. (2018). The protective effect of polyunsaturated fatty acid intake during pregnancy against embryotoxicity of sodium valproate in mice. *Food & Function, 9*(5), 2634–2643. https://doi.org/10.1039/c7fo01604b.

Li, K., Wahlqvist, M. L., & Li, D. (2016). Nutrition, one-carbon metabolism and neural tube defects: A review. *Nutrients, 8*(11). https://doi.org/10.3390/nu8110741.

Li, K., Zhang, X., Pei, L., Chen, G., Liu, J., Wahlqvist, M. L., et al. (2017). High ratios of C20:4n-6/C20:5n-3 and thromboxane B2/6-keto-prostaglandin F1α in placenta are potential risk contributors for neural tube defects: A case-control study in Shanxi Province, China. *Birth Defects Research, 109*(8), 550–563. https://doi.org/10.1002/bdr2.1003.

Mai, C. T., Isenburg, J. L., Canfield, M. A., Meyer, R. E., Correa, A., Alverson, C. J., et al. (2019). National population-based estimates for major birth defects, 2010–2014. *Birth Defects Research, 111*(18), 1420–1435. https://doi.org/10.1002/bdr2.1589.

McKeegan, P. J., & Sturmey, R. G. (2011). The role of fatty acids in oocyte and early embryo development. *Reproduction, Fertility, and Development, 24*(1), 59–67.

Molzer, B., Korschinsky, M., Bernheimer, H., Schmid, R., Wolf, C., & Roscher, A. (1986). Very long chain fatty acids in genetic peroxisomal disease fibroblasts: Differences between the cerebro-hepato-renal (Zellweger) syndrome and adrenoleukodystrophy variants. *Clinica Chimica Acta, 161*(1), 81–90. https://doi.org/10.1016/0009-8981(86)90265-2.

Moncada, S., & Higgs, E. A. (1988). Metabolism of arachidonic acid. *Annals of the New York Academy of Sciences, 522*(1), 454–463. https://doi.org/10.1111/j.1749-6632.1988.tb33385.x.

Niringiyumukiza, J. D., Cai, H., & Xiang, W. (2018). Prostaglandin E2 involvement in mammalian female fertility: Ovulation, fertilization, embryo development and early implantation. *Reproductive Biology and Endocrinology, 16*(1). https://doi.org/10.1186/s12958-018-0359-5.

Nishizuka, Y. (1986). Studies and perspectives of protein kinase C. *Science, 233*(4761), 305–312. https://doi.org/10.1126/science.3014651.

Paige, S. L., Yang, W., Priest, J. R., Botto, L. D., Shaw, G. M., & Collins, R. T. (2019). Risk factors associated with the development of double-inlet ventricle congenital heart disease. *Birth Defects Research, 111*(11), 640–648. https://doi.org/10.1002/bdr2.1501.

Reece, E. A., Wu, Y. K., Wiznitzer, A., Homko, C., Yao, J., Borenstein, M., et al. (1996). Dietary polyunsaturated fatty acid prevents malformations in offspring of diabetic rats. *American Journal of Obstetrics and Gynecology, 175*(4 I), 818–823. Mosby Inc. https://doi.org/10.1016/S0002-9378(96)80005-6.

Rosenquist, T. H., Ratashak, S. A., & Selhub, J. (1996). Homocysteine induces congenital defects of the heart and neural tube: Effect of folic acid. *Proceedings of the National Academy of Sciences of the United States of America, 93*(26), 15227–15232. https://doi.org/10.1073/pnas.93.26.15227.

Shaw, G. M., Carmichael, S. L., Yang, W., & Schaffer, D. M. (2005). Periconceptional dietary intake of Myo-inositol and neural tube defects in offspring. *Birth Defects Research Part A - Clinical and Molecular Teratology, 73*(3), 184–187. https://doi.org/10.1002/bdra.20112.

Shellhaas, C. S., Coffman, T., Dargie, P. J., Killam, A. P., & Helen, H. K. (1997). Intravillous eicosanoid compartmentalization and regulation of placental blood flow. *Journal of the Society for Gynecologic Investigation, 4*(2), 58–63. https://doi.org/10.1016/S1071-5576(97)00008-7.

Siega-Riz, A. M., Olshan, A. F., Werler, M. M., & Moore, C. (2006). Fat intake and the risk of gastroschisis. *Birth Defects Research Part A - Clinical and Molecular Teratology, 76*(4), 241–245. https://doi.org/10.1002/bdra.20249.

Smedts, H. P. M., Rakhshandehroo, M., Verkleij-Hagoort, A. C., De Vries, J. H. M., Ottenkamp, J., Steegers, E. A. P., et al. (2008). Maternal intake of fat, riboflavin and nicotinamide and the risk of having offspring with congenital heart defects. *European Journal of Nutrition, 47*(7), 357–365. https://doi.org/10.1007/s00394-008-0735-6.

Tuvemo, T. (1980). Role of prostaglandins, prostacyclin, and thromboxanes in the control of the umbilical-placental circulation. *Seminars in Perinatology, 4*(2), 91–95.

Wang, Y., Lian, L., Golden, J. A., Morrisey, E. E., & Abrams, C. S. (2007). PIP5KIγ is required for cardiovascular and neuronal development. *Proceedings of the National Academy of Sciences of the United States of America, 104*(28), 11748–11753. https://doi.org/10.1073/pnas.0700019104.

Yang, M., Li, W., Wan, Z., & Du, Y. (2017). Elevated homocysteine levels in mothers with neural tube defects: A systematic review and meta-analysis. *Journal of Maternal-Fetal and Neonatal Medicine, 30*(17), 2051–2057. https://doi.org/10.1080/14767058.2016.1236248.

16

Conjugated linolenic acids and their bioactivities

Gaofeng Yuan

Department of Food Science, College of Food and Medicine, Zhejiang Ocean University, Zhoushan, China

16.1 Introduction

Conjugated fatty acids (CFAs) are the general term for positional and geometric isomers of polyunsaturated fatty acids with conjugated double bonds. CFAs occur as diene, triene, and tetraene, in which the most common conjugated polyenoic acids are octadecanoic and octatrienoic acids, termed as conjugated linoleic acids (CLAs) and conjugated linolenic acids (CLNAs), respectively (Yuan et al., 2014). CFAs have drawn significant attention for their variety of biologically beneficial effects. The health-promoting effects of CFAs were intensively investigated, among which CLA was best characterized and reported in detail (Yuan et al., 2014). The health-promoting effects of CLNAs were comprehensively reviewed in our published paper (Yuan et al., 2014, 2015). In this chapter, we tried to update the recent development in the area of the health-promoting effects of CLNAs (Fig. 16.1).

16.2 Natural sources and utilization of CLNA

CLNA occurs naturally in plant seeds, and a considerable amount of CLNA was found in several plant seeds. Five CLNA isomers occur as major seed oils of several plants: α-eleostearic acid (*cis*-9, *trans*-11, *trans*-13 CLNA, α-ESA) from tung (*Aleurites fordii*), bitter gourd (*Momordica charantia*), and snake gourd seed (*Trichosanthes anguina*), punicic acid (*cis*-9, *trans*-11, *cis*-13 CLNA, and PUA) from pomegranate (*Punica granatum*) and trichosanthes (*Trichosanthes kirilowii*), α-calendic acid (*trans*-8, *trans*-10, *cis*-12 CLNA, and α-CDA) from pot marigold (*Calendula officinalis*), jacaric acid (*cis*-8, *trans*-10, *cis*-12 CLNA, and JA) from jacaranda (*Jacaranda mimosifolia*), and catalpic acid (*trans*-9, *trans*-11, *cis*-13 CLNA, and CA) from catalpa (*Catalpa ovata*).

Unlike CLA, CLNA isomers are present at much higher levels in certain seed oil. However, CLNA isomers from natural sources are mixtures that are difficult to separate from each other. Seed oils rich in CLNA were used in most studies regarding the metabolism and bioactivity; purified CLNA was used in a few in vitro studies. The commercial production of CLNA largely relies on the extraction of seed oils from producer plants at present. Various methods of processing have been carried out to extract CLNA from seeds using different methods of extraction, like solvent extraction, supercritical CO_2 extraction (Liu et al., 2009), ultrasonic-assisted extraction (Tabaraki et al., 2012), and cold press (Khoddami et al., 2014). However, limited natural sources are available. They are, therefore, not suitable for large-scale or widespread production in the future (Holic et al., 2018). One strategy with the potential to obtain CLNAs is to produce them via transgenic plants (Holic et al., 2018). Production of PUA at levels up to 24.8% has been achieved in *Arabidopsis thaliana* (Mietkiewska et al., 2014). Another promising strategy is to produce CLNA by using engineered microorganisms. Production of PUA at levels up to 19.6% (w/w) of total fatty acids was obtained in the metabolically engineered fission yeast *Schizosaccharomyces pombe* (Garaiova et al., 2017). More efforts are needed to obtain a higher concentration of PUA in engineered plants and microorganisms in the future.

16.3 The metabolism of CLNA

CLNA can be converted into *cis*-9,*trans*-11 CLA in Caco-2 cells used as an in vitro model of the human intestinal epithelium (Schneider et al., 2012, 2013). In accordance with these in vitro data, the same conversions of CLNA into CLA were observed in rats, mice, and humans. α-ESA can be metabolized into *cis*-9,*trans*-11 CLA in rats (Tsuzuki et al., 2003, 2006). The majority of α-ESA was slowly absorbed in an unchanged state in the rat intestine and part of the absorbed α-ESA was quickly converted into CLA in the rat intestine in a lipid absorption assay in lymph from the thoracic duct (Tsuzuki et al., 2006). CLA also can be detected in the liver of rats and mice fed with PUA (Koba et al., 2007; Kohno, Suzuki, et al., 2004; Yamasaki et al., 2006). Our study also showed that PUA can be converted into *cis*-9,*trans*-11 CLA in various rat tissues, such as liver, plasma, adipose tissue, kidney, and brain (Yuan, Yuan, & Li, 2009). The incorporation and metabolism of PUA in healthy young humans were also observed (Yuan, Sinclair, Xu, & Li, 2009). In this randomized controlled trial, the test group was supplemented with *trichosanthes* seed kernels containing PUA per day in the form of triacylglycerols for 28 days. The control group was provided with sunflower seed kernels. After the consumption of *trichosanthes* seeds containing PUA per day for 28 days, the proportion of PUA was increased from 0.00% to 0.47% in plasma and 0.00% to 0.37% in red blood cell membranes, respectively. The proportion of *cis*-9,*trans*-11 CLA was increased from 0.05% to 0.23% in plasma and 0.03% to 0.17% in RBCM after 28 days of intervention, respectively (Yuan, Sinclair, Xu, & Li, 2009).

The mechanism of conversion of PUA into *cis*-9,*trans*-11 CLA in vivo is not clear. A Δ13-saturation reaction that converted CLNA into *cis*-9,*trans*-11 CLA in rats and mice was proposed (Tsuzuki, Tokuyama, Igarashi, & Miyazawa, 2004; Tsuzuki, Tokuyama, Igarashi, Nakagawa, et al., 2004). It is possible that PUA was converted into *cis*-9,*trans*-11 CLNA in humans in a similar pathway in animals (Yuan, Sinclair, Xu, & Li, 2009). However, the enzyme that catalyzed the reaction of Δ13-saturation in animals and humans is not identified so far, although there was a presumption suggesting that an NADPH-dependent enzyme which is either a novel enzyme recognizing conjugated trienoic acid or the enzyme active in the leukotriene B4 reductive pathway could carry out this Δ13-saturation reaction in rats and

16.4 CLNA and carcinogenesis

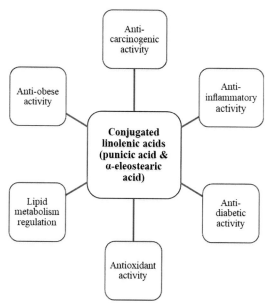

FIG. 16.1 Bioactivities of conjugated linolenic acid isomers.

mice (Tsuzuki et al., 2006; Tsuzuki, Tokuyama, Igarashi, Nakagawa, et al., 2004).

16.4 CLNA and carcinogenesis

16.4.1 In vitro studies

Several studies investigated the cytotoxic effect of isomers of CLNA on various human tumor cell lines and found that alkaline isomerized α-LNA and tung oil fatty acids were cytotoxic to DLD-1, HepG2, A549, MCF-7 (breast), and MKN-7 cell lines (Igarashi & Miyazawa, 2000), PUA, α-ESA, and CA to SV-T2, SV40-transformed mouse fibroblasts, and U-937 (human leukemic cells) (Suzuki et al., 2001), α-ESA and PUA to MDA-MB-231 (an estrogen-insensitive breast cancer cell line) and MDA-ERα7v (an estrogen-sensitive cell line developed from the MDA-MB-231 cells) (Grossmann et al., 2009, 2010), α-ESA and PUA to MCF-7 (Kim et al., 2002; Moon et al., 2010), α-ESA to neuronal PC12, SH-SY5Y, and NG108–15 (Kondo et al., 2010), α-ESA and JA to DLD-1 cells (Shinohara et al., 2012; Tsuzuki, Tokuyama, Igarashi, & Miyazawa, 2004), PUA to LNCaP (Gasmi & Sanderson, 2010), JA and PUA to LNCaP and PC-3 cells (human prostate) (Gasmi & Thomas Sanderson, 2013) and DU 145 (Albrecht et al., 2004; Lansky et al., 2005), and PUA to 3T3-L1 preadipocytes (Chou et al., 2012).

It seems that the position and geometry of three conjugated double bonds of different CLNA isomers affect the cytotoxic activity of CLNA isomers. The cytotoxic activity of four positional and geometrical CLNA isomers was compared and the results indicated that the cytotoxicity of pure α-ESA, PUA, and CA is much greater than that of α-CDA on human leukemic cells (Suzuki et al., 2001). This suggested that the *cis/trans* configuration of 9, 11, 13-CLNA isomers had little effect on their cytotoxic effects because there was little difference in the cytotoxicity of α-ESA, PUA, and CA (Suzuki et al., 2001). However other studies demonstrated conflicting results. CLNA isomers, prepared and fractionated from α-LNA by alkaline treatment, were examined for their growth-inhibitory effects on human tumor cell lines. The results showed that the part consisted of conjugated all-trans trienoic linolenic acid and had stronger growth-inhibitory effects on human tumor cell lines (Igarashi & Miyazawa, 2005). The growth inhibition effects and induction of DNA fragmentation by β-ESA acid and β-CDA in Caco-2 cells were greater than α-ESA and α-CDA with cis configuration (Yasui et al., 2006a). The growth-inhibitory effects of conjugated fatty acids in the cell line HT-29 were investigated and results showed that low concentrations of CLNAs (10 µM) yielded a higher degree of inhibitory effects compared to CLAs. All trans-CFAs were more effective compared to *cis/trans*-CFAs as follows: *trans*-9,*trans*-11, *trans*-13 CLNA ≥ *cis*-9,*trans*-11,*trans*-13 CLNA ≥ *trans*-11,*trans*-13 CLA ≥ *cis*-9,*trans*-11 CLA. The results from these studies suggested that the configuration of conjugated double bonds is important in cytotoxicity and all-trans-CLNA isomers act as more effective tumor growth-inhibitory compounds (Degen et al., 2011). The cytotoxic effects of CLNAs from natural plant sources on DLD-1 were compared and the results indicated that strong cytotoxic effects on DLD-1 human adenocarcinoma cells were obtained with all CLNA isomers (pure PUA, CPA, α-ESA, β-ESA, JA, α-CDA, and β-CDA), but JA had the strongest effect (Shinohara et al., 2012).

On the other hand, the spatial conformation of CLNA plays a key role in the activity of CLNA, and the 3D analysis of structural similarity enabled us to rank geoisomeric fatty acids according to cytotoxic potency, whereas a 2D positional assessment of cis/trans structure did not (Gasmi & Thomas Sanderson, 2013). JA and PUA were the most cytotoxic octadecatrienoic acids in LNCaP and PC-3 cells among JA, PUA, α-CDA, and β-CDA, and spatial conformation cis, trans, cis of JA and PUA was shown to play a key role in the increased potency and efficacy of these two fatty acids in comparison to the other C-18 fatty acids tested (Gasmi & Thomas Sanderson, 2013).

The mechanism of the cytotoxicity of CLNA isomers may involve lipid peroxidation (Igarashi & Miyazawa, 2005; Suzuki et al., 2001). The order of toxicity of the α-ESA, PUA, and CA was consistent with their susceptibility to peroxidation in the aqueous phase supported by the decrease in the cytotoxicity of fatty acids by the addition of butylated hydroxytoluene (Suzuki et al., 2001). Other mechanisms also have been suggested for cytotoxicity activity of CLNA isomers including the increased expression of peroxisome proliferator-activated receptor gamma (PPAR-γ) and the cell cycle arrest genes GADD45 and p53, along with decreased expression of the apoptosis suppressor Bcl-2 (Grossmann et al., 2009; Yasui et al., 2005, 2006a, 2006b). Moreover, CLNA isomers could exert their cytotoxicity activity through several signaling pathways. α-ESA could suppress the proliferation of MCF-7 breast cancer cells via activation of PPAR-γ and inhibition of ERK 1/2 (Moon et al., 2010). It was suggested that PUA has breast cancer inhibitor properties that are dependent on lipid peroxidation and the PKC pathway (Grossmann et al., 2010). α-ESA could act through the MAPK/ERK signaling pathway to modulate the progression of differentiation of 3T3-L1 murine preadipocyte cells (Chou et al., 2012).

16.4.2 In vivo studies

Most animal studies about antitumor effect of CLNA were focused on colon cancer. Pomegranate seed oil (PSO) rich in PUA inhibited the development of azoxymethane-induced colonic aberrant crypt foci in rats (Kohno, Suzuki, et al., 2004). The proposed mechanism of inhibition of AOM-induced colon carcinogenesis in rats included elevation of colonic PPAR-γ expression and increased content of CLA in the lipid composition in colonic mucosa and liver. PSO rich in PUA significantly reduced the incidence and multiplicity of chemically induced skin cancer, potentially through reduced ornithine decarboxylase activity, suggesting that PSO could be a safe and effective chemopreventive agent against skin cancer (Hora et al., 2003).

α-ESA can also suppress AOM-induced colon carcinogenesis in rats (Kohno et al., 2002; Kohno, Yasui, et al., 2004). Dietary feeding with bitter melon seed oil (BGO) for 5 weeks at three dose levels (0.01%, 0.1%, and 1%) caused a significant reduction in the frequency of AOM-induced colonic ACF and a significant reduction in the multiplicity of ACF in rats fed the diet containing 0.01% of BGO (Kohno et al., 2002). In another study, the chemopreventive ability of BGO against colorectal cancer development in rats was confirmed (Kohno, Yasui, et al., 2004). Dietary supplement with BGO rich in α-ESA for 32 weeks significantly lowered the incidence of colonic adenoma and adenocarcinoma induced by AOM and multiplicities of colorectal cancer in rats without causing any adverse effects. α-ESA prepared from tung oil and BGO have a stronger inhibition activity of tumor induced by transplanted DLD-1 human colon cancer cell line in male athymic nude mice CLA (Tsuzuki, Tokuyama, Igarashi, & Miyazawa, 2004). The tumor growth was strongly suppressed in mice of the tung group, compared with other groups, and the effect was associated with lipid peroxidation. However, no anti-carcinogenic activity on 7,12-dimethylbenzanthracene (DMBA)- and 1,2-dimethylhydrazine (DMH)-induced mammary and colon carcinogenesis in female Sprague–Dawley rats was observed (Kitamura et al., 2006).

The mechanism of inhibition of carcinogenesis by CLNA isomers in vivo remained unelucidated since CLA has proved to be a powerful anticarcinogenesis agent in rat mammary carcinogenesis (Belury, 2002; Dilzer & Park, 2012). Therefore, the potential cancer chemopreventive effects of CLNA could be partly due to the presence of CLA isomers derived from CLNA. On the other hand, induction of lipid peroxidation by CLNA isomers was also shown to play a role in their anticarcinogenic activity (Tsuzuki, Tokuyama, Igarashi, & Miyazawa, 2004).

16.5 CLNA and lipid metabolism

16.5.1 CLNA and plasma/serum lipid metabolism

Dyslipidemia, including hypercholesterolemia, hypertriglyceridemia, or their combination, is a major risk factor for cardiovascular diseases (Sengupta et al., 2015). Generally, dyslipidemia is characterized by increased fasting concentrations of total cholesterol, triglycerides, and low-density lipoprotein cholesterol, in conjunction with decreased concentrations of high-density lipoprotein cholesterol (Varady & Jones, 2005). Some animal studies have found that supplementation with CLNAs significantly decreases serum total cholesterol (TC) (Dhar et al., 2006; Koba et al., 2002), apoB-100 (Arao, Yotsumoto, et al., 2004). However, there is no conclusive evidence to confirm the effect of CLNA on lipid profiles in animal models (Table 16.1).

Supplement with 0.5% and 2% of BGO in the diet for 6 weeks significantly reduced plasma free cholesterol levels with a trend toward an increase in high-density lipoprotein cholesterol (HDL-C),

TABLE 16.1 The effect of punicic acid and α-eleostearic acid on lipid metabolism.

Isomer (purity)	Animals/subjects	Dose of supplementation	Study duration	Results	Ref.
α-ESA-enriched BGO (57.7%)	Alloxan-induced diabetes mellitus in rats	0.5% wt diet	6 weeks	Decreased: plasma TC and non-HDL-C	Dhar et al. (2006)
α-ESA-enriched BGO nanocapsules (50.7–52.0%)	Male albino rats with hypercholesterolemia induced by a high-fat diet	50 mg/kg body weight/day	30 days	Decreased: plasma TC, HDL-C, non-HDL-C, and TG Decreased: hepatic TG and TC	Sengupta et al. (2015)
α-ESA-enriched BGO	Male Wistar rats	0.5% and 2% wt diet	6 weeks	Decreased: plasma free cholesterol levels no change in TC	Noguchi et al. (2001)

Continued

TABLE 16.1 The effect of punicic acid and α-eleostearic acid on lipid metabolism—cont'd

Isomer (purity)	Animals/subjects	Dose of supplementation	Study duration	Results	Ref.
α-ESA-enriched BGO (51.1%)	Male albino rats of Charles Foster strain	0.5, 2, and 10% wt diet	4 weeks	No change in plasma TC, HDL-C, and non-HDL-C	Dhar et al. (1999)
PUA-enriched PSO (70%) or α-ESA-enriched tung seed oil (70%)	Male golden Syrian hamsters	1.22–1.27% wt diet	6 weeks	No change in blood cholesterol	Yang et al. (2005)
PUA-enriched PSO (69.0%)	Obese, hyperlipidemic Otsuka Long-Evans Tokushima Fatty (OLETF) rats	1%	2 weeks	No change in serum lipid level Decreased: hepatic TG	Arao, Wang, et al. (2004)
Genetically modified rapeseed oil containing PUA	ICR CD-1 male mice	0.25% wt diet	4 weeks	No change in serum lipid level Decreased: hepatic TG	Koba et al. (2007)
PUA-enriched PSO	ICR CD-1 male mice	0.5% wt diet	4 weeks	No change in serum lipid level Decreased: hepatic TG	Koba et al. (2007)
α-ESA-enriched BGO (54.1%) or PUA-enriched PSO (76.1%)	ICR CD-1 male mice	1% wt diet	6 weeks	No change in plasma lipid Decreased: hepatic TG	Yuan, Sun, Sinclair, and Li (2009)
α-ESA-enriched BGO (50%)	Male C57BL/6JNarl mice fed a high-sucrose diet	1% α-ESA	5 weeks	No change in serum TG and TC Decreased: hepatic TG and TC	Chen et al. (2016)
α-ESA-enriched BGO (50%)	Male C57BL/6J mice with diet-induced obesity	2.5, 5, and 7.5% wt diet	10 weeks	Decreased: 25–37% of hepatic TG and 23% of TC	Chen et al. (2012)
PUA-enriched *Trichosanthes kirilowii* seed kernels (24.26%)	Thirty young healthy volunteers	3 g per day	28 days	No change in TG, TC, HDL-C, and LDL-C	Yamasaki et al. (2006)
PUA-enriched PSO	Fifty-one hyperlipidemic subjects	400 mg of PSO twice daily	4 weeks	No change in serum TC or LDL-C Decreased: TG and the TG: HDL-C ratio in the PSO group as compared with baseline values	Mirmiran et al. (2010)

PSO, pomegranate seed oil; *BGO*, bitter melon seed oil; *PUA*, punicic acid; *α-ESA*, α-eleostearic acid; *TC*, total cholesterol; *TG*, triglycerides; *LDL-C*, low-density lipoprotein cholesterol; *HDL-C*, high-density lipoprotein cholesterol.

but there was no significant change in the TC in rats (Noguchi et al., 2001). PUA significantly decreased apolipoprotein 100 secretion and reduced the uptake of C-14-oleate into newly synthesized cellular triacylglycerol in HepG2 cells as compared with α-LNA (Arao, Yotsumoto, et al., 2004). In another study, the results found that the cis9,trans11,trans13 CLNA isomer was associated with significantly lowering total and HDL-C in diabetic rats (Dhar et al., 2006). BGO nanocapsules also were found to reduce the blood lipids, tissue lipids, and plasma viscosity significantly (Sengupta et al., 2015).

However, other animal studies report controversial results for the hypolipidemic role of CLNA. An early study showed that CLNA didn't affect the cholesterol level (Dhar et al., 1999). After oral administration with 0.5%, 2%, and 10% of BGO for 4 weeks, the concentrations of TC, HDL-C, and non-HDL-C in plasma were similar with control. In another study, the hypocholesterolemic activity of CLNA was compared with α-LNA in hamsters by examining the effects of CLNA, isolated from either PSO or tung seed oil, and α-LNA, isolated from flaxseed oil, on serum cholesterol levels in male hamsters for a period of 6 weeks, and the results found that α-LNA possessed the hypocholesterolemic activity while CLNA had no effect on blood cholesterol, at least not in hamsters (Yang et al., 2005). The serum lipid levels did not get affected after giving supplements rich in PUA in obese hyperlipidemic Otsuka Long-Evans Tokushima fatty rats (Arao, Wang, et al., 2004) and mice (Koba et al., 2007). Similarly, no significant differences in triglycerides (TG), TC, HDL-C, and low-density lipoprotein cholesterol (LDL-C) levels in plasma were found among mice fed a control diet or fed α-ESA or PUA for 6 weeks compared to the control group in our study (Yuan, Sun, Sinclair, & Li, 2009).

A few clinical trials examined the effect of CLNA on serum lipids. No significant change in serum TC and LDL-C was found in our randomized controlled trial (Yuan, Sinclair, Xu, & Li, 2009). A double-blind placebo-controlled randomized clinical trial also observed no significant change in serum cholesterol or LDL-C in hyperlipidemic subjects after supplementing with 400 mg of PSO twice daily for 4 weeks, while TG and the TG:HDL-C ratio were significantly decreased (Mirmiran et al., 2010).

16.5.2 CLNA and hepatic triglyceride accumulation

Nonalcoholic fatty liver disease (NAFLD) is a growing epidemic worldwide characterized by an excessive TG deposition without chronic alcohol consumption (Scorletti & Byrne, 2018). Studies raised the possibility that CLNA attenuated the hepatic triglyceride accumulation in animal models (Table 16.1).

The accumulated hepatic TG in OLETF rats and mice was markedly decreased after supplementing with PSO rich in PUA compared with the control (Arao, Wang, et al., 2004; Koba et al., 2007). Similarly, although the plasma lipid did not get affected, the liver TG levels in mice supplemented with α-ESA or PUA for 6 weeks were significantly decreased compared to the control group (Yuan, Sun, Sinclair, & Li, 2009). A series of studies also investigated the antisteatosis effect of BGO rich in α-ESA in mice. BGO is more effective at attenuating hepatic steatosis than soybean oil, which contains approximately the same amount of PUFAs (Chen et al., 2012; Hsieh et al., 2013). BGO-supplemented mice had 25–37% lower liver TG concentrations and 23% lower liver cholesterol concentrations than the mice fed a high-fat diet for 10 weeks (Chen et al., 2012). In another study, the liver TG and TC concentrations were also significantly reduced by α-ESA administration in mice treated with a high-sucrose diet supplemented with 1% α-ESA for 5 weeks (Chen et al., 2016).

The potential mechanism by which α-ESA exerts the antisteatosis effect could be attributed to that α-ESA increased the cellular NAD+/

NADH ratio, activating PPAR-α, AMPK, and SIRT1 signaling pathways (Chen et al., 2016). α-ESA has been recognized as a potent PPAR-α agonist (Chuang et al., 2006). α-ESA-activated sirtuin 1 deacetylase and AMPK signaling, thus forming a feed-forward PPAR-α/AMPK/sirtuin 1 signaling loop, shifts hepatic lipid metabolism toward catabolism (Chen et al., 2016). Another study investigated the potential mechanism by which α-ESA exerts the antisteatosis effect by using a PPAR-α knockout mouse model (Chang et al., 2016). In this study, the C57BL/6J wild (WD) and PPAR-α knockout (KO) mice were fed a high-fat diet containing BGO (15% soybean oil +15% BGO) or not (30% soybean oil) for 5 weeks. The BGO diet significantly reduced the hepatic triglyceride concentrations, but not in KO mice. This result suggested that BGO-mediated antisteatosis depended on PPAR-α.

16.6 Effect of conjugated linolenic acid on obesity

The prevalence of obesity and its associated comorbidities have grown to epidemic proportions worldwide. Thus, developing safe and effective therapeutic approaches against these widespread and debilitating diseases is important and timely (Bassaganya-Riera, Guri, & Hontecillas, 2011). The effect of CLNA isomers on body weight showed inconsistent outcomes in obese animal models (Table 16.2). CLNA mixtures prepared by alkaline isomerization reduced perirenal adipose tissue weight to a larger extent when compared with linoleic acid, CLA, and linolenic acid in Sprague–Dawley rats (Koba et al., 2002). A PUA-enriched PSO diet also reduced the omental white adipose tissue weights, but not abdominal white adipose tissue weights in obese and hyperlipidemic

TABLE 16.2 The effect of punicic acid and α-eleostearic acid on obesity.

Isomer (purity)	Animals	Dose of supplementation	Study duration	Effects	Ref.
Conjugated linolenic acid mixtures (49.1%)	Male Sprague–Dawley rats	1.0% wt diet	4 weeks	Decreased: perirenal and epididymal adipose tissue weight	Koba et al. (2002)
PUA-enriched PSO	Male OLETF obese rats	1.0% wt diet	2 weeks	Decreased: omental white adipose tissue weight (27%). No change in abdominal white adipose tissue	Arao, Wang, et al. (2004)
PUA-enriched PSO (approximately 80%)	Male ICR CD-1 mice	0.5% wt diet	4 weeks	Decreased: perirenal and epididymal adipose tissue weight	Koba et al. (2007)
Genetically modified rapeseed oil containing PUA	Male ICR CD-1 mice	0.25% wt diet	4 weeks	Decreased: perirenal and epididymal adipose tissue weight	Koba et al. (2007)
PUA-enriched PSO (64.79%)	Male CD-1 mice with high-fat feeding	61.79 mg/d PSO	14 weeks	Decreased: body weight, weight gain	McFarlin et al. (2009)

TABLE 16.2 The effect of punicic acid and α-eleostearic acid on obesity—cont'd

Isomer (purity)	Animals	Dose of supplementation	Study duration	Effects	Ref.
PUA-enriched PSO	Male C57BL/6J mice with diet-induced obesity	1% PSO wt diet	12 weeks	Decreased: body weight, body fat mass	Vroegrijk et al. (2011)
α-ESA-enriched BGO (50%)	Male C57BL/6J mice with diet-induced obesity	7.5% wt diet	5 weeks	Decreased: 21% body fat	Chen et al. (2012)
α-ESA-enriched BGO (50%)	Male C57BL/6J mice with diet-induced obesity	2.5, 5, and 7.5% wt diet	10 weeks	Decreased: 32, 35, and 65% of body fat	Hsieh et al. (2013)
α-ESA-enriched BGO (42.60%)	Male C57BL/6J mice with high-Fat diet-induced obesity	0.1, 0.5, and 1% wt diet	3 weeks	Decreased: body weight, fat index and the adipose sizes	Xu et al. (2016)
α-ESA-enriched BGO	C57BL/6J wild (WD) and PPAR-α knockout (KO) mice with a high-fat diet	15% wt diet	5 weeks	Decreased: contents of retroperitoneal, epididymal, and inguinal fats	Chang et al. (2016)
PUA-enriched PSO (70%) or α-ESA-enriched tung seed oil (70%)	Male golden Syrian hamsters	1.22–1.27% wt diet	6 weeks	No change in body weight	Yang et al. (2005)
α-ESA-enriched BGO (54.1%) or PUA-enriched PSO (76.1%)	Male ICR mice	1% wt diet	6 weeks	No change in body weight, perirenal or epididymal adipose tissues	Yuan, Sun, Sinclair, and Li (2009)
PUA-enriched PSO	Male Wistar rats fed an obesogenic diet	0.5% wt diet	6 weeks	No change in body weight, white adipose tissue or interscapular brown adipose tissue weights	Miranda et al. (2013)

PSO, pomegranate seed oil; *BGO*, bitter melon seed oil; *PUA*, punicic acid; *α-ESA*, α-eleostearic acid.

OLETF rats (Arao, Wang, et al., 2004). Supplementation with PSO or genetically modified rapeseed oil containing PUA decreased the weight of perirenal adipose tissue in ICR CD1 mice in a dose-dependent manner (Koba et al., 2007). Dietary supplementation with 61.79 mg/d of PSO significantly lowered the body weight and weight gain in mice with high-fat feeding, compared with the control (McFarlin et al., 2009). In another study, dietary supplementation with 1% of PSO ameliorated high-fat diet-induced obesity and insulin resistance in mice, independent of changes in food intake or energy expenditure (Vroegrijk et al., 2011). Supplementation with α-ESA-enriched BGO showed it to be more potent than soybean oil in attenuating high-fat diet-induced body fat deposition in mice (Chen et al., 2012; Hsieh et al., 2013).

In contrast, dietary supplementation with 1.22%–1.27% or 1% of CLNA (α-ESA or PUA) for 6 weeks did not significantly change the body weight of hamsters or mice, respectively (Yang et al., 2005; Yuan, Sun, Sinclair, & Li, 2009). Dietary supplementation with 0.5% of PUA did not lead to decreased fat accumulation in adipose tissues, liver, or skeletal muscles when rats were fed an obesogenic diet (Miranda et al., 2013).

The potential mechanism by which CLNA isomers exert the antiobesity effect is not clear. Since cis-9,trans-11 CLA has no anti-adiposity activity (Bhattacharya et al., 2006; Kennedy et al., 2010), the anti-adiposity potential of PUA and α-ESA cannot be attributed to CLA derived from α-ESA in vivo since PUA and α-ESA are proved to be metabolized into cis-9, trans-11 CLA, rather than trans-10, cis-12 CLA (Tsuzuki, Tokuyama, Igarashi, Nakagawa, et al., 2004; Yuan, Sinclair, Zhou, & Li, 2009). PUA, α-ESA and trans-10, cis-12 CLA might share a common metabolic or signaling pathway, leading to a qualitatively similar outcome in the white adipose tissue (Hsieh et al., 2013). Similar to trans-10, cis-12 CLA, CLNA might exert their anti-adiposity effect by the induction of the expression or secretion of cytokines and inhibition of adipogenesis and preadipocyte differentiation through the regulation of PPAR–γ (Chen et al., 2012; Chou et al., 2012; Koba et al., 2002; Lai et al., 2012).

PPAR-γ is a master regulator of adipogenesis as well as a potent modulator of insulin sensitivity, lipogenesis, and adipocyte survival and function (Lai et al., 2012; Siersbæk et al., 2010; Tang & Lane, 2012; Tontonoz & Spiegelman, 2008). The transcriptional activity of PPAR-γ could be mediated by agonist and antagonist. Fatty acids and prostanoids, as the endogenous ligands for PPAR-γ, can bind and activate PPAR-γ (Dussault & Forman, 2000; Kliewer et al., 1997). However, they are weak agonists compared to the strong synthetic thiazolidinedione agonists with robust insulin-sensitizing activities (Kung & Henry, 2012). The transcriptional activity of PPAR-γ is also regulated by post-translational modifications including phosphorylation, SUMOylation, and ubiquitination, providing additional possibilities for fine-tuning (Luconi et al., 2010). BGO and CLNA mixtures were shown to elevate the TNF-α level in C57BL/6J mice with diet-induced obesity and Sprague–Dawley rats (Chen et al., 2012; Koba et al., 2002), respectively, which are known to antagonize PPAR-γ target gene expression (Suzawa et al., 2003). PSO was also shown to inhibit the adipogenesis and differentiation and decrease the protein level of PPAR-γ in 3T3-L1 preadipocytes (Lai et al., 2012). Moreover, sustained activation of ERK/MAPK signaling pathway, accompanied by PPAR-γ phosphorylation, caused by α-ESA in the 3T3-L1 cell differentiation model might not only contribute to apoptosis but also have an inhibitory effect on adipogenesis (Chou et al., 2012).

A neurobiological mechanism of the antiobesity effect of BGO was proposed (Xu et al., 2016). Supplementation with 1 g/kg of BGO in mice fed by a high-fat diet for 3 weeks significantly reversed the obese characteristics. The mechanism of BGO's antiobesity effect may involve the alterations of hypothalamic spine densities, as well as their causative mTOR pathway (Xu et al., 2016).

16.7 Effect of conjugated linolenic acid on type 2 diabetes mellitus

Type 2 diabetes mellitus is one of the most epidemics worldwide and has become a serious threat to public health. The nutritional and dietary interventions have been considered complementary approaches for the treatment of type 2 diabetes mellitus. PSO or PUA could have therapeutic effects in type 2 diabetes mellitus.

Insulin resistance could cause type 2 diabetes mellitus, and the improvement in insulin resistance is associated with the decrease in the risk of developing type 2 diabetes mellitus. A series of studies investigated the effects of PSO or PUA on insulin and glycemic parameters. Incubation of 3T3-L1 adipocyte cells with TNF-α for 24h in the presence of PUA enhanced insulin secretion and protected 3T3-L1 adipocytes from TNF-α-induced insulin resistance (Anusree et al., 2015). Dietary PUA decreased fasting plasma glucose concentrations and improved the glucose-normalizing ability in mice (Hontecillas et al., 2009). Supplementation with 1% PSO in mice fed a high-fat diet for 12 weeks did not affect liver insulin sensitivity but clearly improved peripheral insulin resistance (Vroegrijk et al., 2011). PSO supplementation of 2mL/kg/day on high-fat and high-sucrose (HF/HS) diet-induced obese (DIO) mice for 4 weeks significantly improved insulin sensitivity and reduced fasting blood glucose (Harzallah et al., 2016). Consumption of daily three capsules containing 1g of PSO significantly decreased the within-group fasting blood sugar of obese type 2 diabetic patients (Khajebishak, Payahoo, Alivand, Hamishehkar, et al., 2019).

In addition, CLNA could also have a protective effect against lipid oxidative damage in streptozotocin-induced diabetic rats. Supplementation with PSO or BGO with 0.5% of PUA or 0.5% of α-ESA in streptozotocin-induced diabetic rats for 4 weeks significantly reduced the oxidative stress and lipid peroxidation and restored antioxidant and pro-inflammatory enzymes, such as superoxide dismutase, catalase, and glutathione peroxidase, and reduced glutathione and NO synthase levels in pancreas, blood, and erythrocyte lysate (Saha & Ghosh, 2012). Supplementation with 0.36 and 0.72 mg/kg/daily of PSO in streptozotocin-induced diabetic rats for 3 weeks resulted in a significant increase in glutathione reductase, glutathione peroxidase, and catalase activity and decreased oxidative stress index (Mollazadeh, 2017).

CLNA exerts antidiabetic effects via various mechanisms (Khajebishak, Payahoo, Alivand, & Alipour, 2019). PUA improves glycemic parameters via increasing insulin secretion and upregulation and activation of GLUT4 expression in 3T3-L1 adipocytes (Anusree et al., 2014). Consumption of daily three capsules containing 1g of PSO also significantly increased the GLUT4 gene expression in obese type 2 diabetic patients. GLUT-4 gene expression was increased significantly in the PSO group. PUA of 5, 10, and 30mM improved the insulin resistance of 3T3-L1 adipocytes induced by TNF-α. PUA significantly decreased the phosphorylation of JNK level, the serine phosphorylation at IRS1 residue, and the SOCS3 expression in a dose-dependent manner, thus improving insulin sensitivity in 3T3-L1 adipocytes treated by TNF-α. PUA also ameliorated significantly the upregulation of pro-inflammatory cytokines, suggesting that the anti-inflammatory property of PUA contributes significantly to its insulin-sensitizing potential (Anusree et al., 2018).

16.8 Effect of conjugated linolenic acid on inflammatory bowel diseases

Several in vivo studies assessed the anti-inflammatory effects of PSO or PUA on inflammatory bowel disease (IBD) and the model of necrotizing enterocolitis (NEC) (Table 16.3). Oral administration of pure PUA (400μg/d) or 0.5mL/d of PUA-enriched PSO for 10 days before TNBS injection in a colitis rat model ameliorated the ulceration status and tissue damage, limiting neutrophil activation and lipid peroxidation (Boussetta et al., 2009). Supplementation with 1% of dietary PUA ameliorated spontaneous panenteritis in IL-10$^{-/-}$ model mice of IBD for 42 days and mice with experimental IBD during a 7-day challenge

TABLE 16.3 The effect of punicic acid and α-eleostearic acid on inflammatory bowel diseases.

Isomer (purity)	Animals	Dose of supplementation	Study duration	Results	Ref.
PUA-enriched PSO	Male Wistar rats with TNBS-induced colitis	2% wt diet	10 days	Decreased: ulceration status and tissue damage	Boussetta et al. (2009)
Pure PUA	Male Wistar rats with TNBS-induced colitis	400 µg/d	10 days	Decreased: ulceration status and tissue damage	Boussetta et al. (2009)
PUA-enriched PSO(71%)	IL-10−/− model mice with spontaneous pan-enteritis	1% wt diet	42 days	Decreased: lymphoplasmacytic infiltration Decreased: enlargement of the colonic mucosa	Bassaganya-Riera, DiGuardo, et al. (2011)
PUA-enriched PSO (71%)	C57BL/6J mice with DSS-induced colitis	1% wt diet	42 days	Decreased: experimental IBD	Bassaganya-Riera, DiGuardo, et al. (2011)
PUA-enriched PSO	Neonatal Sprague–Dawley rats with induced NEC	1.5% wt diet	96 h	Decreased: incidence of NEC from 61 to 26% Decreased: necrotizing colitis severity	Coursodon-Boyiddle et al. (2012)
α-ESA-enriched BGO	C57BL/6J mice with DSS-induced colitis	Not mentioned	42 days	Decreased: disease activity Decreased: IBD-related disease phenotypes	Lewis et al. (2011)

PSO, pomegranate seed oil; *BGO*, bitter melon seed oil; *PUA*, punicic acid; *α-ESA*, α-eleostearic acid; *IBD*, inflammatory bowel diseases; *NEC*, necrotizing enterocolitis.

with DSS (Bassaganya-Riera, DiGuardo, et al., 2011). PSO has also been shown to be effective also in a model of NEC. Oral administration with 1.5% of PSO decreased the incidence of NEC from 61% to 26% and severity of necrotizing colitis, protecting the epithelial barrier and preserving the intestinal integrity in the neonatal model of NEC rats (Coursodon-Boyiddle et al., 2012). These results suggested that PUA or PUA-enriched PSO could ameliorate intestinal inflammation and damage.

The underlying mechanisms by which PUA ameliorates experimental IBD are incompletely understood. Similar with *cis*-9, *trans*-11 CLA, PUA was suggested as a potential PPAR-γ agonist (Anusree et al., 2014; Bassaganya-Riera, DiGuardo, et al., 2011; Hontecillas et al., 2009). PUA was shown to robustly bind and activate PPAR-γ, therefore increasing PPAR-γ-responsive gene expression and ameliorating diabetes and gut inflammation (Viladomiu et al., 2013). PUA ameliorated spontaneous panenteritis in IL-10$^{-/-}$ mice and DSS colitis, upregulated Foxp3 expression in T-cell, and suppressed TNF-, but the loss of functional PPAR-γ or -δ impaired these anti-inflammatory effects. The deletion of PPAR-γ in macrophages completely abrogated the amelioration effect of PUA on experimental colitis, whereas the deletion of PPAR-δ or intestinal epithelial cell-specific PPAR-γ decreased its anti-inflammatory efficacy. These results strongly suggested that PUA ameliorates experimental IBD by regulating macrophage and T-cell function through PPAR-γ- and δ-dependent mechanisms (Bassaganya-Riera, DiGuardo, et al., 2011).

α-ESA was also identified as a natural PPAR-γ agonist by using complementary computational and experimental methods and found to be effective in ameliorating disease-associated phenotypes in mice with DSS colitis (Lewis et al., 2011). Activation of PPAR-γ by α-ESA could play an important role in the amelioration of DSS-induced IBD. The anti-inflammatory actions of α-ESA may be both PPAR-γ-dependent and -independent responses that ameliorated the disease activity and intestinal lesions in mice with DSS colitis (Lewis et al., 2011).

Targeting PPAR-γ represents a promising avenue for developing novel prophylactic and therapeutic interventions for IBD (Bertin et al., 2013; Dubuquoy et al., 2006) and obesity (Penumetcha & Santanam, 2012; Tasdelen, 2014). Due to the side effects of full thiazolidinedione agonists of PPAR-γ, there is a demand for naturally occurring PPAR-γ modulators from edible items with minimum adverse effects and high tolerance to the human body (Penumetcha & Santanam, 2012). *Trans*-10, *cis*-12CLA has demonstrated antiobesity effects through regulation of expression and activity of PPAR-γ, which is involved in reducing adipogenesis and lipogenesis and increasing inflammation. CLA (*cis*-9, *trans*-11 CLA or mixtures of *cis*-9, *trans*-11 CLA and *trans*-10, *cis*-12 CLA) was also effective in ameliorating the experimental IBD through activation of PPAR-γ. However, the safety of CLA is still of utmost concern and has been evaluated in numerous animal studies and human clinical trials (Dilzer & Park, 2012). A minority of studies have reported ambiguous or deleterious effects of CLA supplementation with regard to liver functions, milk fat depression, insulin resistance, and oxidative markers (Masters et al., 2002; Ramos et al., 2009; Risérus et al., 2002; Tholstrup et al., 2008). Although the safety of Clarinol and Tonalin TG 80, two oils with approximately 80% of the CLA 50:50 mixture of *cis*-9, *trans* and *trans*-10, *cis*-12 isomers, has been established for the proposed uses and daily doses (3.75 g Clarinol and 4.5 g Tonalin TG 80 corresponding to approximately 3 and 3.5 g of CLA, respectively) for up to 6 months by EFSA Panel on Dietetic Products, Nutrition and Allergies. However, the safety of CLA consumption for periods longer than six months has not been established under the proposed conditions of use (Scientific Opinion, 2012). These observations must be carefully considered, and further investigation is necessary before the widespread use of CLA as a functional food component.

PUA and α-ESA, which were identified as natural agonists of PPAR-γ, have proved beneficial effects on an animal model of intestinal inflammation. PUA and α-ESA also exerted anti-adiposity effect through the regulation of PPAR-γ. Acute toxicological studies have demonstrated that PUA is safe in rats (Meerts et al., 2009). Therefore, these plant-derived natural products are safer and may open the possibility to be used as functional food and nutraceuticals. However, the exact mechanism of PUA and α-ESA exerts their physiological roles, and human interventional studies are necessary to determine their beneficial effects on individuals with obesity or IBD.

CLNA (PUA and α-ESA) play an important role in modulating the expression or activity of PPAR-γ and that could, in turn, be employed as a complementary treatment for obesity and IBD. PUA and α-ESA are identified as natural agonists of PPAR-γ and exert a beneficial effect on the animal model of intestinal inflammation through the activation of PPAR-γ. In addition, PUA and α-ESA might exert their anti-adiposity effect by the induction of cytokine and inhibition of adipogenesis and preadipocyte differentiation through regulation of PPAR-γ.

16.9 Antioxidant activity of CLNA

Plasma lipid peroxidation was significantly lower in rats fed dietary supplementation of 0.5% of α-ESA than control rats (Dhar et al., 1999). The activity of PUA supplemented in the diet of rats at different concentrations was investigated, and it appeared to be efficient as an antioxidant, with maximum antioxidant activity of 0.6% of PUA (Mukherjee et al., 2002). The dietary effect of CLNA on lipid peroxidation in alloxan-induced diabetes mellitus in rats was investigated and the result found that LDL and erythrocyte membrane lipid peroxidation were reduced significantly in rats fed 0.5% of α-ESA (Dhar et al., 2007).

A series of studies in vitro and in vivo conducted by the same group investigated the antioxidant activity of CLNA isomers against chemically induced oxidative stress (Saha, Dasgupta, et al., 2012; Saha & Ghosh, 2009, 2010, 2011; Saha, Patra, & Ghosh, 2012). The antioxidant activity of vegetable oils containing α-ESA and PUA in vitro was evaluated. The results showed that α-ESA and PUA exerted better antioxidant activity at a lower concentration ($125\,mg\,mL^{-1}$) due to better oxidative stability and BGO showed more prominent antioxidant activity than snake gourd oil due to the presence of higher trans content (Saha, Patra, & Ghosh, 2012). The antioxidant efficacy of α-ESA and PUA against arsenic-induced oxidative stress in rats was evaluated (Saha & Ghosh, 2009). The result suggested that α-ESA and PUA increased the activities of superoxide dismutase (SOD), catalase, and glutathione peroxidase and decreased the activity of nitric oxide synthase to a normal level in liver, plasma, and brain (Saha & Ghosh, 2009). In the following studies, the antioxidant activity of α-ESA and PUA against arsenic-induced oxidative stress in rats was further confirmed (Saha & Ghosh, 2010, 2011). However, the antioxidant activity of α-ESA was more predominant than that of PUA in those studies above (Saha & Ghosh, 2009, 2010, 2011). Moreover, α-ESA and PUA (mixture of 1:1, 0.5% and 1.0% of total lipid given for 30 days, respectively) showed a synergistic antioxidant effect against sodium arsenite-induced oxidative stress in the plasma, liver, and brain of rats (Saha, Dasgupta, et al., 2012).

In other studies, the effects of α-LNA and α-ESA (0.5% and 1.0% of total lipid given for each kind of CLNA isomer) against methylmercury-induced oxidative stress were evaluated under in vivo conditions. Results also showed that the activity of antioxidant enzymes of plasma and brain, liver, and kidney tissue and total antioxidant capacity in plasma decreased significantly due to the oxidative stress generated by MeHgCl. Administration of higher doses of both kinds of linolenic acid restored all the activities of antioxidant enzymes and also reduced lipid peroxidation and increased total antioxidant capacity in plasma (Pal & Ghosh, 2012a, 2012b).

However, controversial results for the antioxidant or prooxidant activity of CLNA were reported. Dietary BGO significantly increased the level of plasma hydroperoxides and liver lipid oxidation. A slight but significant increase in hydroperoxides was found in rats fed with 2.0% of BGO. This may be attributed to the lower oxidative stability of α-ESA in BGO (Noguchi et al., 2001). α-ESA- induced lipid peroxidation in DLD-1 cells and transplanted tumors in nude mice (Tsuzuki, Tokuyama, Igarashi, & Miyazawa, 2004). In our clinical study, human subjects supplemented with PUA naturally occurring in trichosanthes seeds exhibited prooxidant activity and increased lipid peroxidation in healthy young humans although the dose used in our study is much lower than the dose used in an animal study (Yuan, Wahlqvist, Yuan, et al., 2009). Similar results were found with other conjugated fatty acids. Supplementation with CLA mixtures at 4.2 g per day increased urinary 8-isoPGF2$_\alpha$ in healthy middle-aged men after 3 months and in middle-aged men with abdominal obesity after 1 month, respectively (Basu, Risérus, et al., 2000; Basu, Smedman, & Vessby, 2000). Other studies also showed that milk or dairy products naturally enriched with CLA can increase lipid peroxidation in humans (Raff et al., 2008; Tholstrup et al., 2008).

Therefore, the antioxidant or prooxidant effect of CLNA in animals and humans is not exclusive. The controversial results obtained from different studies could be due to the dose of CLNA used in animal and human studies. Animal studies have shown that PUA has both prooxidant (at $1.2\,kg^{-1}$ PUA level) and antioxidant (at $6\,kg^{-1}$ PUA level) effects depending on the doses used (Mukherjee et al., 2002; Mukherjee & Bhattacharyya, 2006).

16.10 Conclusion

In this chapter, evidence relating to the physiological role of PUA and α-ESA, such as the anti-carcinogenic, lipid metabolism regulation, anti-inflammatory, anti-obese, and anti-diabetic activities, was reviewed and updated. The available results may provide a potential application for CLNA isomers from natural sources, especially edible plant seeds, as effective functional food ingredients and dietary supplements for the above-mentioned disease management.

Some issues are remained to be resolved before CLNA can be recommended to humans with confidence to improve the health and quality of life, particularly regarding mechanisms and safety concerns. More well-controlled clinical trials with defined subject characteristics, study duration, and doses and preparations on the safety and physiological effects are urgently needed. Moreover, further studies are necessary in order to identify the diversified molecular signaling pathways and the crosstalk among these signaling pathways mediated by CLNA to provide valuable information on the efficacy, specificity, and potential side effects of CLNA.

References

Albrecht, M., Jiang, W., Kumi-Diaka, J., Lansky, E. P., Gommersall, L. M., Patel, A., et al. (2004). Pomegranate extracts potently suppress proliferation, xenograft growth, and invasion of human prostate cancer cells. *Journal of Medicinal Food*, 7(3), 274–283. https://doi.org/10.1089/jmf.2004.7.274.

Anusree, S. S., Nisha, V. M., Priyanka, A., & Raghu, K. G. (2015). Insulin resistance by TNF-α is associated with mitochondrial dysfunction in 3T3-L1 adipocytes and is ameliorated by punicic acid, a PPARγ agonist. *Molecular and Cellular Endocrinology*, 413, 120–128. https://doi.org/10.1016/j.mce.2015.06.018.

Anusree, S. S., Priyanka, A., Nisha, V. M., Das, A. A., & Raghu, K. G. (2014). An in vitro study reveals the nutraceutical potential of punicic acid relevant to diabetes via enhanced GLUT4 expression and adiponectin secretion. *Food & Function*, 5(10), 2590–2601. https://doi.org/10.1039/c4fo00302k.

Anusree, S. S., Sindhu, G., Preetha Rani, M. R., & Raghu, K. G. (2018). Insulin resistance in 3T3-L1 adipocytes by TNF-α is improved by punicic acid through upregulation of insulin signalling pathway and endocrine function, and downregulation of proinflammatory cytokines. *Biochimie*, 146, 79–86. https://doi.org/10.1016/j.biochi.2017.11.014.

Arao, K., Wang, Y. M., Inoue, N., Hirata, J., Cha, J. Y., Nagao, K., et al. (2004). Dietary effect of pomegranate seed oil rich in 9cis, 11trans, 13cis conjugated linolenic acid on lipid metabolism in obese, hyperlipidemic OLETF rats. *Lipids in Health and Disease*, 3. https://doi.org/10.1186/1476-511X-3-24.

Arao, K., Yotsumoto, H., Han, S. Y., Nagao, K., & Yanagita, T. (2004). The 9cis,11trans,13cis isomer of conjugated linolenic acid reduces apolipoprotein B100 secretion and triacylglycerol synthesis in Hep G2 cells. *Bioscience, Biotechnology, and Biochemistry, 68*(12), 2643–2645. https://doi.org/10.1271/bbb.68.2643.

Bassaganya-Riera, J., DiGuardo, M., Climent, M., Vives, C., Carbo, A., Jouni, Z. E., et al. (2011). Activation of PPARγ and δ by dietary punicic acid ameliorates intestinal inflammation in mice. *British Journal of Nutrition, 106*(6), 878–886. https://doi.org/10.1017/S0007114511001188.

Bassaganya-Riera, J., Guri, A. J., & Hontecillas, R. (2011). Treatment of obesity-related complications with novel classes of naturally occurring PPAR agonists. *Journal of Obesity, 2011.* https://doi.org/10.1155/2011/897894.

Basu, S., Risérus, U., Turpeinen, A., & Vessby, B. (2000). Conjugated linoleic acid induces lipid peroxidation in men with abdominal obesity. *Clinical Science, 99*(6), 511–516. https://doi.org/10.1042/CS20000116.

Basu, S., Smedman, A., & Vessby, B. (2000). Conjugated linoleic acid induces lipid peroxidation in humans. *FEBS Letters, 468*(1), 33–36. https://doi.org/10.1016/S0014-5793(00)01193-5.

Belury, M. A. (2002). Inhibition of carcinogenesis by conjugated linoleic acid: Potential mechanisms of action. *Journal of Nutrition, 132*(10), 2995–2998. https://doi.org/10.1093/jn/131.10.2995.

Bertin, B., Dubuquoy, L., Colombel, J. F., & Desreumaux, P. (2013). PPAR-gamma in ulcerative colitis: A novel target for intervention. *Current Drug Targets, 14*(12), 1501–1507. https://doi.org/10.2174/13894501113149990162.

Bhattacharya, A., Banu, J., Rahman, M., Causey, J., & Fernandes, G. (2006). Biological effects of conjugated linoleic acids in health and disease. *Journal of Nutritional Biochemistry, 17*(12), 789–810. https://doi.org/10.1016/j.jnutbio.2006.02.009.

Boussetta, T., Raad, H., Lettéron, P., Gougerot-Pocidalo, M. A., Marie, J. C., Driss, F., et al. (2009). Punicic acid a conjugated linolenic acid inhibits TNFα-induced neutrophil hyperactivation and protects from experimental colon inflammation in rats. *PLoS One, 4*(7). https://doi.org/10.1371/journal.pone.0006458.

Chang, Y. Y., Su, H. M., Chen, S. H., Hsieh, W. T., Chyuan, J. H., & Chao, P. M. (2016). Roles of peroxisome proliferator-activated receptor α in bitter melon seed oil-corrected lipid disorders and conversion of α-eleostearic acid into rumenic acid in C57Bl/6J mice. *Nutrients, 8*(12). https://doi.org/10.3390/nu8120805.

Chen, P. H., Chen, G. C., Yang, M. F., Hsieh, C. H., Chuang, S. H., Yang, H. L., et al. (2012). Bitter melon seed oil-attenuated body fat accumulation in diet-induced obese mice is associated with cAMP-dependent protein kinase activation and cell death in white adipose tissue. *Journal of Nutrition, 142*(7), 1197–1204. https://doi.org/10.3945/jn.112.159939.

Chen, G. C., Su, H. M., Lin, Y. S., Tsou, P. Y., Chyuan, J. H., & Chao, P. M. (2016). A conjugated fatty acid present at high levels in bitter melon seed favorably affects lipid metabolism in hepatocytes by increasing NAD+/NADH ratio and activating PPARα, AMPK and SIRT1 signaling pathway. *The Journal of Nutritional Biochemistry, 33,* 28–35. https://doi.org/10.1016/j.jnutbio.2016.03.009.

Chou, Y. C., Su, H. M., Lai, T. W., Chyuan, J. H., & Chao, P. M. (2012). Cis-9, trans-11, trans-13-conjugated linolenic acid induces apoptosis and sustained ERK phosphorylation in 3T3-L1 preadipocytes. *Nutrition, 28*(7–8), 803–811. https://doi.org/10.1016/j.nut.2011.11.019.

Chuang, C. Y., Hsu, C., Chao, C. Y., Wein, Y. S., Kuo, Y. H., & Huang, C. J. (2006). Fractionation and identification of 9c, 11t, 13t-conjugated linolenic acid as an activator of PPARα in bitter gourd (Momordica charantia L.). *Journal of Biomedical Science, 13*(6), 763–772. https://doi.org/10.1007/s11373-006-9109-3.

Coursodon-Boyiddle, C. F., Snarrenberg, C. L., Adkins-Rieck, C. K., Bassaganya-Riera, J., Hontecillas, R., Lawrence, P., et al. (2012). Pomegranate seed oil reduces intestinal damage in a rat model of necrotizing enterocolitis. *American Journal of Physiology. Gastrointestinal and Liver Physiology, 303*(6), G744–G751. https://doi.org/10.1152/ajpgi.00248.2012.

Degen, C., Ecker, J., Piegholdt, S., Liebisch, G., Schmitz, G., & Jahreis, G. (2011). Metabolic and growth inhibitory effects of conjugated fatty acids in the cell line HT-29 with special regard to the conversion of t11,t13-CLA. *Biochimica et Biophysica Acta - Molecular and Cell Biology of Lipids, 1811*(12), 1070–1080. https://doi.org/10.1016/j.bbalip.2011.08.005.

Dhar, P., Bhattacharyya, D., Bhattacharyya, D. K., & Ghosh, S. (2006). Dietary comparison of conjugated linolenic acid (9 cis, 11 trans, 13 trans) and α-tocopherol effects on blood lipids and lipid peroxidation in alloxan-induced diabetes mellitus in rats. *Lipids, 41*(1), 49–54. https://doi.org/10.1007/s11745-006-5069-7.

Dhar, P., Chattopadhyay, K., Bhattacharyya, D., Roychoudhury, A., Biswas, A., & Ghosh, S. (2007). Antioxidative effect of conjugated linolenic acid in diabetic and non-diabetic blood: An in vitro study. *Journal of Oleo Science, 56*(1), 19–24. https://doi.org/10.5650/jos.56.19.

Dhar, P., Ghosh, S., & Bhattacharyya, D. K. (1999). Dietary effects of conjugated octadecatrienoic fatty acid (9 cis, 11 trans, 13 trans) levels on blood lipids and nonenzymatic in vitro lipid peroxidation in rats. *Lipids, 34*(2), 109–114. https://doi.org/10.1007/s11745-999-0343-2.

Dilzer, A., & Park, Y. (2012). Implication of conjugated linoleic acid (CLA) in human health. *Critical Reviews in Food Science and Nutrition, 52*(6), 488–513. https://doi.org/10.1080/10408398.2010.501409.

Dubuquoy, L., Rousseaux, C., Thuru, X., Peyrin-Biroulet, L., Romano, O., Chavatte, P., et al. (2006). PPARγ as a new therapeutic target in inflammatory bowel diseases. *Gut, 55*(9), 1341–1349. https://doi.org/10.1136/gut.2006.093484.

Dussault, I., & Forman, B. M. (2000). Prostaglandins and fatty acids regulate transcriptional signaling via the peroxisome proliferator activated receptor nuclear receptors. *Prostaglandins and Other Lipid Mediators, 62*(1), 1–13. https://doi.org/10.1016/S0090-6980(00)00071-X.

Garaiova, M., Mietkiewska, E., Weselake, R. J., & Holic, R. (2017). Metabolic engineering of Schizosaccharomyces pombe to produce punicic acid, a conjugated fatty acid with nutraceutic properties. *Applied Microbiology and Biotechnology, 101*(21), 7913–7922. https://doi.org/10.1007/s00253-017-8498-8.

Gasmi, J., & Sanderson, J. T. (2010). Growth inhibitory, antiandrogenic, and pro-apoptotic effects of punicic acid in LNCaP human prostate cancer cells. *Journal of Agricultural and Food Chemistry, 58*(23), 12149–12156. https://doi.org/10.1021/jf103306k.

Gasmi, J., & Thomas Sanderson, J. (2013). Jacaric acid and its octadecatrienoic acid geoisomers induce apoptosis selectively in cancerous human prostate cells: A mechanistic and 3-D structure-activity study. *Phytomedicine, 20*(8–9), 734–742. https://doi.org/10.1016/j.phymed.2013.01.012.

Grossmann, M. E., Mizuno, N. K., Dammen, M. L., Schuster, T., Ray, A., & Cleary, M. P. (2009). Eleostearic acid inhibits breast cancer proliferation by means of an oxidation-dependent mechanism. *Cancer Prevention Research, 2*(10), 879–886. https://doi.org/10.1158/1940-6207.CAPR-09-0088.

Grossmann, M. E., Mizuno, N. K., Schuster, T., & Cleary, M. P. (2010). Punicic acid is an ω-5 fatty acid capable of inhibiting breast cancer proliferation. *International Journal of Oncology, 36*(2), 421–426. https://doi.org/10.3892/ijo-00000515.

Harzallah, A., Hammami, M., Kępczyńska, M. A., Hislop, D. C., Arch, J. R. S., Cawthorne, M. A., et al. (2016). Comparison of potential preventive effects of pomegranate flower, peel and seed oil on insulin resistance and inflammation in high-fat and high-sucrose diet-induced obesity mice model. *Archives of Physiology and Biochemistry, 122*(2), 75–87. https://doi.org/10.3109/13813455.2016.1148053.

Holic, R., Xu, Y., Caldo, K. M. P., Singer, S. D., Field, C. J., Weselake, R. J., et al. (2018). Bioactivity and biotechnological production of punicic acid. *Applied Microbiology and Biotechnology, 102*(8), 3537–3549. https://doi.org/10.1007/s00253-018-8883-y.

Hontecillas, R., O'Shea, M., Einerhand, A., Diguardo, M., & Bassaganya-Riera, J. (2009). Activation of ppar γ and α by punicic acid ameliorates glucose tolerance and suppresses obesity-related inflammation. *Journal of the American College of Nutrition, 28*(2), 184–195. https://doi.org/10.1080/07315724.2009.10719770.

Hora, J. J., Maydew, E. R., Lansky, E. P., & Dwivedi, C. (2003). Chemopreventive effects of pomegranate seed oil on skin tumor development in CD1 mice. *Journal of Medicinal Food, 6*(3), 157–161. https://doi.org/10.1089/10966200360716553.

Hsieh, C. H., Chen, G. C., Chen, P. H., Wu, T. F., & Chao, P. M. (2013). Altered white adipose tissue protein profile in C57BL/6J mice displaying delipidative, inflammatory, and browning characteristics after bitter melon seed oil treatment. *PLoS One, 8*(9). https://doi.org/10.1371/journal.pone.0072917.

Igarashi, M., & Miyazawa, T. (2000). Newly recognized cytotoxic effect of conjugated trienoic fatty acids on cultured human tumor cells. *Cancer Letters, 148*(2), 173–179. https://doi.org/10.1016/S0304-3835(99)00332-8.

Igarashi, M., & Miyazawa, T. (2005). Preparation and fractionation of conjugated trienes from α-linolenic acid and their growth-inhibitory effects on human tumor cells and fibroblasts. *Lipids, 40*(1), 109–113. https://doi.org/10.1007/s11745-005-1365-5.

Kennedy, A., Martinez, K., Schmidt, S., Mandrup, S., LaPoint, K., & McIntosh, M. (2010). Antiobesity mechanisms of action of conjugated linoleic acid. *Journal of Nutritional Biochemistry, 21*(3), 171–179. https://doi.org/10.1016/j.jnutbio.2009.08.003.

Khajebishak, Y., Payahoo, L., Alivand, M., & Alipour, B. (2019). Punicic acid: A potential compound of pomegranate seed oil in type 2 diabetes mellitus management. *Journal of Cellular Physiology, 234*(3), 2112–2120. https://doi.org/10.1002/jcp.27556.

Khajebishak, Y., Payahoo, L., Alivand, M., Hamishehkar, H., Mobasseri, M., Ebrahimzadeh, V., et al. (2019). Effect of pomegranate seed oil supplementation on the GLUT-4 gene expression and glycemic control in obese people with type 2 diabetes: A randomized controlled clinical trial. *Journal of Cellular Physiology, 234*(11), 19621–19628. https://doi.org/10.1002/jcp.28561.

Khoddami, A., Man, Y. B. C., & Roberts, T. H. (2014). Physico-chemical properties and fatty acid profile of seed oils from pomegranate (Punica granatum L.) extracted by cold pressing. *European Journal of Lipid Science and Technology, 116*(5), 553–562. https://doi.org/10.1002/ejlt.201300416.

Kim, N. D., Mehta, R., Yu, W., Neeman, I., Livney, T., Amichay, A., et al. (2002). Chemopreventive and adjuvant therapeutic potential of pomegranate (Punica granatum) for human breast cancer. *Breast Cancer Research and Treatment, 71*(3), 203–217. https://doi.org/10.1023/A:1014405730585.

Kitamura, Y., Yamagishi, M., Okazaki, K., Umemura, T., Imazawa, T., Nishikawa, A., et al. (2006). Lack of chemopreventive effects of α-eleostearic acid on 7,12-dimethylbenz[a]anthracene (DMBA) and 1,2-dimethylhydrazine (DMH)-induced mammary and colon carcinogenesis in female Sprague-Dawley rats. *Food and Chemical Toxicology*, 44(2), 271–277. https://doi.org/10.1016/j.fct.2004.11.021.

Kliewer, S. A., Sundseth, S. S., Jones, S. A., Brown, P. J., Wisely, G. B., Koble, C. S., et al. (1997). Fatty acids and eicosanoids regulate gene expression through direct interactions with peroxisome proliferator-activated receptors α and γ. *Proceedings of the National Academy of Sciences of the United States of America*, 94(9), 4318–4323. https://doi.org/10.1073/pnas.94.9.4318.

Koba, K., Akahoshi, A., Yamasaki, M., Tanaka, K., Yamada, K., Iwata, T., et al. (2002). Dietary conjugated linolenic acid in relation to CLA differently modifies body fat mass and serum and liver lipid levels in rats. *Lipids*, 37(4), 343–350. https://doi.org/10.1007/s11745-002-0901-7.

Koba, K., Imamura, J., Akashoshi, A., Kohno-Murase, J., Nishizono, S., Iwabuchi, M., et al. (2007). Genetically modified rapeseed oil containing cis-9,trans-11,cis-13-octadecatrienoic acid affects body fat mass and lipid metabolism in mice. *Journal of Agricultural and Food Chemistry*, 55(9), 3741–3748. https://doi.org/10.1021/jf063264z.

Kohno, H., Suzuki, R., Noguchi, R., Hosokawa, M., Miyashita, K., & Tanaka, T. (2002). Dietary conjugated linolenic acid inhibits azoxymethane-induced colonic aberrant crypt foci in rats. *Japanese Journal of Cancer Research*, 93(2), 133–142. https://doi.org/10.1111/j.1349-7006.2002.tb01251.x.

Kohno, H., Suzuki, R., Yasui, Y., Hosokawa, M., Miyashita, K., & Tanaka, T. (2004). Pomegranate seed oil rich in conjugated linolenic acid suppresses chemically induced colon carcinogenesis in rats. *Cancer Science*, 95(6), 481–486. https://doi.org/10.1111/j.1349-7006.2004.tb03236.x.

Kohno, H., Yasui, Y., Suzuki, R., Hosokawa, M., Miyashita, K., & Tanaka, T. (2004). Dietary seed oil rich in conjugated linolenic acid from bitter melon inhibits azoxymethane-induced rat colon carcinogenesis through elevation of colonic PPARγ expression and alteration of lipid composition. *International Journal of Cancer*, 110(6), 896–901. https://doi.org/10.1002/ijc.20179.

Kondo, K., Obitsu, S., Ohta, S., Matsunami, K., Otsuka, H., & Teshima, R. (2010). Poly(ADP-ribose) polymerase (PARP)-1-independent apoptosis-inducing factor (AIF) release and cell death are induced by eleostearic acid and blocked by α-tocopherol and MEK inhibition. *Journal of Biological Chemistry*, 285(17), 13079–13091. https://doi.org/10.1074/jbc.M109.044206.

Kung, J., & Henry, R. R. (2012). Thiazolidinedione safety. *Expert Opinion on Drug Safety*, 11(4), 565–579. https://doi.org/10.1517/14740338.2012.691963.

Lai, C. S., Tsai, M. L., Badmaev, V., Jimenez, M., Ho, C. T., & Pan, M. H. (2012). Xanthigen suppresses preadipocyte differentiation and adipogenesis through downregulation of PPARγ and C/EBPs and modulation of SIRT-1, AMPK, and fox O pathways. *Journal of Agricultural and Food Chemistry*, 60(4), 1094–1101. https://doi.org/10.1021/jf204862d.

Lansky, E. P., Harrison, G., Froom, P., & Jiang, W. G. (2005). Pomegranate (Punica granatum) pure chemicals show possible synergistic inhibition of human PC-3 prostate cancer cell invasion across Matrigel™. *Investigational New Drugs*, 23(2), 121–122. https://doi.org/10.1007/s10637-005-5856-7.

Lewis, S. N., Brannan, L., Guri, A. J., Lu, P., Hontecillas, R., Bassaganya-Riera, J., & Bevan, D. R. (2011). Dietary alpha-eleostearic acid ameliorates experimental inflammatory bowel disease in mice by activating peroxisome proliferator-activated receptor-gamma. *PLoS One*, 6(8), e24031.

Liu, G., Xu, X., Hao, Q., & Gao, Y. (2009). Supercritical CO2 extraction optimization of pomegranate (Punica granatum L.) seed oil using response surface methodology. *LWT - Food Science and Technology*, 42(9), 1491–1495. https://doi.org/10.1016/j.lwt.2009.04.011.

Luconi, M., Cantini, G., & Serio, M. (2010). Peroxisome proliferator-activated receptor gamma (PPARγ): Is the genomic activity the only answer? *Steroids*, 75(8–9), 585–594. https://doi.org/10.1016/j.steroids.2009.10.012.

Masters, N., McGuire, M. A., Beerman, K. A., Dasgupta, N., & McGuire, M. K. (2002). Maternal supplementation with CLA decreases milk fat in humans. *Lipids*, 37(2), 133–138. https://doi.org/10.1007/s11745-002-0872-8.

McFarlin, B. K., Strohacker, K. A., & Kueht, M. L. (2009). Pomegranate seed oil consumption during a period of high-fat feeding reduces weight gain and reduces type 2 diabetes risk in CD-1 mice. *British Journal of Nutrition*, 102(1), 54–59. https://doi.org/10.1017/S0007114508159001.

Meerts, I. A. T. M., Verspeek-Rip, C. M., Buskens, C. A. F., Keizer, H. G., Bassaganya-Riera, J., Jouni, Z. E., et al. (2009). Toxicological evaluation of pomegranate seed oil. *Food and Chemical Toxicology*, 47(6), 1085–1092. https://doi.org/10.1016/j.fct.2009.01.031.

Mietkiewska, E., Miles, R., Wickramarathna, A., Sahibollah, A. F., Greer, M. S., Chen, G., et al. (2014). Combined transgenic expression of Punica granatum conjugase (FADX) and FAD2 desaturase in high linoleic acid

Arabidopsis thaliana mutant leads to increased accumulation of punicic acid. *Planta, 240*(3), 575–583. https://doi.org/10.1007/s00425-014-2109-z.

Miranda, J., Aguirre, L., Fernández-Quintela, A., MacArulla, M. T., Martínez-Castaño, M. G., Ayo, J., et al. (2013). Effects of pomegranate seed oil on glucose and lipid metabolism-related organs in rats fed an obesogenic diet. *Journal of Agricultural and Food Chemistry, 61*(21), 5089–5096. https://doi.org/10.1021/jf305076v.

Mirmiran, P., Fazeli, M. R., Asghari, G., Shafiee, A., & Azizi, F. (2010). Effect of pomegranate seed oil on hyperlipidaemic subjects: A double-blind placebo-controlled clinical trial. *British Journal of Nutrition, 104*(3), 402–406. https://doi.org/10.1017/S0007114510000504.

Mollazadeh, H. (2017). Effects of pomegranate seed oil on oxidant/antioxidant balance in heart and kidney homogenates and mitochondria of diabetic rats and high glucose-treated H9c2 cell line. *Avicenna Journal of Phytomedicine, 7*(4), 317–333.

Moon, H. S., Guo, D. D., Lee, H. G., Choi, Y. J., Kang, J. S., Jo, K., et al. (2010). Alpha-eleostearic acid suppresses proliferation of MCF-7 breast cancer cells via activation of PPARγ and inhibition of ERK 1/2. *Cancer Science, 101*(2), 396–402. https://doi.org/10.1111/j.1349-7006.2009.01389.x.

Mukherjee, C., & Bhattacharyya, D. (2006). Dietary effect of punicic acid on oxidative behavior and lipid profiles of brain, heart, liver and kidney tissue lipid of rats. *Journal of Lipid Science and Technology, 38*, 124–128.

Mukherjee, C., Bhattacharyya, S., Ghosh, S., & Bhattacharyya, D. K. (2002). Dietary effects of punicic acid on the composition and peroxidation of rat plasma lipid. *Journal of Oleo Science, 51*(8), 513–522. https://doi.org/10.5650/jos.51.513.

Noguchi, R., Yasui, Y., Suzuki, R., Hosokawa, M., Fukunaga, K., & Miyashita, K. (2001). Dietary effects of bitter gourd oil on blood and liver lipids of rats. *Archives of Biochemistry and Biophysics, 396*(2), 207–212. https://doi.org/10.1006/abbi.2001.2624.

Pal, M., & Ghosh, M. (2012a). Prophylactic effect of alpha-linolenic acid and alpha-eleostearic acid against MeHg induced oxidative stress, DNA damage and structural changes in RBC membrane. *Food and Chemical Toxicology, 50*(8), 2811–2818.

Pal, M., & Ghosh, M. (2012b). Studies on comparative efficacy of α-linolenic acid and α-eleostearic acid on prevention of organic mercury-induced oxidative stress in kidney and liver of rat. *Food and Chemical Toxicology, 50*(3–4), 1066–1072. https://doi.org/10.1016/j.fct.2011.12.042.

Penumetcha, M., & Santanam, N. (2012). Nutraceuticals as ligands of PPAR gamma. *PPAR Research,* 858352. https://doi.org/10.1155/2012/858352.

Raff, M., Tholstrup, T., Basu, S., Nonboe, P., Sørensen, M. T., & Straarup, E. M. (2008). A diet rich in conjugated linoleic acid and butter increases lipid peroxidation but does not affect atherosclerotic, inflammatory, or diabetic risk markers in healthy young men. *Journal of Nutrition, 138*(3), 509–514. https://doi.org/10.1093/jn/138.3.509.

Ramos, R., Mascarenhas, J., Duarte, P., Vicente, C., & Casteleiro, C. (2009). Conjugated linoleic acid-induced toxic hepatitis: First case report. *Digestive Diseases and Sciences, 54*(5), 1141–1143. https://doi.org/10.1007/s10620-008-0461-1.

Risérus, U., Basu, S., Jovinge, S., Fredrikson, G. N., Ärnlöv, J., & Vessby, B. (2002). Supplementation with conjugated linoleic acid causes isomer-dependent oxidative stress and elevated C-reactive protein: A potential link to fatty acid-induced insulin resistance. *Circulation, 106*(15), 1925–1929. https://doi.org/10.1161/01.CIR.0000033589.15413.48.

Saha, S. S., Dasgupta, P., Sengupta, S., & Ghosh, M. (2012). Synergistic effect of conjugated linolenic acid isomers against induced oxidative stress, inflammation and erythrocyte membrane disintegrity in rat model. *Biochimica et Biophysica Acta - General Subjects, 1820*(12), 1951–1970. https://doi.org/10.1016/j.bbagen.2012.08.021.

Saha, S. S., & Ghosh, M. (2009). Comparative study of antioxidant activity of α-eleostearic acid and punicic acid against oxidative stress generated by sodium arsenite. *Food and Chemical Toxicology, 47*(10), 2551–2556. https://doi.org/10.1016/j.fct.2009.07.012.

Saha, S. S., & Ghosh, M. (2010). Ameliorative role of conjugated linolenic acid isomers against oxidative DNA damage induced by sodium arsenite in rat model. *Food and Chemical Toxicology, 48*(12), 3398–3405. https://doi.org/10.1016/j.fct.2010.09.011.

Saha, S. S., & Ghosh, M. (2011). Antioxidant effect of vegetable oils containing conjugated linolenic acid isomers against induced tissue lipid peroxidation and inflammation in rat model. *Chemico-Biological Interactions, 190*(2–3), 109–120. https://doi.org/10.1016/j.cbi.2011.02.030.

Saha, S. S., & Ghosh, M. (2012). Antioxidant and anti-inflammatory effect of conjugated linolenic acid isomers against streptozotocin-induced diabetes. *British Journal of Nutrition, 108*(6), 974–983. https://doi.org/10.1017/S0007114511006325.

Saha, S. S., Patra, M., & Ghosh, M. (2012). In vitro antioxidant study of vegetable oils containing conjugated linolenic acid isomers. *LWT - Food Science and Technology, 46*(1), 10–15. https://doi.org/10.1016/j.lwt.2011.11.008.

Schneider, A. C., Beguin, P., Bourez, S., Perfield, J. W., Mignolet, E., Debier, C., et al. (2012). Conversion of t11t13 CLA into C9t11 CLA in CACO-2 cells and inhibition by sterculic oil. *PLoS One*, 7(3). https://doi.org/10.1371/journal.pone.0032824.

Schneider, A. C., Mignolet, E., Schneider, Y. J., & Larondelle, Y. (2013). Uptake of conjugated linolenic acids and conversion to cis-9, trans-11-or trans-9, trans-11-conjugated linoleic acids in Caco-2 cells. *British Journal of Nutrition*, 109(1), 57–64. https://doi.org/10.1017/S0007114512000608.

Scientific Opinion. (2012). Statement on the safety of the "conjugated linoleic acid (CLA)-rich oils" Clarinol® and Tonalin TG 80 as Novel Food ingredients. In *Vol. 10. EFSA panel on dietetic products*.

Scorletti, E., & Byrne, C. D. (2018). Omega-3 fatty acids and non-alcoholic fatty liver disease: Evidence of efficacy and mechanism of action. *Molecular Aspects of Medicine*, 64, 135–146. https://doi.org/10.1016/j.mam.2018.03.001.

Sengupta, A., Gupta, S. S., Nandi, I., & Ghosh, M. (2015). Conjugated linolenic acid nanoparticles inhibit hypercholesterolemia induced by feeding a high-fat diet in male albino rats. *Journal of Food Science and Technology*, 52(1), 458–464. https://doi.org/10.1007/s13197-013-0974-2.

Shinohara, N., Tsuduki, T., Ito, J., Honma, T., Kijima, R., Sugawara, S., et al. (2012). Jacaric acid, a linolenic acid isomer with a conjugated triene system, has a strong antitumor effect in vitro and in vivo. *Biochimica et Biophysica Acta-Molecular and Cell Biology of Lipids*, 1821(7), 980–988. https://doi.org/10.1016/j.bbalip.2012.04.001.

Siersbæk, R., Nielsen, R., & Mandrup, S. (2010). PPARγ in adipocyte differentiation and metabolism—Novel insights from genome-wide studies. *FEBS Letters*, 584(15), 3242–3249. https://doi.org/10.1016/j.febslet.2010.06.010.

Suzawa, M., Takada, I., Yanagisawa, J., Ohtake, F., Ogawa, S., Yamauchi, T., et al. (2003). Cytokines suppress adipogenesis and PPAR-γ function through the TAK1/TAB1/NIK cascade. *Nature Cell Biology*, 5(3), 224–230. https://doi.org/10.1038/ncb942.

Suzuki, R., Noguchi, R., Ota, T., Abe, M., Miyashita, K., & Kawada, T. (2001). Cytotoxic effect of conjugated trienoic fatty acids on mouse tumor and human monocytic leukemia cells. *Lipids*, 36(5), 477–482. https://doi.org/10.1007/s11745-001-0746-0.

Tabaraki, R., Heidarizadi, E., & Benvidi, A. (2012). Optimization of ultrasonic-assisted extraction of pomegranate (Punica granatum L.) peel antioxidants by response surface methodology. *Separation and Purification Technology*, 98, 16–23. https://doi.org/10.1016/j.seppur.2012.06.038.

Tang, Q. Q., & Lane, M. D. (2012). Adipogenesis: From stem cell to adipocyte. *Annual Review of Biochemistry*, 81, 715–736. https://doi.org/10.1146/annurev-biochem-052110-115718.

Tasdelen, I. (2014). *Modulation of the adipogenic master regulator PPARγ*. Uitgeverij Boxpress.

Tholstrup, T., Raff, M., Straarup, E. M., Lund, P., Basu, S., & Bruun, J. M. (2008). An oil mixture with trans-10, cis-12 conjugated linoleic acid increases markers of inflammation and in vivo lipid peroxidation compared with cis-9, trans-11 conjugated linoleic acid in postmenopausal women. *Journal of Nutrition*, 138(8), 1445–1451. https://doi.org/10.1093/jn/138.8.1445.

Tontonoz, P., & Spiegelman, B. M. (2008). Fat and beyond: The diverse biology of PPARγ. *Annual Review of Biochemistry*, 77, 289–312. https://doi.org/10.1146/annurev.biochem.77.061307.091829.

Tsuzuki, T., Igarashi, M., Komai, M., & Miyazawa, T. (2003). The metabolic conversion of 9,11,13-eleostearic acid (18:3) to 9,11-conjugated linoleic acid (18:2) in the rat. *Journal of Nutritional Science and Vitaminology*, 49(3), 195–200. https://doi.org/10.3177/jnsv.49.195.

Tsuzuki, T., Kawakami, Y., Abe, R., Nakagawa, K., Koba, K., Imamura, J., et al. (2006). Conjugated linolenic acid is slowly absorbed in rat intestine, but quickly converted to conjugated linoleic acid. *Journal of Nutrition*, 136(8), 2153–2159. https://doi.org/10.1093/jn/136.8.2153.

Tsuzuki, T., Tokuyama, Y., Igarashi, M., & Miyazawa, T. (2004). Tumor growth suppression by α-eleostearic acid, a linolenic acid isomer with a cunjugated triene system, via lipid peroxidation. *Carcinogenesis*, 25(8), 1417–1425. https://doi.org/10.1093/carcin/bgh109.

Tsuzuki, T., Tokuyama, Y., Igarashi, M., Nakagawa, K., Ohsaki, Y., Komai, M., et al. (2004). α-Eleostearic acid (9Z11E13E-18:3) is quickly converted to conjugated linoleic acid (9Z11E-18:2) in rats. *Journal of Nutrition*, 134(10), 2634–2639. https://doi.org/10.1093/jn/134.10.2634.

Varady, K. A., & Jones, P. J. H. (2005). Combination diet and exercise interventions for the treatment of dyslipidemia: An effective preliminary strategy to lower cholesterol levels? *Journal of Nutrition*, 135(8), 1829–1835. https://doi.org/10.1093/jn/135.8.1829.

Viladomiu, M., Hontecillas, R., Yuan, L., Lu, P., & Bassaganya-Riera, J. (2013). Nutritional protective mechanisms against gut inflammation. *Journal of Nutritional Biochemistry*, 24(6), 929–939. https://doi.org/10.1016/j.jnutbio.2013.01.006.

Vroegrijk, I. O. C. M., van Diepen, J. A., van den Berg, S., Westbroek, I., Keizer, H., Gambelli, L., et al. (2011). Pomegranate seed oil, a rich source of punicic acid, prevents diet-induced obesity and insulin resistance in mice. *Food and Chemical Toxicology*, 49(6), 1426–1430. https://doi.org/10.1016/j.fct.2011.03.037.

Xu, Y., Xu, L., Chen, X. T., Sun, P., Guo, Q., & Wang, H. L. (2016). Bitter melon seed oil may reduce the adiposity through the hypothalamus mTOR signaling in mice fed a high fat diet. *Journal of Nutrition and Intermediary*

Metabolism, 6, 16–21. https://doi.org/10.1016/j.jnim.2016.04.003.

Yamasaki, M., Kitagawa, T., Koyanagi, N., Chujo, H., Maeda, H., Kohno-Murase, J., et al. (2006). Dietary effect of pomegranate seed oil on immune function and lipid metabolism in mice. *Nutrition, 22*(1), 54–59. https://doi.org/10.1016/j.nut.2005.03.009.

Yang, L., Leung, K. Y., Cao, Y., Huang, Y., Ratnayake, W. M. N., & Chen, Z. Y. (2005). α-Linolenic acid but not conjugated linolenic acid is hypocholesterolaemic in hamsters. *British Journal of Nutrition, 93*(4), 433–438. https://doi.org/10.1079/BJN20041365.

Yasui, Y., Hosokawa, M., Kohno, H., Tanaka, T., & Miyashita, K. (2006a). Growth inhibition and apoptosis induction by all-trans-conjugated linolenic acids on human colon cancer cells. *Anticancer Research, 26*(3 A), 1855–1860.

Yasui, Y., Hosokawa, M., Kohno, H., Tanaka, T., & Miyashita, K. (2006b). Troglitazone and 9cis,11trans,13trans-conjugated linolenic acid: Comparison of their antiproliferative and apoptosis-inducing effects on different colon cancer cell lines. *Chemotherapy, 52*(5), 220–225. https://doi.org/10.1159/000094865.

Yasui, Y., Hosokawa, M., Sahara, T., Suzuki, R., Ohgiya, S., Kohno, H., et al. (2005). Bitter gourd seed fatty acid rich in 9c,11t,13t-conjugated linolenic acid induces apoptosis and up-regulates the GADD45, p53 and PPARγ in human colon cancer Caco-2 cells. *Prostaglandins, Leukotrienes, and Essential Fatty Acids, 73*(2), 113–119. https://doi.org/10.1016/j.plefa.2005.04.013.

Yuan, G., Chen, X., & Li, D. (2014). Conjugated linolenic acids and their bioactivities: A review. *Food & Function, 5*(7), 1360–1368. https://doi.org/10.1039/C4FO00037D.

Yuan, G., Chen, X., & Li, D. (2015). Modulation of peroxisome proliferator-activated receptor gamma (PPAR γ) by conjugated fatty acid in obesity and inflammatory bowel disease. *Journal of Agricultural and Food Chemistry, 63*(7), 1883–1895. https://doi.org/10.1021/jf505050c.

Yuan, G., Sinclair, A. J., Xu, C., & Li, D. (2009). Incorporation and metabolism of punicic acid in healthy young humans. *Molecular Nutrition & Food Research, 53*(10), 1336–1342. https://doi.org/10.1002/mnfr.200800520.

Yuan, G., Sinclair, A. J., Zhou, C., & Li, D. (2009). α-Eleostearic acid is more effectively metabolized into conjugated linoleic acid than punicic acid in mice. *Journal of the Science of Food and Agriculture, 89*(6), 1006–1011. https://doi.org/10.1002/jsfa.3547.

Yuan, G., Sun, H., Sinclair, A. J., & Li, D. (2009). Effects of conjugated linolenic acid and conjugated linoleic acid on lipid metabolism in mice. *European Journal of Lipid Science and Technology, 111*(6), 537–545. https://doi.org/10.1002/ejlt.200800200.

Yuan, G., Wahlqvist, M. L., Yuan, J., Wang, Q., & Li, D. (2009). Effect of punicic acid naturally occurring in food on lipid peroxidation in healthy young humans. *Journal of the Science of Food and Agriculture, 89*(13), 2331–2335. https://doi.org/10.1002/jsfa.3729.

Yuan, G., Yuan, J., & Li, D. (2009). Punicic acid from Trichosanthes kirilowii seed oil is rapidly metabolized to conjugated linoleic acid in rats. *Journal of Medicinal Food, 12*(2), 416–422. https://doi.org/10.1089/jmf.2007.0541.

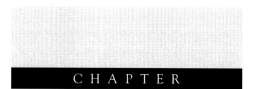

CHAPTER 17

N-3 polyunsaturated fatty acid and homocysteine metabolism

Tao Huang[a,b,c] and Zhenhuang Zhuang[a]

[a]Department of Epidemiology and Biostatistics, School of Public Health, Peking University, Beijing, China [b]Key Laboratory of Molecular Cardiovascular Sciences, Peking University, Ministry of Education, Beijing, China [c]Center for Intelligent Public Health, Institute for Artificial Intelligence, Peking University, Beijing, China

17.1 Introduction

17.1.1 What is homocysteine?

Homocysteine (Hcy) is a sulfur amino acid derived from methionine. De Vigneaud was the first founder of this by-product in 1932 (Clarke et al., 2005). It was demonstrated that vascular diseases are associated with elevated plasma levels of Hcy. Therefore, Hcy gained lots of focus and attention, and methionine metabolism has been extensively investigated. In the circulation of methionine metabolism, methionine is converted to SAM via methionine adenosyltransferase, which is the only methyl-donating pathway in humans (Clarke et al., 1998). This pathway provides methyl groups to activate many biomolecules, such as DNA, creatine, and phospholipids. SAM is demethylated to SAH in these methyltransferase reactions. SAH is hydrolyzed to Hcy in a reversible reaction. Once formed, Hcy is metabolized through two pathways: remethylation and transsulfuration.

Remethylation is the vitamin-dependent pathway, where Hcy is converted back to methionine via the enzyme 5-methyltetrahydrofolate reductase (MTHFR) and the enzyme methionine synthase (MS). Remethylation appears to be the primary modulator of elevated Hcy concentrations (Benito et al., 2006). Transsulfuration requires vitamin B_{12} to convert Hcy to cysteine via a two-step process involving the vitamin B_6-dependent enzyme cystathionine β-synthase (CBS) and cystathionase. Ultimately, cysteine is converted to sulfate and excreted into the urine. In the human body, total Hcy reflects the combined pool of free, reduced, bound, and oxidized forms of Hcy in the blood (Kinsella, Lokesh, & Stone, 1990). Normal tHcy levels range between 5 and 15 μmol/L with elevations of 16–30 μmol/L, 31–100 μmol/L, and >100 μmol/L, classified as mild, moderate, and severe hyperhomocysteinemia (HHcy), respectively (Hu et al., 1999; Li et al., 2007). Life-threatening HHcy is associated with enzymatic defects at various points of Hcy metabolism. Several environmental factors, such as diets and lifestyle, and genetics can cause elevations in Hcy (Olszewski & McCully, 1993). For example, an MTHFR variant (C677T mutation) with reduced enzymatic activity is the most common form of genetic HHcy. Deficiency of B vitamins accounts for the majority of cases of elevated Hcy in the general population (Huang et al., 2011; Van Der Put et al., 1998).

17.1.2 Hyperhomocysteinemia and health consequences

HHcy accounts for the higher prevalence of CVD (Barbosa et al., 2008). HHcy is known to cause multiple disease manifestations: premature occlusive vascular disease (Huang, Yuan, Zhang, Zou, & Li, 2008), progressive arterial stenosis (Klerk et al., 2003), nephritic syndrome, placental vasculopathy, birth defects, dementia, diabetes, and osteoporotic fractures (Blom, 1998; Miriuka et al., 2005). In 1969, McCully demonstrated that Hcy is involved in the pathogenesis of arteriosclerosis (Brattstrom, Israelsson, Jeppsson, & Hultberg, 1988). In general, clinical and epidemiologic studies show an independent association between Hcy levels and CVD, myocardial infarction, and venous thromboembolism. Dinleyici et al. recommended the use of plasma tHcy levels as a risk indicator along with other cardiovascular risk factors for detecting and preventing CVD in diabetic children (Huang et al., 2012). The mechanisms in Hcy-induced vascular disease have been comprehensively investigated and have provided important insights into our understanding of the role of Hcy in CVD (Barbosa et al., 2008).

17.1.3 Brief introduction of nutritional modulation of homocysteine

Plasma Hcy can be lowered with B vitamin supplementation (Clarke et al., 2005). In 1988, Brattström et al. showed that a high dose of folic acid markedly reduced Hcy levels (Brattstrom et al., 1988). Since then, several studies have demonstrated that 0.65–10 mg/d of folic acid alone or together with vitamin B_{12} and/or B_6 reduces the fasting Hcy level by 25%–50%, both in healthy and in subjects with HHcy (Refsum, Ueland, Nygård, & Vollset, 1998). Daily supplemental combination vitamins have been shown to reduce Hcy levels to varying degrees in interventional studies (Clarke et al., 1998). Previous meta-analysis of randomized controlled trials (RCTs) showed that supplemental B vitamin decreased plasma Hcy level and had a protective effect on stroke (Huang, Chen, et al., 2012).

17.2 Epidemiological evidence regarding n-3 PUFAs, genetics, and homocysteine levels

17.2.1 Association between n-3 PUFAs and homocysteine levels

Modification of dietary fat composition has been demonstrated to improve lipid and carbohydrate metabolism, thus decreasing cardiovascular risk (Benito et al., 2006). N-3 polyunsaturated fatty acids (PUFA), especially docosahexaenoic acid (DHA) and eicosapentaenoic acid (EPA), have several beneficial effects on the cardiovascular risk profile (Kinsella et al., 1990). Dietary intake of fish oil leads to increased n-3 PUFA levels in tissues (Hu et al., 1999), which is related to reduced cardiovascular risk via regulating blood pressure, plasma triacylglycerol (TG) levels, and antithrombotic effects. Recently, it was shown that n-3 PUFA was shown to improve Hcy metabolism. Hcy plays an important role in the atherothrombogenic process. The beneficial effects of n-3 PUFA on endothelial function can counteract the endothelial toxicity of Hcy, but only a few short-term studies have been published on the effects of n-3 PUFA on Hcy. Our previous studies reported that plasma phospholipid, n-3 PUFA, was negatively related to plasma Hcy in middle-aged and geriatric hyperlipidemic patients (Li et al., 2007) and in healthy male subjects (Li, Mann, & Sinclair, 2006). High intakes of DHA and EPA have been shown to have beneficial effects on the cardiovascular risk profile (Kinsella et al., 1990). In addition, plasma PL DHA, total n-3 PUFAs, and n-3/n-6 PUFA ratio were also negatively associated with plasma Hcy in healthy Australian male subjects (Li et al., 2006). Increased total n-3 PUFAs and n-3/n-6 PUFA in platelet PL have been associated with decreased plasma Hcy in middle-aged and geriatric hyperlipidemic patients in Hangzhou, China (Li et al., 2007). Over the past two decades, several interventional studies of small sample size and short duration have documented the effects of n-3 PUFAs on plasma Hcy. Previous studies have demonstrated that supplemental n-3 PUFA decreases plasma Hcy in diabetic patients (Zeman et al., 2006), patients with acute myocardial infarction, and men with hyperlipidemia (Olszewski & McCully, 1993). However, the efficacy of n-3 PUFAs on plasma Hcy has not been conclusive (Brude et al., 1999), although our meta-analysis demonstrated the effects of n-3 PUFAs on plasma Hcy levels in RCT (Huang, Zheng, et al., 2011).

17.2.2 Genetics of hyperhomocysteinemia

HHcy is caused by low intake of folate and other B vitamins and genetic factors, including polymorphisms of genes encoding enzymes involved in Hcy remethylation, such as MTHFR, MTR, MTRR, and CBS. Single-nucleotide polymorphisms (SNPs) of the MTHFR gene (MTHFR 677C>T) is a strong determinant of Hcy in individuals with impaired folate status. The 677TT genotype has been described as an independent risk factor for CVD, colorectal neoplasias, and neural tube defects. MTHFR 1298A>C, MTR 2756A>G, MTRR 66A>G, and CBS 844ins68 have been associated with HHcy, neural tube defects, and colorectal cancer. Several other polymorphisms, including CBS 1080C>T and 699C>T, and 67A>G, reduced folate carrier-1 (RFC1) 80G>A, betaine methyltransferase (BHMT) 742G>A, and paraoxonase-1 (PON1) 575A>G have been related to folate or Hcy (Meyer, Fredriksen, & Ueland, 2004; Sunder-Plassmann & Födinger, 2003). The human 5,10-methylenetetrahydrofolate reductase gene (MTHFR, OMIM 607093) is located on chromosome 1p36.3. The product of the MTHFR gene consists of 656 amino acid residues. Two extensively studied polymorphisms in MTHFR are located at nucleotide position 677 (MTHFR 677C>T, rs 1801133) and position 1298 (MTHFR 1298A>C, 1801131). MTHFR 677C>T occurs in exon 4 at the folate-binding site and changes an alanine into a valine residue (A222V). MTHFR 1298A>C is located in exon 7 within the presumptive regulatory domain, changing a glutamic acid into an alanine residue (E429A). MTHFR 677C>T, MTHFR 1298A>C, as well as compound heterozygosity for 1298A>C and 677C>T, are associated with a reduced enzyme activity of 45%, 68%, and 42%, respectively. Over the past decades, compelling studies have demonstrated HHcy and MTHFR 677C>T mutation as risk factors for CVD. The functional polymorphism of the MTHFR gene (MTHFR 677C>T and 1298 A>C) has been shown to be the most frequent genetic cause for mild HHcy. A genome-wide association study of vitamin B6, vitamin B12, folate, and Hcy blood concentrations, MTHFR C677T rs1801133 reached the genome-wide significance ($p_{meta} = 4.36 \times 10^{-13}$). The MTHFR 1298 A>C which is another functional SNP in Hcy metabolism also results in decreased MTHFR activity (Van Der Put et al., 1998). Subjects with MTHFR 1298CC genotype had higher plasma Hcy compared to those with the MTHFR 1298AA genotype. The MTHFR 1298A>C was associated with plasma Hcy. The plasma Hcy was higher in carriers of the 1298 C allele compared with the AA homozygotes and AC heterozygotes. The MTHFR risk genotype 677CT/1298AC is known to be associated with decreased enzyme activity and increased Hcy. Therefore, there appears to be an interaction between these two functional SNPs in regulating plasma Hcy levels. The human methionine synthase gene (MTR, OMIM 156570) is located on chromosome 1q43. The product of the MTR gene consists of 1265 amino acid residues. MTR (EC 2.1.1.13) encodes the enzyme 5-methyltetrahydrofolate-homocysteine methyltransferase. This enzyme, also known as vitamin B12-dependent methionine synthase, catalyzes the final step in methionine biosynthesis. It uses the methyl group from 5-methyltetrahydrofolate for remethylation of Hcy to methionine (Barbosa et al., 2008; Huang et al., 2008). The mutation of MTR is located in a potentially functional domain of the enzyme and shows a decrease in the MTR activity. Therefore, the MTR 2756A>G may lead to increased Hcy levels (Leclerc et al., 1996). Studies showed that the MTR 2756 A>G gene is associated with high Hcy levels. In addition, both fasting and post-methionine load levels decreased with an increasing number of G alleles. Pregnant women with MTR 2756AA had lower vitamin B12 and higher Hcy levels than those with the G carriers in a working male Irish population (Harmon et al., 1999) and healthy adult Canadian controls (Miriuka et al., 2005). The G allele of the MTR gene is a protective factor against increasing Hcy levels (Kim et al., 2007). However, some studies have shown no association between MTR 2756A>G and Hcy. The discrepancy may be due to the sample size and population characteristics; interaction between the MTR 2756A>G and vitamin B12, folate, or other cardiovascular risk factors may also contribute to this difference. For example, one study found that the MTR 2756A>G variant enhanced the severity of CHD related to smoking (Wang, Cai, Cranney, & Wilcken, 1998); the study also documented possible interaction between the MTR 2756A>G polymorphism and MTHFR polymorphisms in Hcy concentration and Hcy-related diseases (Klerk et al., 2003).

17.2.3 Genetic risk, n-3 PUFAs and homocysteine metabolism

The etiology of HHcy is suggested to be multifactorial and includes genetic factors and lifestyle (Refsum et al., 1998). The genetic causes of elevated plasma Hcy include rare inborn errors of Hcy metabolism, such as *CBS* and *MTHFR* (Blom, 1998). Moreover, lifestyle factors also play an important role in the Hcy metabolism. Two-thirds of HHcy in an elderly US population were associated with low plasma/serum concentrations of one or more of B group vitamins in the United States (Selhub et al., 1999). Smoking, drinking (Vinukonda, Shaik Mohammad, Md Nurul Jain, Prasad Chintakindi, & Rama Devi Akella, 2009; Bleich et al., 2001), and physical activity have also been associated with elevated plasma Hcy. Moreover, genetic variants involved in Hcy metabolism may modulate the effect of dietary fatty acids on plasma Hcy in humans. Population studies found that dietary fatty acids interact with MTHFR and MAT1A genetic variants in determining plasma Hcy concentration. Two functional MTHFR variants, 1298A>C and 677C>T, in Boston Puerto Rican adults were associated with hypertension. Importantly, this variant exhibited interactions with intakes of total and n-6 PUFA and the n-3:n-6 PUFA ratio in determining plasma Hcy levels. Moreover, participants with genotypes of 677 TT and 1298AC or CC who had high n-3 PUFA had lower plasma Hcy levels compared with those who had the same genotype but consumed low levels of n-3 PUFA. Therefore, it was suggested that dietary PUFA intake modulates the effect of MTHFR variants on plasma Hcy (Huang et al., 2011). Moreover, the genetic variant MAT1A 3U1510 displayed a significant interaction with the dietary n-3:n-6 PUFA ratio in determining plasma Hcy. The 3U1510G homozygotes had lower plasma Hcy levels than those with major allele homozygotes and heterozygotes (AA +AG) when the n-3:n-6 ratio was >0.09. Two other MAT1A variants (d18777 and i15752) also showed significant interactions with different constituents of dietary fat in influencing Hcy. A population-based study investigated the interactions of *MAT1A* genotypes and dietary fatty acids in modifying plasma Hcy. Subjects were divided into two groups according to the median of dietary fatty acids. There is an interaction between dietary MUFA and *MAT1A* i15752 for plasma Hcy. When dietary MUFA was low (<11.35%/energy/d), plasma Hcy was lower in carriers of the A allele compared to GG subjects. In addition, as total MUFA increased, plasma Hcy levels increased in carriers of the A allele. When total fat intake was low (<31.31%/energy/d), A carriers showed lower plasma Hcy than G homozygotes, while there was no difference between A carriers and noncarriers when total fat intake was high. Furthermore, defects in *MAT1A* which inactivate MAT activity are one cause of HHcy and this may have the consequence of *MAT1A* genotypes and dietary fatty acid interactions. Dietary factors may also alter MAT function, as demonstrated in our earlier animal study which showed that n-3 PUFA upregulated the *MAT* gene expression and enzyme activity (Huang, Wahlqvist, & Li, 2010). These results support the hypothesis that *MAT1A* genotypes may modulate the regulatory effect of n-3 PUFA or n-6 PUFA on Hcy metabolism. In summary, n-3 PUFA intake plays an important role in Hcy metabolism. Previous evidence suggests that interactions between *MAT1A* genetic polymorphisms and dietary fatty acids modulate plasma Hcy concentration. In light of strong evidence that elevated plasma Hcy is an independent risk factor for cardiovascular diseases, understanding the role of dietary factors in the potential amelioration of genetically based risk of HHcy is critical.

17.3 Effects of n-3 PUFAs on homocysteine: Evidence from animal studies and cell culture

17.3.1 Cell culture: n-3 PUFAs regulate homocysteine metabolism

Dietary intake of fish oil rich in n-3 PUFAs increases levels of n-3 PUFA in tissues (Hu et al., 1999) and is associated with reduced incidence of cardiovascular events (Erkkilä, Lichtenstein, Mozaffarian, & Herrington, 2004; Marchioli et al., 2002), blood pressure (Morris, Sacks, & Rosner, 1993), serum/plasma triacylglycerol (TG) levels (Svaneborg et al., 1994), antithrombotic effects, heart rate variability (Christensen, Skou, Madsen, Torring, & Schmidt, 2001), and Hcy. To explain why n-3 PUFA decreases the level of Hcy, studies using cell culture examined the effect of n-3 PUFA on the mRNA expression of genes encoding the critical enzymes involved in methionine metabolism. It was found that n-3 PUFA has been incorporated into the phospholipids of the HepG2 cell membrane. The change in PL fatty acids in the cell membrane is likely to account for the changes in mRNA expression of the critical genes involved in methionine metabolism. Results from cell culture showed that the concentrations of 22:6n-3, 20:5n-3, and 18:3n-3 were significantly increased in the three research groups, respectively ($P<.05$); the levels of n-3 PUFA were also significantly elevated in the three research groups ($P<.05$) when compared with the control group. The expression levels of the MTHFR gene were increased in the DHA group and the ALA group when compared with control; significantly decreased expression of MAT was observed in the three groups compared with control. Furthermore, the level of MAT gene expression was lower in the DHA group than in the ALA group ($P<.05$). Thus, n-3 PUFA affects the rate of SAM synthesis based on the activity of MAT (Selhub, 1999). The resultant decrease in SAM synthesis via MAT would not stimulate SAH production. Furthermore, the lack of recognizable change in SAHH expression helps avoid an increase in Hcy, as the hydrolysis of SAH by the enzyme SAHH is the sole intracellular source of Hcy (Finkelstein, 2000). Cell culture study showed that n-3 PUFA did not change SAHH gene expression. Therefore, a decrease in SAH synthesis resulting from a decreased level of SAM contributes to a reduction in Hcy formation (Selhub, 1999). The potential mechanism is that SAM acts as not only an allosteric inhibitor of MTHFR but also an activator of CBS (Finkelstein & Martin, 1984; Kutzbach & Stokstad, 1971). As such an effector, SAM suppresses the synthesis of N-5-methyltetrahydrofolate, which is an important substrate required for remethylation and promotes the initial reaction of transsulfuration (CBS). In the transsulfuration pathway, Hcy condenses with serine to form cystathionine via CBS (using vitamin B_6 as a cofactor). CBS and CSE are the two important determinants in the transsulfuration pathway. While the result of cell culture did not show the significant effect of n-3 PUFA on the mRNA expression of CBS, the CSE mRNA expression was significantly upregulated by DHA and EPA, and CSE, which is a vitamin B_6-dependent enzyme, catalyzes the conversion of cystathionine into cysteine and H_2S. A previous study found that the enzyme activity and mRNA expression of CSE were upregulated after 8 weeks of tuna oil supplement (Huang et al., 2010). Thus, upregulated CSE mRNA expression expedited the degradation of cystathionine. This means that the transsulfuration reaction will move in a direction beneficial for decreasing Hcy. The findings from cell culture and animal studies suggest that n-3 PUFA may ameliorate hypertension by decreasing Hcy as well as increasing H_2S as a result of the upregulated CSE gene expression. Furthermore, it was speculated that a cis-acting n-3 PUFA-responsive element (n-3 PUFA-RE) may be in the promoter region of n-3 PUFA-regulated genes. To alter gene transcription, a transcription factor (putative n-3 PUFA-binding protein) could bind to n-3 PUFA-RE and block or enhance transcription (Mapper: http://bio.chip.org/mapper). In summary, n-3 PUFA upregulates CSE and MTHFR mRNA expression and downregulates MAT mRNA expression involved in Hcy metabolism. This regulatory effect of n-3 PUFA on critical gene expression is associated with decreased Hcy concentration.

17.3.2 How do n-3 PUFAs regulate the key gene expression involved in homocysteine metabolic pathways?

Population studies found that dietary fatty acids interact with *MTHFR* and *MAT1A* genetic variants in determining plasma Hcy concentration. These results imply the potential mechanisms which may explain the relationship between n-3 PUFA and plasma Hcy levels. To explore the potential mechanisms by which PUFA might regulate Hcy metabolism, an animal study was conducted to investigate the nutritional regulation of different oils rich in PUFA on the mRNA expression of the key gene involved in Hcy metabolism. An animal study suggested that 22:6n-3 decreases plasma Hcy concentration through regulating the critical gene expression and enzyme activity (Huang et al., 2010). Specifically, the animal study showed that plasma PL DHA, EPA, CLA, LA, and ALA were significantly increased in the DHA, EPA, CLA, LA, and ALA groups, respectively, after 8 weeks of treatment. The oils have differently affected plasma Hcy concentration in rats. Plasma Hcy concentration was significantly decreased in DHA and CLA groups, while plasma Hcy concentration was not significantly affected in other groups. In addition, plasma vitamin B_{12} and folate concentration were not significantly affected by treatment groups. mRNA expression of *MTHFR* was significantly upregulated in DHA, EPA, and ALA groups, while downregulated in LA and SO groups. *BHMT* was significantly upregulated in EPA, ALA, and LA groups. *Mat1a* was significantly upregulated in DHA, EPA, ALA, and CLA groups. In addition, *CBS* was significantly upregulated in DHA, EPA, ALA, and CLA groups, while downregulated in LA and SO groups. *PEMT* was significantly upregulated in EPA and ALA groups, while downregulated in SO group. However, different oils did not significantly affect the mRNA expression of *SAHH*. Other critical gene expressions (*Sahh, Bhmt, Cse, Chka, Tyms, Chdh, Gnmt, Mthfs, Mtr, Cept1, Mtrr, Etnk1, and Bad*) which are involved in Hcy metabolism were also regulated by different oils. In an animal study, it was found that plasma Hcy was significantly decreased by tuna oil rich in 22:6n-3. MAT activity was significantly increased and MAT mRNA expression was significantly upregulated by 22:6n-3; CSE mRNA expression was significantly upregulated by 22:6n-3. It was suggested that 22:6n-3 decreases the concentration of Hcy despite increasing MAT activity and upregulating MAT mRNA expression through compensatory CSE mRNA expression, both of which are involved in Hcy metabolism (Huang et al., 2010).

17.4 Experimental epidemiological evidence regarding the effects of n-3 PUFAs on homocysteine metabolism

17.4.1 Effects of supplemental n-3 PUFAs on the levels of homocysteine and cardiometabolic risk factors

A meta-analysis was conducted to determine the effects of n-3 PUFA on plasma Hcy levels in randomized placebo-controlled trials (RCT). This study identified 11 RCT of n-3 PUFA supplementation, reporting results on plasma Hcy in 702 subjects. Seven papers reported a significant Hcy-lowering effect (Benito et al., 2006; Carrero, Lopez-Huertas, Salmeron, Ramos, & Baro, 2006; Carrero et al., 2007; Carrero, López-Huertas, Salmerón, Baró, & Ros, 2005; Grundt, Nilsen, Mansoor, Hetland, & Nordøy, 2003; Pooya et al., 2010; Zeman et al., 2006); two papers showed no change in plasma Hcy, while two papers showed a significant increase in plasma Hcy after the n-3 PUFA supplement. The conflicting results may be due to different durations of treatment and noncomparable populations. The median level of Hcy in Beavers' study population is 2–3 times higher than others (Beavers, Beavers, Bowden, Wilson, & Gentile, 2008). Characteristics of the sample population used in their study, specifically, renal disease, may also help explain why fish oil supplementation had no effect on Hcy levels. Holdt et al. studied the effect of 3 months of fish oil supplementation on Hcy levels in continuous ambulatory peritoneal dialysis patients (Holdt et al., 1996). While the results of this study showed no effect of fish oil supplementation in the reduction of Hcy, it was hypothesized that longer exposure to fish oil might control Hcy levels more effectively. However, a subsequent study revealed that daily administration of 6 capsules of n-3 fatty acids (160 mg of EPA and 100 mg of DHA per capsule) had no effect on Hcy levels even when the researchers extended the fish oil supplementation protocol to 6 months (Beavers et al., 2008). They suggested that potential reasons for the lack of effect of n-3 PUFA on Hcy were related to a dose–response relationship (Beavers et al., 2008). Overall results from meta-analyses showed that the plasma Hcy was significantly decreased ($-1.59\,\mu m/L$ with 95% CI: -2.34, -0.83). These results indicate that high n-3 PUFA supplementation was associated with a decrease in plasma Hcy. The heterogeneity was reduced after excluding Piolot et al. (2003) ($I^2 = 32\%$, P for heterogeneity $= 0.15$) or excluding Zeman et al. (2006) ($I^2 = 45\%$, P for heterogeneity=0.06). In conclusion, this meta-analysis suggests that n-3 PUFA supplementation can decrease plasma Hcy levels. To enable more comprehensive pooled analyses and improve the precision of the effect size estimates, further rigorously designed and conducted long-term randomized controlled trials with larger sample sizes assessing the effect of n-3 PUFA on plasma Hcy are needed. Larger trials, including clinical endpoint trials, of longer duration, are needed to establish the role and mechanisms of n-3 PUFA in plasma Hcy reduction.

17.4.2 Combined effects of supplemental n-3 PUFAs and vitamins on levels of homocysteine and cardiometabolic risk factors

Although several interventional studies of small sample size and short duration have documented the effects of n-3 PUFAs on plasma Hcy, the efficacy of n-3 PUFAs on plasma Hcy level in humans has not been consistently demonstrated (Brude et al., 1999). An interventional study was performed to assess the effects of fish oil and vitamin B_{12} on cardiovascular risk factors in healthy Chinese subjects. It was found that plasma PL fatty acids of 20:5n-3, 22:6n-3, and total n-3 PUFA were increased after 8 weeks of supplementation of fish oil and vitamin B12 +fish oil. Interestingly, plasma PL total saturated fatty acid SFA was also increased, whereas the levels of n-6 PUFA were decreased after 8 weeks of supplementation of fish oil. There was a significant time × treatment interaction for TG, HDL-C, uric acid, and ferritin. Plasma HDL-C level was increased, whereas TG, uric acid, and ferritin concentrations were decreased after 8 weeks of supplementation with fish oil and vitamin B12+fish oil. Plasma glucose concentrations in FO and VitB-12+FO groups were decreased after 8 weeks of supplementation. In addition, plasma ferritin concentration was lowered from 73.5 ± 10.6 pmol/L at baseline to 51.2 ± 10.3 at the end in the FO group and decreased from 82.0 ± 18.6 pmol/L at baseline to 52.9 ± 7.11 at the end in the VitB-12+FO group. Plasma ferritin concentration was significantly lower in the VitB-12+FO group than in the VitB-12 group. There was a significant time-×treatment interaction for plasma concentrations of the VitB-12 and Hcy. In the VitB-12 and VitB-12+FO groups, significant changes in plasma VitB-12 and Hcy were observed during 8 weeks of intervention. Plasma Hcy concentration was reduced from 12.3 ± 1.65 to 9.57 ± 1.05, 12.9 ± 1.45 to 10.4 ± 1.76, and 11.8 ± 1.19 to 7.18 ± 0.61 µmol/L after 8 weeks of supplementation with the VitB-12, fish oil, and VitB-12+fish oil, respectively. The VitB-12, fish oil, and the VitB-12+fish oil supplementation significantly lowered mean plasma Hcy concentrations by 22%, 19%, and 39%, respectively. In summary, supplementation of fish oil alone or in combination with the VitB-12 decreased plasma concentrations of Hcy. Oral supplementation with VitB-12 in combination with fish oil had a synergistic effect on lowering plasma concentrations of Hcy.

17.5 Mechanisms by which n-3 PUFAs reduce homocysteine levels and future research

Previous studies suggested that n-3 PUFA plays an important role in Hcy metabolism (Huang et al., 2012). The potential mechanism responsible for the Hcy-lowering effect of n-3 PUFA has been elucidated during the past years (Huang et al., 2010; Piolot et al., 2003). Piolot reported an interaction of n-3 PUFA and NO on Hcy metabolism in healthy people. They suggested that the reduced Hcy concentrations observed in their study are attributed to possible oxidative stress induction by n-3 PUFA and stimulation of the oxidative catabolism of Hcy (Durand, Prost, Loreau, Lussier-Cacan, &

Blache, 2001). This increased susceptibility to oxidative stress due to n-3 PUFA supplementation is reported (Saedisomeolia, Wood, Garg, Gibson, & Wark, 2009). Furthermore, n-3 PUFA may modulate gene expression of enzyme(s) involved in the formation and metabolism of Hcy (Li et al., 2007). Data from the animal study suggested that n-3 PUFA from fish oil was incorporated into tissue phospholipids (Huang et al., 2010). The changes in the fatty acid composition of liver and lung tissue are related to the activity of enzymes and gene mRNA expression involved in Hcy metabolism. For example, n-3 PUFA from tuna oil upregulates MAT activity and mRNA expression (Huang et al., 2010). Thus, the increased MAT activity and upregulated MAT mRNA expression increased CBS activity and subsequently accelerated the permanent removal of Hcy from the methionine cycle by CBS. In addition, the resultant increase in S-adenosylmethionine synthesis via MAT apparently counterbalanced the increase of SAH, which may upregulate CBS activity and downregulate MTHFR, methionine synthetase, and betaine-homocysteine methyltransferase activity. Moreover, n-3 PUFA from tuna oil upregulates CSE activity and CSE mRNA expression. CSE, which is also a vitamin B_6-dependent enzyme, catalyzes the conversion of cystathionine into cysteine, α-ketobutyrate, taurine, and H_2S and is the rate-limiting enzyme for the synthesis of cysteine from Hcy. Thus, upregulated CSE mRNA expression expedited the degradation of cystathionine. Subsequently, the transsulfuration reaction will move in a direction beneficial for decreasing Hcy. In addition, it was previously reported that MAT1A interacted with PUFA in determining plasma Hcy in humans (Huang, Tucker, et al., 2012), Genetic variant MAT1A 3U1510 displayed significant interaction with dietary n-3:n-6 PUFA ratio in determining plasma Hcy. The 3U1510G homozygotes had significantly lower plasma Hcy concentration than major allele homozygotes and heterozygotes (AA+AG) when the n-3:n-6 ratio was >0.09 (%of total energy). This means that dietary PUFA modules the effect of genetic factors on plasma Hcy, which may help explain the possible mechanism of n-3 PUFA decreasing plasma Hcy (Huang, Tucker, et al., 2012). However, considering the significance of n-3 PUFA in decreasing plasma Hcy levels and protecting CVD, more experiments based on animal, cell culture, and population studies should be conducted to investigate the potential mechanisms by which n-3 PUFA decreases plasma Hcy. In addition, the genetic variation of some critical genes involved among the population could account for the difference in the results of the interventional studies. Therefore, the theory of nutrigenomics should be used to identify the genetic variant-dietary fatty acid interactions in determining plasma Hcy concentration.

17.6 Conclusion

The etiology of HHcy is suggested to be multifactorial, including genetic and lifestyle factors. N-3 PUFA has been demonstrated to play an important role in Hcy metabolism. The potential mechanisms for the Hcy-lowering effect of n-3 PUFA have been comprehensively investigated. Animal study and cell culture suggested that n-3 PUFA was incorporated into tissue phospholipids. The changes in fatty acid composition in tissues may regulate key enzyme activity and gene mRNA expression involved in Hcy metabolism. For example, n-3 PUFA upregulates MAT activity and mRNA expression, which increased CBS activity and subsequently accelerated the removal of Hcy from the methionine metabolic pathways. Furthermore, n-3 PUFA from tuna oil upregulates CSE activity and CSE mRNA expression. Thus, upregulated CSE mRNA expression expedited the degradation of cystathionine which results in a decrease in Hcy levels. However, the genetic variation of some critical genes involved in the methionine cycle may interact with dietary fatty acids in determining Hcy levels. Therefore, the theory of nutrigenomics should be used to identify the genetic variant-dietary fatty acid interactions in determining the plasma Hcy concentration.

References

Barbosa, P. R., Stabler, S. P., Machado, A. L. K., Braga, R. C., Hirata, R. D. C., Hirata, M. H., et al. (2008). Association between decreased vitamin levels and MTHFR, MTR and MTRR gene polymorphisms as determinants for elevated total homocysteine concentrations in pregnant women. *European Journal of Clinical Nutrition, 62*(8), 1010–1021. https://doi.org/10.1038/sj.ejcn.1602810.

Beavers, K. M., Beavers, D. P., Bowden, R. G., Wilson, R. L., & Gentile, M. (2008). Omega-3 fatty acid supplementation and total homocysteine levels in end-stage renal disease patients. *Nephrology, 13*(4), 284–288. https://doi.org/10.1111/j.1440-1797.2008.00934.x.

Benito, P., Caballero, J., Moreno, J., Gutiérrez-Alcántara, C., Muñoz, C., Rojo, G., et al. (2006). Effects of milk enriched with ω-3 fatty acid, oleic acid and folic acid in patients with metabolic syndrome. *Clinical Nutrition, 25*(4), 581–587. https://doi.org/10.1016/j.clnu.2005.12.006.

Bleich, S., Bleich, K., Kropp, S., Bittermann, H. J., Degner, D., Sperkling, W., et al. (2001). Moderate alcohol consumption in social drinkers raises plasma homocysteine levels: A contradiction to the "French paradox"? *Alcohol and Alcoholism, 36*(3), 189–192. https://doi.org/10.1093/alcalc/36.3.189.

Blom, H. J. (1998). Determinants of plasma homocysteine. *The American Journal of Clinical Nutrition, 68*(4), 188–189. https://doi.org/10.1093/ajcn/67.2.188.

Brattstrom, L., Israelsson, B., Jeppsson, J., & Hultberg, B. L. (1988). Folic acid—An innocuous means to reduce plasma homocysteine. *Scandinavian Journal of Clinical and Laboratory Investigation, 48*(3), 215–221.

Brude, I. R., Finstad, H. S., Seljeflot, I., Drevon, C. A., Solvoll, K., Sandstad, B., et al. (1999). Plasma homocysteine concentration related to diet, endothelial function and mononuclear cell gene expression among male hyperlipidaemic smokers. *European Journal of Clinical Investigation, 29*(2), 100–108. https://doi.org/10.1046/j.1365-2362.1999.00419.x.

Carrero, J. J., Fonollá, J., Marti, J. L., Jiménez, J., Boza, J. J., & López-Huertas, E. (2007). Intake of fish oil, oleic acid, folic acid, and vitamins B-6 and E for 1 year decreases plasma C-reactive protein and reduces coronary heart disease risk factors in male patients in a cardiac rehabilitation program. *Journal of Nutrition, 137*(2), 384–390. https://doi.org/10.1093/jn/137.2.384.

Carrero, J. J., López-Huertas, E., Salmerón, L. M., Baró, L., & Ros, E. (2005). Daily supplementation with (n-3) PUFAs, oleic acid, folic acid, and vitamins B-6 and E increases pain-free walking distance and improves risk factors in men with peripheral vascular disease. *Journal of Nutrition, 135*(6), 1393–1399. American Institute of Nutrition https://doi.org/10.1093/jn/135.6.1393.

Carrero, J., Lopez-Huertas, Salmeron, L., Ramos, S. E., & Baro, L. E. (2006). Simvastatin and supplementation with n-3 polyunsaturated fatty acids and vitamins improves claudication distance in a randomized PILOT study in patients with peripheral vascular disease. *Nutrition Research, 26*.

Christensen, J. H., Skou, H. A., Madsen, T., Torring, I., & Schmidt, E. B. (2001). Heart rate variability and n-3 polyunsaturated fatty acids in patients with diabetes mellitus. *Journal of Internal Medicine, 249*(6), 545–552. https://doi.org/10.1046/j.1365-2796.2001.00841.x.

Clarke, R., Brattström, L., Landgren, F., Israelsson, B., Lindgren, A., Hultberg, B., et al. (1998). Lowering blood homocysteine with folic acid based supplements: Meta-analysis of randomised trials. *British Medical Journal, 316*(7135), 894–898. http://www.bmj.com/.

Clarke, R., Frost, C., Sherliker, P., Lewington, S., Collins, R., Brattstrom, L., et al. (2005). Dose-dependent effects of folic acid on blood concentrations of homocysteine: A meta-analysis of the randomized trials. *American Journal of Clinical Nutrition, 82*(4), 806–812. https://doi.org/10.1093/ajcn/82.4.806.

Durand, P., Prost, M., Loreau, N., Lussier-Cacan, S., & Blache, D. (2001). Impaired homocysteine metabolism and atherothrombotic disease. *Laboratory Investigation, 81*(5), 645–672. https://doi.org/10.1038/labinvest.3780275.

Erkkilä, A. T., Lichtenstein, A. H., Mozaffarian, D., & Herrington, D. M. (2004). Fish intake is associated with a reduced progression of coronary artery atherosclerosis in postmenopausal women with coronary artery disease. *American Journal of Clinical Nutrition, 80*(3), 626–632. https://doi.org/10.1093/ajcn/80.3.626.

Finkelstein, J. D. (2000). Pathways and regulation of homocysteine metabolism in mammals. *Seminars in Thrombosis and Hemostasis, 26*(3), 219–225. https://doi.org/10.1055/s-2000-8466.

Finkelstein, J. D., & Martin, J. J. (1984). Methionine metabolism in mammals. Distribution of homocysteine between competing pathways. *Journal of Biological Chemistry, 259*(15), 9508–9513.

Grundt, H., Nilsen, D. W. T., Mansoor, M. A., Hetland, Ø., & Nordøy, A. (2003). Reduction in homocysteine by n-3 polyunsaturated fatty acids after 1 year in a randomised double-blind study following an acute myocardial infarction: No effect on endothelial adhesion properties. *Pathophysiology of Haemostasis and Thrombosis, 33*(2), 88–95. https://doi.org/10.1159/000073852.

Harmon, D. L., Shields, D. C., Woodside, J. V., McMaster, D., Yarnell, J. W. G., Young, I. S., et al. (1999). Methionine synthase D919G polymorphism is a significant but modest determinant of circulating homocysteine concentrations. *Genetic Epidemiology, 17*(4), 298–309. https://doi.org/10.1002/(SICI)1098-2272(199911)17:4<298::AID-GEPI5>3.0.CO;2-V.

Holdt, B., Korten, G., Knippel, M., Lehmann, J. K., Claus, R., Holtz, M., et al. (1996). Increased serum level of total homocysteine in CAPD patients despite fish oil therapy. *Peritoneal Dialysis International, 16*(1), S246–S249. https://doi.org/10.1177/089686089601601s46.

Hu, F. B., Stampfer, M. J., Manson, J. A. E., Rimm, E. B., Wolk, A., Colditz, G. A., et al. (1999). Dietary intake of α-linolenic acid and risk of fatal ischemic heart disease among women. *American Journal of Clinical Nutrition, 69*(5), 890–897. https://doi.org/10.1093/ajcn/69.5.890.

Huang, T., Chen, Y., Yang, B., Yang, J., Wahlqvist, M. L., & Li, D. (2012). Meta-analysis of B vitamin supplementation on plasma homocysteine, cardiovascular and all-cause mortality. *Clinical Nutrition, 31*(4), 448–454. https://doi.org/10.1016/j.clnu.2011.01.003.

Huang, T., Tucker, K. L., Lee, Y. C., Crott, J. W., Parnell, L. D., Shen, J., et al. (2011). Methylenetetrahydrofolate reductase variants associated with hypertension and cardiovascular disease interact with dietary polyunsaturated fatty acids to modulate plasma homocysteine in Puerto Rican adults. *Journal of Nutrition, 141*(4), 654–659. https://doi.org/10.3945/jn.110.134353.

Huang, T., Tucker, K., Lee, Y., Crott, J., Parnell, L., Shen, J., et al. (2012). MAT1A variants modulate the effect of dietary fatty acids on plasma homocysteine concentrations. *Nutrition, Metabolism, and Cardiovascular Diseases*, 362–368. https://doi.org/10.1016/j.numecd.2010.07.015.

Huang, T., Wahlqvist, M. L., & Li, D. (2010). Docosahexaenoic acid decreases plasma homocysteine via regulating enzyme activity and mRNA expression involved in methionine metabolism. *Nutrition, 26*(1), 112–119. https://doi.org/10.1016/j.nut.2009.05.015.

Huang, T., Yuan, G., Zhang, Z., Zou, Z., & Li, D. (2008). Cardiovascular pathogenesis in hyperhomocysteinemia. *Asia Pacific Journal of Clinical Nutrition, 17*(1), 8–16. http://apjcn.nhri.org.tw/server/APJCN/Volume17/vol17.1/Finished/8-16-1020.pdf.

Huang, T., Zheng, J., Chen, Y., Yang, B., Wahlqvist, M. L., & Li, D. (2011). High consumption of Ω-3 polyunsaturated fatty acids decrease plasma homocysteine: A meta-analysis of randomized, placebo-controlled trials. *Nutrition*, 863–867. https://doi.org/10.1016/j.nut.2010.12.011.

Kim, O. J., Hong, S. P., Ahn, J. Y., Hong, S. H., Hwang, T. S., Kim, S. O., et al. (2007). Influence of combined methionine synthase (MTR 2756A > G) and methylenetetrahydrofolate reductase (MTHFR 677C > T) polymorphisms to plasma homocysteine levels in Korean patients with ischemic stroke. *Yonsei Medical Journal, 48*(2), 201–209. https://doi.org/10.3349/ymj.2007.48.2.201.

Kinsella, J. E., Lokesh, B., & Stone, R. A. (1990). Dietary n-3 polyunsaturated fatty acids and amelioration of cardiovascular disease: Possible mechanisms. *American Journal of Clinical Nutrition, 52*(1), 1–28. https://doi.org/10.1093/ajcn/52.1.1.

Klerk, M., Lievers, K. J. A., Kluijtmans, L. A. J., Blom, H. J., Den Heijer, M., Schouten, E. G., et al. (2003). The 2756A>G variant in the gene encoding methionine synthase: Its relation with plasma homocysteine levels and risk of coronary heart disease in a Dutch case-control study. *Thrombosis Research, 110*(2–3), 87–91. https://doi.org/10.1016/S0049-3848(03)00341-4.

Kutzbach, C., & Stokstad, E. L. R. (1971). Mammalian methylenetetrahydrofolate reductase partial purification, properties, and inhibition by S-adenosylmethionine. *BBA - Enzymology, 250*(3), 459–477. https://doi.org/10.1016/0005-2744(71)90247-6.

Leclerc, D., Campeau, E., Goyette, P., Adjalla, C. E., Christensen, B., Ross, M., et al. (1996). Human methionine synthase: cDNA cloning and identification of mutations in patients of the cblG complementation group of folate/cobalamin disorders. *Human Molecular Genetics, 5*(12), 1867–1874. https://doi.org/10.1093/hmg/5.12.1867.

Li, D., Mann, N. J., & Sinclair, A. J. (2006). A significant inverse relationship between concentrations of plasma homocysteine and phospholipid docosahexaenoic acid in healthy male subjects. *Lipids*, 85–89. https://doi.org/10.1007/s11745-006-5074-x.

Li, D., Yu, X. M., Xie, H. B., Zhang, Y. H., Wang, Q., Zhou, X. Q., et al. (2007). Platelet phospholipid n-3 PUFA negatively associated with plasma homocysteine in middle-aged and geriatric hyperlipaemia patients. *Prostaglandins, Leukotrienes, and Essential Fatty Acids, 76*(5), 293–297. https://doi.org/10.1016/j.plefa.2007.02.003.

Marchioli, R., Barzi, F., Bomba, E., Chieffo, C., Di Gregorio, D., Di Mascio, R., et al. (2002). Early protection against sudden death by n-3 polyunsaturated fatty acids after myocardial infarction: Time-course analysis of the results of the Gruppo Italiano per lo studio della Sopravvivenza nell'Infarto Miocardico (GISSI)-Prevenzione. *Circulation, 105*(16), 1897–1903. https://doi.org/10.1161/01.CIR.0000014682.14181.F2.

Meyer, K., Fredriksen, A., & Ueland, P. M. (2004). High-level multiplex genotyping of polymorphisms involved in folate or homocysteine metabolism by matrix-assisted laser desorption/ionization mass spectrometry. *Clinical Chemistry*, *50*(2), 391–402. https://doi.org/10.1373/clinchem.2003.026799.

Miriuka, S. G., Langman, L. J., Evrovski, J., Miner, S. E. S., D'Mello, N., Delgado, D. H., et al. (2005). Genetic polymorphisms predisposing to hyperhomocysteinemia in cardiac transplant patients. *Transplant International*, *18*(1), 29–35. https://doi.org/10.1111/j.1432-2277.2004.00021.x.

Morris, M. C., Sacks, F., & Rosner, B. (1993). Does fish oil lower blood pressure? A meta-analysis of controlled trials. *Circulation*, *88*(2), 523–533. https://doi.org/10.1161/01.CIR.88.2.523.

Olszewski, A. J., & McCully, K. S. (1993). Fish oil decreases serum homocysteine in hyperlipemic men. *Coronary Artery Disease*, *4*(1), 53–60. https://doi.org/10.1097/00019501-199301000-00007.

Piolot, A., Blache, D., Boulet, L., Fortin, L. J., Dubreuil, D., Marcoux, C., et al. (2003). Effect of fish oil on LDL oxidation and plasma homocysteine concentrations in health. *Journal of Laboratory and Clinical Medicine*, *141*(1), 41–49. https://doi.org/10.1067/mlc.2003.3.

Pooya, S., Jalali, M. D., Jazayery, A. D., Saedisomeolia, A., Eshraghian, M. R., & Toorang, F. (2010). The efficacy of omega-3 fatty acid supplementation on plasma homocysteine and malondialdehyde levels of type 2 diabetic patients. *Nutrition, Metabolism, and Cardiovascular Diseases*, *20*(5), 326–331. https://doi.org/10.1016/j.numecd.2009.04.002.

Refsum, H., Ueland, P. M., Nygård, O., & Vollset, S. E. (1998). Homocysteine and cardiovascular disease. *Annual Review of Medicine*, *49*, 31–62. https://doi.org/10.1146/annurev.med.49.1.31.

Saedisomeolia, A., Wood, L. G., Garg, M. L., Gibson, P. G., & Wark, P. A. B. (2009). Lycopene enrichment of cultured airway epithelial cells decreases the inflammation induced by rhinovirus infection and lipopolysaccharide. *Journal of Nutritional Biochemistry*, *20*(8), 577–585. https://doi.org/10.1016/j.jnutbio.2008.06.001.

Selhub, J. (1999). Homocysteine metabolism. *Annual Review of Nutrition*, *19*, 217–246. https://doi.org/10.1146/annurev.nutr.19.1.217.

Selhub, J., Jacques, P. F., Rosenberg, I. H., Rogers, G., Bowman, B. A., Gunter, E. W., et al. (1999). Serum total homocysteine concentrations in the third National Health and Nutrition Examination Survey (1991-1994): Population reference ranges and contribution of vitamin status to high serum concentrations. *Annals of Internal Medicine*, *131*(5), 331–339. https://doi.org/10.7326/0003-4819-131-5-199909070-00003.

Sunder-Plassmann, G., & Födinger, M. (2003). Genetic determinants of the homocysteine level. *Kidney International*, *63*(Suppl. 84), S141–S144. Blackwell Publishing Inc https://doi.org/10.1046/j.1523-1755.63.s84.52.x.

Svaneborg, N., Møller, J. M., Schmidt, E. B., Varming, K., Lervang, H. H., & Dyerberg, J. (1994). The acute effects of a single very high dose of n-3 fatty acids on plasma lipids and lipoproteins in healthy subjects. *Lipids*, *29*(2), 145–147. https://doi.org/10.1007/BF02537154.

Van Der Put, N. M. J., Gabreëls, F., Stevens, E. M. B., Smeitink, J. A. M., Trijbels, F. J. M., Eskes, T. K. A. B., et al. (1998). A second common mutation in the methylenetetrahydrofolate reductase gene: An additional risk factor for neural-tube defects? *American Journal of Human Genetics*, *62*(5), 1044–1051. https://doi.org/10.1086/301825.

Vinukonda, G., Shaik Mohammad, N., Md Nurul Jain, J., Prasad Chintakindi, K., & Rama Devi Akella, R. (2009). Genetic and environmental influences on total plasma homocysteine and coronary artery disease (CAD) risk among South Indians. *Clinica Chimica Acta*, *405*(1–2), 127–131. https://doi.org/10.1016/j.cca.2009.04.015.

Wang, X. L., Cai, H., Cranney, G., & Wilcken, D. E. L. (1998). The frequency of a common mutation of the methionine synthase gene in the Australian population and its relation to smoking and coronary artery disease. *Journal of Cardiovascular Risk*, *5*(5), 289–295. https://doi.org/10.1097/00043798-199810000-00001.

Zeman, M., Žák, A., Vecka, M., Tvrzická, E., Písaříková, A., & Staňková, B. (2006). N-3 fatty acid supplementation decreases plasma homocysteine in diabetic dyslipidemia treated with statin-fibrate combination. *Journal of Nutritional Biochemistry*, *17*(6), 379–384. https://doi.org/10.1016/j.jnutbio.2005.08.007.

CHAPTER

18

Effect of 1,3-diacylglycerol on cardiometabolic risk

Tongcheng Xu and Min Jia

Grain & Oil Engineering Lab, Institute of Agro-food Science and Technology, Shangdong Academy of Agricultural Sciences, Jinan, China

18.1 Introduction

Cardiometabolic risk refers to a series of metabolic and cardiovascular abnormalities, including hypertension, dyslipidemia, insulin resistance, and other symptoms. Most of the patients with these symptoms are accompanied by bad habits, such as irregular eating and little exercise. In addition, poor sleep quality or insufficient sleep time may also increase the occurrence of cardiometabolic risks. Some symptoms of cardiometabolic risk are precursor of many diseases, such as insulin resistance, which makes patients more susceptible to type 2 diabetes. Therefore, studying the mechanism of increased cardiometabolic risk and preventing the occurrence of cardiometabolic risk, thereby reducing the incidence of other related diseases, is an issue that should be paid attention to worldwide.

18.2 The 1,3-diacylglycerol

In recent years, people have paid more and more attention to the quality and safety of edible oils. Diacylglycerol has high processing adaptability, rich in nutritional value, and safe for consumption, which has attracted social attention. Triglycerides are composed of glycerol and 3 fatty acids. The structural lipid formed after one fatty acid (FA) is substituted by a hydroxyl group is called a diacylglycerol. Diacylglycerol is a product obtained by esterification of two molecules of FAs with glycerol. It is a natural component of oils and fats. It can be classified into 1,3-DAG and 1,2-DAG isomers according to the position where the acyl group binds to the hydroxyl group. After 1,3-DAG enters the small intestine, it will be decomposed into glycerol and free fatty acids (FFA) by related enzymes. Glycerol is absorbed by the small intestinal epithelial cells. Most of the FFAs undergo β-oxidation in the mitochondria and are finally decomposed into CO_2 and H_2O for direct release. Therefore, 1,3-DAG in the small intestine lipid decomposition and energy utilization increases, making it difficult to increase the neutral fat in the blood after eating 1,3-DAG (Xu et al., 2018). In this way, continually consumption of 1,3-DAG can reduce body fat accumulation, blood sugar, and cardiometabolic symptoms caused by diseases, such as hyperlipidemia, diabetes, etc. (Yanai et al., 2008).

18.2.1 The source of 1,3-diacylglycerol

The 1,3-DAG is mainly derived from some vegetable oils and is a natural trace component in vegetable oils. In common edible oils and fats, cotton oil and olive oil contain relatively more diacylglycerol, of which 1,3-DAG accounts for about 70% and 1,2-DAG accounts for about 30%. During the metabolism of oil in the human body, a very small amount of 1,3-DAG is produced as an intermediate product, which is combined with other substances or decomposed to participate in the next physiological metabolic process. Although 1,3-DAG is extremely small in nature, it has powerful functions and is widely used in various industries, such as food, medicine, and chemical industries. For example, processing 1,3-DAG into margarine, mayonnaise, etc., as healthy weight loss foods, 1,3-DAG is used as a dispersion medium of active ingredients in medicines in the production of powders and tablets; 1,3-DAG is used to make deodorants, etc. Therefore, in recent years, market and scientific researchers have paid special attention to the preparation process and functional evaluation of 1,3-DAG. The Oil and Fat Professional Branch of Chinese Cereals and Oils Association also proposed that the research and development of 1,3-DAG should be the key direction of oil research in the future.

Currently, 1,3-DAG used in various industries is usually obtained by industrial preparation. The 1,3-DAG preparation methods are mainly divided into two categories: chemical and biological enzymatic method (Pazdur, Geuens, Sels, & Tavernier, 2015). Chemical methods include direct esterification and oil glycerolysis, and biological enzymatic methods include direct esterification, oil glycerolysis, oil alcoholysis, oil hydrolysis, and microbial glycolysis (Zhong et al., 2013). Next, we will briefly describe several commonly used and efficient methods.

18.2.2 Method of preparation of 1,3-diacylglycerol

18.2.2.1 Direct esterification

The direct esterification method uses a catalyst to catalyze the esterification reaction of glycerol and fatty acids to synthesize 1,3-DAG. The direct esterification method is currently the most used method for preparing 1,3-DAG. According to the type of catalyst, it can be divided into chemical and enzymatic synthesis. The direct esterification method can be completed in one step. The reaction time is short and the product purity is high, but the water generated during the reaction must be removed in time to prevent reducing the concentration of the reactant or affecting the activity of the enzyme (Zeng, Qi, Xin, Yang, & Wang, 2015). The purity of DAG prepared by the esterification method is generally about 60%, and the product contains many triglycerides, monoglycerides, and a small amount of FAs and glycerol. In order to obtain higher purity DAG and meet consumer needs, product purification must be carried out. Commonly used purification methods include molecular distillation, supercritical carbon dioxide extraction, and solvent crystallization. This increases the cost of preparation, and it needs to be considered carefully for large-scale production of 1,3-DAG.

18.2.2.2 Selective hydrolysis

Using triglycerides as raw materials, the process of hydrolyzing triglycerides into FAs and glycerol with a specific lipase is called selective hydrolysis, which is the simplest biological enzymatic method for preparing 1,3-DAG.

The above reactions are all bimolecular reactions. The first reaction product is a mixture of diacylglycerols and FAs, which can be separated to obtain diacylglycerols. Therefore, the key to this method is to control the degree of hydrolysis. Excessive hydrolysis is prone to producing too many by-products, and insufficient hydrolysis has a low content of reaction products. Studies have shown that the preparation of 1,3-DAG by hydrolysis of triglycerides as raw materials under the catalysis of lipase can greatly shorten the preparation process. The selective hydrolysis method does not require a large amount of chemical reagents; the process is safe and simple, the output is high, and the obtained product has a pure color and high edible safety. Due to the specificity of the enzyme, there are relatively few by-products produced during the experiment. But, theoretically, to obtain high-yield and high-purity 1,3-DAG through this method, a specific lipase that can specifically hydrolyze the sn-2 ester bond is required. Literatures have mentioned several lipases with high selectivity to the sn-2 ester bond, such as Novozym 435, Lipozyme RM IM, and Lipozyme TL IM (Liu, Wang, Zhao, Zhang, & Zhao, 2011). There is no relevant screening for specific lipase of the sn-2 ester bond.

18.2.2.3 Method of glycolysis

Microbial fermentation refers to the use of natural lipase as catalyst to catalyze the hydrolysis of oils or glycerolysis to synthesize glycerides. Microorganism that can accumulate metabolites as diacylglycerols can be screened out from the soil, and the lipase-catalyzed reaction during the growth of the microorganism can be used to produce 1,3-DAG. In microbial glycolysis, efficient biocatalyst is used to speed up the reaction process, and steps like separation, purification, or fixation of industrial enzymes could be omitted, the production process is simpler and environmental pollution could be reduced. However, this method requires a better understanding of the physiological characteristics of the glycolysis fermentation bacteria.

18.3 Effects of 1,3-diacylglycerol on cardiometabolic risk

18.3.1 The 1,3-diacylglycerol reduces body weight

Fat rich in 1,3-DAG can ameliorate hyperlipidemia, reduce weight and waist circumference, and reduce visceral fat and subcutaneous fat (Prabhavathi Devi et al., 2018). 1,3-DAG can effectively regulate metabolic syndrome, which is beneficial to health. Studies of 1,3-DAG have focused on obesity and energy expenditure (Flickinger & Matsuo, 2003). Compared with the high-TAG oil diet, mice fed with the 1,3-DAG oil diet lost 70% of their body weight after 5 months, and visceral fat, such as epididymis, mesentery, peritoneum, and perirenal fat was also reduced accordingly. Human experiments found that the 1,3-DAG diet group had reduced energy intake, and the weight and fat mass decreased more than the triglyceride group. Experiments showed that 1,3-DAG resynthesizes TAG through the phosphatidic acid pathway and directly shunts fatty acids to the liver for oxidation through the portal vein, which greatly reduces the resynthesis of chylomicrons. In addition, DAG is primarily used for β-oxidation, and the increase in β-oxidation will improve satiety. In clinical trials, β-oxidation of healthy subjects intaking 1,3-DAG oil was significantly higher than that of TAG oil. 1,3-DAG reduces fat synthesis in the liver and increases β-oxidation, thereby reducing the accumulation of subcutaneous and visceral fat. Long-term 1,3-DAG intervention can prevent weight gain and fat deposition and is used as dietary supplements for the treatment of obesity (Maki et al., 2002).

For patients with genetic defects in lipid metabolism, the intake of 1,3-DAG can also reduce their visceral fat. Intake of 1,3-DAG can significantly reduce postprandial serum TAG level, and long-term maintenance of low serum TAG level can reduce visceral fat. Visceral fat obesity is one of the risk factors for diseases, such as diabetes, hyperlipidemia, hypertension, and atherosclerosis. Therefore, 1,3-DAG can significantly improve cardiometabolic diseases and regulate subhealth.

18.3.2 The 1,3-diacylglycerol reduces postprandial lipids

After entering the small intestine, TAG is hydrolyzed into sn-2 monoglyceride (MAG) and two molecules of fatty acids under the action of pancreatic esterase and bile salts. Sn-2 MAG enters the epithelial cells of the small intestine, quickly undergoes an esterification reaction with FAs to synthesize triglycerides, and further forms chylomicrons with cholesterol and proteins, which enter the blood circulation through the lymphatic system (Lee et al., 2020). The resynthesis pathway of triglycerides hydrolysate in the small intestine is called the sn-2 MAG pathway. This pathway reproduces triglycerides very quickly, so the triglyceride intake leads to a rapid postmeal rise in serum triglycerides concentrations (Lu et al., 2020).

Different from TAG metabolism, 1,3-DAG is hydrolyzed into glycerol and two molecules of FFA in the small intestine, absorbed into small intestinal epithelial cells, and then resynthesized into TAG via phospholipid acid (PA) pathway: Glycerol first generates 3-phosphoglycerol (G-3-P) under the action of glycerol kinase (GK) and acyltransferase, then reacts with two molecules of acyl-CoA to generate phosphatidic acid, which is hydrolyzed into 1,2-DAG; 1,2-DAG is further synthesized to TAG. The rate of TAG synthesis is significantly lower than the sn-2 MAG pathway. Studies have shown that, after a long-term intervention with 1,3-DAG in healthy mice, the enzyme activity and mRNA expression levels of three key enzymes, GK, alcohol acyl transferase, and phosphatidic acid phosphatase (PAP) in the small intestinal epithelial cells were significantly increased compared with the TAG group, which further confirmed that the hydrolyzed products of 1,3-DAG were mainly synthesized by the slow PA pathway. Since FFAs are absorbed into the portal vein instead of being resynthesized to TAG in the small intestinal epithelial cells, the serum FFA content increased significantly, while the serum TAG concentration decreased greatly after meals, which is the main way for 1,3-DAG to reduce the postprandial lipids.

18.3.3 The 1,3-diacylglycerol reduces fasting lipids

Hypertriglyceridemia (HTG) is a type of disease caused by impaired serum TAG clearance. It is an important risk factor for cardiometabolic syndrome-related diseases, such as atherosclerosis and hypertension. Active control of hypertriglyceridemia is an important part of the primary prevention of cardiometabolic syndrome-related diseases. Long-term intake of 1,3-DAG significantly reduces fasting serum TAG levels in patients with hypertriglyceridemia and diabetes (Simha, 2020). In addition, the intake of 1,3-DAG can also significantly reduce serum low-density lipoprotein cholesterol (LDL-C) and total cholesterol (TC), and increase high-density lipoprotein cholesterol (HDL-C) and other related indexes of blood lipid metabolism.

Lipoprotein A [Lp(a)], a risk factor for stroke and coronary heart disease, is mainly synthesized in the liver, preventing the dissolution of blood clots in the blood vessels, and accelerating atherosclerosis. The intake of 1,3-DAG can reduce the content of fat in the liver, inhibit the synthesis of Lp(a), and reduce the concentration of Lp(a) in the serum (Saito, Tomonobu, Hase, & Tokimitsu, 2006). Apolipoprotein C (ApoC) is an important structural protein for transporting lipoprotein cholesterol. There are two types of ApoC. ApoC II can improve lipoprotein esterase activity and promote lipid metabolism, while ApoC III can inhibit lipoprotein esterase activity and lead to the increase of lipid levels in the body.

The intake of 1,3-DAG can increase the concentration of serum ApoC II and increase the ratio of ApoC II/ApoC III, thus promoting lipid metabolism and reducing the body's blood lipid level.

The blood lipid-lowering effect of 1,3-DAG is also beneficial to many patients with lipoprotein esterase deficiency. Fatty acid-binding protein 2 (FABP2) is a gene encoding the intestinal FA transporter, which can control the absorption and transport of FA. The intake of 1,3-DAG can significantly reduce the fasting serum total TAG and very low-density lipoprotein cholesterol (VLDL-C) concentration of 54T-FABp2-deficient patients (Wang et al., 2010). Microsomal triglyceride transfer protein (MTP) is another important TAG transfer protein that can catalyze the transfer of TAG and cholesterol. The special structure of 1,3-DAG leads to a significant decrease in the polarity and overall hydrophobicity of its sn-1(3) position, a decrease in the ability to bind to MTP, and a decrease in transport speed, thereby reducing the total serum TAG and VLDL-C concentration of the patient.

In addition to improve blood lipid metabolism-related levels, the intake of 1,3-DAG can also increase the particle size of LDL, reduce the density of HDL, and reduce the risk of cardiometabolic-related diseases.

18.3.4 The 1,3-diacylglycerol improves glucose metabolism

1,3-DAG can significantly improve the related indicators of glucose metabolism in patients with type 2 diabetes, reduce glucose intolerance, and prevent impaired glucose tolerance. The intake of 1,3-DAG stimulates fat oxidation and increases the β-oxidation level of body fat (Murata, Ide, & Hara, 1997). The body obtains more energy through fat oxidation, the liver's gluconeogenic energy supply decreases, and the balance point of liver glycogen storage decreases, thereby reducing blood glucose concentration. Clinical studies have also shown that after the intake of 1,3-DAG, the body's postprandial insulin concentration is significantly lower than that of the TAG group. The decrease in insulin concentration is accompanied by a drop of leptin concentration, as well as leptin receptor. The concentration of leptin is closely related to insulin resistance, which has also been significantly improved (Saito, Hernandez-Ono, & Ginsberg, 2007). In addition, the long-term continuous intervention of 1,3-DAG can improve fasting blood glucose levels, reduce glycosylated hemoglobin concentration, and improve glucose metabolism.

18.4 Metabolism of 1,3-diacylglycerol

18.4.1 Hydrolysis of 1,3-diacylglycerol in vivo

Although 70–80% of food lipid digestion is completed in the small intestine, digestion starts from the stomach. About 10–30% of the ingested lipids are digested in the stomach by gastric lipase, which under acidic conditions (pH 3.0–6.5), relative to the ester bond at the sn-2 position, gastric lipase preferentially cleaves the sn-1,3 position (Kondo, Hase, Murase, & Tokimitsu, 2003). Commonly, TAG can be digested and hydrolyzed into 1,2-DAG and FAs in the stomach and enter the small intestine after being emptied from the stomach. Under the action of enteropancreatic lipase (pancreatic lipase specifically hydrolyzes the ester bonds at sn-1 and sn-3), 2-MAG and FFAs are finally formed, and part of 2-MAG will undergo acyl transfer to form 1-MAG or 3-MAG and will continue to be hydrolyzed into glycerol and FAs.

Similarly, some ester bonds in the ingested 1,3-DAG will be hydrolyzed by gastric lipase at the sn-3 position to form 1-MAG, which will enter the small intestine after gastric emptying and finally be digested and hydrolyzed into 1(3)-MAG, FFA, and glycerol under the action of intestinal pancreatic lipase. Only a small amount of 1(3)-MAG is absorbed from the lumen of the small intestine into mucosal epithelial cells without being hydrolyzed, and the rest is hydrolyzed into glycerol and FFAs, which are also absorbed by mucosal epithelial cells. Except for a small part of the FAs entering the mucosal cells for further synthesis, most of the FAs undergo β-oxidation in mitochondria to provide energy for the human body (Hibi, Takase, Meguro, & Tokimitsu, 2009).

18.4.2 Resynthesis of 1,3-diacylglycerol hydrolysates

The main hydrolysates of 1,3-DAG are 1(3)-MAG, FFA, and glycerol. The hydrolysate is resynthesized after being absorbed by intestinal cells. For 2-MAG, the hydrolysate of TAG in the small intestine, it is rapidly resynthesized into TAG via monoacylglycerol transferase (EC: 2.3.1.22, MGAT), while 1(3)-MAG is processed into TAG and phospholipid at a much slower rate. 1(3)-MAG can also be reesterified into 1,3-DAG in the intestinal mucosa cells (Xu et al., 2018).

Comparing 1-MAG and 2-MAG, the positions of the two bindings to glycerol are different, so there is a big difference as raw material for the resynthesis to neutral fat. The resynthesis progress of the former neutral fat is slowly (Li & Olsen, 2017). This is because MGAT2 and MGAT3 are the key acyl coenzymes used to synthesize DAG. However, the affinity of 1(3)-MAG to MGAT2 is lower than that of 2-MAG, and 1(3)-MAG is not a substrate of MGAT3. The resynthesis of TAG in the small intestine is mainly through the 2-MAG pathway, so the synthesis of TAG is reduced after ingesting 1,3-DAG. Some 1(3)-MAG can be acylated to 1,2(2,3)-DAG, and then TAG can be synthesized by 2-MAG. In addition, FFAs and glycerol can be resynthesized into TAG through the phosphatidic acid (PA) pathway in the small intestinal epithelial cells. Glycerol is converted into G-3-P under the action of GK, and then G-3-P reacts with two molecules of fatty acyl CoA to form phosphatidic acid. Phosphatidic acid is converted into 1,2-DAG by PAP, and 1,2-DAG is converted into TAG under the action of diacylglycerol acyltransferase-2. The TAG formed through the phosphatidic acid pathway is stored in the cell fluid of intestinal cells. This is a slow conversion pool. The stored TAG is then hydrolyzed and reesterified in the microsomes to produce TAG, which is bound to the lymphatic chylomicrons and enters the blood circulation. Another part of 1(3)-MAG is absorbed from the lumen into the mucosal cells without being further hydrolyzed but reesterified into 1,3-DAG in mucosal cells. It can be seen from the unique structure and metabolic characteristics of 1,3-DAG that it has great potential in ameliorating obesity and hyperlipidemia, improving diabetes, and reducing the prevalence of cardiometabolic risk diseases.

18.5 Supplementation of 1,3-diacylglycerol

18.5.1 Cooking oil

The 1,3-DAG is a functional oil with weight loss, which can be absorbed through the lymphatic system or directly through the portal vein. Therefore, 1,3-DAG can be used to produce fat-reducing functional foods and can also be used as household cooking, baking, and food oil substitutes for industrial production. 1,3-DAG are used in baked products, vegetable oil, and other foods, which not only play a nutritional role but also have good stability and flavor. In baking products, the semisolid 1,3-DAG can absorb part of the air in the dough. During the baking process, it is heated and becomes fluffy, which is the characteristic shape and structure of the dough; in addition, the shortened dough composed of 1,3-DAG has good oil retention, easy roll division, and simple demolding, which improves the nutritional value of the finished product and also gives the food a good taste and flavor.

18.5.2 Dietary supplements

The 1,3-DAG can be used as carrier of medicine for cardiovascular diseases. Due to the special structure and metabolic pathway, 1,3-DAG can be directly combined with medicine to accelerate the absorption and release of medicine in the body. When producing medicines, 1,3-DAG can be used as dispersion medium for medicines, which can protect the active ingredients during spray drying.

The 1,3-DAG microcapsules are also used in daily life. Microcapsule technology is also called micro-assembly technology. It uses film-forming materials or polymer materials as wall materials to embed the core material that needs to be protected to form tiny particles. The core material can be fixed, protected, and released in a certain period of time. The 1,3-DAG is insoluble in water, and it has a low absorption rate in the gastrointestinal tract, which limits their application in the food industry. Lipid microencapsulation is currently an effective method to overcome lipid oxidation and nutrient loss. Microcapsules can improve the stability of 1,3-DAG and make up for the deficiency above. The original performance of 1,3-DAG can be optimized while inhibiting lipid oxidation.

In addition, food microemulsions provide a good way to develop 1,3-DAG. Oils are difficult to dissolve in water and have large molecular weights and long molecular chains. Microemulsions can solve these problems well. The solubilization and bioavailability of the microemulsion could be improved by combining the active substance with 1,3-DAG. In addition, in the microemulsion system, the active substances are aggregated into small micelles under the action of surfactants, which reduces the contact with oxygen, plays a protective role on active substances, and greatly improves the oxidation stability of bioactive substances.

18.6 Conclusion

In short, as a natural component of many fats and oils, 1,3-DAG has the functions of improving blood lipids, ameliorating the accumulation of fat in body, and decreasing insulin resistance. This is due to its unique structural and metabolic differences, the 2-MAG synthesis pathway and β-oxidation in the small intestine and the expression of genes related to lipid metabolism are important mechanisms for its function. It plays an active role in treating obesity and hyperlipidemia, improving diabetes, and reducing the prevalence of cardiometabolic risk diseases.

References

Flickinger, B. D., & Matsuo, N. (2003). Nutritional characteristics of DAG oil. *Lipids*, *38*(2), 129–132. https://doi.org/10.1007/s11745-003-1042-8.

Hibi, M., Takase, H., Meguro, S., & Tokimitsu, I. (2009). The effects of diacylglycerol oil on fat oxidation and energy expenditure in humans and animals. *BioFactors*, *35*(2), 175–177. https://doi.org/10.1002/biof.25.

Kondo, H., Hase, T., Murase, T., & Tokimitsu, I. (2003). Digestion and assimilation features of dietary dag in the rat small intestine. *Lipids*, *38*(1), 25–30. https://doi.org/10.1007/s11745-003-1027-7.

Lee, Y.-Y., Tang, T.-K., Phuah, E.-T., Tan, C.-P., Wang, Y., Li, Y., et al. (2020). Production, safety, health effects and applications of diacylglycerol functional oil in food systems: A review. *Critical Reviews in Food Science and Nutrition*, *60*(15), 2509–2525. https://doi.org/10.1080/10408398.2019.1650001.

Li, K., & Olsen, R. E. (2017). Metabolism of sn-1(3)-monoacylglycerol and sn-2-monoacylglycerol in caecal enterocytes and hepatocytes of Brown Trout (*Salmo trutta*). *Lipids*, *52*(1), 61–71. https://doi.org/10.1007/s11745-016-4215-0.

Liu, N., Wang, Y., Zhao, Q., Zhang, Q., & Zhao, M. (2011). Fast synthesis of 1,3-DAG by Lecitase® ultra-catalyzed esterification in solvent-free system. *European Journal of Lipid Science and Technology*, *113*(8), 973–979. https://doi.org/10.1002/ejlt.201000507.

Lu, H., Guo, T., Fan, Y., Deng, Z., Luo, T., & Li, H. (2020). Effects of diacylglycerol and triacylglycerol from peanut oil and coconut oil on lipid metabolism in mice. *Journal of Food Science*, *85*(6), 1907–1914. https://doi.org/10.1111/1750-3841.15159.

Maki, K. C., Davidson, M. H., Tsushima, R., Matsuo, N., Tokimitsu, I., Umporowicz, D. M., et al. (2002). Consumption of diacylglycerol oil as part of a reduced-energy diet enhances loss of body weight and fat in comparison with consumption of a triacylglycerol control oil. *American Journal of Clinical Nutrition*, 76(6), 1230–1236. https://doi.org/10.1093/ajcn/76.6.1230.

Murata, M., Ide, T., & Hara, K. (1997). Reciprocal responses to dietary diacylglycerol of hepatic enzymes of fatty acid synthesis and oxidation in the rat. *British Journal of Nutrition*, 77(1), 107–121. https://doi.org/10.1079/BJN19970013.

Pazdur, Ł., Geuens, J., Sels, H., & Tavernier, S. M. F. (2015). Low-temperature chemical synthesis of high-purity diacylglycerols (DAG) from monoacylglycerols (MAG). *Lipids*, 50(2), 219–226. https://doi.org/10.1007/s11745-014-3980-x.

Prabhavathi Devi, B. L. A., Gangadhar, K. N., Prasad, R. B. N., Sugasini, D., Rao, Y. P. C., & Lokesh, B. R. (2018). Nutritionally enriched 1,3-diacylglycerol-rich oil: Low calorie fat with hypolipidemic effects in rats. *Food Chemistry*, 248, 210–216. https://doi.org/10.1016/j.foodchem.2017.12.066.

Saito, S., Hernandez-Ono, A., & Ginsberg, H. N. (2007). Dietary 1,3-diacylglycerol protects against diet-induced obesity and insulin resistance. *Metabolism, Clinical and Experimental*, 56(11), 1566–1575. https://doi.org/10.1016/j.metabol.2007.06.024.

Saito, S., Tomonobu, K., Hase, T., & Tokimitsu, I. (2006). Effects of diacylglycerol on postprandial energy expenditure and respiratory quotient in healthy subjects. *Nutrition*, 22(1), 30–35. https://doi.org/10.1016/j.nut.2005.04.010.

Simha, V. (2020). Management of hypertriglyceridemia. *BMJ*, 371. https://doi.org/10.1136/bmj.m3109. PMID: 33046451.

Wang, W., Xu, T., Li, X., Zhu, Q., Cheng, A., Du, F., et al. (2010). Effect of diacylglycerol supplementation on fasting serum triacylglycerol concentration: A meta-analysis. *Lipids*, 45(12), 1139–1146. https://doi.org/10.1007/s11745-010-3478-0.

Xu, T., Jia, M., Li, X., Qiu, B., Zhang, Y., Liu, W., et al. (2018). Intake of diacylglycerols and the fasting insulin and glucose concentrations: A meta-analysis of 5 randomized controlled studies. *Journal of the American College of Nutrition*, 37(7), 598–604. https://doi.org/10.1080/07315724.2018.1452168.

Xu, T., Li, J., Zou, J., Qiu, B., Liu, W., Lin, X., et al. (2018). Rat small intestinal mucosal epithelial cells absorb dietary 1,3-diacylglycerol via phosphatidic acid pathways. *Lipids*, 53(3), 335–344. https://doi.org/10.1002/lipd.12030.

Yanai, H., Yoshida, H., Tomono, Y., Hirowatari, Y., Kurosawa, H., Matsumoto, A., et al. (2008). Effects of diacylglycerol on glucose, lipid metabolism, and plasma serotonin levels in lean Japanese. *Obesity*, 16(1), 47–51. https://doi.org/10.1038/oby.2007.46.

Zeng, C.-X., Qi, S.-J., Xin, R.-P., Yang, B., & Wang, Y.-H. (2015). Enzymatic selective synthesis of 1,3-DAG based on deep eutectic solvent acting as substrate and solvent. *Bioprocess and Biosystems Engineering*, 38(11), 2053–2061. https://doi.org/10.1007/s00449-015-1445-0.

Zhong, N., Gui, Z., Xu, L., Huang, J., Hu, K., Gao, Y., et al. (2013). Solvent-free enzymatic synthesis of 1,3-diacylglycerols by direct esterification of glycerol with saturated fatty acids. *Lipids in Health and Disease*, 12(1), 65. https://doi.org/10.1186/1476-511x-12-65.

CHAPTER 19

Palmitoleic acid in health and disease

Jun Tang

Laboratory of Precision Nutrition and Computational Medicine, School of Life Sciences, Westlake University, Hangzhou, China

19.1 Introduction

Palmitoleic acid (16:1n-7) is a 16-carbon monounsaturated fatty acid (MUFA) with a double bond located in the seventh position and can be classified as a cis or trans isomer. The trans-palmitoleic acid (16:1t9) is principally derived from dairy and ruminant fats and represents a very low percentage of total palmitoleic acid, of which the majority is its cis isoform (16:1c9) (Micha et al., 2010). In humans, cis-palmitoleic acid mainly originates from de novo lipogenesis mediated by stearoyl-CoA desaturase-1 (SCD-1), the rate-limiting enzyme catalyzing the synthesis of MUFAs from SFAs. Endogenous synthesis of palmitoleic acid occurs primarily in liver and secondarily in adipose tissue, where it is then incorporated into various lipid fractions such as triacylglycerol (TAG) and phospholipid and eventually transported into circulation for uptake by other organs and tissues to different extents. Palmitoleic acid is widely distributed in various tissues including serum, muscle, liver, and adipose tissues, whereas its concentrations are site- and lipid fraction-specific. For instance, in serum, palmitoleic acid in TAG can occupy over 5% of total FAs, while in free fatty acids (FFAs) around 4%, and in erythrocyte phospholipids only 0.7%. However, concentrations of palmitoleic acid in different lipid fractions in serum are closely correlated, indicating that the changes of endogenous palmitoleic acid might be internally consistent.

Compared with MUFA oleic acid (18:1n-9), which is high in widely consumed olive oil, dietary sources of palmitoleic acid are largely limited. A few foods containing high content of palmitoleic acid include fish oil and macadamia oil, of which palmitoleic acid represents around 7% and 30%, respectively (Wu, Li, & Hildebrand, 2012). Based on the current knowledge, palmitoleic acid is found to be most abundant in the pulp of sea buckthorn, a deciduous shrub cultured mainly in Asia, particularly in Northwest China. The percentage of palmitoleic acid in sea buckthorn pulp oil can vary by different growing areas and plucking times and could be as high as 42% (Fatima et al., 2012). Direct intake of foods containing palmitoleic acid can improve its concentration in the blood. Consumption of macadamia nuts equivalent to 15% energy intake for 4 weeks leads to a significant increase in plasma palmitoleic acid (Garg, Blake, & Wills, 2003), while consumption of fish oil leads to various changes in palmitoleic acid concentration in different lipid fractions (Frigolet & Gutiérrez-Aguilar, 2017).

Expecting for direct dietary sources, indirect dietary factors can also increase palmitoleic acid levels in the body by inducing its endogenous biosynthesis. Carbohydrates are considered to have the strongest correlation with palmitoleic acid concentrations, based on the knowledge that carbohydrate intake can increase de novo lipogenesis. The upregulated SCD-1 gene expression during de novo lipogenesis leads to an increased production of palmitoleic acid. Besides, in the context of hyperlipidemia caused by overnutrition, SCD-1-generated palmitoleic acid, as well as oleic acid, is necessary for the synthesis of TAG and cholesterol esters (Flowers & Ntambi, 2009).

Despite the limited natural sources and complex endogenous metabolism of palmitoleic acid, recent human and animal studies have revealed its biological functions, though findings are inconsistent and even controversial. Here, we continue to summarize existing evidence concerning the effects of palmitoleic acid on metabolic health and underlying mechanisms.

19.2 Is palmitoleic acid a novel lipid hormone?

In fatty acid binding protein-deficient (FABP$^{-/-}$) mice, enhanced de novo lipogenesis in adipose tissue leads to dramatically increased plasma palmitoleic acid. Augmented circulating palmitoleic acid strongly improved muscle insulin sensitivity and reduced hepatosteatosis. Because palmitoleic acid can be released by adipose tissue and exert beneficial effects on metabolic outcomes of distant organs including muscle and liver, which mimics the role of adipokines that mediate the communication between adipose and other tissues, it was defined as the novel lipid hormone "lipokine" (Cao et al., 2008). However, this study did not explain well the null or even opposite role of palmitoleic acid derived from the liver, the main site for biosynthesis of palmitoleic acid. If palmitoleic acid was a lipid hormone transported by circulation, it would exert the same effects on distant organs regardless of where it was derived.

Moreover, the potential of palmitoleic acid as a lipid hormone was also challenged by human studies, where evidence seems to conflict with that from animal studies. In a cross-sectional study of 1926 adults in Costa Rica, palmitoleic acid in adipose tissue was positively associated with obesity, independent of carbohydrate intake, which is generally believed to induce liver synthesis of palmitoleic acid (Gong et al., 2011). Based on this result, it is even speculated that adipose tissue palmitoleic acid may mainly reflect the palmitoleic acid that is synthesized and released by the liver, instead of adipose tissue. In a prospective cohort of 3630 US men and women in the Cardiovascular Health Study, circulating palmitoleic acid is robustly associated with multiple metabolic risk factors but in mixed directions (Mozaffarian et al., 2010a). Similarly, in a population based on 3107 Chinese elderly men and women, erythrocyte palmitoleic acid is associated with an adverse profile of adipokines and inflammatory markers and an increased risk of metabolic syndrome (Zong et al., 2012).

These discrepant findings from animal and human studies raise uncertainties with regard to the potential of palmitoleic acid, which acts as a beneficial lipid hormone. Findings from animal studies are not always applicable to humans, especially when the animal models are set under particular circumstances. In FABP$^{-/-}$ mice, adipose-specific enhanced de novo lipogenesis and increased palmitoleic acid could indeed maintain metabolic homeostasis. However, divergent lifestyle determinants, especially diet or endogenous synthesis, can affect the metabolism and also the role of palmitoleic acid in humans of different health status. Based on the current knowledge, the role of palmitoleic acid in systemic metabolism remains uncertain and needs to be classified by well-designed animal models and randomized controlled trails in humans.

19.3 Effects of palmitoleic acid on metabolic diseases

As a potential lipid hormone, palmitoleic acid has been reported to be closely related to inflammation (Chan et al., 2015), cardiac growth (Foryst-Ludwig et al., 2015), endothelial function (Sarabi, Vessby, Millgård, & Lind, 2001), and also endoplasmic reticulum stress (Akazawa et al., 2010). In humans, circulating and adipose palmitoleic acid are associated with obesity, dyslipidemia, inflammation, insulin sensitivity, and cardiovascular diseases (Okada et al., 2005; Paillard et al., 2008; Stefan et al., 2010; Warensjö, Öhrvall, & Vessby, 2006). However, controversial findings have been found for the roles of endogenous and exogenous palmitoleic acid in chronic metabolic diseases, especially obesity, diabetes, and cardiovascular diseases (Fig. 19.1).

19.3.1 Obesity

Observational studies have investigated the relationship between endogenous palmitoleic acid levels and obesity in different populations. In Canadian adults, serum palmitoleic acid in normal-weight participants was significantly lower in obese participants who were also metabolically unhealthy, but showed no difference with metabolically healthy obese participants, indicating that circulating palmitoleic acid might be associated with metabolic disorders in obese adults (Perreault et al., 2014). However, in a Mediterranean population, both dietary and adipose palmitoleic acid were significantly lower in the morbidly obese group compared with the normal-weight group (Garaulet, Hernandez-Morante, Tebar, & Zamora, 2011). In addition, there was no difference in erythrocyte palmitoleic acid between obese and nonobese women (Cazzola, Rondanelli, Russo-Volpe, Ferrari, & Cestaro, 2004). Unlike the discrepant findings from adults, several observational studies conducted on children from different countries have suggested that palmitoleic acid in different lipid fractions was significantly higher in obese groups compared with that in normal-weight groups (Bermúdez-Cardona & Velásquez-Rodríguez, 2016; Elizondo-Montemayor, Serrano-González, Ugalde-Casas, Cuello-García, & Borbolla-Escoboza, 2011; Gil-Campos et al., 2008; Okada et al., 2005). Though the above-mentioned epidemiological studies seem to support a positive association between circulating palmitoleic acid and obesity, a majority of them could not explain causality due to the

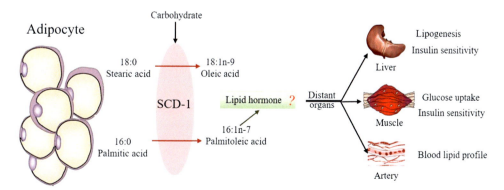

FIG. 19.1 Potential role of palmitoleic acid as a novel lipid hormone in metabolic diseases. Palmitoleic acid can originate from de novo lipogenesis mediated by SCD-1 in humans. Adipose-derived palmitoleic acid has been considered as a novel lipid hormone "lipokine," since animal study demonstrated that palmitoleic acid can affect the metabolism of distant organs such as liver and skeletal muscle.

cross-sectional study design. Besides, potential residual confounding factors involved in race, sex, age, gene, and diet cannot be ruled out and might bias the association toward an unknown direction.

In randomized controlled trails, intake of 1 g palmitoleic acid per day decreased the gastric emptying time and thus affected gastrointestinal transportation and appetite, though no direct effects on body weight were observed (Markey et al., 2011). Similarly, supplementation with palmitoleic acid could increase the secretion of cholecystokinin and reduce food intake in mice (Yang, Takeo, & Katayama, 2013). These studies indicate that appetite could be one pathway for palmitoleic acid contributing to body weight. However, the direct and long-term effects of palmitoleic acid on body weight or obesity are not well established and need to be investigated by further prospective cohort studies and clinical trials.

19.3.2 Diabetes

As a potential lipid hormone, circulating palmitoleic acid is reported to be negatively related to insulin sensitivity or resistance, and risk of diabetes. In a study of 100 white Caucasian subjects, insulin sensitivity was assessed by euglycemic–hyperinsulinemic clamp and oral glucose tolerance tests and was positively associated with circulating palmitoleic acid, of which results are independent of age, sex, and adiposity (Stefan et al., 2010). This finding was consistent with several observational studies demonstrating that serum levels of palmitoleic acid in cholesterol and FFAs were both reported to be inversely associated with insulin resistance (Gertow et al., 2006; Salomaa et al., 1990). However, palmitoleic acid in adipose tissue was found to be inversely associated with insulin sensitivity (Iggman et al., 2010), though included participants were over 70 years old on average, and the association might be of low external validity. In the Cardiovascular Health Study of 3736 US adults, serum trans-palmitoleic acid was associated with a substantial lower incidence of diabetes, and a 0.05% increase in trans-palmitoleic acid in serum can lead to a 28% decrease in incident diabetes (Mozaffarian et al., 2010b). This cohort study suggested a casual effect of circulating trans-palmitoleic acid, the biomarkers of dairy/ruminant fats, on long-term risk of diabetes. Further, rosiglitazone can increase indexes of stearoyl-CoA desaturase activity linked to insulin sensitization independent of peroxisome proliferator-activated receptor-gamma (PPAR-γ), in which process the synthesis of palmitoleic acid by desaturation of palmitic acid was enhanced (Risérus et al., 2005).

Though epidemiological studies demonstrated an inverse association of circulating and adipose palmitoleic acid with insulin resistance or incident type 2 diabetes, the underlying mechanisms remain inconclusive. In line with human studies, animal studies have also found that adipose tissue-released palmitoleic acid increases insulin sensitivity in muscle and suppresses the secretion of monocyte chemoattractant proteins (MCPs) and tumor necrosis factors (TNFs) (Cao et al., 2008). The insulin sensitization effects of palmitoleic were also seen in other animal studies, which further suggested that the activation of GLUT-4 transportation in erythrocytes might be one potential mechanism (Tsuchiya et al., 2010). At the cellular level, palmitoleic acid could promote cell proliferation and secretion (Welters et al., 2006) and reduce endoplasmic reticulum stress and apoptosis (Akazawa et al., 2010). These cellular studies suggest a potential mechanism of palmitoleic acid in diabetes in vitro, but the exact mechanisms should be investigated by studies conducted in vivo.

19.3.3 Cardiovascular diseases

Dietary and circulating saturated, monounsaturated, polyunsaturated and trans-fatty acid have been long proved to be associated with cardiovascular diseases (CVDs). As a MUFA, palmitoleic acid has been reported to be correlated with several risk factors for CVDs including hypertension, serum cholesterol, apolipoprotein, and endothelial function (Sarabi et al., 2001). In a cross-sectional study of 3107 Chinese elderly, erythrocyte palmitoleic acid was positively associated with retinol binding protein 4, blood pressure, total cholesterol, and triglycerides, but negatively associated with serum high-density lipoprotein cholesterol (HDL-C) and adiponectin (Zong et al., 2012). Similarly, a recent case–control study suggested that erythrocyte palmitoleic acid was inversely associated with the prevalence of primary hypertension in Chinese children and adolescents (Tang et al., 2021). Conversely, in a prospective cohort study of 3630 US adults, plasma phospholipid palmitoleic acid was associated with lower serum high-density lipoprotein cholesterol (LDL-C), but associated with higher HDL-C, indicating that palmitoleic acid can beneficially affect blood lipids which are important risk factors for CVDs (Mozaffarian et al., 2010a). Despite the controversial findings with regard to the association between palmitoleic acid and risk factors for CVDs, a prospective nested case–control study further compared cis-trans isomers of palmitoleic acid in the risk of coronary heart diseases (CHD) and found that cis-palmitoleic acid was positively, but the trans-isomer was negatively, associated with the risk of CHD (Djoussé, Matthan, Lichtenstein, & Gaziano, 2012).

Supplementation with palmitoleic acid or enriched diets seems to improve lipid profiles to different extents. Consumption of macadamia nut containing high palmitoleic acid for 3 weeks leads to a dramatic decrease of serum cholesterol and LDL-C in Japanese young women, compared with control groups consuming butter (Hiraoka-Yamamoto et al., 2004). Other randomized controlled trials also showed that 1 month of macadamia nut supplementation could improve serum lipid profiles in both healthy (Curb, Wergowske, Dobbs, Abbott, & Huang, 2000) and hypercholesterolemic (Garg et al., 2003) adults. However, the beneficial effects of palmitoleic acid on serum lipid profiles should be considered as which oil or fatty acid it was compared to. In a 3-week trial conducted in hypercholesterolemic men, supplementation with palmitoleic acid showed no effects on serum LDL-C, but oleic acid significantly decreased serum LDL-C levels, when compared with palmitic acid (Nestel, Clifton, & Noakes, 1994). This finding suggests that palmitoleic acid behaves more like a saturated acid, not a MUFA, in its effect on LDL-C.

The current evidence from both observational studies and clinical trials mainly focuses on CVD risk factors, especially the serum lipid profiles, while the direct effects of palmitoleic acid on risk of CVD have been less investigated. It also should be noted that the potentially beneficial roles of palmitoleic acid varies by what oil or fatty acid had been replaced or compared and by the health status of participants recruited (Table 19.1).

19.4 What are the gaps in evidence that need attention?

As one of the most common MUFAs in nature, palmitoleic acid received far less research attention due to limited dietary sources compared with the oleic acid which is the main constituent of the Mediterranean diet. Based on the evidence from animal studies that it can be released by adipose tissue and exert beneficial effects on distant organs including muscle and liver, palmitoleic acid was considered as a novel lipid hormone "lipokine." Since then, accumulating evidence from animal studies, observational studies, and randomized controlled trails have investigated its roles as a lipid hormone in various metabolism and related chronic diseases. Though palmitoleic acid has been reported to be associated with obesity, diabetes, and CVDs, existing findings are inconsistent and even controversial. Because of the complicated interaction between endogenous synthesis

TABLE 19.1 Evidence with regard to health effects of palmitoleic acid from observational studies and clinical trials.

Author	Study design	Participants	Exposure/intervention	Outcomes	Main conclusion
Cazzola et al. (2004)	Cross-sectional	50 overweight or obese women	Overweight or obese	Fatty acid profiles of erythrocyte membranes	No significant difference was found for 16:1n-7
Garaulet et al. (2011)	Cross-sectional	60 adults of Mediterranean population	Severity of adiposity	Major fatty acid content in subcutaneous and visceral adipose depots	Adipose 16:1n-7 was higher in overweight subjects compared with obese subjects
Gertow et al. (2006)	Cross-sectional	75 Swedish men	Serum and adipose tissue fatty acids profile	Expression levels of acyl-CoA synthase-1 (ACS1) and homeostasis model assessment (HOMA) index	Serum 16:1 predicted ACS1 expression independently of HOMA
Gong et al. (2011)	Cross-sectional	1926 adults in Costa Rica	Adipose tissue 16:1n-7	Obesity	Adipose tissue 16:1n-7 was inversely associated with obesity, but the association was confounded by carbohydrate intake
Iggman et al. (2010)	Cross-sectional	795 adult men	Adipose tissue fatty acid composition	Insulin sensitivity	Adipose tissue 16:1n-7 was negatively associated with insulin sensitivity
Okada et al. (2005)	Cross-sectional	112 children	Plasma 16:1n-7	Indexes of adiposity	Plasma 16:1n-7 content has a significant relationship with abdominal adiposity in obese children
Paillard et al. (2008)	Cross-sectional	134 healthy men	Plasma 16:1n-7	Triglyceridemia and abdominal adiposity	Plasma palmitoleic acid content is an independent marker of both triglyceridemia and abdominal adiposity in men
Perreault et al. (2014)	Cross-sectional	30 adults	Metabolic healthy or unhealthy obesity	Serum total fatty acid composition	Metabolically unhealthy obese participants showed significantly higher serum 16:1n-7 content compared with heathy controls
Salomaa et al. (1990)	Cross-sectional	520 adults	Different health statuses in glucose tolerance	Serum cholesterol esters 16:1n-7 content	Serum cholesterol esters 16:1n-7 was positively associated with insulin resistance

Stefan et al. (2010)	Cross-sectional	100 White Caucasian subjects	The fasting fatty acid pattern in the plasma FFA fraction	Insulin sensitivity	Circulating 16:1n-7 was positively associated with insulin sensitivity
Warensjö et al. (2006)	Cross-sectional	906 Swedish adults	Serum cholesteryl esters fatty acids	Obesity	Serum cholesteryl ester 16:1n-7 was positively associated with obesity
Zong et al. (2012)	Cross-sectional	3107 Chinese elderly men and women	Erythrocyte 16:1n-7	Adipokines, inflammatory markers, and the metabolic syndrome	Erythrocyte palmitoleic acid is associated with an adverse profile of adipokines and inflammatory markers and an increased risk of MetS in this Chinese population
Mozaffarian et al. (2010a)	Prospective cohort	3630 US men and women	Plasma phospholipid 16:1n-7	Risk of metabolic abnormalities and new-onset diabetes	Plasma phospholipid palmitoleic acid was associated with lower serum low-density lipoprotein cholesterol (LDL-C), but associated with higher high-density lipoprotein cholesterol (HDL-C)
Mozaffarian et al. (2010b)	Prospective cohort	3736 US men and women	Plasma phospholipid trans-16:1n-7	Metabolic risk factors and new-onset diabetes	Circulating trans-palmitoleate is associated with lower insulin resistance, presence of atherogenic dyslipidemia, and incident diabetes
Djoussé et al. (2012)	Prospective nested case–control	1000 pairs of incident coronary heart disease (CHD) cases and controls	Cis-16:1n-7 in red blood cell (RBC) membrane	Risk of CHD	RBC membrane cis-16:1n-7 was positively related to CHD
Curb et al. (2000)	Randomized crossover study	30 adults	30-days intervention using a "typical American" diet high in saturated fat (37% energy from fat); an American Heart Association Step 1 diet (30% energy from fat); and a macadamia nut-based monounsaturated fat diet (37% energy from fat) in random order	Serum lipid profiles	The macadamia nut-based diet decreased serum cholesterol and LDL-C levels

Continued

TABLE 19.1 Evidence with regard to health effects of palmitoleic acid from observational studies and clinical trials—cont'd

Author	Study design	Participants	Exposure/intervention	Outcomes	Main conclusion
Markey et al. (2011)	Randomized crossover study	9 healthy, young adults	3 g cinnamon or placebo for 1-day trials	Gastric emptying parameters, postprandial lipemic and glycemic responses, oxidative stress, arterial stiffness, as well as appetite sensations and subsequent food intake	Intake of 1 g palmitoleic acid per day decreased the gastric emptying time and thus affected gastrointestinal transportation and appetite
Hiraoka-Yamamoto et al. (2004)	Randomized controlled trail	71 healthy Japanese women	Coconuts bread, butter bread, or macadamia nut bread for 3 weeks	Weight and serum lipid parameters	A natural diet through intervention with nuts that contain high 16:1n-7 decreased serum total cholesterol and LDL-C levels and reduced body weight in healthy young Japanese women
Nestel et al. (1994)	Randomized controlled trail	34 hypercholesterolemic men	Diets high in palmitic and oleic acid or palmitoleic acid in 3-week periods	Serum lipid profiles	Palmitoleic acid behaves like a saturated and not a MUFA in its effect on LDL-C
Garg et al. (2003)	Intervention study	17 hypercholesterolemic men	4-week period of consuming macadamia nuts	Plasma lipid and homocysteine concentrations	Macadamia nut consumption favorably modifies the plasma lipid profile in hypercholesterolemic men

and diets, the roles of palmitoleic acid as a lipid hormone in metabolism in vivo remain unclear and are largely questioned by human studies. Further studies are warranted to investigate the potential homogenous or discrepant effects of endogenous and exogenous palmitoleic acid on various health outcomes and to elucidate the underlying mechanisms.

References

Akazawa, Y., Cazanave, S., Mott, J. L., Elmi, N., Bronk, S. F., Kohno, S., et al. (2010). Palmitoleate attenuates palmitate-induced Bim and PUMA up-regulation and hepatocyte lipoapoptosis. *Journal of Hepatology*, 52(4), 586–593. https://doi.org/10.1016/j.jhep.2010.01.003.

Bermúdez-Cardona, J., & Velásquez-Rodríguez, C. (2016). Profile of free fatty acids and fractions of phospholipids, cholesterol esters and triglycerides in serum of obese youth with and without metabolic syndrome. *Nutrients*, 8(2). https://doi.org/10.3390/nu8020054.

Cao, H., Gerhold, K., Mayers, J. R., Wiest, M. M., Watkins, S. M., & Hotamisligil, G. S. (2008). Identification of a lipokine, a lipid hormone linking adipose tissue to systemic metabolism. *Cell*, 134(6), 933–944. https://doi.org/10.1016/j.cell.2008.07.048.

Cazzola, R., Rondanelli, M., Russo-Volpe, S., Ferrari, E., & Cestaro, B. (2004). Decreased membrane fluidity and altered susceptibility to peroxidation and lipid composition in overweight and obese female erythrocytes. *Journal of Lipid Research*, 45(10), 1846–1851. https://doi.org/10.1194/jlr.M300509-JLR200.

Chan, K. L., Pillon, N. J., Sivaloganathan, D. M., Costford, S. R., Liu, Z., Théret, M., et al. (2015). Palmitoleate reverses high fat-induced proinflammatory macrophage polarization via AMP-activated protein kinase (AMPK). *Journal of Biological Chemistry*, 290(27), 16979–16988. https://doi.org/10.1074/jbc.M115.646992.

Curb, J. D., Wergowske, G., Dobbs, J. C., Abbott, R. D., & Huang, B. (2000). Serum lipid effects of a high-monounsaturated fat diet based on macadamia nuts. *Archives of Internal Medicine*, 160(8), 1154–1158. https://doi.org/10.1001/archinte.160.8.1154.

Djoussé, L., Matthan, N. R., Lichtenstein, A. H., & Gaziano, J. M. (2012). Red blood cell membrane concentration of cis-palmitoleic and cis-vaccenic acids and risk of coronary heart disease. *American Journal of Cardiology*, 110(4), 539–544. https://doi.org/10.1016/j.amjcard.2012.04.027.

Elizondo-Montemayor, L., Serrano-González, M., Ugalde-Casas, P. A., Cuello-García, C., & Borbolla-Escoboza, J. R. (2011). Plasma phospholipid fatty acids in obese male and female mexican children. *Annals of Nutrition and Metabolism*, 57(3–4), 234–241. https://doi.org/10.1159/000322626.

Fatima, T., Snyder, C. L., Schroeder, W. R., Cram, D., Datla, R., Wishart, D., et al. (2012). Fatty acid composition of developing sea buckthorn (*Hippophae rhamnoides* L.) berry and the transcriptome of the mature seed. *PLoS One*, 7(4). https://doi.org/10.1371/journal.pone.0034099.

Flowers, M. T., & Ntambi, J. M. (2009). Stearoyl-CoA desaturase and its relation to high-carbohydrate diets and obesity. *Biochimica et Biophysica Acta - Molecular and Cell Biology of Lipids*, 1791(2), 85–91. https://doi.org/10.1016/j.bbalip.2008.12.011.

Foryst-Ludwig, A., Kreissl, M. C., Benz, V., Brix, S., Smeir, E., Ban, Z., et al. (2015). Adipose tissue lipolysis promotes exercise-induced cardiac hypertrophy involving the lipokine C16: 1n7-palmitoleate. *Journal of Biological Chemistry*, 290(39), 23603–23615. https://doi.org/10.1074/jbc.M115.645341.

Frigolet, M. E., & Gutiérrez-Aguilar, R. (2017). The role of the novel lipokine palmitoleic acid in health and disease. *Advances in Nutrition*, 8(1), 173–181. https://doi.org/10.3945/an.115.011130.

Garaulet, M., Hernandez-Morante, J. J., Tebar, F. J., & Zamora, S. (2011). Relation between degree of obesity and site-specific adipose tissue fatty acid composition in a Mediterranean population. *Nutrition*, 27(2), 170–176. https://doi.org/10.1016/j.nut.2010.01.004.

Garg, M. L., Blake, R. J., & Wills, R. B. H. (2003). Macadamia nut consumption lowers plasma total and LDL cholesterol levels in hypercholesterolemic men. *Journal of Nutrition*, 133(4), 1060–1063. https://doi.org/10.1093/jn/133.4.1060.

Gertow, K., Rosell, M., Sjögren, P., Eriksson, P., Vessby, B., de Faire, U., et al. (2006). Fatty acid handling protein expression in adipose tissue, fatty acid composition of adipose tissue and serum, and markers of insulin resistance. *European Journal of Clinical Nutrition*, 60(12), 1406–1413. https://doi.org/10.1038/sj.ejcn.1602471.

Gil-Campos, M., Del Carmen Ramírez-Tortosa, M., Larqué, E., Linde, J., Aguilera, C. M., Cañete, R., et al. (2008). Metabolic syndrome affects fatty acid composition of plasma lipids in obese prepubertal children. *Lipids*, 43(8), 723–732. https://doi.org/10.1007/s11745-008-3203-4.

Gong, J., Campos, H., McGarvey, S., Wu, Z., Goldberg, R., & Baylin, A. (2011). Adipose tissue palmitoleic acid and obesity in humans: Does it behave as a lipokine? *American Journal of Clinical Nutrition*, 93(1), 186–191. https://doi.org/10.3945/ajcn.110.006502.

Hiraoka-Yamamoto, J., Ikeda, K., Negishi, H., Mori, M., Hirose, A., Sawada, S., et al. (2004). Serum lipid effects of a monounsaturated (palmitoleic) fatty acid-rich diet based on macadamia nuts in healthy, young japanese women. *Clinical and Experimental Pharmacology and Physiology*, 31(2), S37–S38. https://doi.org/10.1111/j.1440-1681.2004.04121.x.

Iggman, D., Ärnlöv, J., Vessby, B., Cederholm, T., Sjögren, P., & Risérus, U. (2010). Adipose tissue fatty acids and insulin sensitivity in elderly men. *Diabetologia*, 53(5), 850–857. https://doi.org/10.1007/s00125-010-1669-0.

Markey, O., McClean, C. M., Medlow, P., Davison, G. W., Trinick, T. R., Duly, E., et al. (2011). Effect of cinnamon on gastric emptying, arterial stiffness, postprandial lipemia, glycemia, and appetite responses to high-fat breakfast. *Cardiovascular Diabetology*, 10. https://doi.org/10.1186/1475-2840-10-78.

Micha, R., King, I. B., Lemaitre, R. N., Rimm, E. B., Sacks, F., Song, X., et al. (2010). Food sources of individual plasma phospholipid trans fatty acid isomers: The cardiovascular health study. *American Journal of Clinical Nutrition*, 91(4), 883–893. https://doi.org/10.3945/ajcn.2009.28877.

Mozaffarian, D., Cao, H., King, I. B., Lemaitre, R. N., Song, X., Siscovick, D. S., et al. (2010a). Circulating palmitoleic acid and risk of metabolic abnormalities and new-onset diabetes. *American Journal of Clinical Nutrition*, 92(6), 1350–1358. https://doi.org/10.3945/ajcn.110.003970.

Mozaffarian, D., Cao, H., King, I. B., Lemaitre, R. N., Song, X., Siscovick, D. S., et al. (2010b). Trans-palmitoleic acid, metabolic risk factors, and new-onset diabetes in U.S. adults: A cohort study. *Annals of Internal Medicine*, 153(12), 790–799. https://doi.org/10.7326/0003-4819-153-12-201012210-00005.

Nestel, P., Clifton, P., & Noakes, M. (1994). Effects of increasing dietary palmitoleic acid compared with palmitic and oleic acids on plasma lipids of hypercholesterolemic men. *Journal of Lipid Research*, 35(4), 656–662.

Okada, T., Furuhashi, N., Kuromori, Y., Miyashita, M., Iwata, F., & Harada, K. (2005). Plasma palmitoleic acid content and obesity in children. *American Journal of Clinical Nutrition*, 82(4), 747–750. https://doi.org/10.1093/ajcn/82.4.747.

Paillard, F., Catheline, D., Duff, F. L., Bouriel, M., Deugnier, Y., Pouchard, M., et al. (2008). Plasma palmitoleic acid, a product of stearoyl-coA desaturase activity, is an independent marker of triglyceridemia and abdominal adiposity. *Nutrition, Metabolism, and Cardiovascular Diseases*, 18(6), 436–440. https://doi.org/10.1016/j.numecd.2007.02.017.

Perreault, M., Zulyniak, M. A., Badoud, F., Stephenson, S., Badawi, A., Buchholz, A., et al. (2014). A distinct fatty acid profile underlies the reduced inflammatory state of metabolically healthy obese individuals. *PLoS One*, 9(2). https://doi.org/10.1371/journal.pone.0088539.

Risérus, U., Tan, G. D., Fielding, B. A., Neville, M. J., Currie, J., Savage, D. B., et al. (2005). Rosiglitazone increases indexes of stearoyl-CoA desaturase activity in humans: Link to insulin sensitization and the role of dominant-negative mutation in peroxisome proliferator-activated receptor-γ. *Diabetes*, 54(5), 1379–1384. https://doi.org/10.2337/diabetes.54.5.1379.

Salomaa, V., Ahola, I., Tuomilehto, J., Aro, A., Pietinen, P., Korhonen, H. J., et al. (1990). Fatty acid composition of serum cholesterol esters in different degrees of glucose intolerance: A population-based study. *Metabolism*, 39(12), 1285–1291. https://doi.org/10.1016/0026-0495(90)90185-F.

Sarabi, M., Vessby, B., Millgård, J., & Lind, L. (2001). Endothelium-dependent vasodilation is related to the fatty acid composition of serum lipids in healthy subjects. *Atherosclerosis*, 156(2), 349–355. https://doi.org/10.1016/S0021-9150(00)00658-4.

Stefan, N., Kantartzis, K., Celebi, N., Staiger, H., Machann, J., Schick, F., et al. (2010). Circulating palmitoleate strongly and independently predicts insulin sensitivity in humans. *Diabetes Care*, 33(2), 405–407. https://doi.org/10.2337/dc09-0544.

Tang, J., Yang, B., Yan, Y., Tong, W., Zhou, R., Zhang, J., et al. (2021). Palmitoleic acid protects against hypertension by inhibiting NF-κB-mediated inflammation. *Molecular Nutrition & Food Research*, 2001025. https://doi.org/10.1002/mnfr.202001025.

Tsuchiya, Y., Hatakeyama, H., Emoto, N., Wagatsuma, F., Matsushita, S., & Kanzaki, M. (2010). Palmitate-induced down-regulation of sortilin and impaired GLUT4 trafficking in C2C12 Myotubes. *Journal of Biological Chemistry*, 285(45), 34371–34381. https://doi.org/10.1074/jbc.M110.128520.

Warensjö, E., Öhrvall, M., & Vessby, B. (2006). Fatty acid composition and estimated desaturase activities are associated with obesity and lifestyle variables in men and women. *Nutrition, Metabolism, and Cardiovascular Diseases*, 16(2), 128–136. https://doi.org/10.1016/j.numecd.2005.06.001.

Welters, H. J., Diakogiannaki, E., Mordue, J. M., Tadayyon, M., Smith, S. A., & Morgan, N. G. (2006). Differential protective effects of palmitoleic acid and cAMP on caspase activation and cell viability in pancreatic β-cells exposed to palmitate. *Apoptosis*, 11(7), 1231–1238. https://doi.org/10.1007/s10495-006-7450-7.

Wu, Y., Li, R., & Hildebrand, D. F. (2012). Biosynthesis and metabolic engineering of palmitoleate production, an important contributor to human health and sustainable industry. *Progress in Lipid Research*, 51(4), 340–349. https://doi.org/10.1016/j.plipres.2012.05.001.

Yang, Z. H., Takeo, J., & Katayama, M. (2013). Oral administration of omega-7 palmitoleic acid induces satiety and the release of appetite-related hormones in male rats. *Appetite*, 65, 1–7. https://doi.org/10.1016/j.appet.2013.01.009.

Zong, G., Ye, X., Sun, L., Li, H., Yu, Z., Hu, F. B., et al. (2012). Associations of erythrocyte palmitoleic acid with adipokines, inflammatory markers, and the metabolic syndrome in middle-aged and older Chinese. *American Journal of Clinical Nutrition*, 96(5), 970–976. https://doi.org/10.3945/ajcn.112.040204.

CHAPTER 20

Ximenynic acid and its bioactivities

Fang Cai[a], Dhanushka Hettiarachchi[b], Xiaojie Hu[c], Anish Singh[d], Yandi Liu[b], and Bruce Sunderland[b]

[a]School of Life Sciences, Guizhou Normal University, Guiyang, China [b]School of Pharmacy, Curtin Health Innovation Research Institute, Curtin University, Perth, WA, Australia [c]College of Life Science, Linyi University, Linyi, China [d]Institute of Nutrition & Health, Qingdao University, Qingdao, China

20.1 Introduction

Ximenynic acid (*trans*-11-octadecen-9-ynoic acid, 18:2Δ9a,11 t), also known as santalbic acid, is an octadeca-carbon-conjugated enynic acid. It was first discovered in the *Santalum album* seed oil named santalbic acid by Madhuranath in 1938 (Madhuranath & Manjunath, 1938), and then, it was found in three species of *Ximenia* and was called ximenynic acid by Lighthelmin 1950 (Lighthelm & Schwartz, 1950). At first, it was considered to be a non-conjugated octadecatrienoic acid (Madhuranath & Manjunath, 1938). Gunstone later found that it was identical to ximenynic acid with many similar chemical features (Gunstone & Mcgee, 1954). Subsequently, ximenynic acid was discovered in many plants, the majority of them belonging to species of the Opiliaceae, Olacaceae, and Santalaceae (Aitzetmuller, 2012). Most of natural ximenynic acid exists in the seed oil of these three species, such as sandalwood seed oil and Ximenia kernel oil (Aitzetmuller, 2012).

Ximenynic acid has been found out many biological activities, although it is not a necessary fatty acid for humans and animals. What is the most interesting to researchers is its anti-inflammatory activity. It showed strong effects on arachidonic acid metabolism pathway by selective inhibition of COX-1 (Cai et al., 2016) and restraining 5-LOX products such as leukotriene B4 (Croft et al., 1987). Interestingly, COX-1 and 5-LOX are both closely associated with inflammation pathways. Considering the strong relationship of inflammation with tumor development (Grivennikov et al., 2010), ximenynic acid has been shown to have a potential anticancer activity (Cai et al., 2016). On the other hand, its effects on fatty acid metabolism also have caught the researchers' attention. Ximenynic acid has shown an inhibitory activity against FADS2 (Cai et al., 2016) (the key enzyme of the fatty acid synthesis pathway) and is a potent agonist on FFA1 (GPR40) (Christiansen et al., 2015), which have been link to the diabetic pathway (Itoh et al., 2003; Walle et al., 2019).

Besides, sandalwood seed oil (containing 33% ximenynic acid) was found its activity of ameliorating insulin resistance by mediating JNK/NF-κB and PI3K/AKT pathways (Zhang et al., 2021). Other medical applications of ximenynic acid include its antimicrobial (Jones et al., 1995; Vadnere et al., 2017), antifungal (Jones et al., 1995; Vadnere et al., 2017) and larvicidal activities (Mavundza et al., 2016). Ximenynic acid has also been applied in the industry, especially in the cosmetic industry.

Ximenynic acid is attracting more and more attention with the in-depth study of its functions. Therefore, the demand for ximenynic acid continues growing with the discovery of its virtues. Natural ximenynic acid can be easily extracted from the plant by different methods, such as recrystallization under low temperature, thin-layer chromatography (TLC), and high-performance liquid chromatography (HPLC). However, extraction of natural ximenynic acid from these rare plants cannot meet the increasing needs. In this case, synthesis of ximenynic acid is an alternative option.

Here we reviewed the bioactives, application, distribution, and main preparation methods for ximenynic acid. Whether the biosynthesis pathways or multiple activities of ximenynic acid, the underlying mechanism is being disclosed but far from complete. Further research is needed.

20.2 Bioactivities, functions, and applications of ximenynic acid

20.2.1 Effect of ximenynic acid on fatty acid metabolism

Although ximenynic acid is not an essential fatty acid, it is a traditional food for Aboriginals, so its metabolism in vivo is worth pursuing. Liu and Longmore analyzed the metabolism of ximenynic acid in ARC mice (Liu & Longmore, 1997). They found that 16:1n-7/16:0 and 18:1n-9/18:0 fatty acid ratios significantly increased in the adipose tissue of the sandalwood seed oil-fed mice ($P < 0.05$), implying that ximenynic acid could affect Δ9-desaturase enzyme activity to convert 18:0 into 18:1n-9. In contrast, the arachidonic acid content in the sandalwood seed oil group decreased compared with the control group. It suggested that ximenynic acid acted as a substrate to inhibit the conversion of 18:2n-6 to arachidonic acid. However, docosahexaenoic acid (DHA) content in the sandalwood seed oil group was higher than in the control group. It indicated that ximenynic acid might promote the biosynthesis of DHA. After feeding mice with sandalwood seed oil, ximenynic acid only existed in adipose tissue, with a low content (0.3–3%).

The metabolism of ximenynic acid in rats was similar to that in mice. Li et al. fed male SD rats with a diet containing 10% different oils (Li et al., 2013). The ratio of 18:1n-9 in the sandalwood seed oil group was higher in rat adipose tissue and liver lipids than in other groups except for the olive oil group. Sandalwood seed oil increased the DHA level in total tissue and phospholipids fatty acid composition of rats' liver. Notably, sandalwood seed oil also significantly increased the total polyunsaturated fatty acids (PUFA) compared with olive oil and safflower oil groups in adipose tissue, liver tissue, and phospholipids. Furthermore, sandalwood seed oil decreased the n-6: n-3 PUFA ratio in the three samples compared with soybean oil, olive oil and safflower oil (Li et al., 2013). These studies showed that sandalwood seed oil can increase n-3 fatty acid levels in rats and mice tissues, but whether it is caused directly by ximenynic acid is unknown.

To investigate whether ximenynic acid can increase the proportion of n-3 PUFA in animal tissues, we did in vitro and in vivo studies on the metabolism of sandalwood seed oil and ximenynic acid metabolism in mice or HepG2 cells (Cai, Li, et al., 2016). It is known that oleic acid and ximenynic acid are the main components of sandalwood seed oil, and olive oil is primarily composed of oleic acid. Besides, the structure of ximenynic acid is similar to oleic acid. Therefore, this study could scientifically reflect the actual impact of sandalwood seed oil or ximenynic acid on fatty acid metabolism. We found that sandalwood seed oil increased n-3 levels in the liver of mice that was consistent with the previous reports (Li et al., 2013). However, in vitro experiments showed that ximenynic acid could not increase n-3 levels in HepG2 cells. Furthermore, ximenynic acid even significantly inhibited the expression of FADS2 (a key enzyme of PUFA synthesis) at the transcriptional level and translational level in HepG2. Thus, they hypothesized that ximenynic acid could not improve n-3 fatty acid levels but linolenic acid (precursor to DHA) in sandalwood seed oil was likely the key factor to increase n-3 fatty acid levels in animal tissues.

20.2.2 Effect of ximenynic acid on diabetes

Diabetes is one of the severe non-communicable diseases threatening human health. Around 463 million people worldwide had diabetes in 2019, and the number keeps climbing (Saeedi et al., 2019). Whether ximenynic acid can improve diabetes has always been an urgent problem to be solved. Sandalwood leaves can stimulate glucose uptake in some reports. It might relate to ximenynic acid (Gulati et al., 2015). In addition, another 18-carbon acetylenic acid (6-octadecynoic acid), which has an antibacterial activity, also has a potential in treating diabetes (Ohtera et al., 2013). Furthermore, Christiansen et al. reported the effect of ximenynic acid on FFA1 and FFA4 in HEK 293 cells (Christiansen et al., 2015). They found that ximenynic acid has a potent agonism on FFA1 (pEC50: 5.33; Emax: 56%), whereas it has a partial agonism on FFA4 (pEC50: 5.00; Emax: 39%) (Christiansen et al., 2015). Potency (pEC50) and efficacy (Emax) values of FFA1 and FFA4 upon ximenynic acid treatment were detected by a Ca^+ mobilization assay and beta-arrestin-2 interaction BRET assay. FFA1 expression in pancreatic beta cells, and FFA4 in the intestinal tract, fat, and macrophage cells, are all associated with incretin secretion (Hara et al., 2014). Besides, the FFA1 agonist is also a practical drug target for increased insulin secretion in type 2 diabetes clinical trials (Burant et al., 2012; Mancini & Poitout, 2013).

Recently, we also found that ximenynic acid inhibited the expression of FADS2 (Cai et al., 2020). FADS2 encodes Δ-6 desaturase, a rate-limiting enzyme involved in synthesizing long-chain polyunsaturated fatty acids (Glaser et al., 2010). However, according to a clinical study, FADS2 gene expression was increased in the NAFLD (non-alcoholic fatty liver disease) patients' liver (Walle et al., 2019). In addition, the Δ-6 desaturase activity was increased in these patients, and FADS2 methylation level was lower than in ordinary people (Walle et al., 2019). The methylation changes at some sites of the FADS2 gene are associated with metabolic diseases such as type 2 diabetes mellitus (Yao et al., 2015). That is to say, ximenynic acid as an agonist of FFA1 and a partial agonist of FFA4, and also inhibits the expression of Δ-6 desaturase; both are related to improving diabetic function. Therefore, it is supposed that ximenynic acid may have a potential antidiabetic activity.

To further study the relationship between sandalwood seed oil and type 2 diabetes, a feeding experiment was carried out by feeding rats with sandalwood seed oil (containing 33% ximenynic acid) (Zhang et al., 2021). The rats were fed with a high-fat and high-sugar diet to induce a rat model of obesity and insulin resistance, and treated with different edible oils and sandalwood seed oil. The results showed that sandalwood seed oil effectively prevented glucose intolerance and hyperglycemia, and reduced insulin resistance. Furthermore, the PI3K/Akt insulin signaling pathway, involved in insulin resistance, was activated in sandalwood seed oil group. However, in addition to ximenynic acid, sandalwood seed oil also contained 45.7% 18:1n-9 and 4.5% 18:3n-3. Therefore, there is no direct evidence that ximenynic acid contributes to improving the insulin resistance function. Whether ximenynic acid can prevent and treat diabetes still needs to be further verified by in vivo and in vitro experiments.

20.2.3 Anti-inflammatory activities of ximenynic acid

The discovery of the anti-inflammatory activity of ximenynic acid has been related to the habit of aboriginal people using sandalwood seeds. Western Australian Aboriginals used the seeds to treat arthritis with therapeutic effects by topical application or oral injection for a long time (Liu & Longmore, 1996), that aroused the interest of scientific researchers. As early as the 1990s, The impact of ximenynic acid in the bioconversion of arachidonic acid to prostaglandin E2B was investigated on sheep vesicular gland microsomes, and ximenynic acid showed a moderate inhibition effect (IC50: 39 µM) on sheep vesicular gland microsomes (Nugteren & Christ-Hazelhof, 1987). Subsequently, ximenynic acid also inhibited some inflammation cytokines like leukotriene B_4 (IC50: 60 µM), thromboxane B_2, and 6-ketoprostaglandin $F_{1\alpha}$ production of rat peritoneal leukocytes in dose-dependent patterns (Croft et al., 1987). Besides, ximenynic acid showed 40–50% inhibition of phospholipase activity at 100 µM. It showed that a higher dose of ximenynic acid will contribute to phospholipase inhibition and reduction release of inflammatory cytokines (Croft et al., 1987).

Anti-inflammatory activity of ximenynic acid is often used ximenynic acid-rich seed oil as the research object for in vivo study. After feeding with 15% sandalwood seed oil for 4 weeks, a minor exotic fatty acid derivative was detected and named furanoid fatty acid (8,-11-epoxy-8,11-octadecadienoic) in the total liver lipids of the fed mice (Liu & Longmore, 1996). It was assumed that the exotic fatty acid might be biosynthesized from ximenynic acid, which competitively inhibited the biosynthesis from arachidonic acid to PGE_2 (Liu & Longmore, 1996). The sandalwood seed oil also significantly decreased the concentrations of PGF_{2a}, PGE_2, TXB_2, and LTB_4 in rats' plasma and liver compared with soybean oil and safflower oil (Li et al., 2013). It indicated that ximenynic acid could stimulate n-3 PUFA production and promote an anti-inflammatory activity in rats. The anti-inflammatory activity of ximenynic acid also displayed in the metabolic disorder rats after sandalwood seed oil intervention. Sandalwood seed oil strikingly decreased the obese rats' serum levels of pro-inflammatory factors IL-1β, IL-6, and TNF-α compared to the control (Zhang et al., 2021). Further investigation of its anti-inflammatory mechanisms revealed that sandalwood seed oil downregulated the rats' liver JNK/NF-κB inflammatory signaling pathway (Zhang et al., 2021).

Inflammation is not only responsible for certain diseases, such as arthritis, but also contributes to a variety of diseases, including metabolic syndrome, cardiovascular disease (CVD), cancer, diabetes, non-alcoholic fatty liver disease (NAFLD), and neurodegenerative diseases, etc. (Furman et al., 2019). Together, ximenynic acid has unique anti-inflammatory properties, including acute inflammation and chronic inflammation. Considering the close link between inflammation and many diseases, the anti-inflammatory activities of ximenynic acid may be benefit to many chronic diseases.

20.2.4 Anticancer activities of ximenynic acid

Acetylenic lipids have shown many activities due to their unique structure, and their anticancer activity has attracted much attention. More than 300 natural and synthetic acetylenic lipids - had been reviewed their cytotoxicity and anticancer activities, many acetylenic acids among them show cancer suppression activity by inhibiting COXs pathways (Dembitsky, 2006). COXs are essential enzymes in arachidonic acid metabolism, which generate many inflammatory substances (Khanapure et al., 2007). Given that cancer cancer progression is closely linked with inflammation responses (Grivennikov et al., 2010), COX pathways play a crucial role in carcinogenesis (Imig & Hammock, 2009). Aspirin, for example, is a famous COX inhibitor and has shown an excellent anticancer activity (Cuzick et al., 2009).

Some seeds of *Olacaceae* species which contain ximenynic acid have showed anticancer activity. For example, methanol extract of *Olax subscorpioidea* seed had a remarkable inhibitory effect on prostate cancer and leukemia cells (Kuete et al., 2011). *Ximenia caffra* (*X. caffra*) seed oil can significantly suppress the proliferation of Caco-2 and HEK-293 cells (Chivandi, Cave, et al., 2012). But they cannot draw the conclusion on the anticancer effect of ximenynic acid due to the mixture of seed oil. To address this question, we performed an *in vitro* experiment using purified ximenynic acid. We found the potent inhibition of ximenynic acid on cell proliferation in HCT116 cells. The cell cycle was tightly arrested at G1-S phase, and cell apoptosis was promoted after ximenynic acid treatment (Cai, Chen, et al., 2016). Furthermore, our study showed the cytotoxic effect of ximenynic acid on HepG2 cells through inhibiting cell proliferation and inducing apoptosis in a dose-dependent manner (Cai et al., 2016). In addition, ximenynic acid affected the cell cycle distribution by G0/G1 arrest. Interestingly, ximenynic acid selectively inhibited COX-1 activity rather than COX-2 (Cai et al., 2016). It suggested that the anticancer activity of ximenynic acid was correlated with the selective inhibition on COX-1. Remarkably, ximenynic acid also inhibited several angiogenesis factors in HepG2 cells (Cai et al., 2016). As a COX-1-selective inhibitor, ximenynic acid may also have a suppression activity for other malignancies, such as colon and breast cancer.

As discussed above, ximenynic acid is an agonist of FFA1 and a partial agonist of FFA4 (Christiansen et al., 2015). FFA4 is not just related to anti-inflammatory, insulin sensitization activities (Oh et al., 2010), but also can activate GRP120 and promote angiogenesis and migration of cancer cells (Wu et al., 2013). In all, the anticancer activity of ximenynic acid might involve COXs pathways and the agonist activity against FFA1 and FFA4. Currently, the underlying mechanism remains unknown.

20.2.5 Antimicrobial and larvicidal activities of ximenynic acid

Except of the anti-inflammatory and anticancer activities mentioned above, many natural acetylenic fatty acids also show antimicrobial properties (Kuklev et al., 2013). As crushed sandalwood seeds were used to treat skin lesions by Australian aborigines, which might be related to the antimicrobial activity of ximenynic acid (Jones et al., 1995). Ten kinds of *S. acuminatum* (quandong) extracts was tested their antibacterial activities (Jones et al., 1995), then found that ximenynic acid and its sodium or potassium salts showed a strong inhibition activity on Gram-positive bacteria such as *Staphylococcus aureus* and *Staphylococcus epidermidis* in a dose-dependent manner. But they were inactive toward Gram-negative bacteria (Jones et al., 1995). Besides, ximenynic acid was also found to be sensitive to two other Gram-positive bacteria, *Mycobacterium bovis* BCG (MICs: 25 μg/mL) and recombinant *Mycobacterium intracellulare* (MICs: >100 μg/mL) (Shawar et al., 1997). However, ethanol extracts from ximenynic acid-enriched Santalum album seeds showed no activities against Gram-positive (*B. subtilis*, *S. aureus*) and Gram-negative bacteria (*P. aeruginosa*, *E. coli*) (Patil et al., 2011). In addition, the result was consistent with recent study by using ethanol extract of *Santalum album* seeds (Vadnere et al., 2017). However, in the later study, the petroleum ether extract of *Santalum album* seeds was significantly inhibited some Gram-positive (*B. subtilis*, *S. aureus*) and Gram-negative (*P. aeruginosa*, *E. coli*) bacteria, which was speculatively attributed to the ximenynic acid in the petroleum ether extract but not in ethanol extract (Vadnere, Md, Lodhi and Patil, 2017). It indicates that ximenynic acid might have a broad antibacterial activity, and which is summarized in Table 20.1.

There are a number of studies that focus on the antifungal activity of ximenynic acid (Table 20.2). Jone et al. revealed that ximenynic acid could significantly inhibit pathogenic fungal growth in a dose-dependent manner, and the salts of ximenynic acid had better antifungal efficacies (Jones et al., 1995). *Olax subscorpioidea* fruit organic extracts have moderate inhibition on three yeast strains, *Cryptococcus neoformans* (MIC of 0.39 mg/mL), *Candida parapsilosis* (MIC: 0.39 mg/mL), *Candida lusitaniae* (MIC: 0.19 mg/mL), and a strong inhibition against the growth of *Candida albicans* (MIC: 0.097 mg/mL) and *Candida tropicalis* (MIC: 0.048 mg/mL) (Dzoyem et al., 2014). Animal studies have assessed the effects of *Olax subscorpioidea* fruit organic extracts on *C. albicans* infected rats. Oral administration with the extract significantly decreased the fungal load (colony-forming units per milliliter: cfu/mL) of blood in a dose- and time-dependent manner compared with the control group (Dzoyem et al., 2014). But it was still unclear which effective compounds of the extracts contributed to the antifungal activity. Later, the petroleum ether extract of *S. album* seeds, primarily containing ximenynic acid, could inhibit certain fungi. On this ground, they hypothesized that

TABLE 20.1 Antibacterial activity of ximenynic acid.

Susceptible	Product	MIC (μg/mL)	Ref.
Gram-positive			
Staphylococcus aureus	Ximenynic acid	22	Jones et al. (1995)
	Sodium santalbate	250	Jones et al. (1995)
Staphylococcus epidermidis	Ximenynic acid	N/A	Jones et al. (1995)
Recombinant *Mycobacterium bovis* BCG (rBCG)	Ximenynic acid	2.5×10^4	Shawar et al. (1997)
Recombinant *Mycobacterium intracellulare*	Ximenynic acid	10	Shawar et al. (1997)
Bacillus subtilis	Ximenynic acid	78.125	Vadnere et al. (2017)
S. aureus	Ximenynic acid	156.25	Vadnere et al. (2017)
Gram-negative			
Escherichia coli	Ximenynic acid	Ineffective	Jones et al. (1995)
	Ximenynic acid	625	Vadnere et al. (2017)
Escherichia cloacae	Ximenynic acid	Ineffective	Jones et al. (1995)
Enterobacter aerogenes	Ximenynic acid	Ineffective	Jones et al. (1995)
Serratia marcescens	Ximenynic acid	Ineffective	Jones et al. (1995)
Pseudomonas aeruginosa	Ximenynic acid	Ineffective	Jones et al. (1995)
	Ximenynic acid	19.331	Vadnere et al. (2017)
Proteus vulgaris	Ximenynic acid	Ineffective	Jones et al. (1995)

MIC, minimum inhibitory concentration; N/A, not mentioned; Ref., reference.

TABLE 20.2 Antifungal activity of ximenynic acid.

Susceptible	Product	IC50 (mg/mL)	Ref.
Microsporum canis	Ximenynic acid	≤ 20	Jones et al. (1995)
	Sodium santalbate	≤ 10	Jones et al. (1995)
Microsporum gypseum	Ximenynic acid	< 20	Jones et al. (1995)
	Sodium santalbate	< 25	Jones et al. (1995)
Trichophyton rubrum	Ximenynic acid	<10	Jones et al. (1995)
	Sodium santalbate	<20	Jones et al. (1995)
Trichophyton mentagrophytes	Ximenynic acid	<10	Jones et al. (1995)
	Sodium santalbate	≤20	Jones et al. (1995)
Epidermophyton floccosum	Ximenynic acid	<20	Jones et al. (1995)
	Sodium santalbate	≤10	Jones et al. (1995)

Susceptible	Product	MIC (mg/mL)	Ref.
Candida albicans	*Olax subscorpioidea* extract	0.097	Dzoyem et al. (2014)
	Ximenynic acid	0.039	Vadnere et al. (2017)
Cryptococcus neoformans	*Olax subscorpioidea* extract	0.39	Dzoyem et al. (2014)
Candida tropicalis	*Olax subscorpioidea* extract	0.048	Dzoyem et al. (2014)
Candida krusei	*Olax subscorpioidea* extract	1.56	Dzoyem et al. (2014)
Candida parapsilosis	*Olax subscorpioidea* extract	0.39	Dzoyem et al. (2014)
Candida lusitaniae	*Olax subscorpioidea* extract	0.19	Dzoyem et al. (2014)
Candida guilliermondii	*Olax subscorpioidea* extract	0.78	Dzoyem et al. (2014)
Candida glabrata	*Olax subscorpioidea* extract	1.56	Dzoyem et al. (2014)

MIC, minimum inhibitory concentration; *Ref.*, reference.

this antifungal activity was related to ximenynic acid (Vadnere et al., 2017).

Trypanosoma cruzi (*T. cruzi*) is the pathogen of South American trypanosomiasis, and an estimated 7 million people worldwide are infected with *T. cruzi*, mainly in Latin America (de Fuentes-Vicente et al., 2018). *Porcelia macrocarpa* (Annonaceae), a native plant of Brazil, ximenynic acid was successfully isolated from its flower. And the extracted ximenynic acid had a significant inhibitory effect on the Trypomastigote forms of *T. cruzi* (IC50 was about 60 µM) (Londero et al., 2018). This exciting finding is vital for the development of Brazil's local drugs. However, ximenynic acid showed no significant effect on the plasma membrane potential of *T. cruzi*. It suggests that it may have other mechanisms for its insecticidal activity.

In addition to microbial activity, ximenynic acid was also found to have some larvicidal function. Ximenynic acid extraction from *Olax dissitiflora* bark was evaluated the larvicidal effect against *Anopheles arabiensis* mosquitoes, and showed an intense larvicidal activity with an

EC50 value of 62.17 μg/mL and had a powerful synergistic effect with exocarpic acid (with an EC50 value of 17.31 μg/mL) (Mavundza et al., 2016). *Anopheles arabiensis mosquitoes* is a considerable vector of malaria in South Africa, where malaria is still rife. The larvicidal activity of ximenynic against larvae of *Anopheles arabiensis mosquitoes* may potentially decrease the incidence of malaria.

20.2.6 Applications in the cosmetic industry

Consumers increasingly favor natural or organic cosmetics, and therefore many natural extracts such as vegetable oils are also the primary material of the cosmetic industry. Ximenynic acid-rich seed oil from Ximenia or sandalwood seed is traditionally used for skincare. For example, *Santalum acuminatum* kernel oil has been used in the treatment of skin diseases and hair care (Lim, 2013). *Ximenia caffra* seed oil has been used to soften and care for the chapped skin (Eliton Chivandi et al., 2008). Ximenia oil was also nontoxic to human keratinocytes at a high concentration of 10 g/mL, indicating that the oil is safe for the skin (Satoto et al., 2019).

Ximenynic acid, one of the main components of these seed oils, has also been found in skincare properties. In vitro assay also found that ximenynic acid could significantly inhibit collagenase activity, indicating that ximenynic acid might have a potential anti-aging activity (Shivatare et al., 2020b). A double-blind half-face trial of ethyl ximenynate on eyelid skin showed an improvement of the skin condition (skin dryness and roughness, and eye puffiness) after 4 weeks of treatment. Besides, it also showed effects of anti-wrinkle and improvement of skin microcirculation (Sparavigna et al., 2014). Another clinical trial indicated that ximenynic acid had some beneficial effects on improving blood circulation. Volunteers who used a cream containing 0.5% ximenynic acid increased the blood flow (Vermaak et al., 2011). Therefore, ximenynic acid can protect the skin as a barrier and increase capillary blood flow, and could be a good ingredient for cosmetic products to assist against aging and environmental skin damage.

Another important application of ximenynic acid in the cosmetics industry is its hair-care function, which may also be related to its microvascular activity. When applied topically over a long time, a patent claimed that ximenynic acid or its esters could promote the skin's microvascular circulation and reduce sebum secretion, which aids in hair care (Bombardelli et al., 1997). Another patent also claimed that ximenynic acid and other active ingredients were contributed to prevent hair loss due to the anti-inflammatory activity (Kapoor et al., 2019; Kumar et al., 2019). Combining the micro-vasculokinetic and antiseborrheic properties, ximenynic acid may potentially prevent hair loss and dry skin (Hettiarachchi et al., 2010).

In the cosmetic industry, ximenynic acid is also used as a skin softener, emollient, conditioner, hair oil, and an ingredient of lipsticks and lubricants (Lall & Kishore, 2014). In addition, it has been applied in soap manufacturing as a substrate as well (Rezanka & Sigler, 2007). The synthesized sodium salt has efficient cleansing (detergent) action (Narayana & Rao, 1982). Besides, it can be applied as a softener in the leather industry (Chivandi, Davidson, & Erlwanger, 2012). With the increasing understanding of the properties of ximenynic acid, it may be developed for more practical applications in the cosmetic industry.

20.2.7 Other applications

Ximenynic acid is often used in other industrial and agricultural fields in the form of seed oil. In addition to making soap, sandalwood seed oil can be used as a raw material for surface-active products as well. Its reaction products of gelatin, diethanolamine, or sodium had an excellent foaming ability and foam stability (Shankaranarayana & Parthasarathi, 1986). It was also found that ximenynic acid was the perfect raw material for surfactants; its sodium salts have good foaming and cleaning properties (Narayana & Rao, 1982).

In the paint and dye industry, sandalwood seed oil can play an important role. For example, sandalwood seed oil is applied in the natural media dyeing process for its high unsaturated fatty acids and acetylenic fatty acids content. Too much saturated fatty acid is easy to obtain a high level of unsaponifiable and then affects cotton thread's dyeing efficiency (Cunningham et al., 2011). Ximenynic acid-rich seed oil may also be suitable as a desiccant for paints and inks because the oxidation rate of the conjugated fatty acids is increased compared with that of the non-conjugated fatty acids (Baud, 2018).

Furthermore, ximenynic acid has a special conjugated ene-yne structure, making it very reactive and arousing the interest of the chemical industry. Ximenynic acid can be oxidized easily to other compounds, such as methyl 9(10)-oxooctadec-*trans*-11-enoates (Pasha & Ahmad, 1993). Oxidation reactions of ximenynic acid with selenium dioxide/TBHP in aqueous dioxane produced 6% of methyl 8-oxo-octadec-11(E)Z-en-9-ynoate and 70% methyl 8-hydroxy-octadec-11E-en-9-ynoate, which are regiospecific products (Jie et al., 1997). Epoxidation of the double bond of methyl ximenynate with potassium peroxomonosulfate gives rise to methyl 11,12-E-epoxy-octadec-9-ynoate (Jie & Pasha, 1998), which can also generate many derivatives (Lie Ken Jie et al., 2003). Ximenynic acid could be converted to methyl 9-*cis*,11-*trans* octadecadienoate-9,10-d_2 (CLA-d_2) using the Lindlar-catalyzed reduction for further metabolism studies and oxidation (Adlof, 1999). Lewis acid-induced addition reactions of carbocations to conjugated enyne of methyl ximenynate gave many branched and long-chain compounds (Biermann et al., 2000).

In addition, ximenynic acid-rich seed oil still has other uses. Sandalwood seed oil, for example, could react with zinc chloride to obtain a black plastic solid, which was an ideal material for insulating tape (Kumar et al., 2019). *Ximenia caffra* seed oil could soften leather, and lubricate agricultural machinery (Maroyi, 2016). Together, ximenynic acid or seed oil rich in ximenynic acid still has vast space for exploration in the future applications.

20.3 Safety of ximenynic acid

As a kind of unique natural unique polyunsaturated fatty acid, the safety of ximenynic acid has also aroused many concerns. The brine shrimp assay is a simple bioassay for cytotoxicity testing with compounds or extracts of brine shrimp (Meyer et al., 1982). Cantrell et al. separated ximenynic acid from the seed oil of *Olax subscorpioidea oliv* by reverse preparative HPLC and analyzed its activity against brine shrimp (Cantrell et al., 2003). The LC50 of ximenynic acid against *Artemia salina* was 26.3 µg/ml, much lower than the positive control (cycloheximide, LC50 = 40 µg/mL) (Cantrell et al., 2003). It indicates that ximenynic acid is a low toxic substance against brine shrimp. Besides, the brine shrimp assay is used chiefly to detect environmental pollution. But whether ximenynic acid is harmful to mammals needs further study.

A feeding rat's trial first examined ximenynic acid's safety in mammals with a fat diet (containing 34.1% ximenynic acid) for 10–20 days (Jones et al., 1994). It showed that ximenynic acid was detected in the adipose tissue, skeletal muscle, heart, and liver, not in the brain. But the P-450 activity in the hepatic microsomal cytochrome of the 20 days' group was significantly increased over the control (Jones et al., 1994). Several years later, further studies were carried out to identify the relationship between ximenynic acid and P-450 activity (Jones et al., 1999). After feeding the SD rats with sandalwood seed oil or sandalwood kernels, more than 99% of ximenynic acid can be absorbed. Furthermore, ximenynic acid significantly increased the activities of hepatic cytochrome P450 and cytochrome P450 4A. In addition, methyl ximenynate could also increase cytochrome P450A in kidney and liver microsomes (Jones et al., 1999).

Cytochrome P450 (P450) enzymes are involved in many drug metabolisms, which can catalyze multiple reactions, and reduce the toxicity of compounds (Guengerich, 2008). However, activation of P450s does not necessarily indicate that its reaction substrates are harmful to the body. For example, arachidonic acid can also be metabolized by cytochrome P450 4A and 2C in the kidney, but its reaction products play an essential role in regulating renal tubule and vascular functions (Maier & Roman, 2001). Although ximenynic acid has some effects on the activity of hepatic cytochrome P450 and cytochrome P450 4A, the metabolism of ximenynic acid does not seem to be harmful in animal studies (Jones et al., 1994, 1999).

There are no clinical trials to report whether ximenynic acid is beneficial or harmful to humans. However, ximenynic acid-rich seeds like sandalwood or Ximenia, have been a traditional food for local people for a long time. Archeologists have discovered several stone tools in the Australian Murray Darling Basin, which specially used to break up the local sandalwood seeds, suggesting that the Aborigines consumed sandalwood seeds from ancient times (Pardoe et al., 2019). Moreover, the Quandong kernels are also a prevalent local food (Lim, 2013). In Africa, Ximenia seeds, also rich in ximenynic acid, are a portion of traditional food and products and are widely used (Urso et al., 2016). All these indicate that ximenynic acid may have low or no toxicity to the human body. However, modestly, clinical trials should be performed to confirm the safety of ximenynic acid.

20.4 Physical characteristics and natural distribution

20.4.1 Structure and identification of ximenynic acid

Ximenynic acid is an 18-carbon polyunsaturated fatty acid with a triple bond and a double bond at C9 and C11positions, respectively. These two unsaturated bonds form a conjugated alkyne system, which becomes the characteristic structure of ximenynic acid. The majority of natural ximenynic acid has a *trans* structure, and the *cis* structure is very few (Spitzer et al., 1991). Crystals of ximenynic acid are white and very thin plates, with an oblong shape. X-ray examination showed that they are triclinic crystals, with a melting point of 38–40°C (Gunstone & Mcgee, 1954; Tesche, 1954). This means that ximenynic acid is solid at room temperature, unlike common polyunsaturated fatty acids.

A great deal of literature has reported structural features of ximenynic acid. UV spectra showed that there was a typical absorption peak at about 229 nm, indicating a conjugated alkyne structure in ximenynic acid. Besides, its infrared absorption peak at 955 cm^{-1} also shows the trans double-bond structure (Gunstone & Mcgee, 1954). The ^{1}H NMR spectrum of ximenynic acid showed a doublet at 5.48 ppm, J 15 Hz, and a double-triplet at 6.05 ppm, J1 15 Hz, J2 7.5 Hz (Fig. 20.1A and B), which indicates the trans-alkenic protons of a conjugated enyne system. Compared with ^{13}C NMR (Fig. 20.1C), the DEPT 135 spectrum (Fig. 20.1D) of ximenynic acid does not show two singlets (at 79.30 and 88.51 ppm) assigned to the acetylenic carbon atoms; another disappeared peak at 180.36 ppm means the absence of carbon atom of carboxyl group; the two upward peaks at 110.91 and 143.11 ppm indicate the olefinic carbon atoms; the upward peak at 14.09 ppm shows a methyl group carbon atom; the remaining 12 downward peaks reveal a methylene carbon

20.4 Physical characteristics and natural distribution

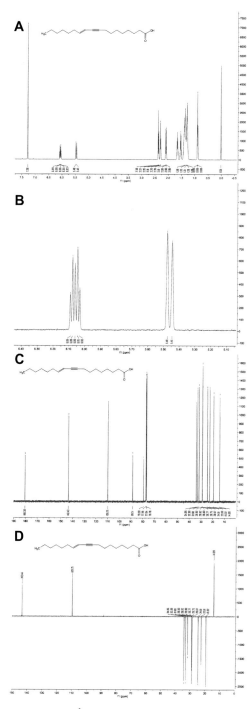

FIG. 20.1 NMR spectrum of ximenynic acid. (A) ^{1}H NMR spectrum of ximenynic acid, (B) The enlarged doublet (5.48 ppm, J 15 Hz) and double-triplet (6.05 ppm, J1 15 Hz) of ^{1}H NMR spectrum of ximenynic acid, (C) ^{13}C NMR of ximenynic acid, (D) DEPT 135 spectrum of ximenynic acid.

atom. These NMR results were consistent with the previous reports (Liu & Longmore, 1996; Vickery et al., 1984).

Mass spectrum of methyl ximenynate showed the molecular ion peak (m/z 292, C19H32O2) (Vickery et al., 1984) and iron of m/z 261 (M-CH3O) (Liu et al., 1996). Besides m/z 292 and 261 (M-31), the fragments of m/z 164 [H-(CH=CH)2-CH=CH(CH2)5CH3]+ and m/z 150 [CH2=C=CHCH=CH(CH2)5CH3]+ indicates a triple bond between C9 and C10 of ximenynic acid structure (Spitzer et al., 1991). Furthermore, the intensive fragment of m/z 79 (C6H7)+ was assigned over one double or a triple bond in the structure of ximenynic acid (Liu et al., 1996), which was consistent with the result reported by Butaud (Butaud et al., 2008). Although trans-ximenynic acid is abundant in nature, its isomer, the cis-ximenynic acid, was also found in the seed oil of *Santalum spicatum* with a tiny proportion (Liu et al., 1996). GC/MS analysis of a 4,4-dimethyloxazolyne derivative (DMOX) mixture of sandalwood seed oil showed two peaks with similar mass spectra, which were in keeping with trans-ximenynic acid (RT: 38.51 min) and cis-ximenynic acid (RT: 36.33 min) (Liu et al., 1996).

20.4.2 The distribution of ximenynic acid in nature

Ximenynic acid is primarily distributed in the root, stem, leaf, and seed in three species of Opiliaceae, Olacaceae, and Santalaceae, and it is the most abundant in seed oil (Bulock & Smith, 1963). However, the content of ximenynic acid in seeds is constantly changing with the development of seeds. For example, the increase of ximenynic acid and oleic acid is accompanied by the decrease of other fatty acids during sandalwood seed development. The content of ximenynic acid can also be affected by different years, areas, and methods of extraction (Hettiarachchi et al., 2012). The following table summarizes most of the reports on ximenynic acid content. It is the most abundant in the Santalaceae family (1%–95%) (Table 20.3), followed by Olacaceae (0.17%–63%) and Opiliaceae families (5%–55.4%) (Table 20.4).

20.5 Preparation methods of natural ximenynic acid

20.5.1 Low-temperature crystallization

As mentioned above, most natural ximenynic acid exists in the form of triglycerides in plant seed oil. For instance, *Santalum spicatum* R.Br. seed oil contains ximenynic acid, oleic acid, palmitic acid, stearic acid, and other fatty acids (Hettiarachchi et al., 2010). Seed oil can be extracted from the kernel by various methods, such as solvent extraction (Pasha & Ahmad, 1993) and supercritical carbon dioxide extraction (Hettiarachchi et al., 2013). Ximenynic acid can be easily isolated from the seed oil using low-temperature crystallization (Lighthelm & Schwartz, 1950). Natural oils such as sandalwood seed oil need to be converted to free fatty acids or fatty acid methyl esters to improve the extraction efficiency of ximenynic acid. First, to get free fatty acids, the seed oil should be hydrolyzed and the saponified solution (1 M KOH/EtOH) should be acidified (pH 1). Ximenynic acid can be crystallized from the free fatty acids using hexane at -20 to $-25°C$ (Hopkins et al., 1969; Liu et al., 1996). After several times of recrystallization, the pure ximenynic acid can be obtained as white flakes (Hopkins et al., 1969; Liu et al., 1996). Another method for the isolation of ximenynic acid is to precipitate the compound with urea-methanol solution and then recrystallize the urea complex with light petroleum or acetone-purified ximenynic acid (Crombie & Griffin, 1958; Hatt et al., 1959). The urea adduct method is suitable for the separation of polyunsaturated fatty acid (PUFA) from saturated fatty

TABLE 20.3 The contents of ximenynic acid in Santalaceae family.

Plant species	Plant part	XA content	Ref.	Plant species	Plant part	XA content	Ref.
Acanthosyris spinescens	Seed	1%	Hopkins et al. (1968)	Leptomeria acida	Root, stem	N/A	Hatt, Meisters, Triffett, and Wailes (1967)
Buckleya distichophylla	Seed	12%	Hopkins et al. (1969)	Leptomeria aphylla	Seed	19.50%	Hatt et al. (1960)
Buckleya lanceolata	Seed	9%	Hopkins et al. (1969)	Osyris alba L.	Seed	57.1%–64%	Hopkins et al. (1969), Mikolajczak, Earle, and Wolff (1963)
Cervantesia tomentosa	Seed	13.10%	Aitzetmuller (2012)	Pyrularia edulis	Seed	1.43%	Zhang et al. (1989)
Choretrum pauciflorum	Root, stem, leaf	N/A	Hatt et al. (1967)	Pyrularia pubera	Seed	10%–30.5%	Hopkins et al. (1968, 1969)
Choretrum glomeratum	Root (wood)	N/A	Hatt et al. (1967)	Santalum album	Seed	75%–95%	Aitzetmuller (2012), Butaud et al. (2008), Gunstone and Russell (1955), Hopkins et al. (1969), Jie et al. (1996), Morris and Marshall (1966)
Colpoon compressum	seed	72.59%	Aitzetmuller (2012)	Santalum acuminatum	Seed	32.6%–52.5%	Aitzetmuller (2012), Badami and Patil (1980), Hatt and Schoenfeld (1956), Hopkins et al. (1969), Jones et al. (1994), Morris and Marshall (1966)
Comandra pallida A. DC.	Seed	43%	Mikolajczak et al. (1963)	Santalum spicatum	Seed	31.72%–40%	Aitzetmuller (2012), Hatt and Schoenfeld (1956), Hettiarachchi et al. (2010), Hettiarachchi et al. (2012), Hopkins et al. (1969), Liu, Longmore, Boddy, and Fox (1997), Liu, Longmore, and Kailis (1997), Liu et al. (1996)

Continued

TABLE 20.3 The contents of ximenynic acid in Santalaceae family—cont'd

Plant species	Plant part	XA content	Ref.	Plant species	Plant part	XA content	Ref.
Exocarpos sparteus	Seed	69.70%	Aitzetmuller (2012)	Santalum obtusifolium	Seed	71.50%	Aitzetmuller (2012)
Exocarpus stricta	Seed	N/A	Hatt et al. (1959)	Santalum insulare	Seed	64%–86%	Butaud et al. (2008)
Exocarpus aphyllus	Seed	67.50%	Aitzetmuller (2012)	Santalum murrayanum	Seed	45%–47.48%	Aitzetmuller (2012), Hatt and Schoenfeld (1956)
Exocarpus cupressiformis	Seed	16.7%–53.2%	Aitzetmuller (2012), Badami and Patil (1980)	Santalum lanceolatum	Seed	46%	Butaud et al. (2008)
Geocaulon lividum	Seed	37.50%	Hopkins et al. (1969)	Santalum yasi	Seed	83%	Hopkins et al. (1969)
Henslowia queenslandiae	Stem	N/A%	Hatt et al. (1967)	Thesium humile	Seed	42%	Hopkins et al. (1969)
Jodina rhombifolia	Seed	20.3%–55%	Hopkins et al. (1969), Spitzer, Bordignon, Schenkel, and Marx (1994)				

XA, ximenynic acid; Ref., references.

TABLE 20.4 The contents of ximenynic acid in Olacaceae and Opiliacea family.

Plant species (Olacaceae)	Plant part	XA content	Ref.	Plant species (Opiliaceae)	Plant part	XA content	Ref.
Curupira tefeensis	Seed	N/A	Spitzer et al. (1991)	*Agonandra brasiliensis*	Seed	18.80%	Aitzetmuller (2012)
Dulacia candida	Root	N/A	Shawar et al. (1997)	*Agonandra excelsa*	Seed	5%–8.9%	Aitzetmuller (2012)
Heisteria silvanii	Seed	3.50%	Spitzer, Tomberg, Hartmann, and Aichholz (1997)	*Agonandra silvatica*	Seed	4.8%–7.6%	Aitzetmuller (2012)
Olax dissitiflora	Bark	N/A	Mavundza et al. (2016)	*Agonandra racemosa*	Seed	25.80%	Aitzetmuller (2012)
Olax benthamiana	Seed	63%	Aitzetmuller (2012)	*Cansjera rheedei*	Seed	55.40%	Aitzetmuller (2012)
Olax subscorpioidea.	Seed	N/A	Cantrell et al. (2003)	*Opilia amentacea*	Seed	7.60%	Aitzetmuller (2012)
Ximenia americana var. *microphylla*	Seed	21.90%	Ligthelm et al. (1954)				
X. americana Linn	Root (bark)	N/A	Hatt et al. (1967)	**Plant species (Annonaceae)**			
	Seed	6.30%	Mikolajczak et al. (1963)				
Ximenia caffra	Seed	24.30%	Ligthelm et al. (1954)	*Porcelia macrocarpa*	Flower	N/A	Londero et al. (2018)
Ximenia caffra var. *natalensisg*	Seed	22%	Ligthelm et al. (1954)				
Heisteria acuminata	Seed	7.50%	Aitzetmuller (2012)				
Ongokea go re	Seed	1%	Aitzetmuller (2012)				
Malania oleifera	Seed	0.17%	Aitzetmuller (2012)				

XA, ximenynic acid; Ref., references; N/A, not mentioned.

acids or mono-unsaturated fatty acids, and thus is widely used for the separation of ximenynic acid.

20.5.2 Chromatography

Chromatography is a common technique for separating fatty acids. It is based on the different distribution coefficients of different fatty acids in the stationary and mobile phases. The elution rate of fatty acids is mainly related to the length of the carbon chain, unsaturation, and particular structures. The acetylenic link can affect the elution rate markedly, contributing to separating ximenynic acid from other olefin acids (Crombie et al., 1955). In addition to the conjugated enyne system, the extra double bond can increase the Rf value (retention factor value) of ximenynic acid and may contribute to separation from other acetylenic acids (Ballance & Crombie, 1958).

Besides, simple chromatographic methods such as paper chromatographic (Ballance & Crombie, 1958) and thin-layer chromatography (TLC) (Mavundza et al., 2016) are also used to separate ximenynic acid. Ximenynic acid can be isolated by means of paper chromatography, which uses paper as a carrier, through paraffin/ 90% acetic acid with an Rf of 0.59 (Ballance & Crombie, 1958). TLC separates mixed samples using a substrate coated on a plate as the stationary phase and a suitable solvent as the mobile phase. Pure ximenynic acid can be obtained by multiple TLC (silica plates, 20 × 20 cm) separations of the extract from *O. dissitiflora* bark with elution system of hexane: ethyl acetate solution (7:3) (Mavundza et al., 2016).

Column chromatography is another widely used separation method for ximenynic acid. It only requires simple equipment and can increase ximenynic acid production. Alumina was used as a filler in the early days (Ligthelm et al., 1954), but today the columns are mostly filled with silica gel. The eluent can be pure light petroleum (Ligthelm et al., 1952) and benzene (Narayana & Rao, 1982), but usually they are used in combination, or with more solvents for gradient elution, e.g., hexane and diethyl ether (1%–5%) (Smith et al., 1991). The De Vries column is applied to separate ximenynic acid elution by ether-light petroleum (1:49) (Hopkins et al., 1968).

An improved method with gradient elution is the reverse-phase partition chromatography. Columns can be packed with water-repellent kieselguhr (Crombie et al., 1955) or Hyflo Supercel with gradient eluent of acetone-water solution (40%–45%) (Hatt et al., 1960). Nowadays, C18 silica (60 Å pore size) is also used as the stationary phase, and acetone: isopropyl alcohol (65:35) as the mobile phase (Hettiarachchi, 2014). In this way, several fractions can be obtained, and some of them contain over 91% ximenynic acid triacylglycerol (Hettiarachchi, 2014).

Along with the development of chromatography, high-performance liquid chromatography (HPLC) has contributed to the compound's separation and purification, with a decrease in complexity and improvement of purity. Reverse-phase HPLC is usually used to separate ximenynic acid. The preparative HPLC can directly or be combined with column chromatography to separate ximenynic acid. For instance, ximenynic acid fraction can be harvested from the seed extract of *Olax subscorpioidea* through gradient elution with MeOH: H_2O by reverse-phase silica gel column chromatography. Then, it can be further purified by HPLC using acetonitrile: H_2O (8:2) (Cantrell et al., 2003). Highly refined methyl ximenynate (>98%) can also be obtained directly by preparative reverse-phase HPLC, using acetonitrile as the elution solvent (Adlof, 1999).

HPLC can be used in conjunction with a UV detector to detect the purity of ximenynic acid according to its UV absorption (Hettiarachchi, 2014). Thus, it can omit the preprocessing step and improve the efficiency compared with the GC method. Besides, high-performance thin-layer chromatography (HPTLC) is a novel method for ximenynic acid purity detection. The mobile and stationary phases were toluene: chloroform: methanol: formic acid, and silica gel aluminum plate (Shivatare et al., 2020a). This method can indirectly reflect the ximenynic acid content in sandalwood seed oil by detecting the oil optical density and calculating the peak area of linear regression (Shivatare et al., 2020a).

20.5.3 Supercritical chromatography

Supercritical fluid extraction (SFE) is a technique that extracts a specific component from a liquid or solid phase by using the different solubility of the substance in the supercritical or non-supercritical state. The extensive application of SFE benefits from the standard supercritical fluid CO_2, which makes this technique safer than the organic extraction method. High-purity ximenynic acid can be obtained when SFE combined with other technologies. For example, 95% of ximenynic acid can be separated by a supercritical chromatography system, which consists of a column filled with about 50 g of silica and uses CO_2 as a carrier (Catchpole et al., 2013). The combination of supercritical chromatography and UV detector allowed a better separation of ximenynic acid (Montañés et al., 2017). Also, particle size and the stationary phase of the supercritical chromatography column are the most critical parameters for separating high-purity ximenynic acid. For example, a Greensep silica gel column of 5 µm can be used to separate ximenynic acid with purity greater than 99.5% (Montañés et al., 2017).

20.5.4 Triximenynin extraction

Natural ximenynic acid exists in the form of triglycerides. For example, sandalwood seed oil mainly contains three forms of triglycerides (TAGs), namely, triximenynin with three ximenynic molecules (XXX), triglyceride with two ximenynic acid molecules and one oleic molecule (XXO/XOX), and triglyceride with two oleic molecules and one ximenynic acid molecule (OOX/OXO) (Liu, Longmore, Boddy, & Fox, 1997). Triximenynin and glyceryl triximenynate can also be isolated from sandalwood seed oil. Three fractions were obtained from *S. album* seed oil using preparative silica TLC, and the most polar fraction contained only glyceryl triximenynate (Jie et al., 1996). The hexane/diethyl ether/acetic acid (70:30:1) has been used as a developing solution to separate the sandalwood oil (Liu, Longmore, Boddy, & Fox, 1997). They got five bands, one of which ($R_f = 0.58$) was identified by GC/MS as triximenynin with a purity of about 99.9% (Liu, Longmore, Boddy, & Fox, 1997). Recently, a new structure of OOX was separated by enantiomeric liquid chromatography-mass spectrometry from the TAGs of sandalwood seed oil (Palyzová & Řezanka, 2020). The oil was separated into three peaks using chiral-LC/MS with the ratio of 3:2:14: sn- OXiO, sn- XiOO, and sn- OOXi, and was found that ximenynic acid was more common in the sn-3 position of TAG (Palyzová & Řezanka, 2020).

20.6 Synthesis of ximenynic acid

20.6.1 The chemical synthesis of ximenynic acid

Given the limited natural ximenynic acid resources, chemical synthesis is an alternative way to prepare ximenynic acid. The de novo synthesis of ximenynic acid has been reported over the past several decades. The main procedures start with the Reformatsky reaction of propargyl bromide and heptaldehyde, followed by several steps of deacylation, chain elongation, and hydrolysis. Pure *trans*-ximenynic acid can be obtained by urea fractionation of the reaction end-product (Crombie & Jacklin, 1955, 1957).

There are other more common and easier approaches for ximenynic acid synthesis. These usually start from ricinoleic acid or its derivatives, and then go through several desaturation reactions to produce a ximenynic acid mixture (Fig. 20.2). One of the important intermediate products is methyl ricinoleate, as it can be easily dehydrated to obtain methyl ximenynate (Grigor et al., 1954). Ximenynic acid can also be synthesized from castor oil that is used as the prime chemical material and is directly chlorinated with ricinstearolic acid without esterification to obtain a methyl ricinstearolate intermediate, which can reduce the total synthesis steps and cut costs (Wang et al., 2012).

20.6.2 The biosynthesis of ximenynic acid

Although the reports on the biosynthesis of ximenynic acid are not too many, it is a promising research direction for the preparation of ximenynic acid, as it is much cleaner and safer than many other methods. The research on the biosynthesis of ximenynic acid has a long history, it was studied by using the isotope tracer method as early as 1960s. Ximenynic acid's carbon chain could be partly derived from acetate when *S. acuminatum* was incubated with acetate-1-^{14}C for 12 weeks (Bulock & Smith,

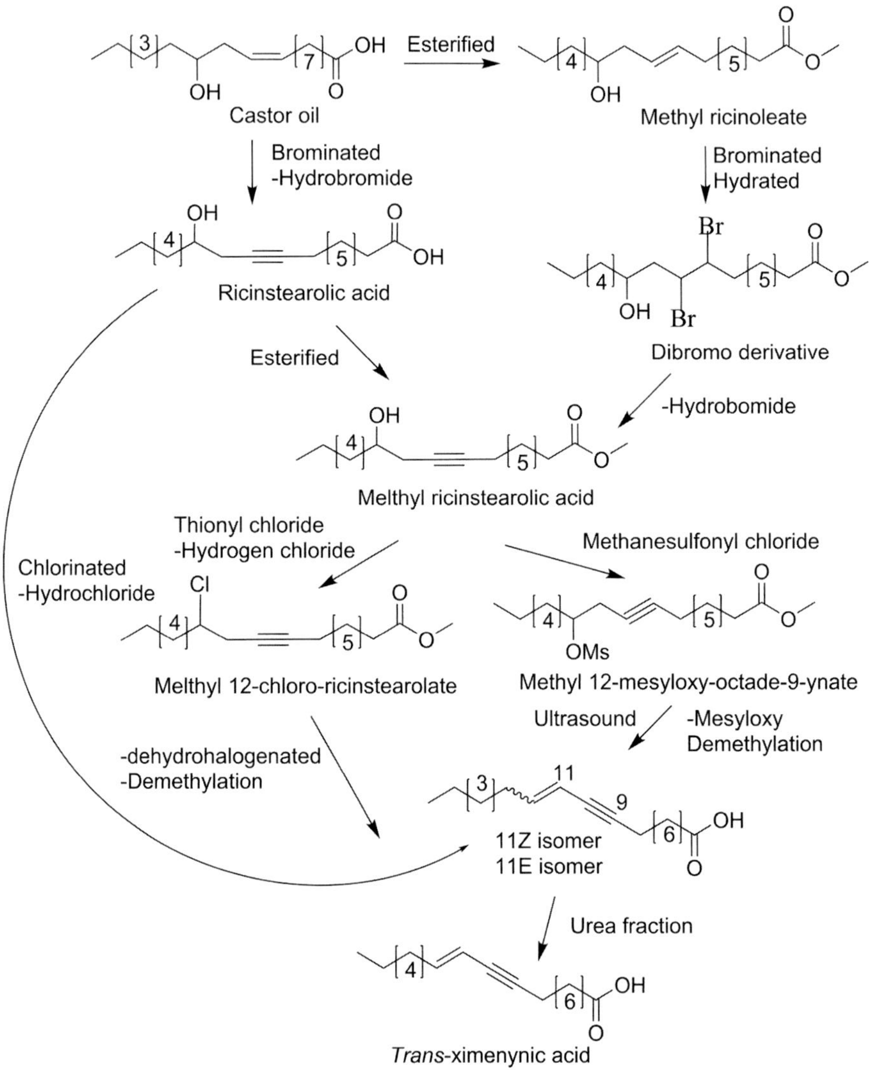

FIG. 20.2 The chemical synthesis procedures of ximenynic acid from coaster oil. Oms, mesyloxy.

1963), but the formation process of ximenynic acid's unsaturated bond is still not clear. Besides, this study focused on the fatty acids' changes during the germination of sandalwood seeds by isotope tracer in vitro, but not seed formation, the biosynthesis mechanisms of ximenynic acid in plants remains unclear.

The biosynthesis of ximenynic acid's unsaturated bons might have two paths, synthesis followed with the carbon chain or after the formation of long chain fatty acids (Bulock & Smith, 1963). Although previous isotopic tracer experiments could not accurately determine the synthesis process of ximenynic acid's alkyne bond, it was found that the ^{14}C was first integrated into the saturated fatty acids, and later found in acetylenic acids (Bulock & Smith, 1963). Apart from that, radioisotopic studies of the synthesis of another similar-structured acid, crepenynic acid (18:2Δ9c,12a), showed that its acetylenic bond was formed by dehydrogenation of the long chain fatty acid (Haigh et al., 1968). The biosynthesis of ximenynic acid might also dominate by dehydrogenation from the carboxyl direction and desaturation of the olefinic bond to the acetylene bond. Therefore, ximenynic acid might be converted by other fatty acids in plants. Firstly, it has been proposed that ximenynic acid is derived from stearolic acid by the sequential dehydrogenation process (Hopkins & Chisholm, 1968) or by isomerization of 18:2(9a, 12t); the latter is involved in desaturation from stearolic acid (Morris & Marshall, 1966). Then, ximenynic acid may come from oleic acid which intermediates the synthesis of linolenic (Hatt & Schoenfeld, 1956). Fatty acid composition of seed oil changed significantly during sandalwood seed development, ximenynic acid and oleic acid increased overtly along with proportional decrease of other fatty acids, and conjugated linoleic acid might be an active intermediate in formation of ximenynic acid from oleic acid (Liu et al., 1997). By the way, ximenynic acid may also be a transition product during forming other acetylenic acids from oleic acid by desaturation, a-oxidation, and hydroxylation (Hopkins et al., 1968).

The biosynthesis of ximenynic acid needs participation of many enzymes. The formation of *Santalum album* L. seed oil is associated with Ca^{2+}-dependent protein kinase (CDPK) during the seed maturation period, and was that CDPK can regulate sandalwood seed oil accumulation and biogenesis (Anil et al., 2003). Furthermore, Delta-12 fatty acid desaturases (FADs) were found in some plant families, and were suggested to be involved in the acetylenic bond formation of plant fatty acids (Okada et al., 2013).

Considering the very high expression of Santalaceae FAD2 genes in the seed of *E. cupressiformis* (Okada et al., 2013), these genes may play an important role in forming ximenynic acid. What enzymes catalyze ximenynic acid's alkyne bond formation has set off discussions. Research has suggested that ximenynic acid alkynyl group is formed through stearolic acid pathway (Minto & Blacklock, 2008). Stearolic acid might be the intermediate product of ximenynic acid synthesis pathway in plant. This point was supported by widely distribution of stearolic acid in several Santalaceae plants which also rich in ximenynic acid (Badami & Patil, 1980; Morris & Marshall, 1966). Therefore, the unsaturated bond formation process of ximenynic acid may be formed by dehydrogenation to an alkyne bond at C-9 position and then an alkene bond at C-11. Santalaceae FAD2 demonstrated not only Δ12-desaturation activity of oleic acid, but also *trans*-Δ11-desaturation and *trans*-Δ12-desaturation activities of stearolic acid (Okada et al., 2013). However, Santalaceae FAD enzymes did not show Δ9-acetylenase activity (Okada et al., 2013). It indicated that ximenynic acid could be produced directly by *trans*-Δ11-desaturation of stearolic acid and might also by isomerization of *trans*-12-octadecen-9-ynoic acid from *trans*-Δ12-desaturation of stearolic acid, rather than Δ9-desaturation of conjugated linoleic acid. In other words, Santalaceae FAD2 produced ximenynic acid by *trans*-Δ11-desaturation of stearolic acid rather than conjugated linoleic acid (Okada et al., 2013), which was consistent with the proposal that stearolic acid was from the Δ9-acetylenase of oleic acid (Minto & Blacklock, 2008). However, the Δ9-acetylenase activity was not found in Santalaceae FAD enzymes (Okada et al., 2013). These results suggest that ximenynic acid synthesis may originate from oleic acid by undergoing two intermedia including stearolic acid and conjugated linoleic acid (Fig. 20.3).

20.7 Conclusion and future studies of ximenynic acid

Ximenynic acid has been studied for more than 80 years and displays many physiological and biological functions (Fig. 20.4). First, reports have shown that ximenynic acid can affect the metabolic pathway of polyunsaturated fatty acids. Ximenynic acid inhibited the expression

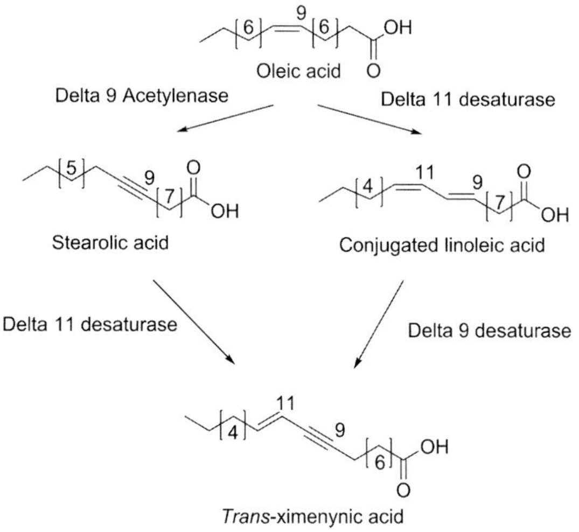

FIG. 20.3 The hypothesis of biosynthesis of ximenynic acid from oleic acid.

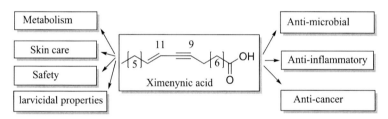

FIG. 20.4 The bioactivities of ximenynic acid.

of FADS2 in vitro and possessed an agonist activity on long-chain fatty acid receptors FFA1/FFA4, and both showed a potential regulation of insulin secretion. Subsequently, ximenynic acid-rich sandalwood seed oil improved insulin resistance in rats by modulating JNK/NF-κB inflammatory and PI3K/Akt pathways. Whether ximenynic acid is beneficial for metabolic disease needs to be validated further.

Furthermore, ximenynic acid possesses a potent anti-inflammatory activity that has been reported in vitro and in vivo experiments. It can inhibit phospholipase activity and decrease the levels of inflammatory factors in rats. It also selectively inhibits the COX-1 activity in HepG2 cells. Given the close relationship between inflammation and cancer development, ximenynic acid also showed the potential inhibition of angiogenesis of a HepG2 cell line.

Another point of research is the antimicrobial and larvicidal activity of ximenynic acid. As is often the case of acetylenic fatty acids, the antimicrobial activity of ximenynic acid is also effective, showing a potent inhibition of Gram-positive bacteria and some pathogenic fungi. Thus, ximenynic acid-rich kernel is also commonly used by local people to treat epidermal inflammation. Beyond that, the larvicidal activity of ximenynic acid against *Anopheles arabiensis* mosquitoes indicated the potential application to prevent malaria.

The significant application of ximenynic acid is in the cosmetic industry. Clinical trials have demonstrated that ximenynic acid can increase capillary blood flow, which may be a reason for its anti-aging, anti-hair loss, and protecting environment damaged skin. This application is essential for the production of sandalwood trees and the long-term research of ximenynic acid.

With its increasing demand in medicine, cosmetic, and other industries, the preparation methods of ximenynic acid are worthy of attention. This paper reviewed the distribution, separation, and purification of natural ximenynic acid. We also introduced the chemical synthesis and biosynthesis of ximenynic acid. The common purification methods include low-temperature crystallization, urea embedding, column chromatography, HPLC, and new supercritical chromatography. All these methods can obtain high-purity ximenynic acid, but the efficiencies are different. The combination of these methods may achieve higher recovery rates and purity. For example, supercritical chromatography technique augments the separation efficiency by selecting unsaturated bonds into a stationary phase and a special number of carbon atoms. Natural ximenynic acid only exists in several rare plant species that cannot meet the rapidly increasing demand. Therefore, the synthesis of ximenynic acid also deserves great attention. However, most of the methods we mentioned above are based on toxic organic reagents with lower yields. More efficient and less polluting techniques need to be developed to isolate ximenynic acid in the future.

Since discovering ximenynic acid, researchers have been enthusiastic about its natural distribution, purification, and chemical synthesis, with relatively few studies on its physiological activities. As a unique conjugated octadecenynoic acetylenic acid whose structure is similar to conjugated linoleic acid, ximenynic acid has good physiological functions to be explored. Although there is a long history of ximenynic acid, it still failed to give enough propaganda.

References

Adlof, R. (1999). The lindlar-catalyzed reduction of methyl santalbate: A facile preparation of methyl 9-cis,11-trans-Octadecadienoate-9,10-d2. *Journal of the American Oil Chemists' Society*, 76(3), 301–304. https://doi.org/10.1007/s11746-999-0235-8.

Aitzetmuller, K. (2012). Santalbic acid in the plant kingdom. *Plant Systematics and Evolution*, 298(9), 1609–1617. https://doi.org/10.1007/s00606-012-0678-5.

Anil, V. S., Harmon, A. C., & Rao, K. S. (2003). Temporal association of ca(2+)-dependent protein kinase with oil bodies during seed development in Santalum album L.: Its biochemical characterization and significance. *Plant & Cell Physiology*, 44(4), 367–376.

Badami, R. C., & Patil, K. B. (1980). Structure and occurrence of unusual fatty acids in minor seed oils. *Progress in Lipid Research*, 19(3–4), 119–153. https://doi.org/10.1016/0163-7827(80)90002-8.

Ballance, P. E., & Crombie, W. M. (1958). Paper chromatography of saturated and unsaturated fatty acids. *Biochemical Journal*, 69, 632–640.

Baud, S. (2018). Seeds as oil factories. *Plant Reproduction*, 31(3), 213–235. https://doi.org/10.1007/s00497-018-0325-6.

Biermann, U., Lützen, A., Lie Ken Jie, M. S. F., & Metzger, J. O. (2000). Regioselective cationic 1,2- and 1,4-additions forming carbon−carbon bonds to methyl Santalbate, a conjugated Enyne. *European Journal of Organic Chemistry*, 2000(17), 3069–3073.

Bombardelli, E., Cristoni, A., & Morazzoni, P. (1997). *Combinations of vasoactive substances with fatty acids to prevent hair loss*. Google Patents.

Bulock, J. D., & Smith, G. N. (1963). Acetylenic fatty acids in seeds and seedlings of sweet Quandong. *Phytochemistry*, 2(3), 289–296.

Burant, C. F., Viswanathan, P., Marcinak, J., Cao, C., Vakilynejad, M., Xie, B., et al. (2012). TAK-875 versus placebo or glimepiride in type 2 diabetes mellitus: A phase 2, randomised, double-blind, placebo-controlled trial. *Lancet*, 379(9824), 1403–1411. https://doi.org/10.1016/S0140-6736(11)61879-5.

Butaud, J. F., Raharivelomanana, P., Bianchini, J. P., & Gaydou, E. M. (2008). Santalum insulare Acetylenic fatty acid seed oils: Comparison within the Santalum genus. *Journal of the American Oil Chemists' Society, 85*(4), 353–356. https://doi.org/10.1007/s11746-008-1196-z.

Cai, F., Chen, S., Yang, J., Zhang, X., Zou, Z., & Li, D. (2016). The antitumor activity of ximenynic acid on HCT116 cells and its mechanism. *Acta Nutrimenta Sinica, 6*(38), 566–571.

Cai, F., Li, J., Liu, Y., Zhang, Z., Hettiarachchi, D. S., & Li, D. (2016). Effect of ximenynic acid on cell cycle arrest and apoptosis and COX-1 in HepG2 cells. *Molecular Medicine Reports, 14*(6), 5667–5676. https://doi.org/10.3892/mmr.2016.5920.

Cai, F., Liu, Y., Hettiarachichi, D. S., Wang, F., Li, J., Sunderland, B., et al. (2020). Ximenynic acid regulation of n-3 PUFA content in liver and brain. *Lifestyle Genom, 13*(2), 64–73. https://doi.org/10.1159/000502773.

Cantrell, C. L., Berhow, M. A., Phillips, B. S., Duval, S. M., Weisleder, D., & Vaughn, S. F. (2003). Bioactive crude plant seed extracts from the NCAUR oilseed repository. *Phytomedicine, 10*(4), 325–333. https://doi.org/10.1078/094471103322004820.

Catchpole, O., Tallon, S., Dyer, P., Montanes, F., Moreno, T., Vági, E., et al. (2013). Integrated supercritical fluid extraction and bioprocessing. *American Journal of Biochemistry and Biotechnology, 8*(4), 263–287.

Chivandi, E., Cave, E., Davidson, B. C., Erlwanger, K. H., Moyo, D., & Madziva, M. T. (2012). Suppression of Caco-2 and HEK-293 cell proliferation by Kigelia africana, Mimusops zeyheri and Ximenia caffra seed oils. *In Vivo, 26*(1), 99–105.

Chivandi, E., Davidson, B. C., & Erlwanger, K. H. (2008). A comparison of the lipid and fatty acid profiles from the kernels of the fruit (nuts) of Ximenia caffra and Ricinodendron rautanenii from Zimbabwe. *Industrial Crops and Products, 27*(1), 29–32. https://doi.org/10.1016/j.indcrop.2007.06.002.

Chivandi, E., Davidson, B. C., & Erlwanger, K. H. (2012). Red sour plum (Ximenia caffra) seed: A potential nonconventional energy and protein source for livestock feeds. *International Journal of Agriculture and Biology, 14*(4), 149.

Christiansen, E., Watterson, K. R., Stocker, C. J., Sokol, E., Jenkins, L., Simon, K., et al. (2015). Activity of dietary fatty acids on FFA1 and FFA4 and characterisation of pinolenic acid as a dual FFA1/FFA4 agonist with potential effect against metabolic diseases. *British Journal of Nutrition, 113*(11), 1677–1688. https://doi.org/10.1017/S000711451500118X.

Croft, K. D., Beilin, L. J., & Ford, G. L. (1987). Differential inhibition of thromboxane B2 and leukotriene B4 biosynthesis by two naturally occurring acetylenic fatty acids. *Biochimica et Biophysica Acta, 921*(3), 621–624. https://doi.org/10.1016/0005-2760(87)90091-9.

Crombie, W. M., Comber, R., & Boatman, S. G. (1955). The estimation of unsaturated fatty acids by reversed-phase partition chromatography. *The Biochemical Journal, 59*(2), 309–316.

Crombie, L., & Griffin, B. P. (1958). Lipids .7. Synthesis of 8-hydroxyoctadec-cis-11 and trans-11-En-9-ynoic acid—The status of natural 8-hydroxyximenynic acid. *Journal of the Chemical Society*, 4435–4444.

Crombie, L., & Jacklin, A. G. (1955). Lipids .2. Total synthesis of ricinoleic acid. *Journal of the Chemical Society*, 1740–1748. https://doi.org/10.1039/Jr9550001740.

Crombie, L., & Jacklin, A. G. (1957). 310. Lipids. Part V. Total synthesis of ximenynic acid, homoricinstearolic acid, and two fatty hydroxy-acids with allenic sidebranches. *Lipids*, 1622–1631. https://doi.org/10.1039/jr9570001622.

Cunningham, A., Maduarta, I. M., Howe, J., Ingram, W., & Jansen, S. (2011). Hanging by a thread: Natural metallic mordant processes in traditional Indonesian textiles. *Economic Botany, 65*(3), 241–259. https://doi.org/10.1007/s12231-011-9161-4.

Cuzick, J., Otto, F., Baron, J. A., Brown, P. H., Burn, J., Greenwald, P., et al. (2009). Aspirin and non-steroidal anti-inflammatory drugs for cancer prevention: An international consensus statementAspirin and non-steroidal anti-inflammatory drugs for cancer prevention: An international consensus statement. *The Lancet Oncology, 10*(5), 501–507. https://doi.org/10.1016/S1470-2045(09)70035-X.

de Fuentes-Vicente, J. A., Gutiérrez-Cabrera, A. E., Flores-Villegas, A. L., Lowenberger, C., Benelli, G., Salazar-Schettino, P. M., et al. (2018). What makes an effective Chagas disease vector? Factors underlying Trypanosoma cruzi-triatomine interactions. *Acta Tropica, 183*, 23–31. https://doi.org/10.1016/j.actatropica.2018.04.008.

Dembitsky, V. (2006). Anticancer activity of natural and synthetic acetylenic lipids. *Lipids, 41*(10), 883–924. https://doi.org/10.1007/s11745-006-5044-3.

Dzoyem, J. P., Tchuenguem, R. T., Kuiate, J. R., Teke, G. N., Kechia, F. A., & Kuete, V. (2014). In vitro and in vivo antifungal activities of selected Cameroonian dietary spices. *BMC Complementary and Alternative Medicine, 14*, 58. https://doi.org/10.1186/1472-6882-14-58.

Furman, D., Campisi, J., Verdin, E., Carrera-Bastos, P., Targ, S., Franceschi, C., et al. (2019). Chronic inflammation in the etiology of disease across the life span. *Nature Medicine, 25*(12), 1822–1832. https://doi.org/10.1038/s41591-019-0675-0.

Glaser, C., Heinrich, J., & Koletzko, B. (2010). Role of FADS1 and FADS2 polymorphisms in polyunsaturated fatty acid metabolism. *Metabolism, 59*(7), 993–999. https://doi.org/10.1016/j.metabol.2009.10.022.

Grigor, J., Macinnes, D., & Mclean, J. (1954). The synthesis of Ximenynic acid. *Chemistry & Industry, 36*, 1112–1113.

Grivennikov, S. I., Greten, F. R., & Karin, M. (2010). Immunity, inflammation, and cancer. *Cell*, *140*(6), 883–899. https://doi.org/10.1016/j.cell.2010.01.025.

Guengerich, F. P. (2008). Cytochrome p450 and chemical toxicology. *Chemical Research in Toxicology*, *21*(1), 70–83. https://doi.org/10.1021/tx700079z.

Gulati, V., Gulati, P., Harding, I. H., & Palombo, E. A. (2015). Exploring the anti-diabetic potential of Australian aboriginal and Indian Ayurvedic plant extracts using cell-based assays. *BMC Complementary and Alternative Medicine*, *15*(1), 8. https://doi.org/10.1186/s12906-015-0524-8.

Gunstone, F. D., & Mcgee, M. A. (1954). Santalbic acid. *Chemistry & Industry*, *36*, 1112.

Gunstone, F. D., & Russell, W. C. (1955). Fatty acids. 3. The constitution and properties of santalbic acid. *Journal of the Chemical Society*, 3782–3787.

Haigh, W. G., Morris, L. J., & James, A. T. (1968). Acetylenic acid biosynthesis in Crepis rubra. *Lipids*, *3*(4), 307–312. https://doi.org/10.1007/BF02530929.

Hara, T., Ichimura, A., & Hirasawa, A. (2014). Therapeutic role and ligands of medium- to long-chain fatty acid receptors. *Frontiers in Endocrinology (Lausanne)*, *5*, 83. https://doi.org/10.3389/fendo.2014.00083.

Hatt, H. H., Meisters, A., Triffett, A. C., & Wailes, P. C. (1967). Acetylenic acids from fats of Olacaceae and Santalaceae. V. A spectroscopic survey of somatic fats of additional species. *Australian Journal of Chemistry*, *20*(10), 2285–2289.

Hatt, H. H., & Schoenfeld, R. (1956). Some seed fats of the santalaceae family. *Journal of the Science of Food and Agriculture*, *7*(2), 130–133. https://doi.org/10.1002/jsfa.2740070207.

Hatt, H. H., Triffett, A. C. K., & Wailes, P. C. (1959). Acetylenic acids from fats of Santalaceae and Olacaceae—Seed and root oils of exocarpus-Cupressiformis Labill. *Australian Journal of Chemistry*, *12*(2), 190–195.

Hatt, H. H., Triffett, A. C. K., & Wailes, P. C. (1960). Acetylenic acids from fats of the Olacaceae and Santalaceae. IV. The occurrence of octadeca-trans-11, trans-13-dien-9-ynoic acid in plant lipids. *Australian Journal of Chemistry*, *13*(4), 488–497.

Hettiarachchi, D. S. (2014). *Pharmaceutical evaluation of Western Australian sandalwood seed oil*. Curtin University.

Hettiarachchi, D. S., Liu, Y. D., Boddy, M. R., Fox, J. E. D., & Sunderland, V. B. (2013). Contents of fatty acids, selected lipids and physicochemical properties of Western Australian sandalwood seed oil. *Journal of the American Oil Chemists' Society*, *90*(2), 285–290.

Hettiarachchi, D. S., Liu, Y., Fox, J., & Sunderland, B. (2010). Western Australian sandalwood seed oil: New opportunities. *Lipid Technology*, *22*(2), 27–29. https://doi.org/10.1002/lite.200900071.

Hettiarachchi, D. S., Liu, Y. D., Jose, S., Boddy, M. R., Fox, J. E. D., & Sunderland, B. (2012). Assessment of Western Australian sandalwood seeds for seed oil production. *Australian Forestry*, *75*(4), 246–250.

Hopkins, C. Y., & Chisholm, M. (1968). A survey of the conjugated fatty acids of seed oils. *Journal of the American Oil Chemists Society*, *45*(3), 76–182. https://doi.org/10.1007/BF02915346.

Hopkins, C. Y., Chisholm, M. J., & Cody, W. J. (1969). Fatty acid components of some Santalaceae seed oils. *Phytochemistry*, *8*(1), 161–165.

Hopkins, C. Y., Jevans, A. W., & Chisholm, M. J. (1968). Acetylenic fatty acids of Pyrularia Pubera seed oil. *Journal of the Chemical Society C: Organic*, *19*, 2462–2465.

Imig, J. D., & Hammock, B. D. (2009). Soluble epoxide hydrolase as a therapeutic target for cardiovascular diseases. *Nature Reviews. Drug Discovery*, *8*(10), 794–805. https://doi.org/10.1038/nrd2875.

Itoh, Y., Kawamata, Y., Harada, M., Kobayashi, M., Fujii, R., Fukusumi, S., et al. (2003). Free fatty acids regulate insulin secretion from pancreatic beta cells through GPR40. *Nature*, *422*(6928), 173–176. http://www.ncbi.nlm.nih.gov/pubmed/12629551.

Jie, M. S., & Pasha, M. K. (1998). Epoxidation reactions of unsaturated fatty esters with potassium peroxomonosulfate. *Lipids*, *33*(6), 633–637.

Jie, M. S., Pasha, M. K., & Ahmad, F. (1996). Ultrasound-assisted synthesis of santalbic acid and a study of triacylglycerol species in Santalum album (Linn.) seed oil. *Lipids*, *31*(10), 1083–1089.

Jie, M. S., Pasha, M. K., & Alam, M. S. (1997). Oxidation reactions of acetylenic fatty esters with selenium dioxide/tert-butyl hydroperoxide. *Lipids*, *32*(10), 1119–1123.

Jones, G. P., Birkett, A., Sanigorski, A., Sinclair, A. J., Hooper, P. T., Watson, T., et al. (1994). Effect of feeding quandong (Santalum acuminatum) oil to rats on tissue lipids, hepatic cytochrome P-450 and tissue histology. *Food and Chemical Toxicology*, *32*(6), 521–525.

Jones, G. P., Rao, K. S., Tucker, D. J., Richardson, B., Barnes, A., & Rivett, D. E. (1995). Antimicrobial activity of Santalbic acid from the oil of Santalum-Acuminatum (Quandong). *International Journal of Pharmacognosy*, *33*(2), 120–123.

Jones, G. P., Watson, T. G., Sinclair, A. J., Birkett, A., Dunt, N., Nair, S. S., et al. (1999). Santalbic acid from quandong kernels and oil fed to rats affects kidney and liver P450. *Asia Pacific Journal of Clinical Nutrition*, *8*(3), 211–215.

Kapoor, S., Nailwal, N., Kumar, M., & Barve, K. (2019). Recent patents and discovery of anti-inflammatory agents from marine source. *Recent Patents on Inflammation & Allergy Drug Discovery*, *13*(2), 105–114. https://doi.org/10.2174/1872213X13666190426164717.

Khanapure, S. P., Garvey, D. S., Janero, D. R., & Letts, L. G. (2007). Eicosanoids in inflammation: Biosynthesis, pharmacology, and therapeutic frontiers. *Current Topics in Medicinal Chemistry, 7*(3), 311–340.

Kuete, V., Krusche, B., Youns, M., Voukeng, I., Fankam, A. G., Tankeo, S., et al. (2011). Cytotoxicity of some Cameroonian spices and selected medicinal plant extracts. *Journal of Ethnopharmacology, 134*(3), 803–812.

Kuklev, D. V., Domb, A. J., & Dembitsky, V. M. (2013). Bioactive acetylenic metabolites. *Phytomedicine, 20*(13), 1145–1159. https://doi.org/10.1016/j.phymed.2013.06.009.

Kumar, Y., Subrata, M., & Jagatpati, T. (2019). A short review on white sandalwood (Santalum album L.). *International Journal of Scientific Research and Reviews, 08*, 73–136.

Lall, N., & Kishore, N. (2014). Are plants used for skin care in South Africa fully explored? *Journal of Ethnopharmacology, 153*(1), 61–84.

Li, G., Singh, A., Liu, Y., Sunderland, B., & Li, D. (2013). Comparative effects of sandalwood seed oil on fatty acid profiles and inflammatory factors in rats. *Lipids, 48*(2), 105–113. https://doi.org/10.1007/s11745-012-3752-4.

Lie Ken Jie, M. S. F., Lau, M. M. L., Lam, C. N. W., Alam, M. S., Metzger, J. O., & Biermann, U. (2003). Novel halo-oxo-allenic fatty ester derivatives from epoxidized methyl santalbate (methyl trans-11-octadecen-9-ynoate). *Chemistry and Physics of Lipids, 125*(2), 93–101. https://doi.org/10.1016/s0009-3084(03)00071-9.

Lighthelm, S. P., & Schwartz, H. M. (1950). The isolation of a conjugated unsaturated acid from the oil from Ximenia-Caffra Kernels. *Journal of the American Chemical Society, 72*(4), 1868. https://doi.org/10.1021/Ja01160a539.

Ligthelm, S. P., Horn, D. H. S., Schwartz, H. M., & Von Holdt, M. M. (1954). A chemical study of the fruits of three south African Ximenia species, with special reference to the kernel oils. *Journal of the Science of Food and Agriculture, 5*(6), 281–288.

Ligthelm, S. P., Schwartz, H. M., & Vonholdt, M. M. (1952). The chemistry of Ximenynic acid. *Journal of the Chemical Society*, 1088–1093.

Lim, T. K. (2013). *Edible medicinal and non-medicinal plants. In Santalum acuminatum. Vol. 5*. Netherlands: Springer. https://doi.org/10.1007/978-94-007-5653-3_43.

Liu, Y. D., & Longmore, R. B. (1996). A biotransformation product of ximenynic acid and its significance. *Proceeding of the Nutrition Society of Australia, 20*, 203.

Liu, Y. D., & Longmore, R. B. (1997). Dietary sandalwood seed oil modifies fatty acid composition of mouse adipose tissue, brain, and liver. *Lipids, 32*(9), 965–969. https://doi.org/10.1007/s11745-997-0125-x.

Liu, Y. D., Longmore, R. B., Boddy, M. R., & Fox, J. E. D. (1997). Separation and identification of triximenynin from Santalum spicatum R Br. *Journal of the American Oil Chemists' Society, 74*(10), 1269–1272. https://doi.org/10.1007/s11746-997-0056-6.

Liu, Y. D., Longmore, R. B., & Fox, J. E. D. (1996). Separation and identification of ximenynic acid isomers in the seed oil of Santalum spicatum RBr as their 4,4-dimethyloxazoline derivatives. *Journal of the American Oil Chemists Society, 73*(12), 1729–1731. https://doi.org/10.1007/Bf02517979.

Liu, Y. D., Longmore, R. B., & Kailis, S. G. (1997). Proximate and fatty acid composition changes in developing sandalwood (Santalum spicatum) seeds. *Journal of the Science of Food and Agriculture, 75*(1), 27–30.

Londero, V. S., da Costa-Silva, T. A., Gomes, K. S., Ferreira, D. D., Mesquita, J. T., Tempone, A. G., et al. (2018). Acetylenic fatty acids from Porcelia macrocarpa (Annonaceae) against trypomastigotes of Trypanosoma cruzi: Effect of octadec-9-ynoic acid in plasma membrane electric potential. *Bioorganic Chemistry, 78*, 307–311. https://doi.org/10.1016/j.bioorg.2018.03.025.

Madhuranath, M., & Manjunath, B. (1938). Chemical examination of the oil from the seeds of Santalum album (Linn). *Journal of the Indian Chemical Society, 15*, 389–392.

Maier, K. G., & Roman, R. J. (2001). Cytochrome P450 metabolites of arachidonic acid in the control of renal function. *Current Opinion in Nephrology and Hypertension, 10*(1), 81–87. https://doi.org/10.1097/00041552-200101000-00013.

Mancini, A. D., & Poitout, V. (2013). The fatty acid receptor FFA1/GPR40 a decade later: How much do we know? *Trends in Endocrinology and Metabolism, 24*(8), 398–407. https://doi.org/10.1016/j.tem.2013.03.003.

Maroyi, A. (2016). Ximenia caffra Sond. (Ximeniaceae) in sub-Saharan Africa: A synthesis and review of its medicinal potential. *Journal of Ethnopharmacology, 184*, 81–100. https://doi.org/10.1016/j.jep.2016.02.052.

Mavundza, E. J., Chukwujekwu, J. C., Maharaj, R., Finnie, J. F., Van Heerden, F. R., & Van Staden, J. (2016). Identification of compounds in Olax dissitiflora with larvacidal effect against Anopheles arabiensis. *South African Journal of Botany, 102*, 1–3.

Meyer, B. N., Ferrigni, N. R., Putnam, J. E., Jacobsen, L. B., Nichols, D. E., & McLaughlin, J. L. (1982). Brine shrimp: A convenient general bioassay for active plant constituents. *Planta Medica, 45*(05), 31–34. https://doi.org/10.1055/s-2007-971236.

Mikolajczak, K. L., Earle, F. R., & Wolff, I. A. (1963). The acetylenic acid in Comandra pallida and Osyris alba seed oils. *Journal of the American Oil Chemists Society, 40*(8), 342–343. https://doi.org/10.1007/BF02631553.

Minto, R. E., & Blacklock, B. J. (2008). Biosynthesis and function of polyacetylenes and allied natural products. *Progress in Lipid Research, 47*(4), 233–306. https://doi.org/10.1016/j.plipres.2008.02.002.

Montañés, F., Tallon, S., & Catchpole, O. (2017). Isolation of non-methylene interrupted or Acetylenic fatty acids from seed oils using semi-preparative supercritical chromatography. *Journal of the American Oil Chemists' Society*, 94(7), 981–991. https://doi.org/10.1007/s11746-017-2999-6.

Morris, L. J., & Marshall, M. O. (1966). Occurrence of Stearolic acid in Santalaceae seed oils. *Chemistry & Industry*, 11, 460.

Narayana, K. H. S., & Rao, G. S. K. (1982). Sodium santalbate-dimethyl sulfate inclusion complex. *Journal of the American Oil Chemists' Society*, 59(5), 240–241. https://doi.org/10.1007/BF02582185.

Nugteren, D. H., & Christ-Hazelhof, E. (1987). Naturally occurring conjugated octadecatrienoic acids are strong inhibitors of prostaglandin biosynthesis. *Prostaglandins*, 33(3), 403–417.

Oh, D. Y., Talukdar, S., Bae, E. J., Imamura, T., Morinaga, H., Fan, W., et al. (2010). GPR120 is an omega-3 fatty acid receptor mediating potent anti-inflammatory and insulin-sensitizing effects. *Cell*, 142(5), 687–698. https://doi.org/10.1016/j.cell.2010.07.041.

Ohtera, A., Miyamae, Y., Nakai, N., Kawachi, A., Kawada, K., Han, J., et al. (2013). Identification of 6-octadecynoic acid from a methanol extract of Marrubium vulgare L. as a peroxisome proliferator-activated receptor gamma agonist. *Biochemical and Biophysical Research Communications*, 440(2), 204–209. https://doi.org/10.1016/j.bbrc.2013.09.003.

Okada, S., Zhou, X. R., Damcevski, K., Gibb, N., Wood, C., Hamberg, M., et al. (2013). Diversity of Delta12 fatty acid desaturases in Santalaceae and their role in production of seed oil acetylenic fatty acids. *The Journal of Biological Chemistry*, 288, 32405–32413.

Palyzová, A., & Řezanka, T. (2020). Separation of triacylglycerols containing allenic and acetylenic fatty acids by enantiomeric liquid chromatography-mass spectrometry. *Journal of Chromatography A*, 1623. https://doi.org/10.1016/j.chroma.2020.461161.

Pardoe, C., Fullagar, R., & Hayes, E. (2019). Quandong stones: A specialised Australian nut-cracking tool. *PLoS One*, 14(10). https://doi.org/10.1371/journal.pone.0222680, e0222680.

Pasha, M. K., & Ahmad, F. (1993). Synthesis of oxygenated fatty-acid esters from Santalbic acid Ester. *Lipids*, 28(11), 1027–1031. https://doi.org/10.1007/Bf02537126.

Patil, V., Vadnere, G. P., & Patel, N. (2011). Absence of antimicrobial activity in alcoholic extract of Santalum album Linn. *Journal of Pharmaceutical Negative Results*, 2(2), 107–109. https://doi.org/10.4103/0976-9234.90224.

Rezanka, T., & Sigler, K. (2007). Identification of very long chain unsaturated fatty acids from Ximenia oil by atmospheric pressure chemical ionization liquid chromatography-mass spectroscopy. *Phytochemistry*, 68(6), 925–934. https://doi.org/10.1016/j.phytochem.2006.11.034.

Saeedi, P., Petersohn, I., Salpea, P., Malanda, B., Karuranga, S., Unwin, N., et al. (2019). Global and regional diabetes prevalence estimates for 2019 and projections for 2030 and 2045: Results from the international Diabetes federation Diabetes Atlas, 9(th) edition. *Diabetes Research and Clinical Practice*, 157. https://doi.org/10.1016/j.diabres.2019.107843, 107843.

Satoto, G., Fernandes, A., Saraiva, N., Santos, F., Santos de Almeida, T., & Araújo, M. E. M. (2019). An overview on the properties of Ximenia oil used as cosmetic in Angola. *Biomolecules*, 10(1), 18. https://doi.org/10.3390/biom10010018.

Shankaranarayana, K. H., & Parthasarathi, K. (1986). Surface active products from sandal seed oil. *Journal of the American Oil Chemists' Society*, 63(11), 1473–1474.

Shawar, R. M., Humble, D. J., vanDalfsen, J. M., Stover, C. K., Hickey, M. J., Steele, S., et al. (1997). Rapid screening of natural products for antimycobacterial activity by using luciferase-expressing strains of Mycobacterium bovis BCG and mycobacterium intracellulare. *Antimicrobial Agents and Chemotherapy*, 41(3), 570–574.

Shivatare, R. S., Musale, R., Lohakare, P., Patil, D., Choudhary, D., Ganu, G., et al. (2020a). In vitro antioxidant activity and stability indicating high-performance thin-layer chromatographic method for Ximenynic acid in Santalum Album seed extract. *Asian Journal of Pharmaceutics*, 14(1), 9–16.

Shivatare, R., Musale, R., Lohakare, P., Patil, D., Choudhary, D., Ganu, G., et al. (2020b). Isolation, identification and characterization of Ximenynic acid with anti-aging activity from Santalum Album. *International Journal of Research in Pharmaceutical Sciences*, 11, 1394–1399. https://doi.org/10.26452/ijrps.v11i2.2005.

Smith, G. N., Taj, M., & Braganza, J. M. (1991). On the identification of a conjugated diene component of duodenal bile as 9z, 11e-Octadecadienoic acid. *Free Radical Biology and Medicine*, 10(1), 13–21.

Sparavigna, A., Tenconi, B., De Ponti, I., & Guglielmini, G. (2014). Evaluation of the activity and tolerability of a cosmetic treatment for the periocular area on the aging face: Controlled clinical and instrumental evaluation vs. Placebo. *Cosmetics*, 1(2), 105.

Spitzer, V., Bordignon, S. A.de L., Schenkel, E. P., & Marx, F. (1994). Identification of nine acetylenic fatty acids, 9-hydroxystearic acid and 9,10-epoxystearic acid in the seed oil of Jodina rhombifolia hook et arn. (Santalaceae). *Journal of the American Oil Chemists' Society*, 71(12), 1343–1348.

Spitzer, V., Marx, F., Maia, J. G., & Pfeilsticker, K. (1991). Curupira tefeensis II: Occurrence of acetylenic fatty acids. *Fat Science Technology*, 93(5), 169–174. https://doi.org/10.1002/lipi.19910930502.

Spitzer, V., Tomberg, W., Hartmann, R., & Aichholz, R. (1997). Analysis of the seed oil of *Heisteria silvanii* (Olacaceae)—a rich source of a novel C-18 acetylenic fatty acid. *Lipids*, 32(11), 1189–1200.

Tesche, O. A. (1954). The crystal structure of Ximenynic acid. *Acta Crystallographica*, 7(11), 737–739.

Urso, V., Signorini, M. A., Tonini, M., & Bruschi, P. (2016). Wild medicinal and food plants used by communities living in mopane woodlands of southern Angola: Results of an ethnobotanical field investigation. *Journal of Ethnopharmacology*, 177, 126–139. https://doi.org/10.1016/j.jep.2015.11.041.

Vadnere, G., Md, U., Lodhi, S., & Patil, V. (2017). Phytochemical investigation and in vitro antimicrobial screening of santalum album seeds extracts. *International Journal of Pharmacy and Pharmaceutical Sciences*, 9, 117. https://doi.org/10.22159/ijpps.2017v9i11.21216.

Vermaak, I., Kamatou, G. P. P., Komane-Mofokeng, B., Viljoen, A. M., & Beckett, K. (2011). African seed oils of commercial importance—Cosmetic applications. *South African Journal of Botany*, 77(4), 920–933. https://doi.org/10.1016/j.sajb.2011.07.003.

Vickery, J. R., Whitfield, F. B., Ford, G. L., & Kennett, B. H. (1984). Ximenynic acid in Santalum-Obtusifolium seed oil. *Journal of the American Oil Chemists Society*, 61(5), 890–891. https://doi.org/10.1007/Bf02542158.

Walle, P., Männistö, V., de Mello, V. D., Vaittinen, M., Perfilyev, A., Hanhineva, K., et al. (2019). Liver DNA methylation of FADS2 associates with FADS2 genotype. *Clinical Epigenetics*, 11(1), 10. https://doi.org/10.1186/s13148-019-0609-1.

Wang, L. T., Li, J. B., & Xue, X. W. (2012). Concise synthesis of Ximenynic acid. *Synthetic Communications*, 42(23), 3540–3543. https://doi.org/10.1080/00397911.2011.585443.

Wu, Q., Wang, H., Zhao, X., Shi, Y., Jin, M., Wan, B., et al. (2013). Identification of G-protein-coupled receptor 120 as a tumor-promoting receptor that induces angiogenesis and migration in human colorectal carcinoma. *Oncogene*, 32(49), 5541–5550. https://doi.org/10.1038/onc.2013.264.

Yao, M., Li, J., Xie, T., He, T., Fang, L., Shi, Y., et al. (2015). Polymorphisms of rs174616 in the FADS1-FADS2 gene cluster is associated with a reduced risk of type 2 diabetes mellitus in northern Han Chinese people. *Diabetes Research and Clinical Practice*, 109(1), 206–212. https://doi.org/10.1016/j.diabres.2015.03.009.

Zhang, H., Gao, X., Li, K., Liu, Y., Hettiarachichi, D. S., Sunderland, B., et al. (2021). Sandalwood seed oil ameliorates hepatic insulin resistance by regulating the JNK/NF-κB inflammatory and PI3K/AKT insulin signaling pathways. *Food & Function*, 12(5), 2312–2322. https://doi.org/10.1039/D0FO03051A.

Zhang, J. Y., Yu, X. J., Wang, H. Y., Liu, B. N., Yu, Q. T., Huang, Z. H., et al. (1989). Location of triple bonds in the fatty acids from the kernel oil of *Pyrularia edulis* by GC-MS of their 4,4-dimethyloxazoline derivatives. *Journal of the American Oil Chemists Society*, 66(2), 256–259.

CHAPTER 21

Application of phytosterols in management of plasma cholesterol

Wen-Sen He[a] and Zhen-Yu Chen[b]

[a]School of Food and Biological Engineering, Jiangsu University, Zhenjiang, Jiangsu, China [b]School of Life Sciences, The Chinese University of Hong Kong, Shatin, New Territories, China

21.1 Introduction

Cardiovascular diseases (CVDs) are currently the number one cause of death globally (World Health Organization, 2017). In 2016, approximately 17.9 million people died of CVDs, accounting for 31% of total deaths globally (World Health Organization, 2017) and 40% in China (Hu et al., 2018). Hyperlipidemia characterized by elevation of plasma total cholesterol (TC), low-density lipoprotein cholesterol (LDL-C), and triacylglycerol (TAG) and reduction of high-density lipoprotein cholesterol (HDL-C) is one of the principal risk factors for CVDs (Kaur & Myrie, 2020). Successful management of hyperlipidemia is the most predominant approach to reducing the risk of CVDs. Phytosterols (or plant sterols) are a class of biologically active compounds naturally occurring in plants, primarily comprising of beta-sitosterol, stigmasterol, campesterol, and brassicasterol. Cholesterol and phytosterols share a similar basic chemical structure, but they differ in the geometry of the hydrophobic carbon side chain (Fig. 21.1) (He, Zhu, & Chen, 2018). Phytosterols and their derivatives have exhibited numerous health benefits in humans, including cholesterol reduction (Cedó, Farràs, Lee-Rueckert, & Escolà-Gil, 2019), antiobesity (Ghaedi et al., 2019), antioxidation (Wang, Hicks, & Moreau, 2002), antiinflammation (Hu, Zhuo, Fang, Zhang, & Feng, 2017), anticancer (Suttiarporn et al., 2015), neuroprotection (Raju et al., 2021), cardiovascular protection (Gylling et al., 2014), and other activities (Rong, Xu, & Li, 2016). This chapter is mainly to update the current knowledge regarding the cholesterol-reducing benefits of phytosterols and their derivatives in both animal studies and clinical trials and to explore the associated underlying molecular mechanisms. In addition, the structure diversity and sources of dietary phytosterols as well as the current commercial applications of phytosterols will be reviewed.

21.2 Structure diversity and sources of dietary phytosterols

Sterols are the basic components of eukaryotic cells and are mainly responsible for regulation on the fluidity of cell membrane. On the

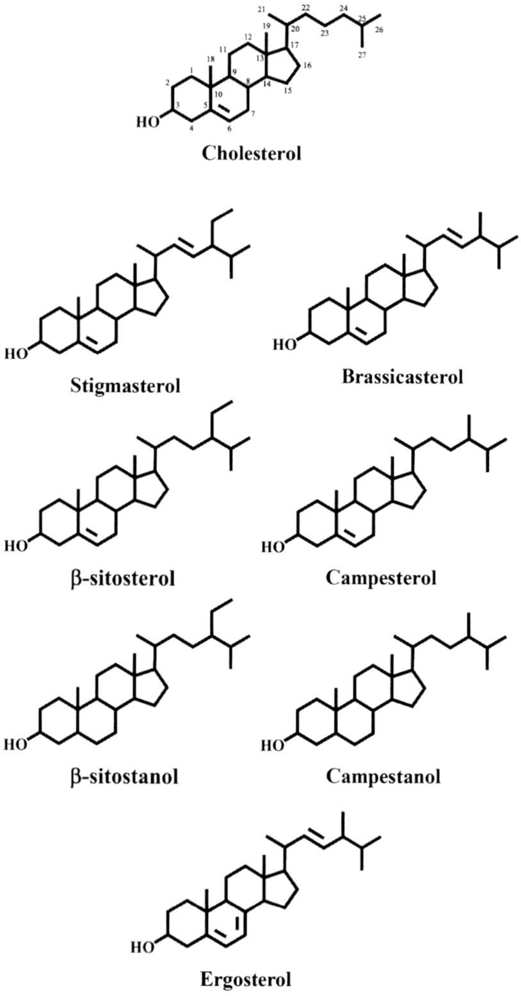

FIG. 21.1 Sterols from different sources in nature.

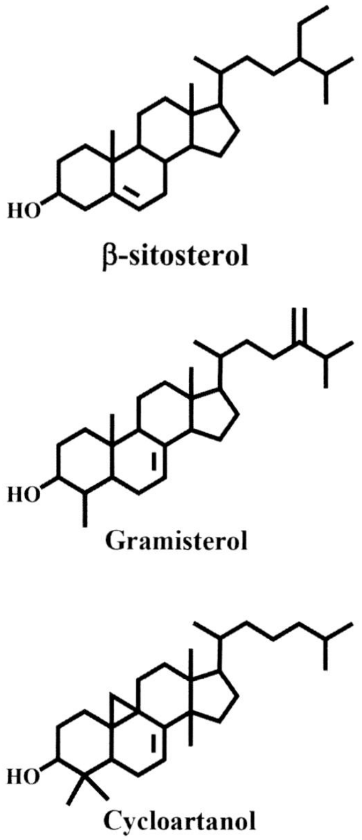

FIG. 21.2 Typical 4-desmethyl sterols, 4-monomethyl sterols, and 4,4-dimethyl sterols.

basis of their origin, sterols in plants are classified as phytosterols, while sterol in mammals is named cholesterol and that in fungus is called ergosterol (Fig. 21.1). These sterols share a similar basic skeleton (steroid nucleus) but they differ in the length and unsaturation of the side chains (He et al., 2018). Structurally, sterols can be divided into three categories according to the numbers of methyl group attached to the C-4 position of the steroid core: 4-desmethyl sterols, 4-monomethyl sterols, and 4,4-dimethyl sterols (Fig. 21.2).

In general, 4-monomethyl sterols and 4,4-dimethyl sterols are the biosynthetic intermediates acting as precursor of 4-desmethyl sterols (Darnet & Schaller, 2019). Gramisterol is the typical example of 4-monomethyl sterols, while cycloartenol and cycloartanol are representatives of 4,4-dimethyl sterols (Moreau, Whitaker, & Hicks, 2002). Beta-sitosterol, stigmasterol, campesterol, brassicasterol, cholesterol, or ergosterol belongs to 4-desmethyl sterols (Figs. 21.1 and 21.2). These subtle differences in structure determine the extremely diverse types of sterols. It is estimated that there are more than 1700 sterols in nature with 250 phytosterols being fully characterized (Moreau et al., 2018). Of these natural sterols, beta-sitosterol, campesterol, and stigmasterol are the three most abundant phytosterols, accounting for 65%, 30%, and 3% of total dietary sterols, respectively (Kaur & Myrie, 2020).

Phytosterols are mainly found in legumes, nuts, grains, fruits, and vegetables and their by-products (Wang et al., 2018). Industrially, the deodorized distillate produced by the refining process of vegetable oil is the main source of phytosterols. In addition, tall oil, a by-product of the paper industry, is another important source of phytosterols (He et al., 2018). Among dietary sources, vegetable oils contain a large amount of phytosterols (Wang et al., 2018). The contents of phytosterols in different vegetable oils are shown in Table 21.1. Phytosterols naturally exist in either free or conjugate form (Figs. 21.1–21.3). The former contains a free hydroxyl group at the C-3 position, whereas in the latter, hydroxyl group is generally bonded with a sugar moiety or conjugated with an organic acid. The common conjugated sterols mainly consist of fatty acid sterol esters (esterified to fatty acids), sterol phenolates (esterified to phenolic acids, such as ferulic acid), sterol glycosides, and acylated sterol glycosides (Fig. 21.3). Phytostanols (plant stanols) are the saturated form of phytosterols. In general, phytosterols contain one or two double bonds at the C-5 position of the sterol ring and/or the C-22 position of the side chain, whereas phytostanols do not have any double bonds on the side chain (Fig. 21.1). Sitostanol

TABLE 21.1 Phytosterol content in different vegetable oils (mg/100g).

Oils	Stigmasterol	β-Sitosterol	Campesterol	Total sterols
Rice bran oil	106.0	493.3	175.9	775.2
Corn oil	32.6	266.3	191.7	490.6
Flaxseed oil	53.5	237.5	112.1	403.1
Perilla seed oil	10.5	318.6	18.7	347.8
Safflower oil	25.4	168.3	50.0	243.7
Grape seed oil	24.9	145.5	39.0	209.4
Pumpkin seed oil	1.3	182.3	2.3	185.9
Peony seed oil	ND	148.6	5.9	154.5
Torreya grandis seed oil	5.9	109.3	20.0	135.2
Walnut oil	17.5	75.1	23.1	115.7
Sea buckthorn seed oil	ND	104.7	ND	104.7
Evening primrose oil	29.2	44.0	18.2	91.4
Almond oil	2.5	34.6	9.6	46.7
Camellia oil	9.6	18.5	7.1	35.2

ND, not detected.
From Yang, R., Zhang, L., Li, P., Yu, L., Mao, J., Wang, X., & Zhang, Q. (2018). A review of chemical composition and nutritional properties of minor vegetable oils in China. Trends in Food Science and Technology, 74, 26–32.

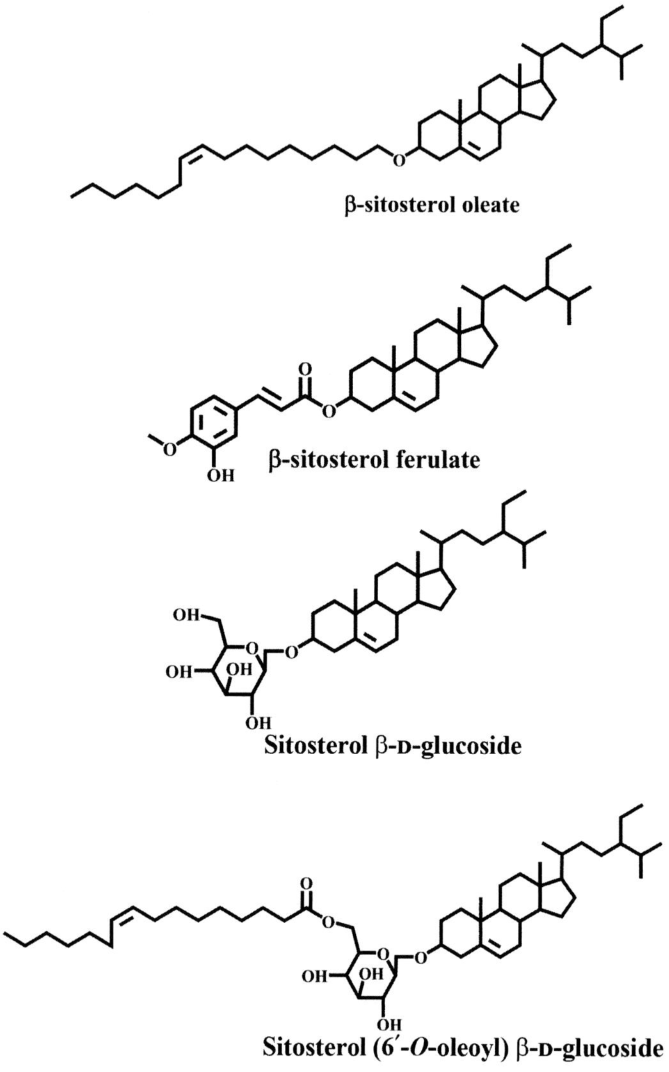

FIG. 21.3 The main conjugated forms of sterols in nature.

β-sitosterol oleate

β-sitosterol ferulate

Sitosterol β-D-glucoside

Sitosterol (6′-O-oleoyl) β-D-glucoside

and campestanol are the two most abundant phytostanols (Kaur & Myrie, 2020). The contents of phytostanols in nature are very low, accounting for about 2% of the total sterols. Phytostanols are usually prepared by hydrogenation of phytosterols.

Most of the existing studies on sterols have focused on 4-desmethyl sterols (phytosterols) with a few studies concentrating on 4-monomethyl sterols and 4,4′-dimethyl sterols. In addition, current related research mainly focuses on the efficacy, processing, and utilization of free and esterified sterols. However, limited information is available on other forms of sterols, such as sterol phenates, sterol glycosides, and acylated sterol glycosides.

21.3 Cholesterol-lowering effects

Of the various biological activities of phytosterols, the most studied is their cholesterol-reducing activity. Such benefit was first reported in the early 1950s by Peterson (1951), who fed soybean sterols to the chicks and found that soy sterols significantly reduced plasma and hepatic cholesterol (Peterson, 1951). This cholesterol-reducing activity of phytosterols was further demonstrated in rabbits and humans by Pollak (1953a, 1953b). Since then, a great number of animal and clinical trials regarding the cholesterol-reducing activity of phytosterols have been reported.

21.3.1 Animal studies

The cholesterol-lowering properties of phytosterols have been performed in different animal models, but the results showed some subtle differences. In general, the mice are the most commonly used animal models as they have the advantages of well-known genetic background, easy handling, and relatively low cost (Solati & Moghadasian, 2015). However, the mouse is not a good choice for studying cholesterol-lowering properties as the cholesterol absorption is very limited in mice (Solati & Moghadasian, 2015). In C57BL/6J wild-type mice, phytosterol consumption did not show any cholesterol-reducing trend (Rideout, Harding, & Jones, 2010). Similar results were observed in a recent study investigating the role of ergosterol in the alleviation of hyperlipidemia (He, Cui, Li, Rui, & Tong, 2020). Apolipoprotein E (Apo E) is a critical lipoprotein for the degradation of chylomicrons, and its deficiency can lead to excessive accumulation of cholesterol in the blood (Solati & Moghadasian, 2015). In this regard, phytosterols were effective in reducing plasma cholesterol in Apo $E^{-/-}$ mice, but not in their wild-type counterparts (Moghadasian et al., 2001). In Apo $E^{-/-}$ mice, the reduction in plasma cholesterol was accompanied by a marked increase in hepatic HMG-CoA reductase (HMGCR) activity and fecal sterol excretion, suggesting cholesterol-lowering activity of phytosterols in Apo $E^{-/-}$ mice was mediated by decreasing cholesterol absorption and promoting cholesterol excretion (Moghadasian et al., 2001). The lipoprotein receptor (LDL-R) is responsible for the removal of plasma cholesterol from the circulation. LDL-R knockout (LDL $R^{-/-}$) mice are very sensitive to cholesterol and are prone to atherosclerosis (Solati & Moghadasian, 2015). Supplementation of phytosterols led to a significant reduction in both plasma and arterial cholesterol in LDL $R^{-/-}$ mice (Bombo et al., 2013). Meanwhile, plasma phytosterol concentration in phytosterol-fed mice was significantly higher than that of the control group. However, no significant difference was observed in the arterial wall between the two groups (Bombo et al., 2013). Supplementation of phytosterols not only reduced plasma cholesterol but also decreased atherosclerotic lesion area (Bombo et al., 2013). Although feeding phytosterols caused an increase in the concentration of plasma phytosterols, they did not lead to accumulation of phytosterols in the arterial wall, thus preventing the development of atherosclerotic lesions (Bombo et al., 2013).

Hamsters are a good animal model for studying cholesterol metabolism as they are sensitive to dietary cholesterol and hypercholesterolemia is easily induced (Zhang et al., 2009). In addition, hamsters possess lipoprotein profiles close to humans, and they synthesize and metabolize cholesterol in a manner similar to humans (Zhang et al., 2009). Currently, numerous studies have utilized hamsters as an animal model to investigate the cholesterol-reducing potency of phytosterols and their esters. When male hamsters were fed with high cholesterol diets containing 0%, 0.1%, and 0.2% soybean germ phytosterols, respectively, for 6 wk (Zhu et al., 2019), plasma cholesterol was dependently reduced, and the underlying mechanism was likely through inhibiting cholesterol absorption and enhancing bile excretion (Zhu et al., 2019). Similarly, the regulatory effects of soybean-derived sterols (0%, 0.1%, 0.5%, vs 1%) on cholesterol metabolism and gut microbiota were investigated in hamsters (Li et al., 2019). The excellent cholesterol-lowering properties of soybean sterols were positively associated with the changes of the gut microbiota (Li et al., 2019). Furthermore, similar results were observed for wood pulp-derived sterols when using hamsters as animal models (Wang et al., 2018). Supplementation of 0.5%, 1.0%, or 5.0% beef tallow phytosterol esters in diets for 4 wk decreased cholesterol absorption, hepatic cholesterol, and plasma non-HDL-C levels in a dose-dependent manner (Guderian, Rasmussen, Wray, Dussault, & Carr, 2007). Additionally, tallow phytosterol esters showed a higher cholesterol-reducing activity than that of their respective counterparts, phytosterols and fatty acids (Guderian et al., 2007). To explore the role of hydrolysis in cholesterol-lowering effects of phytosterol esters, male Syrian hamsters were fed with diets containing 5% sterol stearate esters, 5% sterol palmitate esters, 5% sterol oleate esters, 5% sterol stearate ethers, or 3% free sterols plus 2% sunflower oil, respectively, for 4 wk (Carden, Hang, Dussault, & Carr, 2015). Of these test compounds, the hydrolysis ratio of sterol oleate esters approached above 88%, while those of sterol stearate esters, sterol palmitate esters, and sterol stearate ethers were below 5%. Correlation analyses showed that the hydrolysis percentage was negatively associated with cholesterol absorption, but it positively correlated to the cholesterol-lowering effects of phytosterol esters (Carden et al., 2015).

Similar to hamsters, rabbits are also a common animal model for studying cholesterol metabolism because they are very sensitive to cholesterol in diets and can rapidly develop severe hypercholesterolemia and atherosclerosis (Lozano, Arias-Mutis, Calvo, Chorro, & Zarzoso, 2019). Most importantly, rabbits offer a unique feature of lipoprotein similar to humans (Lozano et al., 2019). New Zealand white rabbits were used to investigate the inhibitory effect of plant stanols fatty acid esters at different doses on cholesterol absorption (Xu et al., 2001). In this study, among the four doses (0.33%, 0.66%, 1.2%, and 2.4%) of plant stanol fatty acid esters tested, plasma cholesterol concentrations were significantly reduced by 50% when the dose of stanol esters was 1.2%. But such reductions did not further increase when the dose exceeded 1.2%. Correspondingly, the cholesterol absorption was decreased from 73.0% to 43.8% after the addition of 1.2% stanol esters. Increasing the dose of stanol esters to 2.4% did not further reduce cholesterol absorption. Additionally, 1.2% stanol esters unexpectedly decreased HMG-CoA reductase activity and LDL-R-mediated binding (Xu et al., 2001). In this rabbit model, the most effective dose of stanol esters that effectively inhibited cholesterol absorption and significantly reduced plasma cholesterol concentration was 1.2% (Xu et al., 2001). Similarly, male New Zealand White rabbits were used as an animal model to examine the effects of sitostanol at the doses of 0.01%, 0.2%, and 0.8% on plasma lipid levels, coronary artery plaque formation and lecithin: cholesterol acyl transferase (LCAT) activity (Ntanios, Jones, & Frohlich, 1998). Only 0.8% sitostanol significantly reduced plasma levels of TC and very-low-density lipoprotein cholesterol (VLDL-C). Moreover, the hamsters received 0.8% sitostanol showed notably less plaque accretion in coronary arteries and ascending aorta when compared with that of the other groups (the control, 0.01% sitostanol, 0.2% sitostanol). However, dietary sitostanol at 0.8% increased the fractional esterification rate of free cholesterol, but it did not alter LCAT activity, which indicated that sitostanol reduced plasma cholesterol unlikely by changing the LCAT activity. In the heterozygous Watanabe heritable hyperlipidemic rabbits, dietary stanol esters (1.7%, 3.4%, w/w) and sterol esters (3.4%, w/w) derived from rapeseed oil significantly reduced plasma TC, LDL-C, and aortic cholesterol (Schroder et al., 2009). Concomitantly, campesterol, sitosterol, and brassicasterol were detected in the plasma, and campesterol was detected in the aorta.

Apart from these animal models described above, other animal models such as rats and chickens have also been used for investigating the cholesterol-reducing activity of phytosterols and phytostanols. Numerous studies in different experimental animals have provided a lot of information regarding safety, cholesterol-reducing efficacy, and proper dosage of phytosterols and phytostanols, which pave the way for conducting clinical research.

21.3.2 Clinical studies

The cholesterol-lowering activity of phytosterols and phytostanols has been clinically investigated. In the 1950s, phytosterols derived from tall oil were developed and marketed by Eli Lilly as a drug Cytellin™ to reduce plasma cholesterol in hypercholesterolemic individuals (Moreau et al., 2002). The cholesterol-lowering efficacy and safety of this product have been confirmed by many clinical studies. However, poor dispersibility and low bioactivity of phytosterols resulted in the unreliability of cholesterol-lowering effects of Cytellin. Such therapeutic effects could only be achieved by taking a large amount (at least 25 g/d) of this product clinically. Nevertheless, a high-dose intake of this product led to an increase in plasma phytosterol concentration, which might cause estrogenic or atherogenic effects. In this regard, this product was ultimately withdrawn from the market. In recent years, with the growing interest in functional foods, the use of phytosterols and phytostanols to reduce serum cholesterol levels has regained tremendous interest. Many factors, including daily intake dose, food matrix, type and contents of fat, occasion and frequency of intake, and chemical forms (free versus esterified sterol or stanol) can affect the cholesterol-lowering activity of phytosterols (Table 21.2).

21.3.2.1 Dose response

The effects of different doses on the cholesterol-lowering efficacy of phytosterols have been conducted to determine the optimal intake dose of phytosterols. The effects of phytosterols intakes at doses of 59, 459, and 2059 mg/d on cholesterol metabolism were evaluated (Racette et al., 2010). Three groups of participants with plasma LDL-C levels between 100 and 189 mg/dL received a diet lacking phytosterols plus different volumes of beverage containing phytosterols for 4 wk. At the moderate dose (459 mg/d) of intake, LDL-C was reduced by 5.0% ($P=.07$), and at a high dose (2059 mg/d), LDL-C reduction was 8.9% ($P<.05$). In addition, phytosterols consumption in moderate and high doses significantly increased the cholesterol excretion in feces (36% vs 74%) and bile acid (38% vs 77%) and decreased the intestinal cholesterol absorption rate (10% vs 25%). Most importantly, the cholesterol-reducing effect of phytosterols was dose-dependent (Racette et al., 2010). Such findings were also observed in several meta-analyses of randomized controlled studies (Demonty et al., 2009; Rouyanne, Johanna, & Eike, 2014). In a meta-analysis including 59 studies with 95 strata (AbuMweis, Barake, & Jones, 2008), phytosterols intakes ranged from 0.3 g/d to 9.0 g/d. Of these doses, the minimum (−0.25 mmol/L; 95% CI: −0.32, −0.18) and maximum (−0.42 mmol/L; 95% CI: −0.46, −0.39) of LDL-C-lowering effects of phytosterols were attained by consuming <1.5 g/d and >2.5 g/d phytosterols, respectively. For intakes of 1.5–2.0 g/d and 2.1–2.5 g/d, the average reductions in LDL-C were −0.29 mmol/L and 0.32 mmol/L, respectively (AbuMweis et al., 2008). A meta-analysis including 124 studies with 201 strata (Rouyanne et al., 2014)

TABLE 21.2 Characteristics and results of 12 included randomized controlled trials.

Study design	No. of subjects (M/F)	Population	Dose	Duration	Sample/matrix	Comparison	Effect	References
Placebo-controlled crossover	18	Volunteers (LDL-C: 100–189 mg/dL), 18–80 y	0.46, 2.06 g/d	4 wk	Sterols/beverage	59 mg/d	↓ LDL-C 5.0%, 8.9%	Racette et al. (2010)
Double-blind crossover	39	Mildly hypercholesterolemic subjects, 18–65 y	2.5 g/d, one versus three meals	4 wk	Stanol esters/margarines or shortenings	Placebo	↓ LDL-C 0.29 vs 0.31 mmol/L	Plat, van Onselen, van Heugten, and Mensink (2000)
Double-blind parallel	184 (81/103)	Moderate hypercholesterolemic subjects, 57 ± 2 y	3 g/d	4 wk	Sterol esters/yogurt with or without a meal	Placebo drink	↓ LDL-C 9.3–9.5% (meal) vs 5.1–6.9% (without meal)	Doornbos, Meynen, Duchateau, van der Knaap, and Trautwein (2006)
Double-blind parallel	119	Mildly to moderately hypercholesterolemic volunteers, 25–60 y	2 g/d	4 wk	Stanols/biscuit	Control biscuits	↓ TC 4.9%, ↓ LDL-C 6.1%	Kriengsinyos, Wangtong, and Komindr (2015)
Double-blind crossover	25	Healthy volunteers, 39.2 ± 2.9 y	0.15, 0.3 g/meal	—	Sterols/corn oil	Sterol-free corn oil	↓ cholesterol absorption 12.1%, 27.9%	Ostlund, Racette, Okeke, and Stenson (2002)
Double-blind crossover	63 (25/38)	Healthy subjects, 42 ± 11 y	1.82 g/d	3 wk	Sterols/margarine	Control margarine	↓ TC 3.4%, ↓ LDL-C 5.4%, ↑ HDL-C 3.4%	Mussner et al. (2002)
Double-blind crossover	53 (22/31)	Hypercholesterolemic patients, 58 ± 12 y	1.6 g/d	2 months	Sterols/spread	Control spread	↓ TC 5.5%, ↓ LDL-C 7.7%	Nigon et al. (2001)
Double-blind crossover	53 (22/31)	Hypercholesterolemic patients, 58 ± 12 y	1.6 g/d	2 months	Sterols/spread with fibrate	Control spread	↓ TC 8.5%, ↓ LDL-C 11.1%	Nigon et al. (2001)
Double-blind controlled trial	159 (85/74)	Normocholesterolemic participants, 19–79 y	2 g/d	3 wk	Sterols/soya drink	Placebo soya drink	↓ LDL-C 5.9%	Chau et al. (2020)
Double-blind trial	99 (72/27)	Mild hypercholesterolemia, 25–60 y	2 g/d	4 wk	Sterols/functional black tea	Placebo	↓ TC 5.6%, ↓ LDL 8.7%	Orem et al. (2017)

Design	N	Subjects	Dose	Duration	Intervention	Control	Results	Reference
Double-blind parallel	32 (16/16)	Hypercholesterolemic adults	3 g/d	4 wk	Sterol esters/capsule	Placebo capsule	↓ LDL 11%, ↓ LDL/HDL 10%	Carr, Stanek Krogstrand, Schlegel, and Fernandez (2009)
Single-blind crossover	22	Hypercholesterolemic subjects	2.4 g/d	4 wk	Sterol esters, stanols/bread, breakfast cereal	Placebo foods	↓ LDL-C 13.6%, 8.3%	Nestel, Cehun, Pomeroy, Abbey, and Weldon (2001)
Single-blind crossover	15	Hypercholesterolemic subjects	2.4 g/d	4 wk	Sterol esters/dairy spread	Spread	↓ LDL-C 12.2%	Nestel et al. (2001)
Randomized crossover trial	47	Mild-to-moderately hypercholesterolemic individuals	2 g/d	4 wk	Free sterols vs sterol esters/yogurt	Placebo	↓ TC 7.7%, 6.3%, ↓ LDL-C 11.7%, 11.6%	Shaghaghi, Harding, and Jones (2014)

Characteristics and results of 12 included randomized controlled trials.

demonstrated that daily intake of 0.6–3.3 g phytosterols could lower LDL cholesterol concentration by 6–12% and the average phytosterols dose of 2.1 g/d resulted in a significant LDL-C reduction of 8.1% (Rouyanne et al., 2014). These observations are consistent with the current recommended intake dose of phytosterols by National Cholesterol Education Program Adult Treatment Panel III.

21.3.2.2 Lipid characteristics and age of subjects

The cholesterol-lowering efficacy of phytosterols was positively associated with the baseline characteristics of subjects' blood lipids. The absolute LDL-C reduction of phytosterols in subjects with a high baseline level was higher than that of subjects with normal or borderline levels (−0.37 vs −0.28 mmol/L) (AbuMweis et al., 2008). Likewise, phytosterols exhibited a marked difference in LDL-C reductions for subjects with high and normal plasma TC levels (−0.45 vs −0.37 mmol/L) (Wu, Fu, Yang, Zhang, & Han, 2009). A meta-analysis carried out reported greater absolute LDL-C reductions of phytosterols in subjects with higher baseline LDL-C levels (Demonty et al., 2009). Nevertheless, phytosterols do elicit LDL-C reductions in subjects with hyperlipidemia and normal blood lipids.

Furthermore, the absolute reduction in LDL-C caused by phytosterols and phytostanols increased with the age of subjects (Katan et al., 2003). For example, the absolute LDL-C reductions produced by phytosterols and phytostanols were 8, 11, 12, 15, and 16 mg/dL in subjects with the age-groups of 4–6, 20–29, 30–39, 40–49, and 50–60 years, respectively (Katan et al., 2003). However, no significant difference was observed in relative LDL-C reduction among all age-groups because the baseline value of LDL-C level increases with age. Hence, the relative efficacy of phytosterols as a percentage of reduction in lowering LDL-C is not affected by age, suggesting that all subjects at different ages would benefit from supplementation of phytosterols.

21.3.2.3 Intake frequency and occasion

The effects of different intake frequencies on the cholesterol-lowering efficacy of phytostanol esters were directly compared (Plat et al., 2000). There was no significant difference in LDL-C reductions when phytostanol esters were consumed one meal a day and three meals a day (Plat et al., 2000). It was therefore concluded that intake frequency seems not to affect the cholesterol-lowering efficacy of phytostanols. However, consuming phytosterols ≥2 times a day (1.81 g/d) caused a greater LDL-C reduction when compared with taking once a day (1.76 g/d) (Demonty et al., 2009). Likewise, the reduction in LDL-C levels caused by two to three times daily intake of phytosterols was higher (0.34 vs 0.14 mmol/L) than that of one intake at breakfast (AbuMweis et al., 2008). Such results supported that intake frequency was one of the factors affecting the cholesterol-lowering efficacy of phytosterols.

Additionally, the effects of intake occasion (breakfast versus lunch or dinner) on the cholesterol-lowering efficacy of phytosterols were also assessed (AbuMweis et al., 2008). Interestingly, once-a-day intake in the morning resulted in an absolute reduction in LDL-C level by 0.14 mmol/L, while that in the afternoon or with a main meal significantly reduced LDL-C by 0.30 mmol/L. The exact reason for the difference in cholesterol-lowering effects caused by the intake of phytosterols at different intake occasions is not clear. One explanation is related to a circadian rhythm of cholesterol absorption, but there is currently no evidence that cholesterol absorption is lower in the morning (Trautwein, Vermeer, Hiemstra, & Ras, 2018). Another explanation is associated with the stimulation of bile flow caused by food intake, because food intake is an important cause of bile flow to form micelles. The food provided for breakfast is relatively limited, so the interference of phytosterols in cholesterol absorption is not sufficient (Trautwein et al., 2018). Several studies have pointed out the importance of phytosterols intake in a main meal (Doornbos et al., 2006; Kriengsinyos et al., 2015). Phytosterol-enriched yogurt with a meal caused a significantly greater reduction in TC and LDL-C when it was compared to taking this yogurt before breakfast (Doornbos et al., 2006). And the decrease in LDL-C (8.9%) and LDL/HDL ratio (11.4%) of taking phytostanol biscuits with a meal was much higher than that of not eating other foods (Kriengsinyos et al., 2015). These findings emphasized the importance of intake occasions when consuming phytosterols.

21.3.2.4 Food matrix type

Phytosterols and their esters have been incorporated into various types of foods, such as fat spreads and dairy products. To date, a large number of clinical studies have investigated the cholesterol-lowering effects of phytosterols in different food systems. The most suitable matrix for phytosterols is considered to be fat-rich foods because fat can enhance the solubility of phytosterols. In health subjects, sterol-free corn oil exhibited a $38.0 \pm 10.2\%$ higher cholesterol absorption than normal corn oil containing 0.77% phytosterols (Ostlund et al., 2002). When corn oil phytosterols were added back to sterol-free corn oil at a concentration of 150 or 300 mg/test meal, the absorption of cholesterol was reduced by $12.1 \pm 3.7\%$ and $27.9 \pm 9.1\%$, respectively (Ostlund et al., 2002). A randomized, double-blind, cross-over study investigating the effects of phytosterol ester-enriched margarine on the lipid status in mild-to-moderate hypercholesterolemia demonstrated that phytosterol esters at a dose of 1.82 g/d produced a significant improvement in lipoprotein profile of plasma TC (-3.4%, $P < .005$), LDL-C (-5.4%, $P < .001$), HDL-C ($+13.4\%$, $P < .05$), apolipoprotein B (-4.0%, $P < .005$), and LDL-C/HDL-C ratio (-7.8%, $P < .001$) (Mussner et al., 2002). Consumption of low-dose phytosterol esters can improve the lipid status in mild-to-moderate hypercholesterolemia. It is especially beneficial for subjects with high dietary cholesterol, energy, total fat, and saturated fatty acid intake and subjects with high intestinal cholesterol absorption. Therefore, daily intake of margarine rich in phytosterol esters can reduce the risk of atherosclerosis in subjects with mild-to-moderate hypercholesterolemia. Another similar study also demonstrated that plant sterol-enriched margarine was a useful adjunctive treatment for patients with hypercholesterolemia (Nigon et al., 2001). Apart from fat-based foods, low-fat- or nonfat-based foods are also good carriers for phytosterols and their cholesterol-lowering effects have been confirmed (Chau et al., 2020; Orem et al., 2017). In a randomized and double-blind trial, consumption of phytosterol-enriched soya drink with phytosterols at a dose of 2 g/d elicited a significant LDL-C reduction by 5.96% (95% CI, -8.91%, -3.00%) (Chau et al., 2020). In subjects with mild hypercholesterolemia, daily intake of functional black tea with 2 g phytosterols for 4 wk significantly reduced plasma concentrations of TC and LDL-C by 5.6% and 8.7%, respectively. Likewise, phytosterol-enriched orange juice, vegetable juice, yogurt, beverage, milk, and milk tea could effectively reduce plasma cholesterol levels (AbuMweis et al., 2008; Demonty et al., 2009).

Several meta-analyses of randomized controlled trials (RCTs) have evaluated the cholesterol-lowering efficacy of phytosterols added into different food matrixes. In an early meta-analysis of 59 studies including >4500 participants, the effects of different food matrixes on the cholesterol-reducing efficacy of phytosterols were investigated (AbuMweis et al., 2008). These food formats consisted of margarine, yogurt, salad dressing, chocolate bars, orange juice, dairy spread, beverage, soft cheese, meat, croissants, muffins, mayonnaise, vegetable oil, and milk. The overall pooled estimation found that phytosterol-fortified foods led to a decrease in LDL-C by an average of

0.31 mmol/L (95% CI, −0.35 to −0.27, $P < .0001$). In contrast, phytosterols exhibited a stronger cholesterol-lowering effect when fortified with fat spreads, mayonnaise, salad dressings, milk, and yogurt than other foods (such as croissants and muffins, orange juice, nonfat beverages, cereal bars, and chocolate). Such findings highlight the importance of food matrixes and appropriate formulations in the application of phytosterols.

However, in other meta-analysis studies, there was no significant difference in the cholesterol-lowering efficacy of phytosterols when they were incorporated in different food matrices. The effects of phytosterols/stanols on plasma cholesterol concentrations were systematically assessed through meta-analysis, and no significant difference was observed between fat-based and nonfat-based food formats or between diary and nondairy foods (Demonty et al., 2009). Furthermore, the effects of three predominant fats from soybean/sunflower (SS), rapeseed/canola (RC) oils, and animal fats on hypocholesterolemic activities of phytosterol-fortified foods were studied in a recent meta-analysis of 32 studies including 2157 subjects (Ferguson, Stojanovski, MacDonald-Wicks, & Garg, 2016). Phytosterol-enriched food formats mainly involved margarine, yogurt, butter, milk, and cheese, and their daily intake ranged from 1.5 to 4 g. All fat types exhibited excellent cholesterol-lowering efficacy. Specifically, the overall pooled TC and LDL-C were significantly reduced by 6.4% (95% CI: −7.3, −5.5; $P < .001$) and 9.3% (95% CI: −10.4, −8.2; $P < .001$), respectively. In terms of LDL-C reduction, RC fat type was more effective than SS fat type (Ferguson et al., 2016). An explanation may be ascribed to the differences in fatty acid profiles since RC spreads provided higher amounts of MUFA and n-3 PUFA, which might facilitate the incorporation of phytosterols into the micelle and thereby enhance the affinity of phytosterols for solubilization into the micelle.

21.3.2.5 *Phytosterols versus phytostanols*

Phytostanols and phytosterols have similar chemical structures, and the difference only exists in the absence or presence of double bonds. It is worth mentioning that phytosterols exhibit a higher bioavailability than phytostanols, indicating a potential difference in displacement of cholesterol in the intestinal micelles. This raises the question of whether there is a difference in the efficacy of the two forms. In an early meta-analysis of 41 studies (Katan et al., 2003), the average LDL-C reduction of phytostanols (−10.1%, 2.5 g/d) was not significantly distinct from that of phytosterols (−9.7%, 2.3 g/d). A meta-analysis of 14 randomized controlled trials evaluated the effects of phytosterols and phytostanols at doses of 0.6–2.5 g/d on healthy and hypercholesterolemia patients and demonstrated that the cholesterol-reducing efficacy of both was not statistically different (Talati, Sobieraj, Makanji, Phung, & Coleman, 2010). Based on these reports, both phytostanols and phytosterols are equally effective in reducing plasma cholesterol.

Nevertheless, a meta-analysis including 113 published trials and one unpublished trial reported a statistical difference in LDL-C reduction between phytostanols and phytosterols (Musa-Veloso, Poon, Elliot, & Chung, 2011). The maximum relative LDL-C reduction was 16.4% for phytostanols, which was significantly greater than 8.3% for phytosterols (Musa-Veloso et al., 2011). The reason for the significant difference in cholesterol-lowering efficacy between the two still remains inconclusive. Despite having similar chemical structures, they differ in absorption and metabolism. For example, the absorption rate of phytosterols in the body is 0.4–3.5%, while that of phytostanols is even lower (0.02–0.3%) (Calpe-Berdiel, Escolà-Gil, & Blanco-Vaca, 2009). In addition, phytostanols can reduce plasma phytosterol concentration, but its mechanism of action is still unclear (Musa-Veloso et al., 2011).

21.3.2.6 Free versus esterified phytosterols

Esterification of phytosterols with fatty acids can improve their lipid solubility, thereby promoting their entry into micelles. The cholesterol-lowering efficacy of esterified phytosterols has been consistently confirmed in animal and clinical studies (Carr et al., 2009; Guderian et al., 2007). However, to date, clinical studies that directly compare the effects of free and esterified phytosterols on reducing plasma cholesterol are still limited. A study investigating the efficacy of phytosterol esters versus free phytostanols in reducing cholesterol in hypercholesterolemic subjects demonstrated that the LDL-C reductions for phytosterol esters and phytostanols were 13.6% and 8.3%, respectively (Nestel et al., 2001). Although the reduction of LDL cholesterol in phytosterol esters was greater than that in phytostanols, the difference was not statistically significant. In another head-to-head study, water dispersible phytosterols (free form) and phytosterol esters elicited similar reductions in serum TC (7.7% versus 6.3%) and LDL-C (11.7% vs 11.6%) levels when incorporated into yogurt (Shaghaghi et al., 2014). An RCT meta-analysis in adults further supported these findings (Demonty et al., 2009). Overall, the current evidences suggest that free and esterified phytosterols have equivalent cholesterol-lowering effects.

21.4 Cholesterol-lowering mechanisms

The cholesterol-lowering effect of phytosterols has long been demonstrated in vivo and in vitro. However, their underlying mechanism of action has not been fully elucidated so far. Several mechanisms for the cholesterol-lowering efficacy of phytosterols have been recommended. Of them, inhibition on intestinal cholesterol absorption is the first proposed mechanism for phytosterols to lower plasma cholesterol. Cholesterol absorption is an extremely complicated process controlled by cholesterol dissolution of intestine lumen, cholesterol uptake of enterocytes, and assembling and transportation of chylomicrons (Fig. 21.4). Cholesterol absorbed in the intestine includes exogenous and endogenous sources, the former coming from diets and the latter being from bile secretion. As well-known, cholesterol can be only absorbed by intestinal enterocytes after being incorporated into dietary mixed micelles owing to its water insolubility. As the structural analogs of cholesterol, phytosterols competed with dietary cholesterol for incorporating into dietary mixed micelles. Phytosterols have higher hydrophobicity than cholesterol and therefore exhibit a higher affinity for mixed micelles and preferentially enter the mixed micelles (Ikeda, Tanabe, & Sugano, 1989). The capability of mixed micelles to accommodate sterols is limited, thereby resulting in the reduction of cholesterol solubilization in the presence of phytosterols (Brown, Hang, Dussault, & Carr, 2010). In vitro trials demonstrated that phytosterols caused a decrease in cholesterol concentrations in bile salts micelles (Brown et al., 2010; Matsuoka, Kajimoto, Horiuchi, Honda, & Endo, 2010). In rats that added 0.5% cholesterol plus 0.5% sitosterol to their diet, the cholesterol concentrations in the micellar phase were reduced by 24% compared to rats that added 0.5% cholesterol to the diet (Ikeda et al., 1989). In healthy human subjects, injecting phytostanol esters into the duodenum reduced the solubility of cholesterol in micelles and ultimately inhibited intestinal cholesterol absorption (Nissinen, Gylling, Vuoristo, & Miettinen, 2002). These findings indicate that the inhibitory effect of phytosterols on cholesterol absorption is largely achieved by interfering with micellar cholesterol incorporation. Another potential mechanism explaining the inhibition of intestinal cholesterol absorption is the co-crystallization of phytosterols and cholesterol (Cedó et al., 2019). Both phytosterols and cholesterol are sparingly soluble in oil and fats. When coexisted, phytosterols

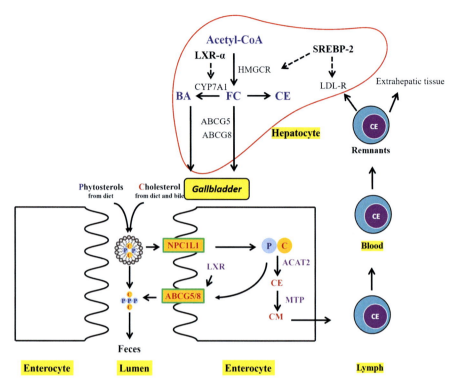

FIG. 21.4 The process of intestinal cholesterol absorption and hepatic cholesterol metabolism and possible sites of action of cholesterol-lowering activity of phytosterols. *C*, cholesterol; *P*, phytosterols; *BA*, bile acids; *FC*, free cholesterol; *CE*, cholesterol ester; *NPC1L1*, Niemann-Pick C1-like 1; *ACAT2*, acyltransferase-2; *LXR*, liver X receptor; *ABCG5/8*, adenosine triphosphate binding cassette G5/8; *CM*, chylomicrons; *MTP*, microsomal triglyceride transport protein; *LXR-α*, liver X receptor alpha; *LDL-R*, low-density lipoprotein receptor; *HMGCR*, HMG-CoA reductase; *SREBP-2*, sterol regulatory element binding protein-2; *CYP7A1*, cholesterol 7α-hydroxylase.

and cholesterol easily formed insoluble mixed crystals in the intestinal lumen with being directly excreted with feces. Therefore, the absorption of cholesterol was greatly reduced in the intestinal enterocytes.

Cholesterol absorbed in the intestine includes exogenous and endogenous sources, the former coming from diets and the latter being from bile secretion. As well-known, cholesterol can be only absorbed by intestinal enterocytes after being incorporated into dietary mixed micelles owing to its water insolubility. As the structural analogs of cholesterol, phytosterols competed with dietary cholesterol for incorporating into dietary mixed micelles. Phytosterols have higher hydrophobicity than cholesterol and therefore exhibit a higher affinity for mixed micelles and preferentially enter the mixed micelles (Ikeda et al., 1989). The capability of mixed micelles to accommodate sterols is limited, thereby resulting in the reduction of cholesterol solubilization in the presence of phytosterols (Brown et al., 2010). In vitro trials demonstrated that phytosterols caused a decrease in cholesterol concentrations in bile salts micelles (Brown et al., 2010; Matsuoka et al., 2010). In rats that added 0.5% cholesterol plus 0.5% sitosterol to their diet, the cholesterol concentrations in the micellar phase were reduced by 24% compared to rats that added

0.5% cholesterol to the diet (Ikeda et al., 1989). In healthy human subjects, injecting phytostanol esters into the duodenum reduced the solubility of cholesterol in micelles and ultimately inhibited intestinal cholesterol absorption (Nissinen et al., 2002). These findings indicate that the inhibitory effect of phytosterols on cholesterol absorption is largely achieved by interfering with micellar cholesterol incorporation. Another potential mechanism explaining the inhibition of intestinal cholesterol absorption is the co-crystallization of phytosterols and cholesterol (Cedó et al., 2019). Both phytosterols and cholesterol are sparingly soluble in oil and fats. When coexisted, phytosterols and cholesterol easily formed insoluble mixed crystals in the intestinal lumen with being directly excreted with feces. Therefore, the absorption of cholesterol was greatly reduced in the intestinal enterocytes.

Cholesterol absorption from the intestinal lumen to the lymph is a multistep process including at least three steps as follows (Fig. 21.4). Firstly, cholesterol that liberated from the micelles crossed the brush border membrane of the epithelium with NPC1L1 as an influx transporter. The unesterified phytosterols were returned into intestinal lumen with ABCG5/8 as an efflux transporter (Smet, Mensink, & Plat, 2012; Trautwein et al., 2003). Secondly, cholesterol that enters the enterocytes is re-esterified in mucosal cells in the presence of ACAT-2 (Smet et al., 2012; Trautwein et al., 2003). Thirdly, cholesterol esters, triacylglycerols, and Apo B-48 were assembled into chylomicrons by MTP for entering lymphatic system. Each process may be affected by phytosterols (Smet et al., 2012; Trautwein et al., 2003).

Current studies have demonstrated that phytosterols are poorly absorbed in the enterocytes, because their intestinal absorption requires NPC1L1 as a transporter (Jia, Betters, & Yu, 2011). NPC1L1 is mainly responsible for the transfer of cholesterol molecule to the surface of the brush border membrane of the small intestine mucosa of enterocytes through endocytosis (Fig. 21.4) (Smet et al., 2012; Trautwein et al., 2003). It has been suggested that cholesterol-lowering activity of phytosterols is also possibly mediated by downregulating the intestinal NPC1L1 expression and subsequently decreasing the entry of cholesterol into enterocytes (Jesch, Seo, Carr, & Lee, 2009). In FHs 74 Int cells, sitosterol caused a nearly 50% decrease in mRNA expression of NPC1L1 and a significant decrease in NPC1L1 protein expression (Jesch et al., 2009). Similarly, stigmasterol or sitosterol significantly reduced the expression of NPC1L1 in HepG2 cells, indicating that phytosterols may also inhibit the absorption of cholesterol in hepatic cells (Park & Carr, 2013). However, such findings cannot be confirmed in hamsters and mice (Calpe-Berdiel et al., 2005; Jain et al., 2008; Plösch et al., 2006).

ABCG5/8 is the target gene of LXR, and its expression is regulated by LXR (Fig. 21.4) (Smet et al., 2012; Trautwein et al., 2003). Some studies have shown that some sterols such as sitosterol, stigmasterol, or their derivatives acting as LXR ligands can activate the expression of ABCG5/8 (Kaneko et al., 2003; Yang et al., 2004). However, phytosterol intake also did not cause transcriptional changes in intestinal ABCG5 and ABCG8 (Calpe-Berdiel et al., 2005; Jain et al., 2008; Plösch et al., 2006). It is worth mentioning that phytosterols caused similar reductions of intestinal cholesterol absorption in both wild-type and ABCG5- and ABCG5/8-deficient mice (Calpe-Berdiel, Escolà-Gil, & Blanco-Vaca, 2007; Plösch et al., 2006). Similarly, in wild-type and LXRαβ-deficient mice, consumption of phytosterols significantly reduced the absorption of intestinal cholesterol and no significant difference was observed between the two (Cedó et al., 2017). Therefore, it is inconclusive that the cholesterol absorption-inhibiting effect is mediated by altering the expression of enterocyte sterol transporters such as ABCG5, ABCG8, and NPC1L1.

After entering the enterocytes, cholesterol is re-esterified into cholesterol esters (Smet et al., 2012; Trautwein et al., 2003). In this step, ACAT-2 is a key rate-limiting enzyme, which directly affects the absorption of cholesterol in the intestine. Since phytosterols are poor substrates of ACAT-2, they can occupy available active sites (Temel, Gebre, Parks, & Rudel, 2003). It has been suggested that phytosterols may reduce the esterification of cholesterol in the enterocytes by reducing ACAT-2 expression or affecting ACAT activity and ultimately reduce cholesterol absorption. In the rabbits fed on a high-cholesterol diet, sitosterol caused a significant reduction in ACAT-2 activity in the jejunum and ileum (Field & Mathur, 1983). In addition, the transcription expressions of ACAT-2 in the intestine were also observed in the hamsters supplemented with 0.1% sitosterol and stigmasterol (Liang et al., 2011). Such findings were further demonstrated in Caco-2 cells, in which different phytosterols showed the inhibition effects on ACAT-2 expression (Yuan, Zhang, Jia, Xie, & Shen, 2020). These results suggest that the cholesterol-lowering activity of phytosterols is likely associated with the alterations of ACAT-2 gene expression.

In addition, MTP is a lipid transfer protein necessary for the synthesis and secretion of chylomicrons in small intestinal cells (Smet et al., 2012; Trautwein et al., 2003). MTP can promote the transport of triacylglycerols, cholesterol esters, and phospholipids on both sides of the membrane and plays an important role in lipid metabolism. Dietary intake of 0.1% sitosterol and 0.1% stigmasterol could significantly reduce the level of MTP mRNA in the small intestine of golden hamsters (Liang et al., 2011). These changes should be further confirmed in related gene (ACAT-2, MTP) knockout animal models. Therefore, the inhibition of intestinal cholesterol absorption caused by phytosterols may be achieved by interfering with the synthesis of chylomicrons.

In addition to inhibiting the absorption of intestinal cholesterol, phytosterols may also regulate the synthesis of cholesterol in the body (Fig. 21.4). Cholesterol synthesis mainly occurs in the liver, and HMG-CoA reductase is the rate-limiting enzyme in this process. To date, reports on the effect of phytosterols on HMG-CoA reductase activity are still inconsistent. Some studies demonstrated the inhibition effect of phytosterols on HMG-CoA reductase activity (Batta, Xu, Honda, Miyazaki, & Salen, 2006). Stigmasterol significantly reduced the HMG-CoA reductase activity by 44% and 77% in Wistar and the WKY rats, respectively (Batta et al., 2006). Similar reduction in HMG-CoA reductase activity was observed in the albino rats fed ergosterol (Moselhy, Kamal, Kumosani, & Huwait, 2016). However, our recent studies observed significant feedback increase in the mRNA expressions of hepatic HMG-CoA reductase in the rats or mice fed ergosterol or its linolenate (He et al., 2019, 2020). In line with our studies, similar alterations were also reported in the mice supplemented with stigmasterol and β-sitosterol (Feng et al., 2018).

Reverse cholesterol transport (RCT) pathway is the most important way to remove cholesterol. In this regard, phytosterols likely alter the expressions of cholesterol excretion-related transport proteins and rate-limiting enzymes of bile acid synthesis pathway, thereby promoting cholesterol excretion. In peripheral cells, ABCA1 mediates the outflow of cholesterol in the form of HDL-C and is taken up by SR-BI into the liver. Cholesterol transported to the liver is mainly excreted in two ways as follows. One is that cholesterol is converted into bile acid under the action of CYP7A1 or CYP27A1 and then stored in the gallbladder (Fig. 21.4). The other is that cholesterol is directly secreted out of liver cells under the action of ABCG5/8 and then excreted into the intestinal lumen under the transport of bile. In SHRSP and WKY rats, phytosterols feeding significantly increased the mRNA expressions of hepatic ABCA1, ABCG5, and CYP27A1 (Chen, Gruber, Pakenham, Ratnayake, & Scoggan, 2009). Algal sterols at a dose of 0.30 g/kg caused a significant decrease of plasma cholesterol concentration in Syrian golden hamsters fed a high cholesterol diet, accompanied by a significant increase in hepatic LDL-R expression level (Chen, Jiao, Jiang, Bi, & Chen, 2014). Consistently, phytostanol esters caused a significant increase of LDL-R at the transcriptional levels in human mononuclear blood cells by 43% (Plat & Mensink, 2002).

The hepatobiliary pathway of cholesterol elimination through fecal excretion predominates in maintaining cholesterol homeostasis. However, disrupting bile cholesterol secretion does not influence fecal neutral sterol excretion (Kruit et al., 2005). This indicates the existence of a nonbiliary route to eliminate cholesterol. Transintestinal cholesterol excretion (TICE) refers to the process of cholesterol transfer from circulating plasma through the enterocytes directly to the intestinal lumen (Van Der Velde, Brufau, & Groen, 2010). It has recently been proposed as a potential target to investigate the mechanism of cholesterol-lowering activity of phytosterols. Brufau et al. demonstrated that phytosterols stimulate cholesterol excretion through such a nonbiliary pathway (Brufau, Kuipers, Lin, Trautwein, & Groen, 2011). It was found that the ABCG5/8 heterodimer played a vital role in this process. Feeding phytosterols caused an expected significant increase in fecal neutral sterol excretion in wild-type mice, but such increase was greatly reduced in ABCG5 knockout mice (Brufau et al., 2011). In addition, cholesterol excretion caused by phytosterols through the TICE pathway increased six times in wild-type mice, while it only increased 3.5 times in ABCG5 knockout mice (Brufau et al., 2011). Nakano et al. further found that phytosterols entered the brush border membrane and quickly returned into the lumen and cholesterol transporters in the brush border membrane participated in this process (Nakano et al., 2018). However, the molecular target of phytosterols on the brush border membrane is still unclear. It was speculated that the efflux of cholesterol would increase as phytosterols enter the brush border membrane (Nakano et al., 2018).

21.5 Commercial applications and regulated policy

A large number of animal experiments and clinical studies have confirmed the safety and cholesterol-lowering effects of phytosterols, phytostanols, and their related esters. Based on these evidences, most countries such as the United States, China, the European Union, Canada, and Japan have approved the use of phytosterols, phytostanols, and their esters in foods (National Health Commission of the People's Republic of China, n.d.; Moreau et al., 2018; Zawistowski & Jones, 2015). Some countries also allow people to declare cholesterol-lowering activity as a healthy claim on food labels when phytosterols are added (Moreau et al., 2018; Zawistowski & Jones, 2015).

Benecol margarine produced by Raisio Company in Finland in 1995 was the first food to add phytostanol esters (Zawistowski & Jones, 2015). In July 2000, the European Commission (EC) approved sterol esters as a novel food ingredient and allowed them to be added to yellow fat spreads (Zawistowski & Jones, 2015). In 2004, EC further expanded the application of phytosterols, phytostanols, and their esters in foods. These foods include milk beverages, milk products containing fruits and/or cereals, semi-skimmed and skimmed milk, yogurt products, fermented milk beverages, soy beverages, fat spreads, salad dressings, hot sauce and cheese products, black wheat bread, edible oil, mayonnaise, and rice beverages (Zawistowski & Jones, 2015). In 2009, EC approved a health statement stating that the intake of phytosterols, phytostanol, and their esters was positively correlated with the reduction of plasma cholesterol and negatively associated with the risk of coronary heart disease (CHD) (Zawistowski & Jones, 2015). The foods containing phytosterols, phytostanols, and their esters are allowed to make such claims regarding their cholesterol-lowering effects. However, they must provide at least 2 g of phytosterols or stanols per day.

In 1998, the US Food and Drug Administration (FDA) updated the "Generally Recognized as Safe" (GRAS) confirmation procedure (Moreau et al., 2018). Based on the new rule, two phytosterol-rich vegetable fat spreads, namely Benecol and Take Control produced by Raisio and Unilever, respectively, were allowed to enter the US market. Moreover, phytosterols were allowed to apply in various food categories such as dairy products, bakery and cereal products, oils, salad dressings, and juices (Zawistowski & Jones, 2015). In 2000, the FDA issued an interim final rule (IFR), which approved a health claim that foods containing phytosterols or their esters reduce the risk of CHD (Moreau et al., 2018). In 2010, FDA further issued a proposed rule to amend the IFR (Zawistowski & Jones, 2015). Based on the new rule, a daily intake of 2 g phytosterols was considered necessary to reduce the risk of CHD.

In 2008, the Ministry of Health of China approved the use of phytostanol esters (National Health Commission of the People's Republic of China, n.d.). As a novel food ingredient, they were allowed to be used in vegetable oils, vegetable butters, margarines, dairy products, vegetable protein drinks, condiments, salad dressings, mayonnaise, fruit juices, macaroni, noodles, and instant cereals. It also stipulated that the maximum intake of phytostanol esters should not exceed 5 g/d. Foods with added phytostanol esters are not suitable for pregnant women and children under 5 years old. In March 2010, the Ministry of Health issued an announcement stating that phytosterols and their esters were allowed to be used in food as novel food ingredients (National Health Commission of the People's Republic of China, n.d.). This announcement did not clearly limit the scope of food allowed, but it stipulated that phytosterols and their esters could not be added to the foods for infants and babies. The maximum intake of phytosterols and their esters for subjects should not exceed 2.4 g/d and 3.9 g/d, respectively. In this regard, phytosterols are generally made using the fractions from soybean oil or tall oil as raw materials through saponification, extraction, crystallization, and other processes. Phytosterol esters are mainly prepared by esterification of phytosterols and sunflower oil fatty acids.

In addition to the above-mentioned countries or organizations, most other countries/regions have also approved the use of phytosterols or their esters in foods and have issued corresponding regulatory regulations (Zawistowski & Jones, 2015). However, the application of phytosterols or their esters in different countries or regions varies greatly. For example, there are many types of foods supplemented with phytosterols in the European market, but there are relatively few such foods available in the Asia-Pacific market.

21.6 Conclusive remarks and future perspectives

To date, the potential molecular mechanisms of phytosterols and their esters for lowering plasma cholesterol have begun to be confirmed or elucidated. Current evidences highlight the importance of phytosterols or their esters in reducing blood cholesterol concentration. Supplementation of phytosterols or their esters in diets has been considered an important strategy to prevent the event of CHD. Therefore, the application of phytosterols or their esters in various foods should be widely popularized worldwide. It should point out that the current studies mainly concentrate on 4-desmethyl sterols and their fatty acid esters. The efficacy of other sterols such as 4-monomethyl sterols or 4,4'-dimethyl sterols or other sterol derivatives such as sterol phenolates and their related application should be the subject of future studies.

References

National Health Commission of the People's Republic of China (n.d.). http://www.nhc.gov.cn/sps/zcwj2/zcwj.shtml.

World Health Organization. (2017). Cardiovascular Diseases (CVDs). https://www.who.int/news-room/factsheets/detail/cardiovascular-diseases-(cvds) 2017.

AbuMweis, S. S., Barake, R., & Jones, P. J. H. (2008). Plant sterols/stanols as cholesterol lowering agents: A meta-analysis of randomized controlled trials. *Food & Nutrition Research, 52*. https://doi.org/10.3402/fnr.v52i0.1811.

Shaghaghi, M. A., Harding, S. V., & Jones, P. J. H. (2014). Water dispersible plant sterol formulation shows improved effect on lipid profile compared to plant sterol esters. *Journal of Functional Foods, 6*(1), 280–289. https://doi.org/10.1016/j.jff.2013.10.017.

Batta, A. K., Xu, G., Honda, A., Miyazaki, T., & Salen, G. (2006). Stigmasterol reduces plasma cholesterol levels and inhibits hepatic synthesis and intestinal absorption in the rat. *Metabolism, Clinical and Experimental, 55*(3), 292–299. https://doi.org/10.1016/j.metabol.2005.08.024.

Bombo, R. P. A., Afonso, M. S., Machado, R. M., Lavrador, M. S. F., Nunes, V. S., Quintão, E. R., et al. (2013). Dietary phytosterol does not accumulate in the arterial wall and prevents atherosclerosis of LDLr-KO mice. *Atherosclerosis, 231*(2), 442–447. https://doi.org/10.1016/j.atherosclerosis.2013.10.015.

Brown, A. W., Hang, J., Dussault, P. H., & Carr, T. P. (2010). Phytosterol ester constituents affect micellar cholesterol solubility in model bile. *Lipids, 45*(9), 855–862. https://doi.org/10.1007/s11745-010-3456-6.

Brufau, G., Kuipers, F., Lin, Y., Trautwein, E. A., & Groen, A. K. (2011). A reappraisal of the mechanism by which plant sterols promote neutral sterol loss in mice. *PLoS One, 6*(6). https://doi.org/10.1371/journal.pone.0021576, e21576.

Calpe-Berdiel, L., Escolà-Gil, J. C., & Blanco-Vaca, F. (2007). Are LXR-regulated genes a major molecular target of plant sterols/stanols? *Atherosclerosis, 195*(1), 210–211. https://doi.org/10.1016/j.atherosclerosis.2006.11.042.

Calpe-Berdiel, L., Escolà-Gil, J. C., & Blanco-Vaca, F. (2009). New insights into the molecular actions of plant sterols and stanols in cholesterol metabolism. *Atherosclerosis, 203*(1), 18–31. https://doi.org/10.1016/j.atherosclerosis.2008.06.026.

Calpe-Berdiel, L., Escolà-Gil, J. C., Ribas, V., Navarro-Sastre, A., Garcés-Garcés, J., & Blanco-Vaca, F. (2005). Changes in intestinal and liver global gene expression in response to a phytosterol-enriched diet. *Atherosclerosis, 181*(1), 75–85. https://doi.org/10.1016/j.atherosclerosis.2004.11.025.

Carden, T. J., Hang, J., Dussault, P. H., & Carr, T. P. (2015). Dietary plant sterol esters must be hydrolyzed to reduce intestinal cholesterol absorption in hamsters. *Journal of Nutrition, 145*(7), 1402–1407. https://doi.org/10.3945/jn.114.207662.

Carr, T. P., Stanek Krogstrand, K. L., Schlegel, V. L., & Fernandez, M. L. (2009). Stearate-enriched plant sterol esters lower serum LDL cholesterol concentration in normo- and hypercholesterolemic adults. *Journal of Nutrition, 139*(8), 1445–1450. https://doi.org/10.3945/jn.109.106328.

Cedó, L., Farràs, M., Lee-Rueckert, M., & Escolà-Gil, J. C. (2019). Molecular insights into the mechanisms underlying the cholesterol-lowering effects of phytosterols. *Current Medicinal Chemistry, 26*(37), 6704–6723. https://doi.org/10.2174/0929867326666190822154701.

Chau, Y. P., Cheng, Y. C., Sing, C. W., Tsoi, M. F., Cheng, V. K. F., Lee, G. K. Y., et al. (2020). The lipid-lowering effect of once-daily soya drink fortified with phytosterols in normocholesterolaemic Chinese: A double-blind randomized controlled trial. *European Journal of Nutrition, 59*(6), 2739–2746. https://doi.org/10.1007/s00394-019-02119-w.

Chen, Q., Gruber, H., Pakenham, C., Ratnayake, W. M. N., & Scoggan, K. A. (2009). Dietary phytosterols and phytostanols alter the expression of sterol-regulatory genes in SHRSP and WKY inbred rats. *Annals of Nutrition and Metabolism, 55*(4), 341–350. https://doi.org/10.1159/000252350.

Chen, J., Jiao, R., Jiang, Y., Bi, Y., & Chen, Z. Y. (2014). Algal sterols are as effective as β-sitosterol in reducing plasma cholesterol concentration. *Journal of Agricultural and Food Chemistry, 62*(3), 675–681. https://doi.org/10.1021/jf404955n.

Darnet, S., & Schaller, H. (2019). Metabolism and biological activities of 4-methyl-sterols. *Molecules, 24*. https://doi.org/10.3390/molecules24030451, 451.

Demonty, I., Ras, R. T., Van Der Knaap, H. C. M., Duchateau, G. S. M. J. E., Meijer, L., Zock, P. L., et al. (2009). Continuous dose-response relationship of the LDL-cholesterol-lowering effect of phytosterol intake. *Journal of Nutrition, 139*(2), 271–284. https://doi.org/10.3945/jn.108.095125.

Doornbos, A. M. E., Meynen, E. M., Duchateau, G. S. M. J. E., van der Knaap, H. C. M., & Trautwein, E. A. (2006). Intake occasion affects the serum cholesterol lowering of a plant sterol-enriched single-dose yoghurt drink in mildly hypercholesterolaemic subjects. *European Journal of Clinical Nutrition, 60*(3), 325–333. https://doi.org/10.1038/sj.ejcn.1602318.

Feng, S., Dai, Z., Liu, A. B., Huang, J., Narsipur, N., Guo, G., et al. (2018). Intake of stigmasterol and β-sitosterol alters lipid metabolism and alleviates NAFLD in mice fed a high-fat western-style diet. *Biochimica et Biophysica Acta - Molecular and Cell Biology of Lipids, 1863*(10), 1274–1284. https://doi.org/10.1016/j.bbalip.2018.08.004.

Ferguson, J. J. A., Stojanovski, E., MacDonald-Wicks, L., & Garg, M. L. (2016). Fat type in phytosterol products influence their cholesterol-lowering potential: A systematic review and meta-analysis of RCTs. *Progress in Lipid Research*, 64, 16–29. https://doi.org/10.1016/j.plipres.2016.08.002.

Field, F. J., & Mathur, S. N. (1983). β-Sitosterol: Esterification by intestinal acylcoenzyme A: Cholesterol acyltransferase (ACAT) and its effect on cholesterol esterificaton. *Journal of Lipid Research*, 24(4), 409–417.

Ghaedi, E., Varkaneh, H. K., Rahmani, J., Mousavi, S. M., Mohammadi, H., Fatahi, S., et al. (2019). Possible anti-obesity effects of phytosterols and phytostanols supplementation in humans: A systematic review and dose–response meta-analysis of randomized controlled trials. *Phytotherapy Research*, 33(5), 1246–1257. https://doi.org/10.1002/ptr.6319.

Guderian, D. M., Rasmussen, H. E., Wray, C. A., Dussault, P. H., & Carr, T. P. (2007). Cholesterol-lowering properties of plant sterols esterified with beef tallow fatty acids in hamsters. *Nutrition Research*, 27(5), 283–288. https://doi.org/10.1016/j.nutres.2007.03.006.

Gylling, H., Plat, J., Turley, S., Ginsberg, H. N., Ellegård, L., Jessup, W., et al. (2014). Plant sterols and plant stanols in the management of dyslipidaemia and prevention of cardiovascular disease. *Atherosclerosis*, 232(2), 346–360. https://doi.org/10.1016/j.atherosclerosis.2013.11.043.

He, W. S., Cui, D., Li, L., Rui, J., & Tong, L. T. (2020). Plasma triacylglycerol-reducing activity of ergosterol linolenate is associated with inhibition of intestinal lipid absorption. *Journal of Functional Foods*, 64. https://doi.org/10.1016/j.jff.2019.103686, 103686.

He, W. S., Cui, D., Li, L., Tong, L. T., Rui, J., Li, H., et al. (2019). Cholesterol-reducing effect of ergosterol is modulated via inhibition of cholesterol absorption and promotion of cholesterol excretion. *Journal of Functional Foods*, 57, 488–496. https://doi.org/10.1016/j.jff.2019.04.042.

He, W. S., Zhu, H., & Chen, Z. Y. (2018). Plant sterols: Chemical and enzymatic structural modifications and effects on their cholesterol-lowering activity. *Journal of Agricultural and Food Chemistry*, 66(12), 3047–3062. https://doi.org/10.1021/acs.jafc.8b00059.

Hu, S., Gao, R., Liu, L., Zhu, M., Wang, W., & Wang, Y. (2018). Summary of the 2018 report on cardiovascular diseases in China (in Chinese). *Chinese Circulation Journal*, 34, 209–220.

Hu, Q., Zhuo, Z., Fang, S., Zhang, Y., & Feng, J. (2017). Phytosterols improve immunity and exert anti-inflammatory activity in weaned piglets. *Journal of the Science of Food and Agriculture*, 97(12), 4103–4109. https://doi.org/10.1002/jsfa.8277.

Ikeda, I., Tanabe, Y., & Sugano, M. (1989). Effects of sitosterol and sitostanol on micellar solubility of cholesterol. *Journal of Nutritional Science and Vitaminology*, 35(4), 361–369. https://doi.org/10.3177/jnsv.35.361.

Jain, D., Ebine, N., Jia, X., Kassis, A., Marinangeli, C., Fortin, M., et al. (2008). Corn fiber oil and sitostanol decrease cholesterol absorption independently of intestinal sterol transporters in hamsters. *Journal of Nutritional Biochemistry*, 19(4), 229–236. https://doi.org/10.1016/j.jnutbio.2007.02.012.

Jesch, E. D., Seo, J. M., Carr, T. P., & Lee, J. Y. (2009). Sitosterol reduces messenger RNA and protein expression levels of Niemann-Pick C1-like 1 in FHs 74 Int cells. *Nutrition Research*, 29(12), 859–866. https://doi.org/10.1016/j.nutres.2009.10.016.

Jia, L., Betters, J. L., & Yu, L. (2011). Niemann-Pick C1-Like 1 (NPC1L1) protein in intestinal and hepatic cholesterol transport. *Annual Review of Physiology*, 73, 239–259. https://doi.org/10.1146/annurev-physiol-012110-142233.

Kaneko, E., Matsuda, M., Yamada, Y., Tachibana, Y., Shimomura, I., & Makishima, M. (2003). Induction of intestinal ATP-binding cassette transporters by a phytosterol-derived liver X receptor agonist. *Journal of Biological Chemistry*, 278(38), 36091–36098. https://doi.org/10.1074/jbc.M304153200.

Katan, M. B., Grundy, S. M., Jones, P., Law, M., Miettinen, T., & Paoletti, R. (2003). Efficacy and safety of plant stanols and sterols in the management of blood cholesterol levels. *Mayo Clinic Proceedings*, 78(8), 965–978. https://doi.org/10.1016/s0025-6196(11)63144-3.

Kaur, R., & Myrie, S. B. (2020). Association of dietary phytosterols with cardiovascular disease biomarkers in humans. *Lipids*, 55(6), 569–584. https://doi.org/10.1002/lipd.12262.

Kriengsinyos, W., Wangtong, A., & Komindr, S. (2015). Serum cholesterol reduction efficacy of biscuits with added plant stanol ester. *Cholesterol*, 2015. https://doi.org/10.1155/2015/353164, 353164.

Kruit, J. K., Plösch, T., Havinga, R., Boverhof, R., Groot, P. H. E., Groen, A. K., et al. (2005). Increased fecal neutral sterol loss upon liver X receptor activation is independent of biliary sterol secretion in mice. *Gastroenterology*, 128(1), 147–156. https://doi.org/10.1053/j.gastro.2004.10.006.

Li, X., Zhang, Z., Cheng, J., Diao, C., Yan, Y., Liu, D., et al. (2019). Dietary supplementation of soybean-derived sterols regulates cholesterol metabolism and intestinal microbiota in hamsters. *Journal of Functional Foods*, 59, 242–250. https://doi.org/10.1016/j.jff.2019.05.032.

Liang, Y. T., Wong, W. T., Guan, L., Tian, X. Y., Ma, K. Y., Huang, Y., et al. (2011). Effect of phytosterols and their oxidation products on lipoprotein profiles and vascular function in hamster fed a high cholesterol diet. *Atherosclerosis*, 219(1), 124–133. https://doi.org/10.1016/j.atherosclerosis.2011.06.004.

Cedó, L., Santos, D., Ludwig, I. A., Silvennoinen, R., García-León, A., Kaipiainen, L., et al. (2017). Phytosterol-mediated inhibition of intestinal cholesterol absorption in mice is independent of liver X receptor. *Molecular Nutrition & Food Research*, 61. https://doi.org/10.1002/mnfr.201700055, 1600055.

Lozano, W. M., Arias-Mutis, O. J., Calvo, C. J., Chorro, F. J., & Zarzoso, M. (2019). Diet-induced rabbit models for the study of metabolic syndrome. *Animals*, 9. https://doi.org/10.3390/ani9070463, 463.

Matsuoka, K., Kajimoto, E., Horiuchi, M., Honda, C., & Endo, K. (2010). Competitive solubilization of cholesterol and six species of sterol/stanol in bile salt micelles. *Chemistry and Physics of Lipids*, 163(4–5), 397–402. https://doi.org/10.1016/j.chemphyslip.2010.03.006.

Moghadasian, M. H., Nguyen, L. B., Shefer, S., Salen, G., Batta, A. K., & Frohlich, J. J. (2001). Hepatic cholesterol and bile acid synthesis, low-density lipoprotein receptor function, and plasma and fecal sterol levels in mice: Effects of apolipoprotein E deficiency and probucol or phytosterol treatment. *Metabolism, Clinical and Experimental*, 50(6), 708–714. https://doi.org/10.1053/meta.2001.23303.

Moreau, R. A., Nyström, L., Whitaker, B. D., Winkler-Moser, J. K., Baer, D. J., Gebauer, S. K., et al. (2018). Phytosterols and their derivatives: Structural diversity, distribution, metabolism, analysis, and health-promoting uses. *Progress in Lipid Research*, 70, 35–61. https://doi.org/10.1016/j.plipres.2018.04.001.

Moreau, R. A., Whitaker, B. D., & Hicks, K. B. (2002). Phytosterols, phytostanols, and their conjugates in foods: Structural diversity, quantitative analysis, and health-promoting uses. *Progress in Lipid Research*, 41(6), 457–500. https://doi.org/10.1016/S0163-7827(02)00006-1.

Moselhy, S. S., Kamal, I. H., Kumosani, T. A., & Huwait, E. A. (2016). Possible inhibition of hydroxy methyl glutaryl CoA reductase activity by nicotinic acid and ergosterol: As targeting for hypocholesterolemic action. *African Health Sciences*, 16(1), 319–324. https://doi.org/10.4314/ahs.v16i1.42.

Musa-Veloso, K., Poon, T. H., Elliot, J. A., & Chung, C. (2011). A comparison of the LDL-cholesterol lowering efficacy of plant stanols and plant sterols over a continuous dose range: Results of a meta-analysis of randomized, placebo-controlled trials. *Prostaglandins, Leukotrienes, and Essential Fatty Acids*, 85(1), 9–28. https://doi.org/10.1016/j.plefa.2011.02.001.

Mussner, M. J., Parhofer, K. G., Von Bergmann, K., Schwandt, P., Broedl, U., & Otto, C. (2002). Effects of phytosterol ester-enriched margarine on plasma lipoproteins in mild to moderate hypercholesterolemia are related to basal cholesterol and fat intake. *Metabolism, Clinical and Experimental*, 51(2), 189–194. https://doi.org/10.1053/meta.2002.29988.

Nakano, T., Inoue, I., Takenaka, Y., Ikegami, Y., Kotani, N., Shimada, A., et al. (2018). Luminal plant sterol promotes brush border membranetolumen cholesterol efflux in the small intestine. *Journal of Clinical Biochemistry and Nutrition*, 63(2), 102–105. https://doi.org/10.3164/jcbn.17116.

Nestel, P., Cehun, M., Pomeroy, S., Abbey, M., & Weldon, G. (2001). Cholesterol-lowering effects of plant sterol esters and non-esterified stanols in margarine, butter and low-fat foods. *European Journal of Clinical Nutrition*, 55(12), 1084–1090. https://doi.org/10.1038/sj.ejcn.1601264.

Nigon, F., Serfaty-Lacrosniére, C., Beucler, I., Chauvois, D., Neveu, C., Giral, P., et al. (2001). Plant sterol-enriched margarine lowers plasma LDL in hyperlipidemic subjects with low cholesterol intake: Effect of fibrate treatment. *Clinical Chemistry and Laboratory Medicine*, 39(7), 634–640. https://doi.org/10.1515/CCLM.2001.103.

Nissinen, M., Gylling, H., Vuoristo, M., & Miettinen, T. A. (2002). Micellar distribution of cholesterol and phytosterols after duodenal plant stanol ester infusion. *American Journal of Physiology - Gastrointestinal and Liver Physiology*, 282(6), G1009–G1015. https://doi.org/10.1152/ajpgi.00446.2001.

Ntanios, F. Y., Jones, P. J. H., & Frohlich, J. J. (1998). Dietary sitostanol reduces plaque formation but not lecithin cholesterol acyl transferase activity in rabbits. *Atherosclerosis*, 138(1), 101–110. https://doi.org/10.1016/S0021-9150(98)00008-2.

Orem, A., Alasalvar, C., Vanizor Kural, B., Yaman, S., Orem, C., Karadag, A., et al. (2017). Cardio-protective effects of phytosterol-enriched functional black tea in mild hypercholesterolemia subjects. *Journal of Functional Foods*, 31, 311–319. https://doi.org/10.1016/j.jff.2017.01.048.

Ostlund, R. E., Racette, S. B., Okeke, A., & Stenson, W. F. (2002). Phytosterols that are naturally present in commercial corn oil significantly reduce cholesterol absorption in humans. *American Journal of Clinical Nutrition*, 75(6), 1000–1004. https://doi.org/10.1093/ajcn/75.6.1000.

Park, Y., & Carr, T. P. (2013). Unsaturated fatty acids and phytosterols regulate cholesterol transporter genes in Caco-2 and HepG2 cell lines. *Nutrition Research*, 33(2), 154–161. https://doi.org/10.1016/j.nutres.2012.11.014.

Peterson, D. W. (1951). Effect of soybean sterols in the diet on plasma and liver cholesterol in chicks. *Proceedings of the Society for Experimental Biology and Medicine*, 78(1), 143–147. https://doi.org/10.3181/00379727-78-19002.

Plat, J., & Mensink, R. P. (2002). Effects of plant stanol esters on LDL receptor protein expression and on LDL receptor and HMG-CoA reductase mRNA expression in mononuclear blood cells of healthy men and women. *FASEB Journal: Official Publication of the Federation of American Societies for Experimental Biology*, 16(2), 258–260. https://doi.org/10.1096/fj.01-0653fje.

Plat, J., van Onselen, E. N. M., van Heugten, M. M. A., & Mensink, R. P. (2000). Effects on serum lipids, lipoproteins and fat soluble antioxidant concentrations of consumption frequency of margarines and shortenings enriched with plant stanol esters. *European Journal of Clinical Nutrition*, 54(9), 671–677. https://doi.org/10.1038/sj.ejcn.1601071.

Plösch, T., Kruit, J. K., Bloks, V. W., Huijkman, N. C. A., Havinga, R., Duchateau, G. S. M. J. E., et al. (2006).

Reduction of cholesterol absorption by dietary plant sterols and stanols in mice is independent of the Abcg5/8 transporter. *Journal of Nutrition*, *136*(8), 2135–2140. https://doi.org/10.1093/jn/136.8.2135.

Pollak, O. J. (1953a). Reduction of blood cholesterol in man. *Circulation*, *7*(5), 702–706. https://doi.org/10.1161/01.CIR.7.5.702.

Pollak, O. J. (1953b). Successive prevention of experimental hypercholesteremia and cholesterol atherosclerosis in the rabbit. *Circulation*, *7*(5), 696–701. https://doi.org/10.1161/01.CIR.7.5.696.

Racette, S. B., Lin, X., Lefevre, M., Spearie, C. A., Most, M. M., Ma, L., et al. (2010). Dose effects of dietary phytosterols on cholesterol metabolism: A controlled feeding study. *American Journal of Clinical Nutrition*, *91*(1), 32–38. https://doi.org/10.3945/ajcn.2009.28070.

Raju, D., Sarmistha, M., Chayan, A. M., Fatimah, O. D., Abdul, H. M., Min, C. S., et al. (2021). Phytosterols: Targeting neuroinflammation in neurodegeneration. *Current Pharmaceutical Design*, *27*(3), 383–401. https://doi.org/10.2174/1381612826666200628022812.

Rideout, T. C., Harding, S. V., & Jones, P. J. H. (2010). Consumption of plant sterols reduces plasma and hepatic triglycerides and modulates the expression of lipid regulatory genes and de novo lipogenesis in C57BL/6J mice. *Molecular Nutrition & Food Research*, *54*(1), S7–S13. https://doi.org/10.1002/mnfr.201000027.

Rong, S., Xu, R., & Li, W. (2016). Phytosterols and dementia. *Plant Foods for Human Nutrition*, *71*, 347–354.

Rouyanne, T. R., Johanna, M. G., & Eike, A. T. (2014). LDL-cholesterol-lowering effect of plant sterols and stanols across different dose ranges: A meta-analysis of randomised controlled studies. *British Journal of Nutrition*, *112*, 214–219. https://doi.org/10.1017/s0007114514000750.

Schroder, M., Fricke, C., Pilegaard, K., Poulsen, M., Wester, I., Lütjohann, D., et al. (2009). Effect of rapeseed oil-derived plant sterol and stanol esters on atherosclerosis parameters in cholesterol-challenged heterozygous Watanabe Heritable hyperlipidaemic rabbits. *British Journal of Nutrition*, *102*(12), 1740–1751. https://doi.org/10.1017/S0007114509991206.

Smet, E. D., Mensink, R. P., & Plat, J. (2012). Effects of plant sterols and stanols on intestinal cholesterol metabolism: Suggested mechanisms from past to present. *Molecular Nutrition & Food Research*, *56*(7), 1058–1072. https://doi.org/10.1002/mnfr.201100722.

Solati, Z., & Moghadasian, M. H. (2015). Use of animal models in plant sterol and stanol research. *Journal of AOAC International*, *98*(3), 691–696. https://doi.org/10.5740/jaoacint.SGESolati.

Suttiarporn, P., Chumpolsri, W., Mahatheeranont, S., Luangkamin, S., Teepsawang, S., & Leardkamolkarn, V. (2015). Structures of phytosterols and triterpenoids with potential anti-cancer activity in bran of black non-glutinous rice. *Nutrients*, *7*(3), 1672–1687. https://doi.org/10.3390/nu7031672.

Talati, R., Sobieraj, D. M., Makanji, S. S., Phung, O. J., & Coleman, C. I. (2010). The comparative efficacy of plant sterols and stanols on serum lipids: A systematic review and meta-analysis. *Journal of the American Dietetic Association*, *110*(5), 719–726. https://doi.org/10.1016/j.jada.2010.02.011.

Temel, R. E., Gebre, A. K., Parks, J. S., & Rudel, L. L. (2003). Compared with Acyl-CoA: Cholesterol O-acyltransferase (ACAT) 1 and lecithin: Cholesterol acyltransferase, ACAT2 displays the greatest capacity to differentiate cholesterol from sitosterol. *Journal of Biological Chemistry*, *278*(48), 47594–47601. https://doi.org/10.1074/jbc.M308235200.

Wang, T., Hicks, K. B., & Moreau, R. (2002). Antioxidant activity of phytosterols, oryzanol, and other phytosterol conjugates. *Journal of the American Oil Chemists' Society*, *79*, 1201–1206. https://doi.org/10.1007/s11746-002-0628-x.

Trautwein, E. A., Duchateau, G. S. M. J. E., Lin, Y., Mel'nikov, S. M., Molhuizen, H. O. F., & Ntanios, F. Y. (2003). Proposed mechanisms of cholesterol-lowering action of plant sterols. *European Journal of Lipid Science and Technology*, *105*(3–4), 171–185. https://doi.org/10.1002/ejlt.200390033.

Trautwein, E. A., Vermeer, M. A., Hiemstra, H., & Ras, R. T. (2018). LDL-cholesterol lowering of plant sterols and stanols—Which factors influence their efficacy? *Nutrients*, *10*. https://doi.org/10.3390/nu10091262, 1262.

Van Der Velde, A. E., Brufau, G., & Groen, A. K. (2010). Transintestinal cholesterol efflux. *Current Opinion in Lipidology*, *21*(3), 167–171. https://doi.org/10.1097/MOL.0b013e3283395e45.

Wang, M., Huang, W., Hu, Y., Zhang, L., Shao, Y., Wang, M., et al. (2018). Phytosterol profiles of common foods and estimated natural intake of different structures and forms in China. *Journal of Agricultural and Food Chemistry*, *66*(11), 2669–2676. https://doi.org/10.1021/acs.jafc.7b05009.

Wu, T., Fu, J., Yang, Y., Zhang, L., & Han, J. (2009). The effects of phytosterols/stanols on blood lipid profiles: A systematic review with meta-analysis. *Asia Pacific Journal of Clinical Nutrition*, *18*(2), 179–186. http://apjcn.nhri.org.tw/server/APJCN/Volume18/vol18.2/Finished/5_1398_179-186.pdf.

Xu, G., Salen, G., Shefer, S., Tint, G. S., Nguyen, L. B., Batta, A. K., et al. (2001). Plant stanol fatty acid esters inhibit cholesterol absorption and hepatic hydroxymethyl glutaryl coenzyme A reductase activity to reduce plasma levels in rabbits. *Metabolism, Clinical and Experimental*, *50*(9), 1106–1112. https://doi.org/10.1053/meta.2001.25664.

Yang, C., Yu, L., Li, W., Xu, F., Cohen, J. C., & Hobbs, H. H. (2004). Disruption of cholesterol homeostasis by plant sterols. *Journal of Clinical Investigation, 114*(6), 813–822. https://doi.org/10.1172/JCI22186.

Yuan, L., Zhang, F., Jia, S., Xie, J., & Shen, M. (2020). Differences between phytosterols with different structures in regulating cholesterol synthesis, transport and metabolism in Caco-2 cells. *Journal of Functional Foods, 65*, 103715.

Zawistowski, J., & Jones, P. (2015). Regulatory aspects related to plant sterol and stanol supplemented foods. *Journal of AOAC International, 98*(3), 750–756. https://doi.org/10.5740/jaoacint.SGEZawistowski.

Zhang, Z., Wang, H., Jiao, R., Peng, C., Wong, Y. M., Yeung, V. S. Y., et al. (2009). Choosing hamsters but not rats as a model for studying plasma cholesterol-lowering activity of functional foods. *Molecular Nutrition & Food Research, 53*(7), 921–930. https://doi.org/10.1002/mnfr.200800517.

Zhu, H., Chen, J., He, Z., Hao, W., Liu, J., Kwek, E., et al. (2019). Plasma cholesterol-lowering activity of soybean germ phytosterols. *Nutrients, 11*. https://doi.org/10.3390/nu11112784, 2784.

CHAPTER 22

Lipids in breast milk and formulas

Jin Sun[a], Ce Qi[a], and Renqiang Yu[b]

[a]Institute of Nutrition and Health, Qingdao University, Qingdao, China [b]Department of Neonatology, The Affiliated Wuxi Maternity and Child Health Care Hospital of Nanjing Medical University, Wuxi, China

Abbreviation

ALA	α-linolenic acid
ARA	arachidonic acid
BSSL	bile salt-stimulated lipase
DHA	docosahexaenoic acid
EPA	eicosapentaenoic acid
FA	fatty acid
LA	linoleic acid
MCFA	medium-chain fatty acid
MFG	milk fat globules
MLCT	medium- and long-chain triacylglycerol
OPL	oleoylpalmitoyl-linoleoylglycerol
OPO	dioleoyl-palmitoylglycerol
PUFA	polyunsaturated fatty acid
TAGs	triacylglycerols

22.1 Introduction

Total lipids are the most variable macronutrient in human milk, with sample concentrations varying between approximately 2 and 100 g/L, increasing throughout a feed, changing throughout the day, and typically increasing throughout lactation (Mitoulas et al., 2002). Lipids in human milk and formula provide 45%–55% of the total energy for infants in the first 6 months of life. Triacylglycerol (TAG) represent 98% of breast milk lipids with a specific fatty acid (FA) profile and structure. The minor fraction of breast milk lipids consists predominantly of diacylglycerols, monoacylglycerols, free FAs, phospholipids, sphingolipids, and cholesterol. These components are anchored into the milk fat globules (MFGs), with phospholipids forming the bulky membrane and TAG the core. Lipid composition is strongly influenced by the stage of lactation, dietary habits, genetics, and individual conditions. Regiodistribution of FAs in TAG has a significant influence on their bioavailability.

Research to date has focused on the biological properties of these FAs, from the short-chain FAs to the long-chain polyunsaturated FAs (PUFAs). Many studies have revealed that these FAs arise in milk from the maternal diet and are subsequently metabolized in maternal tissues. Specific lipids ensure the correct development of the child in the prenatal, postnatal, and lactation stages and have a significant impact on health outcomes. Milk lipids are sources of PUFAs, including linoleic n-6 (18:2n-6, LA) and α-linolenic n-3 acids (18:3n-3, ALA), 20:4n-6, 20:5n-3, and 22:6n-3, which are required for numerous physiological functions. These milk lipids are a source of energy for the cells, the principal building material of cell membranes, and the precursors of important metabolic compounds, such as prostacyclins, prostaglandins, thromboxanes, and leukotrienes. Specific lipids, such as medium-chain FAs (MCFAs) and sphinganine, also play a role in the development of gut microbiota in infants.

Traditionally, a mixture of vegetable fats, bovine milk fat, algae oil, and fish oil are used for infant formula. In recent decades, several human milk fat substitutes, especially sn-2 palmitate, have been successfully developed and commercialized as energy supplements, sources of essential FAs, and more recently as nutritional supplements in infant formula. Clinical studies have demonstrated the safety and potential benefits of different sources of bovine milk fat globule membrane or its components in infant formula (Fontecha et al., 2020; Niklas & Bo, 2015). Despite the technological advances, the composition of these formulas is significantly different from that of human milk.

In this chapter, we first present the state-of-the-art knowledge about human milk lipids and then provide an introduction of the recent progress in the studies of lipids in infants' formula.

22.2 Composition of breast milk lipids

22.2.1 Physical structure of milk fat globule

Lipids are incompatible with aqueous systems in breast milk. However, no phase separation occurs due to an emulsifier, MFG membrane that reduces the interfacial tension.

Human milk fat is present mainly in the form of MFG (Fig. 22.1). The FGM decreases the lipid-serum interface to very low values, 1–2.5 mN/m, preventing immediate flocculation and coalescence of the globules as well as protecting them from enzymatic activity. Triacylglycerols, the predominant component of human milk fat, are present in the core of MFG. However, polar lipids present in the trilayer membrane include phospholipids, glycosphingolipids, and cholesterol. Phospholipids comprise approximately 30% of the total lipid weight of MFG membrane, the three most prominent being sphingomyelin, phosphatidylcholine, and phosphatidylethanolamine, which together represent up to 85% of total phospholipids. The inner side of the MFG membrane consists of a layer of unstructured lipoproteins acquired within the secretory cells as the triglycerides move from the site of synthesis in the rough endoplasmic reticulum in the basal region of the cell toward the apical membrane (Fig. 22.1).

During milk secretion, intracellular triglyceride droplets are secreted into the milk as plasma membrane bilayer-coated structures by a process that is distinct from the classical secretory pathway used for lipid secretion by hepatocytes and enterocytes (Mather & Keenan, 1998). This process forms the three-layer membrane structure of MFG (Fig. 22.1).

22.2.2 Fatty acid

The FA profiles of human milk are affected by the stage of lactation. We investigated the FA composition (% of total FA) in human milk at three lactating stages from three regions in China and the relationship with maternal dietary intake during lactation (Jiang et al., 2016). Total saturated FA remained stable during lactation, ranging from 34.26% to 35.48%, but MCFAs (C10:0 and C12:0) showed a lower percentage in colostrum compared with those in transitional and mature milk. Total monounsaturated FAs increased significantly from colostrum (34.50%) to transitional milk (37.06%). The amount of PUFA was the highest in colostrum (~29.58%). Docosahexaenoic acid (DHA, C22:6n-3) and arachidonic acid (ARA, 20:4n-6) are the two most important PUFAs in BM. A survey of 65 studies on the composition of human milk from 2474

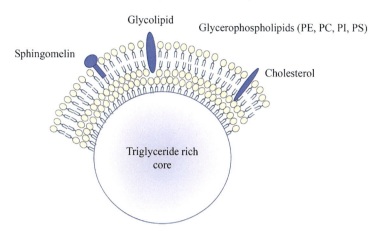

FIG. 22.1 Different types of lipids in milk fat globules.

women worldwide, indicated a mean DHA content of 0.32% (wt/wt; range 0.06%~1.4%) and a higher ARA mean content of 0.47% (0.24%~1.0%) (Brenna et al., 2007).

Another study examined the fatty profiles of breast milk samples from 103 healthy volunteers during colostrum, transitional, and mature stages by multicomponent analysis (Qi et al., 2018). Orthogonal partial least squares discriminant analysis clearly revealed that the breast milk FA profile is dependent on the lactation period. The FA profile of colostrum is significantly different from that of transitional ($R^2X=0.531$) and maturation milk ($R^2X=0.473$), and it also shows greater individual variation (Fig. 22.2). Cluster analysis of the fat composition of each stage showed that the dominant FAs shared by each stage include C12:0, C14:0, C16:1 n-7, C18:0, C16:0, C18:1n-9, C18:2n-6 (LA), C22:6n-3, and C20:4n-6. Both transitional and mature milk contain C18:3n-3 (ALA) and C10:0.

Dietary patterns differed across the various geographical regions of China, which could underlie the differences in the FA profile of human milk. In our study, the samples from Hangzhou, Lanzhou, and Beijing showed obvious region-specific differences regarding monounsaturated FAs and PUFAs (Jiang, Wu, et al., 2016). However, there were no significant differences between the three regions in the composition of total saturated FAs. Mothers from Hangzhou had the highest amount of C22:6n-3 in their milk, indicating the specific characteristics of the coastal region regarding diet and other factors. The Chinese Center for Disease Control and Prevention has developed a regional human milk composition data bank based on the analysis of samples from 11 provinces, municipalities, or autonomous regions (Yin & Yang, 2016). FA profiles were analyzed in samples taken on postpartum day 42 ($n=660$). Based on the distribution characteristics of the FA profile, these samples were clearly divided according to the sampling areas, and the vertical mirror image of PLS-DA corresponds to the Chinese map (Fig. 22.3). Large variation of FA content in maternal milk was also found across different populations of the world. Special concern is necessary for both the quality and total amount of fat intake of pregnant and lactating mothers (Bahreynian, Feizi, & Kelishadi, 2020).

The positioning of the FAs on the TAG glycerol backbone is particularly important because after ingestion, pancreatic and bile salts stimulate lipases, preferentially hydrolyzing the FA ester bonds at the Sn-1 and Sn-3 positions, resulting in two free FA and one Sn-2 monoglyceride. Using

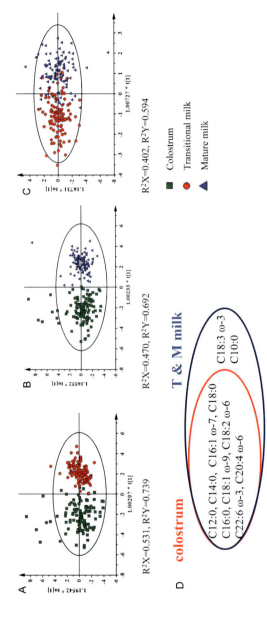

FIG. 22.2 Orthogonal partial least squares discriminant analysis (PLS-DA) (A, B, C) of breast milk FA profile and specific FAs (D). R2X indicates the difference between the two lactation periods, and R2Y indicates individual variation.

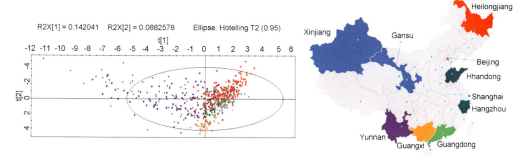

FIG. 22.3 Vertical mirror image of PLS-DA of the FA profile of breast milk samples taken on postpartum day 42 from different regions of China.

liquid chromatography-ion mobility-mass spectrometry, 205 regioisomers of TAGs have been identified in breast milk (George et al., 2020). This study also identified numerous TAGs containing odd chains, which may derive from FA dairy intake. Through HPLC-atmospheric pressure chemical ionization mass spectrometry, it was found that colostrum contained more TAGs with three long-chain FAs (LLL type), whereas the relative content of TAGs containing MCFAs was considerably higher in transitional and mature milk. Nearly half of the TAG molecules in breast milk contained MCFA, among which 12:0 was the most abundant (Yuan et al., 2019). MCFAs predominated in human milk as MLCT, and especially MLL-type palmitic acid was the major saturated FA of human milk, and the majority (70%) of it was thought to reside in the Sn-2 position of TAGs (Breckenridge, Marai, & Kuksis, 1969). In human milk, dioleoyl-palmitoylglycerol (OPO) and oleoylpalmitoyl-linoleoylglycerol (OPL) are the two most abundant TAG, the main regioisomers of which are 1,3-dioleoyl-2-palmitoylglycerol (rac-OPO) and 1-oleoyl-2-palmitoyl-3-linoleoylglycerol (rac-OPL), respectively (Kallio, Nylund, Boström, & Yang, 2017). Samples from many cities, such as Wuxi, contained more OPL than OPO (Yuan et al., 2019). In samples from European countries, such as Denmark, Spain, Finland, or Italy, the major TAG was OPO (Gastaldi et al., 2011).

22.2.3 Phospholipids and complex minor constituents

22.2.3.1 Phospholipids

A smaller portion of milk FAs (0.2%–2%) is esterified in the form of phospholipids and polar lipids. Polar lipids have a fundamental role in milk production and the emulsification of fat in water. Milk phospholipids can be divided into two major classes, glycerophospholipids and sphingolipids, according to the type of alcohol backbone (glycerol or sphingosine). The main phospholipids contained in mammalian milk and dairy products are distributed into five major classes: three predominant (62%–80%) (phosphatidylethanolamine, phosphatidylcholine, and sphingomyelin) and two minor compounds (12%–15%) (phosphatidylinositol, phosphatidylinositol; phosphatidylserine, and phosphatidylserine) (Cilla, Diego Quintaes, Barberá, & Alegría, 2016). The content of mature milk in different types of phospholipids varies and depends on the detection method and sample source (Table 22.1). Overall, sphingomyelin is the most abundant, followed by phosphatidylethanolamine and phosphatidylcholine. The average concentration of the individual phospholipids classes (phosphatidylinositol, phosphatidylethanolamine, phosphatidylcholine, and phosphatidylserine) was highest in the colostrum and decreased during the lactational

TABLE 22.1 Phospholipid composition of mature milk (mg/100 g).

Phospholipids	16 1	17 1	15 2	183
PI	1.1	1.07	0.74	n.d.
PS	1.4	n.d.	1.74	n.d.
PE	6.8	7.49	4.6	2.524
PC	6.0	5.08	2.6	5.996
SM	8.5	8.47	6.54	10.761

Phospholipids were quantified by HPLC-ELSD1, HPLC-MS 2, and HILIC-ESI-IT-TOF-MS3.

period, with the exception of that of sphingomyelin whose levels in the colostrum and transitional milk were much lower than those measured in the mature milk (Ma et al., 2017).

22.2.3.2 Sterols

MFG membrane contains cholesterol and other sterols (cholesterol precursors such as desmosterol, lathosterol, and lanosterol, which participate in the biosynthesis of cholesterol, and plant sterols such as campesterol, stigmasterol, and β-sitosterol, which originate exclusively from the mother's diet), which have been identified in small concentrations in human milk (10–24 mg per 100 mL). Cholesterol is important for the development of the nervous system and synthesis of hormones and vitamin D. Its synthesis might be downregulated in children and adults who were breastfed during infancy (Wong, Hachey, Insull, Opekun, & Klein, 1993). Cholesterol content in human milk slightly decreased from 13.1 mg/100 g in 1 month to 11.3 mg/100 g 120 days after delivery (Beggio, Cruz-Hernandez, Golay, Lee, & Giuffrida, 2018).

22.2.3.3 Fat-soluble nutrients

Vitamin A and vitamin E are two essential nutrients for growth and development of newborns. These vitamins are naturally present in human milk and play a significant role in the offspring's antioxidant status. In addition, carotenes have provitamin A and antioxidant activities (Debier & Larondelle, 2005). The alpha-tocopherol and retinol concentrations in breast milk decreased from the colostrum to mature milk over the course of lactation. These were highest in the colostrum (146.9 and 612.6 μg per 100 g) and lowest in mature milk (59.5 and 177.1 μg per 100 g). There was a significant positive correlation between the retinol and α-tocopherol contents. Neither vitamin A nor vitamin E was correlated with maternal dietary intake during lactation (Jiang et al., 2016).

22.2.4 Source of breast milk lipids

22.2.4.1 Medium-chain and long-chain FAs

FAs in human milk derive from mobilization of the maternal endogenous stores, from synthesis in the liver or breast tissue, and from the mother's diet (Innis, 2007). De novo FA synthesis is responsible only for the production of medium-chain FAs (8–14 carbons), such as caprylic acid (8:0), capric acid (10:0), lauric acid (12:0), and myristic acid (14:0) (Neville & Picciano, 1997). The human mammary gland responds to changes in dietary macronutrients by altering the de novo synthesis of MCFA and glycerol. The individual and total FA (C6–C14) were higher during feeding on a high-carbohydrate diet compared with a high-fat diet (Mohammad, Sunehag, & Haymond, 2014). De novo FA synthesis of MCFAs in the mammary gland is catalyzed by the enzyme FA synthase (Suburu et al., 2014). Deletion of FA synthase gene has been shown to hinder development and induce premature involution of the lactating mammary gland and significantly decrease medium- and long-chain FAs and total FA contents in the milk (Suburu et al., 2014).

22.2.4.2 Long-chain polyunsaturated FAs

Long-chain FAs (>16 carbons) in milk lipids are obtained through transport from the serum following lipoprotein lipase-mediated release from serum triglycerides (Neville & Picciano, 1997). LPL transcript and activity levels in mouse mammary glands increase dramatically at the end of pregnancy in conjunction with the increased de novo FA synthesis (McManaman, 2009). More than 50% of the milk FAs derive directly from the diet (Innis, 2014). Dietary α-linolenic acid (ALA) can be rapidly transported into milk without changing during lactation and reach peak levels approximately 12 h after intake (Fidler, Sauerwald, Pohl, Demmelmair, & Koletzko, 2000). Approximately 30% of milk linoleic acid derives directly from dietary intake, whereas approximately 70% originates from maternal body fat stores. This process buffers the short-term variation in the maternal dietary supply of the parent's essential FA and provides the infant with a relatively stable parent's essential FA supply. However, long-term changes in dietary supply will also modify maternal body fat stores and thereby explain the observed marked changes over time (Ailhaud et al., 2006). ALA may be endogenously converted to eicosapentaenoic acid (EPA) and then to DHA. There was no significant association between dietary EPA and DHA intake during the postpartum period and their concentrations in human milk. However, dietary intake of these two FAs during the third trimester of pregnancy was directly related to the content of these FAs in mature human milk (Silva et al., 2005). Therefore, maternal endogenous stores have a greater influence on breast milk FA composition than the estimated dietary intake during the postpartum period. The tissue levels in women during lactation are directly related to the reserve capacity and metabolic utilization of FAs (synthesis, oxidation, and transport). Hence, the maternal diet and metabolism of FAs in women during lactation seem to be the most important factors affecting DHA concentration in human milk.

22.3 Composition of formulas in lipids

22.3.1 Fatty acid and triacylglycerol profile

Infant formulas are generally produced by mixing skimmed milk and whey to approximate the amino acid content of human milk with a 60:40 whey-to-casein ratio. Lactose is then added to standardize the lactose concentration in the human milk range. Infant formulas mainly consist of vegetable oils such as palm oil, soybean oil, rapeseed oil, and coconut oil, among others, and are enriched with vitamins, minerals, and essential amino acids. The recommendations for infant formula lipids have always been established on the basis of human milk FA composition, which is still considered as the "gold standard." However, infant formula can only mimic the general composition of the 20th-century human milk FAs, and its basic composition includes 34%–47% of saturated FAs (palmitic acid: 17%–25% of total FAs), approximately 31%–43% monounsaturated FAs (oleic acid: 26%–36%), approximately 12%–26% n-6 PUFA, and approximately 0.8% 0.3.6% n-3 PUFA (Delplanque, Gibson, Koletzko, Lapillonne, & Strandvik, 2015) (Table 22.2). LA and ALA should be provided in proper quantities and proportions (LA/ALA ratio). Considering the dramatic increase in the LA/ALA ratio of human milk (reflecting mother's dietary changes) (Qi et al., 2018), caution should be exercised about the definition of a "gold standard" in terms of n-6 and n-3 PUFA. However, LA as an "essential FA," which means that a minimum intake is necessary to avoid reproduction deficiency or atopic diseases. Infant formulas blended with dairy fat, with naturally low LA levels (2%), could be a solution to reduce LA levels and improve the LA/ALA ratio for better bioconversion to

TABLE 22.2 Fatty acid composition of human milk, cow's milk, and infant formulas (% of total FAs).

Fatty acid	Breast milk	Blend of dairy and vegetable oil	Vegetable formula (palm)	Vegetable formula + coco oil
C4:0	ND	0.6–0.7		ND
C6:0	0.03–0.79	0.6		0.1
C8:0	0.08–0.61	0.4		1.0–1.5
C10:0	0.72–1.71	1.1–1.2		0.9–1.3
C12:0	2.31–6.74	1.3–1.6		7.8–11.5
14:0	3.98–8.67	5.0–5.5		4.0–5.5
C16:0	16.6–25	16.5–20.4	26.1–29.5	18.2–25.4
C18:0	3.39–6.89	5.4–6.1	3.3–4.1	3.5–4.0
C18:1 n-9	26.5–35.6	39.1–41.2	42.3–45.5	28.4–40.8
C18:2 n-6	10.1–24,3	15.6–16.3	16.8–17.8	13.3–18.5
C18:3 n-6	0.06–0.23			
C20:4 n-6	0.45–0.86			
C22:4 n-6	0.04–0.47			
C18:3 n-3	0.67–1.9	2.4–2.5	1.9–3.4	1.6–2.4
C18:4 n-3	0.23–0.68	0.04–0.08		
C20:3 n-3	0.05–0.4			
C20:5 n-3	0.06–0.33	ND–0.1		
C22:5 n-3	0.16–0.54	0.03		
C22:6 n-3	0.09–1.03			
Ratio LA/ALA	3.45–11.9	6.2–6.7	4.9–9.4	5.5–10.6
added DHA		0.2–0.3	0.2–0.3	
added ARA		0.1–0.6	0.1–0.6	

From Delplanque, B., Gibson, R., Koletzko, B., Lapillonne, A., & Strandvik, B. (2015). Lipid Quality in Infant Nutrition: Current Knowledge and Future Opportunities. Journal of Pediatric Gastroenterology and Nutrition 16(1): 8–17. https://doi.org/10.1097/MPG.0000000000000818.

DHA. In addition, breast milk contains very low levels of DHA and ARA (20:4n-6) (0.1%–1% and 0.4%–0.9%, respectively) and some infant formulas contain added ARA and DHA (Table 22.2). Infant formulas based on vegetable oils lack cholesterol, some MCFAs, and triglycerides carrying palmitic acid at the sn2 position, etc. However, some of these components could be provided by the addition of specific oils or products (e.g., coconut for MCFAs).

Although the total FA composition of human milk may be matched during the commercial preparation of infant formulas, the fat that derives from vegetable oils possesses a different positional distribution of FAs compared to human milk. The MCFAs naturally present in human milk are medium- and long-chain triacylglycerols (MLCTs), especially TAG with one MCFA and two long-chain FAs (MLL type), whereas the plant oil formula contained higher proportions of TAG with three MCFAs (MMM type) and goat's milk formula contained higher proportions of TAG with two MCFAs and one long-chain FA (MML type) (Yuan, Qi, et al., 2019). The significantly higher 12:0-MLL content compared with all infant formulas was a feature of human milk.

In human milk, OPO and OPL are the two most abundant TAGs. To mimic human milk, much attention has been paid to supplement rac-OPO in infant formulas. rac-OPO is allowed as a nutrient fortifier supplement in commercial infant formulas in China, which results in a higher formula price for the formulas compared with those that are not labeled as rac-OPO formulas. The predominant regioisomers of OPO and PPO in infant formulas labeled as containing rac-OPO were rac-OPO (approximately 70%) and rac-PPO (above 95%), while in those not labeled as rac-OPO were rac-OOP (65.24e100%) and rac-POP (approximately 90%) (Chen et al., 2019).

DHA is often added to infant formulas to meet the nutritional requirements of formula-fed infants (Table 22.2). Bovine milk and human milk contain DHA-TAG of smaller molecular sizes (728–952 Da), whereas many infant formulas samples contain species of a broader mass range (from 728 to 1035 Da) (Liu, Cocks, & Rochfort, 2016).

22.3.2 Phospholipids and minor constituents

In vegetable fat-based infant formula, phospholipids are provided by lecithin, derived from either sunflower seeds or soybeans (Delplanque et al., 2015). They are also provided by residual bovine milk fat from skimmed milk powder. Phospholipids from skimmed milk powder also account for the presence of sphingomyelin, which cannot be provided from plant-based fat blends. The levels of phospholipids vary among infant formulas, which consist mostly of phosphatidylcholine, sphingomyelin, and PE, with lower levels of phosphatidylinositol and phosphatidylserine. Sphingomyelin were the dominant phospholipids in human milk, whereas phosphatidylcholine and phosphatidylinositol were the dominant phospholipids in infant formulas. The mean diameter of MFG in infant formulas was much smaller than that found in human milk (200 nm vs. 5.63 μm). Significant differences were observed between human milk and infant formulas with regard to phospholipids, suggesting that more research is needed to develop means to achieve the human phospholipids profile in infant formulas (He et al., 2019).

Although bovine milk fat contains higher levels, approximately 300 mg/L, of cholesterol, infant formulas only contain 0–4 mg/L of cholesterol. Infant formulas based on a blend of vegetable fats and bovine milk fat contain, on average, 0.185 mg/L and 0.927 of cholesterol, respectively (Claumarchirant, Matencio, Sanchez-Siles, Alegría, & Lagarda, 2015). The infant formulas contain low concentrations of cholesterol that mostly originates from the small amount of milk fat in skimmed milk. This implies that the addition of bovine milk fat is very low in infant formulas.

22.3.3 Sources of formulas lipids

22.3.3.1 *Vegetable oils and animal fat*

Natural vegetable oil is an important source of human milk fat because all FAs in human milk fat are also present in different vegetable oils. Their yields are large and inexpensive. Due to the lack of ingredients of animal origin, they easily obtain an International Halal Certificate (namely Halal Food Certificate) and comply with the regulations of different countries and nations. Therefore, all oils used in infant formulas contain a certain proportion of vegetable oil (usually a mixture of several vegetable oils). The blends of vegetable oils used in infant formulas were selected to match the excellent absorption by the infant. However, the FA profiles of these oils differ considerably from those of human milk fat, except for the absence of long-chain PUFA. Palm oil and its low melting fraction, palm olein, a relatively inexpensive source of palmitic acid, are added to many infant formulas in amounts that mimic the palmitic acid content of human milk (Koo, Hockman, Koo, & Dow, 2006). However, the positional distribution of individual FAs on the triacylglyceride molecules, which affects fat absorption, differs between these vegetable oils and human milk fat.

22.3.3.2 Marine oils and microbial oils

Marine fish, including salmon, tuna, and halibut, are a rich and conventional source to produce EPA and DHA. Cold-water marine fish contain larger proportions of DHA oil. Their lipid content is approximately 20% of their dry weight, which may reach up to 50%. However, fish oil may contain chemical contaminants such as mercury and have a pungent smell (Bajpai, 2017). Marine algae are a more remarkable source of DHA due to large coastal deposition, although they contain low levels of lipids (Bajpai, 2017). Microalgae can reach much higher levels of EPA and DHA content compared with other possible sources. Heterotrophic microalgae are well established as an alternative source of DHA and are added to infant formula. DHA in algal and fish oils does not have a strong positional specificity. DHA was better absorbed by infants fed the formula containing algal oils than those fed the formula containing fish oil.

Oils derived from microbial sources are named microbial oils, unicellular oils, or single-cell oils. It has been proposed that single-cell oils used for infant formula production should derive from nonpathogenic microorganisms and be free of contaminating substances (Koletzko & Sinclair, 1999).

22.3.3.3 Human milk fat substitutes

When compared to various other naturally occurring lipids, human milk fats are significantly different. For example, the majority of palmitic acid in human milk is in sn-2 position of OPO or OPL, which is different from that in other mammalian milk fats and vegetable oils. The development of sn-2 palmitates, primarily OPO, was another breakthrough in current infant formula science. FA distribution modification on the TAGs was made possible by specialized enzymes and their usage at the industrial scale. The first sn-2 palmitate was introduced to the market as Betapol® and was developed by IOI Loders Croklaan. Its first usage in infant formulas dates to 1995.

The most typical type of MLCT in human milk is MLM, in which MCFAs are esterified at the sn-1,3 positions and long-chain FAs at the sn-2 position. MLM-type MLCT can act as an effective carrier of long-chain FAs compared to the other types. Compared with the physical mixture of MCTs and LCTs, MLCTs display greater control over the release of MCFAs into the bloodstream (Koh et al., 2010). Some researchers are trying different methods and substrates to synthesize MLCT. MLCT-rich structured lipids (SLs) can be synthesized by lipase-catalyzed inter-esterification of single-cell oils derived ARA with MCTs in a solvent-free system (Korma et al., 2018). Through Lipozyme RM IM lipase-catalyzed esterification, MLCT can be synthesized from glycerol and mixtures of capric and oleic acid (Koh et al., 2010).

Fat droplets have a mode diameter of 0.4 μm, based on volume, and proteins are the main emulsifiers of fat droplets. This results in a stable and reproducible product with a long shelf life, but with a fat droplet architecture strongly different from that in human milk, which affects lipolysis (Bourlieu et al., 2015). However, human MFG is difficult to mimic in infant formula because of its highly complex structure and variable composition. Gallier et al. developed a method to mimic the emulsified state of human milk. Larger fat droplets were obtained by adding bovine milk phospholipids to 1.5% of total fat and modified processing procedures (Gallier et al., 2015).

22.4 Breast milk and formula lipid nutrition

22.4.1 Digestion of breast milk fat in the infant gastrointestinal tract

As the pH drops below 5.5, the MFG membrane structure becomes less stable and tends to favor aggregation and coalescence of lipid particles. The breakdown of the membrane protein coating by gastric proteases promotes the release of trapped fat globules from the clot matrix into the digesta (Ye, Cui, Dalgleish, & Singh, 2016). Fat digestion begins in the stomach through gastric lipase, which is secreted by the chief cells of the gastric mucosa located in the fundus and body of the stomach. Excretion of gastric lipase is well developed in infants, and its activity is similar to that observed in adults (Fig. 22.4) (DiPalma et al., 1991). Following a meal, gastric pH increases to approximately 6–6.5, which is most suitable for gastric lipase, but decreases over time together with a reduction in gastric volume to create optimal conditions for lipid hydrolysis (Yu, Zheng, & Li, 2014). Therefore, the lipolytic activity of gastric lipases is essential for infant fat digestion. It hydrolyzes the sn-3 position of a triglyceride with a higher rate for medium-chain triglycerides (Ransac et al., 1990). As gastric lipolysis continues, natural emulsifiers are generated from breast milk, primarily free FAs and some monoacylglycerols as well as surface-active phospholipids from the gastric mucosal barrier (Bernhard, Postle, Rau, & Freihorst, 2001).

Compared with adults, the secretion of colipase-dependent pancreatic triglyceride lipase and bile acids is immature in the first months of life. After consuming evaporated milk or modified formula, the duodenal bile salts of infants drop to approximately 1 mmol/L, which is below the critical micelle concentration of 2 mmol/L (Lavy, Silverberg, & Davidson, 1971). In early infancy, pancreatic triglyceride lipase in the duodenum is insufficiently low in pancreatic lipase-related protein 2, and bile salt-stimulated lipase (BSSL) from the pancreas and milk is the dominant lipase for fat digestion in the small intestine

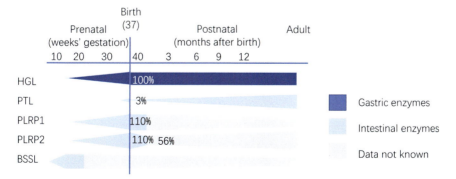

FIG. 22.4 Expression of enzymes in infants relative to adults is involved in lipid digestion in the gastrointestinal tract. *BSSL*, bile salt-stimulated lipase; *HGL*, human gastric lipase; *PTL*, pancreatic triglyceride lipase; *PLRP1*, pancreatic lipase-related protein 1; *PLRP2*, pancreatic lipase-related protein 2. *Modified from McClean, P. & Weaver, L. T. (1993). Ontogeny of human pancreatic exocrine function. Archives of Disease in Childhood 68(1 Spec No), 62–65. https://doi.org/10.1136/adc.68.1_spec_no.62.*

(Lindquist & Hernell, 2010). Pancreatic triglyceride lipase alone cannot efficiently hydrolyze an intralipid emulsion or native MFG unless these emulsions are partially hydrolyzed by other lipases. Pre-digestion of human milk in the stomach may therefore increase the ability of pancreatic lipase-related protein 2 and BSSL, the latter secreted from both the mammary gland into milk and the exocrine pancreas, to further digest lipids from milk in the duodenum (Fig. 22.4) (Johnson, Ross, Miller, Xiao, & Lowe, 2013). BSSL is activated by primary bile salts and can hydrolyze a broad range of substrates including cholesteryl esters, retinol esters, triacylglycerols, diacylglycerols, monoacylglycerols, phospholipids, and ceramide. It is important to hydrolyze the glycerol esters of long-chain PUFAs, such as C22:6n-3 and C20:4n-6. BSSL is more active against medium- and long-chain triglycerides than pancreatic lipase-related protein 2. The lipolytic products self-assemble into various lipid-crystalline structures depending on their molar ratio relative to bile salts (Nilsson & Duan, 2006).

In the gut, breast milk sphingomyelin is first degraded to ceramide through the activity of the alkaline sphingomyelinase, and ceramide is further degraded to sphingosine by a neutral ceramidase, and finally, sphingosine is absorbed by the enterocytes (Nilsson & Duan, 2006).

22.4.2 Formation of calcium–FA soap complexes

In human milk, most of the calcium (~79%) is found in the soluble (whey) fraction. Ionized long-chain FAs will accumulate at the oil–water interface and can complex with local free Ca^{2+} in a 1:2M ratio to form a layer of crystalline calcium-FA soap (Torcello-Gómez, Boudard, & Mackie, 2018). In adults, the pH of the small intestine ranges from weakly acidic to neutral (duodenum: 5.0–7.4; jejunum: 5.5–7.7; ileum: 6.6–7.9), whereas in infants, the pH approaches neutrality (duodenum: 6.4; jejunum: 6.6; ileum: 6.9). The presence of bicarbonate and higher pH leads to a higher proportion of ionized FAs, enhancing FA soap formation and lipolysis (Bandali, Wang, Lan, Rogers, & Shapses, 2016). The majority of insoluble FA soap formation occurs in the distal small intestine. As the gut matures over time and bile salt concentrations increase, the absorption of saturated FAs will be significantly improved and therefore less will be available for soap formation.

22.4.3 Physiology and health role of human milk lipids

22.4.3.1 Breast milk lipids and gut microbiota

The high concentration of MCFA and the presence of sphingomyelin are unique to human milk. Sphingosine has antimicrobial effects against a series of bacteria, including *Escherichia coli* and *Staphylococcus aureus*. Lauric acid also has antimicrobial effects against a number of bacteria, including the species of *Fusobacterium*, *Clostridium*, *Salmonella*, and *Listeria* (Fischer et al., 2012). In addition, oleic acid has been found to stimulate the growth of several *Lactobacillus* species (Williams & Fieger, 1946). Addition of 50mM or higher concentrations of MCFA in cultured gut bacteria increased the relative abundance of lactic acid-producing genera, including *Lactobacillus* and *Bifidobacterium*. For *Bifidobacterium*, the same effect was also observed in the presence of a mixture containing long-chain FA and sphingosine. On the contrary, the relative abundance of Enterobacteriaceae was significantly decreased in the presence of both lipid mixtures (Nejrup et al., 2015). A study on mice revealed that the type of emulsifier as well as the type of oil consumed during intestinal colonization influences the resulting microbial community structure 14 days after inoculation (Nejrup, Licht, & Hellgren, 2017). This may influence the overall metabolic activity of the bacterial community.

MCFA and sphingomyelin in breast milk might have functional effects on the establishment of the gut microbiota in early life.

22.4.3.2 Lipid intake in early life, and later obesity risk and metabolic health

Early life nutrition plays a key role in infant growth and development and has a programming effect related to the appearance of future noncommunicable diseases, such as obesity and diabetes (Koletzko et al., 2019). Breast milk of overweight mothers contained increased saturated FAs and n-6:n-3 ratio and decreased ALA, DHA, and monounsaturated FAs (Mäkelä, Linderborg, Niinikoski, Yang, & Lagström, 2013). Infant BMI-for-age at 6 months of age was inversely associated with colostrum n-6 (e.g., AA) and n-3 (e.g., DHA) FAs and positively associated with the n-6:n-3 ratio (De La Garza Puentes et al., 2019). Results of the INFAT study showed that dietary intervention significantly reduced the breast milk n-6/n-3 long-chain PUFA ratio. Early breast milk DHA, EPA, and n-3 LC PUFAs at 6 weeks postpartum were positively related to the sum of four skinfold thickness measurements at age 1. And human milk ARA and n-6 long-chain PUFAs at 6 weeks postpartum were negatively associated with weight, BMI, and lean body mass up to 4 months postpartum (Much et al., 2013).

22.4.3.3 Milk lipids on the development of the nervous system

Phospholipids are also vital nutrients that play an important role in brain development. Higher levels of breast milk sphingomyelin were significantly associated with higher rates of change in verbal development in the first 2 years of life (Schneider et al., 2019).

Dietary supply of PUFAs is essential for infant brain development and function. Nearly 60% of the dry weight of the human brain consists of lipids, and approximately 35% of the lipids in the gray matter are long-chain PUFA. The most abundant long-chain PUFA in the neuronal membrane is ARA and DHA, which rapidly accumulates in the human brain during the first 1000 days, supporting the rapid increase in brain volume. Infant cognition was positively influenced by breast milk linoleic acid, n-6 PUFAs, ALA, DHA, and n-3 long-chain PUFAs and negatively affected by the n-6:n-3 ratio (De La Garza Puentes et al., 2019). A study that included samples of 28 countries revealed that breast milk DHA makes a highly significant contribution to math scores (Lassek & Gaulin, 2015). The DHA:ARA ratio of human milk is around 1:1.5, based on the mean concentrations of these LC PUFAs worldwide (Brenna et al., 2007). A proper balance between DHA and ARA is essential for optimal cognitive development. For supplementation in infant formulas, the recommendations state that DHA:ARA can range from 1:1 to 1.

22.5 Conclusion

In recent years, great progress has been made in the study of MFG. As the functional importance of MFG is gradually revealed, milk-derived MFGM will be gradually applied to infant formula as a potential supplement. With population studies of different sizes, we now know that geography or diet is a key factor in the composition of FAs in breast milk. At the same time, FA differences also lead to more complex triglyceride composition in breast milk. This suggests that in terms of FAs, there is a need for personalized formula for babies in different regions. It is necessary to establish a more ideal formula standard of triglyceride in breast milk. Seeking suitable sources or developing synthetic technology is the bottleneck problem of transforming breast milk triglyceride nutrition into industrial application. In terms of digestion, recent advances have shown that (1) BSSL provided by breast milk is an important active protein for infants to digest lipids. Gastric esterase is very important for babies. (2) Because MCFA has bactericidal activity, it will have an impact on the composition of intestinal flora. (3) The n-3 LC PUFAs affect brain development and are also associated with the incidence of obesity.

References

Ailhaud, G., Massiera, F., Weill, P., Legrand, P., Alessandri, J. M., & Guesnet, P. (2006). Temporal changes in dietary fats: Role of n-6 polyunsaturated fatty acids in excessive adipose tissue development and relationship to obesity. *Progress in Lipid Research*, 45(3), 203–236. https://doi.org/10.1016/j.plipres.2006.01.003.

Bahreynian, M., Feizi, A., & Kelishadi, R. (2020). Is fatty acid composition of breast milk different in various populations? A systematic review and meta-analysis. *International Journal of Food Sciences and Nutrition*, 71(8), 909–920. https://doi.org/10.1080/09637486.2020.1746958.

Bajpai, V. K. (2017). Availability and functionality of omega-3 in diversified marine algae. *Indian Journal of Geo-Marine Sciences*, 46(7), 1239–1244. http://nopr.niscair.res.in/bitstream/123456789/42258/1/IJMS%2046(7)%201239-1244.pdf.

Bandali, E., Wang, Y., Lan, Y., Rogers, M., & Shapses, S. A. (2016). The influence of dietary fat and intestinal pH on calcium bioaccessibility: An in vitro study. *Food & Function*, 9.

Beggio, M., Cruz-Hernandez, C., Golay, P. A., Lee, L. Y., & Giuffrida, F. (2018). Quantification of total cholesterol in human milk by gas chromatography. *Journal of Separation Science*, 41(8), 1805–1811. https://doi.org/10.1002/jssc.201700833.

Bernhard, W., Postle, A. D., Rau, G. A., & Freihorst, J. (2001). Pulmonary and gastric surfactants. A comparison of the effect of surface requirements on function and phospholipid composition. In *Vol. 129. Comparative biochemistry and physiology—A molecular and integrative physiology* (pp. 173–182). Elsevier Inc. https://doi.org/10.1016/S1095-6433(01)00314-2. Issue 1.

Bourlieu, C., Ménard, O., De La Chevasnerie, A., Sams, L., Rousseau, F., Madec, M. N., et al. (2015). The structure of infant formulas impacts their lipolysis, proteolysis and disintegration during in vitro gastric digestion. *Food Chemistry*, 182, 224–235. https://doi.org/10.1016/j.foodchem.2015.03.001.

Breckenridge, W., Marai, L., & Kuksis, A. (1969). Triglyceride structure of human milk fat. *Canadian Journal of Biochemistry*, 47, 761–769.

Brenna, J. T., Varamini, B., Jensen, R. G., Diersen-Schade, D. A., Boettcher, J. A., & Arterburn, L. M. (2007). Docosahexaenoic and arachidonic acid concentrations in human breast milk worldwide. *American Journal of Clinical Nutrition*, 85(6), 1457–1464. https://doi.org/10.1093/ajcn/85.6.1457.

Chen, Y., Zhang, X., Li, D., Yi, H., Xu, T., Li, S., et al. (2019). Fatty acid and triacylglycerol comparison of infant formulas on the Chinese market. *International Dairy Journal*, 95, 35–43. https://doi.org/10.1016/j.idairyj.2019.02.017.

Cilla, A., Diego Quintaes, K., Barberá, R., & Alegría, A. (2016). Phospholipids in human Milk and infant formulas: Benefits and needs for correct infant nutrition. *Critical Reviews in Food Science and Nutrition*, 56(11), 1880–1892. https://doi.org/10.1080/10408398.2013.803951.

Claumarchirant, L., Matencio, E., Sanchez-Siles, L. M., Alegría, A., & Lagarda, M. J. (2015). Sterol composition in infant formulas and estimated intake. *Journal of Agricultural and Food Chemistry*, 63(32), 7245–7251. https://doi.org/10.1021/acs.jafc.5b02647.

De La Garza Puentes, A., Alemany, A. M., Chisaguano, A. M., Goyanes, R. M., Castellote, A. I., Torres-Espínola, F. J., et al. (2019). The effect of maternal obesity on breast milk fatty acids and its association with infant growth and cognition-the PREOBE follow-up. *Nutrients*, 11(9). https://doi.org/10.3390/nu11092154.

Debier, C., & Larondelle, Y. (2005). Vitamins A and E: Metabolism, roles and transfer to offspring. *British Journal of Nutrition*, 93(2), 153–174. https://doi.org/10.1079/BJN20041308.

Delplanque, B., Gibson, R., Koletzko, B., Lapillonne, A., & Strandvik, B. (2015). Lipid quality in infant nutrition: Current knowledge and future opportunities. *Journal of Pediatric Gastroenterology and Nutrition*, 16(1), 8–17. https://doi.org/10.1097/MPG.0000000000000818.

DiPalma, J., Kirk, C. L., Hamosh, M., Colon, A. R., Benjamin, S. B., & Hamosh, P. (1991). Lipase and pepsin activity in the gastric mucosa of infants, children, and adults. *Gastroenterology*, 101(1), 116–121. https://doi.org/10.1016/0016-5085(91)90467-Y.

Fidler, N., Sauerwald, T., Pohl, A., Demmelmair, H., & Koletzko, B. (2000). Docosahexaenoic acid transfer into human milk after dietary supplementation: A randomized clinical trial. *Journal of Lipid Research*, 41(9), 1376–1383.

Fischer, C. L., Drake, D. R., Dawson, D. V., Blanchette, D. R., Brogden, K. A., & Wertz, P. W. (2012). Antibacterial activity of sphingoid bases and fatty acids against gram-positive and gram-negative bacteria. *Antimicrobial Agents and Chemotherapy*, 56(3), 1157–1161. https://doi.org/10.1128/AAC.05151-11.

Fontecha, J., Brink, L., Wu, S., Pouliot, Y., Visioli, F., & Jiménez-Flores, R. (2020). Sources, production, and clinical treatments of milk fat globule membrane for infant nutrition and well-being. *Nutrients*, 12(6). https://doi.org/10.3390/nu12061607.

Gallier, S., Vocking, K., Post, J. A., Van De Heijning, B., Acton, D., Van Der Beek, E. M., et al. (2015). A novel infant milk formula concept: Mimicking the human milk fat globule structure. *Colloids and Surfaces B: Biointerfaces*, 136, 329–339. https://doi.org/10.1016/j.colsurfb.2015.09.024.

Gastaldi, D., Medana, C., Giancotti, V., Aigotti, R., Dal Bello, F., & Baiocchi, C. (2011). HPLC-APCI analysis of triacylglycerols in milk fat from different sources. *European Journal of Lipid Science and Technology*, 113(2), 197–207. https://doi.org/10.1002/ejlt.201000068.

George, A. D., Gay, M. C. L., Wlodek, M. E., Trengove, R. D., Murray, K., & Geddes, D. T. (2020). Untargeted lipidomics using liquid chromatography-ion mobility-mass spectrometry reveals novel triacylglycerides in human milk. *Scientific Reports*, 10(1). https://doi.org/10.1038/s41598-020-66235-y.

He, Y., Wu, T., Sun, H., Sun, P., Liu, B., Luo, M., et al. (2019). Comparison of fatty acid composition and positional distribution of microalgae triacylglycerols for human milk fat substitutes. *Algal Research*, 37, 40–50. https://doi.org/10.1016/j.algal.2018.11.004.

Innis, S. M. (2007). Human milk: Maternal dietary lipids and infant development. *Proceedings of the Nutrition Society*, 66(3), 397–404. https://doi.org/10.1017/S0029665107005666.

Innis, S. M. (2014). Impact of maternal diet on human milk composition and neurological development of infants. *American Journal of Clinical Nutrition*, 99(3). https://doi.org/10.3945/ajcn.113.072595.

Jiang, J., Wu, K., Yu, Z., Ren, Y., Zhao, Y., Jiang, Y., et al. (2016). Changes in fatty acid composition of human milk over lactation stages and relationship with dietary intake in Chinese women. *Food & Function*, 7(7), 3154–3162. https://doi.org/10.1039/c6fo00304d.

Jiang, J., Xiao, H., Wu, K., Yu, Z., Ren, Y., Zhao, Y., et al. (2016). Retinol and α-tocopherol in human milk and their relationship with dietary intake during lactation. *Food & Function*, 7(4), 1985–1991. https://doi.org/10.1039/c5fo01293g.

Johnson, K., Ross, L., Miller, R., Xiao, X., & Lowe, M. E. (2013). Pancreatic lipase-related protein 2 digests fats in human milk and formula in concert with gastric lipase and carboxyl ester lipase. *Pediatric Research*, 74(2), 127–132. https://doi.org/10.1038/pr.2013.90.

Kallio, H., Nylund, M., Boström, P., & Yang, B. (2017). Triacylglycerol regioisomers in human milk resolved with an algorithmic novel electrospray ionization tandem mass spectrometry method. *Food Chemistry*, 233, 351–360. https://doi.org/10.1016/j.foodchem.2017.04.122.

Koh, S. P., Tan, C. P., Lai, O. M., Arifin, N., Yusoff, M. S. A., & Long, K. (2010). Enzymatic synthesis of medium- and long-chain triacylglycerols (MLCT): Optimization of process parameters using response surface methodology. *Food and Bioprocess Technology*, 3(2), 288–299. https://doi.org/10.1007/s11947-008-0073-y.

Koletzko, B., Godfrey, K. M., Poston, L., Szajewska, H., Van Goudoever, J. B., De Waard, M., et al. (2019). Nutrition during pregnancy, lactation and early childhood and its implications for maternal and long-term child health: The early nutrition project recommendations. *Annals of Nutrition and Metabolism*, 74(2), 93–106. https://doi.org/10.1159/000496471.

Koletzko, B., & Sinclair, A. (1999). Long-chain polyunsaturated fatty acids in diets for infants: Choices for recommending and regulating bodies and for manufacturers of dietary products. *Lipids*, 34(2), 215–220. https://doi.org/10.1007/s11745-999-0356-x.

Koo, W. W. K., Hockman, E. M., Koo, W. W. K., & Dow, M. (2006). Palm Olein in the fat blend of infant formulas: Effect on the intestinal absorption of calcium and fat, and bone mineralization. *Journal of the American College of Nutrition*, 25(2), 117–122. https://doi.org/10.1080/07315724.2006.10719521.

Korma, S. A., Zou, X., Ali, A. H., Abed, S. M., Jin, Q., & Wang, X. (2018). Preparation of structured lipids enriched with medium- and long-chain triacylglycerols by enzymatic interesterification for infant formula. *Food and Bioproducts Processing*, 107, 121–130. https://doi.org/10.1016/j.fbp.2017.11.006.

Lassek, W. D., & Gaulin, S. J. C. (2015). Maternal milk DHA content predicts cognitive performance in a sample of 28 nations. *Maternal & Child Nutrition*, 11(4), 773–779. https://doi.org/10.1111/mcn.12060.

Lavy, U., Silverberg, M., & Davidson, M. (1971). Role of bile acids in fat absorption in low birth weights infants. *Pediatric Research*, 5(8), 387.

Lindquist, S., & Hernell, O. (2010). Lipid digestion and absorption in early life: An update. *Current Opinion in Clinical Nutrition and Metabolic Care*, 13(3), 314–320. https://doi.org/10.1097/MCO.0b013e328337bbf0.

Liu, Z., Cocks, B. G., & Rochfort, S. (2016). Comparison of molecular species distribution of DHA-containing triacylglycerols in milk and different infant formulas by liquid chromatography-mass spectrometry. *Journal of Agricultural and Food Chemistry*, 64(10), 2134–2144. https://doi.org/10.1021/acs.jafc.5b05920.

Ma, L., MacGibbon, A. K. H., Jan Mohamed, H. J. B., Loy, S. L., Rowan, A., McJarrow, P., et al. (2017). Determination of phospholipid concentrations in breast milk and serum using a high performance liquid chromatography–mass spectrometry–multiple reaction monitoring method. *International Dairy Journal*, 71, 50–59. https://doi.org/10.1016/j.idairyj.2017.03.005.

Mäkelä, J., Linderborg, K., Niinikoski, H., Yang, B., & Lagström, H. (2013). Breast milk fatty acid composition differs between overweight and normal weight women: The STEPS study. *European Journal of Nutrition*, 52(2), 727–735. https://doi.org/10.1007/s00394-012-0378-5.

Mather, I. H., & Keenan, T. W. (1998). Origin and secretion of milk lipids. *Journal of Mammary Gland Biology and Neoplasia*, 3(3), 259–273. https://doi.org/10.1023/A:1018711410270.

McManaman, J. L. (2009). Formation of milk lipids: A molecular perspective. *Future Lipidology*, 4(3), 391–401. https://doi.org/10.2217/CLP.09.15.

Mitoulas, L. R., Kent, J. C., Cox, D. B., Owens, R. A., Sherriff, J. L., & Hartmann, P. E. (2002). Variation in fat, lactose and protein in human milk over 24h and throughout the first year of lactation. *British Journal of Nutrition*, 88(1), 29–37. https://doi.org/10.1079/BJNBJN2002579.

Mohammad, M. A., Sunehag, A. L., & Haymond, M. W. (2014). De novo synthesis of milk triglycerides in humans. *American Journal of Physiology - Endocrinology and Metabolism*, 306(7), E838–E847. https://doi.org/10.1152/ajpendo.00605.2013.

Much, D., Brunner, S., Vollhardt, C., Schmid, D., Sedlmeier, E. M., Brüderl, M., et al. (2013). Breast milk fatty acid profile in relation to infant growth and body composition: Results from the INFAT study. *Pediatric Research*, 74(2), 230–237. https://doi.org/10.1038/pr.2013.82.

Nejrup, R. G., Bahl, M. I., Vigsnæs, L. K., Heerup, C., Licht, T. R., & Hellgren, L. I. (2015). Lipid hydrolysis products affect the composition of infant gut microbial communities in vitro. *British Journal of Nutrition*, 114(1), 63–74. https://doi.org/10.1017/S0007114515000811.

Nejrup, R. G., Licht, T. R., & Hellgren, L. I. (2017). Fatty acid composition and phospholipid types used in infant formulas modifies the establishment of human gut bacteria in germ-free mice. *Scientific Reports*, 7(1), 1–11.

Neville, M. C., & Picciano, M. F. (1997). Regulation of milk lipid secretion and composition. *Annual Review of Nutrition*, 17, 159–184. https://doi.org/10.1146/annurev.nutr.17.1.159.

Niklas, T., & Bo, M. (2015). Comment on 'Safety and tolerance evaluation of milk fat globule membrane-enriched infant formulas: A randomized controlled multicenter non-inferiority trial in healthy term infants.'. *Clinical Medicine Insights. Pediatrics*, 9, 63–64.

Nilsson, A., & Duan, R. D. (2006). Absorption and lipoprotein transport of sphingomyelin. *Journal of Lipid Research*, 47(1), 154–171. https://doi.org/10.1194/jlr.M500357-JLR200.

Qi, C., Sun, J., Xia, Y., Yu, R., Wei, W., Xiang, J., et al. (2018). Fatty acid profile and the sn-2 position distribution in triacylglycerols of breast milk during different lactation stages. *Journal of Agricultural and Food Chemistry*, 66(12), 3118–3126. https://doi.org/10.1021/acs.jafc.8b01085.

Ransac, S., Rogalska, E., Gargouri, Y., Deveer, A. M. T. J., Paltauf, F., De Haas, G. H., et al. (1990). Stereoselectivity of lipases. I. Hydrolysis of enantiomeric glyceride analogues by gastric and pancreatic lipases, a kinetic study using the monomolecular film technique. *Journal of Biological Chemistry*, 265(33), 20263–20270.

Schneider, N., Hauser, J., Oliveira, M., Cazaubon, E., Mottaz, S. C., O'Neill, B. V., et al. (2019). Sphingomyelin in brain and cognitive development: Preliminary data. *eNeuro*, 6(4). https://doi.org/10.1523/ENEURO.0421-18.2019.

Silva, M. H. L., Silva, M. T. C., Brandão, S. C. C., Gomes, J. C., Peternelli, L. A., & Franceschini, S. D. C. C. (2005). Fatty acid composition of mature breast milk in Brazilian women. *Food Chemistry*, 93(2), 297–303. https://doi.org/10.1016/j.foodchem.2004.09.026.

Suburu, J., Shi, L., Wu, J., Wang, S., Samuel, M., Thomas, M. J., et al. (2014). Fatty acid synthase is required for mammary gland development and milk production during lactation. *American Journal of Physiology - Endocrinology and Metabolism*, 306(10), E1132–E1143. https://doi.org/10.1152/ajpendo.00514.2013.

Torcello-Gómez, A., Boudard, C., & Mackie, A. R. (2018). Calcium alters the interfacial organization of hydrolyzed lipids during intestinal digestion. *Langmuir*, 34(25), 7536–7544. https://doi.org/10.1021/acs.langmuir.8b00841.

Williams, V. R., & Fieger, E. A. (1946). Oleic acid as a growth stimulant for *Lactobacillus casei*. *The Journal of Biological Chemistry*, 166(1), 335–343.

Wong, W. W., Hachey, D. L., Insull, W., Opekun, A. R., & Klein, P. D. (1993). Effect of dietary cholesterol on cholesterol synthesis in breast-fed and formula-fed infants. *Journal of Lipid Research*, 34(8), 1403–1411.

Ye, A., Cui, J., Dalgleish, D., & Singh, H. (2016). The formation and breakdown of structured clots from whole milk during gastric digestion. *Food & Function*, 7(10), 4259–4266. https://doi.org/10.1039/c6fo00228e.

Yin, S. A., & Yang, Z. Y. (2016). An on-line database for human milk composition in China. *Asia Pacific Journal of Clinical Nutrition*, 25(4), 818–825. https://doi.org/10.6133/apjcn.092015.47.

Yu, G., Zheng, Q. S., & Li, G. F. (2014). Similarities and differences in gastrointestinal physiology between neonates and adults: A physiologically based pharmacokinetic modeling perspective. *The AAPS Journal*, 16(6), 1162–1166. https://doi.org/10.1208/s12248-014-9652-1.

Yuan, T., Qi, C., Dai, X., Xia, Y., Sun, C., Sun, J., et al. (2019). Triacylglycerol composition of breast Milk during different lactation stages. *Journal of Agricultural and Food Chemistry*, 67(8), 2272–2278. https://doi.org/10.1021/acs.jafc.8b06554.

Yuan, T., Zhang, H., Wang, X., Yu, R., Zhou, Q., Wei, W., et al. (2019). Triacylglycerol containing medium-chain fatty acids (MCFA-TAG): The gap between human milk and infant formulas. *International Dairy Journal*, 99. https://doi.org/10.1016/j.idairyj.2019.104545.

Index

Note: Page numbers followed by *f* indicate figures and *t* indicate tables.

A

ABCG5/8, 343
Addiction, 64
Alanine aminotransferase (ALT), 136–138
Alpha-linolenic acid (ALA), 51
Ameliorate cancer cachexia, 100–101
Ameliorate chemotherapy resistance, 99–100
Aminotransferase (AST), 136–138
AMP-activated protein kinase (AMPK), 142–143
Anticancer activities, 306–307
Antifungal activity, 309*t*
Anti-inflammatory activities, 306
Anti-inflammatory response, 183
Antimicrobial and larvicidal activities, 307–310, 308*t*
Antioxidant activity of, 264–265
Anxiety disorders, 59–60
Apoptosis, 85–86
Arachidonic acid, 33–35
Aspartate aminotransferase (AST), 138–140
Asthma, 148–149
Atherogenesis, 196–198
Atherogenic postprandial phenotype, 194–196
Attention-deficit/hyperactivity disorder (ADHD), 60–61
Autism spectrum disorder (ASD), 63

B

Beckwith-Wiedemann syndrome, 243
Benecol margarine, 345–346
Biosynthesis, 319–321
Bipolar disorders (BDs), 62
Birth defects
   animal studies, 245
   eicosanoid
      composition, 244
      metabolism, 246
   fatty acids, 244
   inositol, 244–245
   mechanism, 245–247
   protein kinase C (PKC), 246–247
   risk in human studies, 244–245
Blood lipids, 128–129
Blood pressure, dietary supplements of lipids on, 169–173
Body weight, 287–288
Brain
   anatomical regions, 30–31
   arachidonic acid, 33–35
   brain anatomical regions, 30–31
   contrast lipid content, 29–30
   diversity of lipids, 27–29
   docosahexaenoic acid (DHA), 27–28, 32–33
   eicosanoids, 34–35
   exogenous/dietary agents on, 36–40
      cholesterol, 37
      ethanol, 36–37
      lipid peroxidation, 37–38
      methyl mercury (MeHg), 39–40
      microparticulate plastic, 39
      plasticizers and microparticulate plastics, 38–39
      reactive oxygen species (ROS), 37–38
      saturated fat-enriched diets, 37
      thyroid hormones (THs), 39
      traumatic brain injury (TBI), 38
   fatty acids, 29–30
   galactosphingolipids, 29
   gangliosides, 28–29
   G-coupled membrane proteins, 28
   hypermetabolism, 34–35
   inositol phospholipids, 29
   lipid mediators, 29
   lipids metabolism in, 51–53, 52*f*
   lipids synthesized
      fatty acid transport, 35–36
      14C-labeled polyunsaturated fatty acids, 35–36
      uptake from blood, 35
   mass spectrometry techniques, 31–32
   membrane lipids, 29
   myelin, 28–29
   oligodendrocytes, 28
   omega-3 PUFA deficiency, 34–35
   phosphatidylcholine (PC), 28
   phosphatidylserine, 28–29
   n-3 polyunsaturated fatty acids (PUFAs), 32
   polyunsaturated fatty acids (PUFAs), 30–31
   properties, 32–35
   saturated fatty acids, 32
   specialized lipid mediators (SPMs), 33
   sphingomyelin, 29
   unsaturated fatty acids, 32
BRD4 inhibitor, 98–99
Breast cancer
   epidemiological evidence, 111–114
      dietary lipids exposure timing, 113–114
      different fatty acid types, 113
      fat intake, 112–113
   n-3 PUFA, 114–121
      epidemiological evidence, 114–116
      Faecalibacterium, 119–120
      fish fat intake, 117–118*t*
      long non-coding RNA (lncRNA) regulation, 116–119
      mechanisms, 116–121

Breast milk
  composition of, 354–359
    fat-soluble nutrients, 358
    fatty acid, 354–357, 355f
    milk fat globule, 354, 355f
    phospholipids, 357–358, 358t
    sterols, 358
  formula lipid nutrition, 363–365
    digestion, infant gastrointestinal tract, 363–364
    FA soap complexes, 364
    formation of calcium, 364
    gut microbiota, 364–365
    metabolic health, 365
    nervous system, 365
    obesity risk, 365
  formulas composition
    fatty acid, 359–361
    formulas lipids, sources of, 361–363
    human milk fat substitutes, 362–363
    marine oils, 362
    microbial oils, 362
    minor constituents, 361
    phospholipids, 361
    triacylglycerol profile, 359–361
    vegetable oils and animal fat, 361–362
  milk fat globules (MFGs), 353
  polyunsaturated FAs (PUFAs), 353–354
  source of
    long-chain polyunsaturated FAs, 358–359
    medium-chain and long-chain FAs, 358
  triacylglycerols (TAGs), 353

C

Cancer
  fatty acid, 217–218
  fatty acid synthase (FASN), 218–219
  4-hydroxynonenal (HNE), 219
  lipid peroxidation metabolites on cancer development, 219
Carcinogenesis
  pomegranate seed oil (PSO), 254
  in vitro studies, 253–254
  in vivo studies, 254–255
Cardiometabolic disorder, 173–175

Cardiometabolic health
  dietary fat and
    fat content on weight, 78
    fat-to-carbohydrate ratios, 76–78
    food sources, 75
    gut microbiota, 79–80
    higher fat content, 79, 79f
    microbial metabolites, 79–80
    trends in, 75–76
    types of, 75
Cardiovascular disease (CVD), 5–7, 136, 193, 204–205, 211–212, 329
  association between ceramides, 216
  association between eicosanoids, 216–217
Cell proliferation, 85–86
Cholesterol, 37
Cholesterol-lowering effects
  age of subjects, 338
  animal studies, 333–335
  clinical studies, 335–341
  dose response, 335–338
  food matrix type, 339–340
  free versus esterified phytosterols, 341
  intake frequency and occasion, 338–339
  lipid characteristics, 338
  phytostanols, 340
Chronic kidney disease, 10
Chronic obstructive pulmonary disease (COPD), 147, 153–154
Chylomicron (CM), 197f
Cis-PUFA, 6
Cognition, 8–9
Colorectal cancer (CRC), 91–101
Conjugated fatty acids (CFAs), 251
Conjugated linolenic acids (CLNAs)
  antioxidant activity of, 264–265
  bioactivities of, 253f
  carcinogenesis
    pomegranate seed oil (PSO), 254
    in vitro studies, 253–254
    in vivo studies, 254–255
  conjugated fatty acids (CFAs), 251
  inflammatory bowel diseases, 261–264, 262t
  lipid metabolism
    hepatic triglyceride accumulation, 257–258
    plasma/serum lipid metabolism, 255–257, 255–256t
  metabolism of, 252–253

  natural sources, 251–252
  obesity, 258–260, 258–259t
  type 2 diabetes mellitus, 260–261
  utilization, 251–252
Contrast lipid content, 29–30
Cooking oil, 290
Coronary heart disease (CHD), 345–346
Cosmetic industry, 310
C-reactive protein, 19–21
Crohn's disease (CD), 233–234
Cross-sectional and prospective studies, 14–17
Cystathionine β-synthase (CBS), 273–274
Cytochrome P450, 182

D

Dementia, 61–62
Deoxyguanine (dG), 14
Depression, 9, 56–59
Diabetes mellitus, 7
1,3-diacylglycerol, cardiometabolic risk, 287–288
  body weight, 287–288
  definition, 285–287
  direct esterification, 286
  fasting lipids, 288–289
  glucose metabolism, 289
  glycerol, 285
  glycolysis method, 287
  hypertriglyceridemia (HTG), 288
  metabolism, 289–290
    hydrolysis of, 289–290
    resynthesis of, 290
  postprandial lipids, 288
  selective hydrolysis, 286–287
  source of, 286
  supplementation, 290–291
    cooking oil, 290
    dietary supplements, 291
Dietary Approaches to Stop Hypertension (DASH), 165
Dietary fats, 199
  fat content on weight, 78
  fat-to-carbohydrate ratios, 76–78
  food sources, 75
  gut microbiota, 79–80
  higher fat content, 79, 79f
  microbial metabolites, 79–80
  trends in, 75–76
  types of, 75
Dietary fatty acid, 14

Dietary lipids, 111–112
    cardiovascular disease (CVD), 5
    categories, 2
    cholesterol, 2
    cis-PUFA, 6
    dietary monounsaturated fat intake, 6
    dietary polyunsaturated fat intake, 6–10
        cancers, 7–8
        cardiovascular diseases, 6–7
        chronic kidney disease, 10
        cognition, 8–9
        depression, 9
        diabetes mellitus, 7
        inflammation, 10
        nonalcoholic fatty liver disease (NAFLD), 9–10
        respiratory diseases, 8
        risk factors, 6–7
    dietary total fat intake, 3–5
    exposure timing, 113–114
    high-density lipoprotein cholesterol (HDL-C), 3
    homeostasis model assessment for insulin resistance (HOMA-IR), 5
    human health, 3–5
    lipoprotein cholesterol (LDL-C), 3
    longitudinal cohort-based relationship of case-control/cross-sectional studies, 180–181
    high blood pressure, 175–180
    nonpolar lipids, 2
    palm oil, 5
    plant/vegetable seed oil and animal fat, 2
    polar lipids, 2
    randomized controlled trials (RCTs), 5
    total cholesterol (TC), 3
    triacylglycerol (TG), 2
Dietary monounsaturated fat intake, 6
Dietary n–3 lipids, antihypertensive effects of, 181–185
Dietary polyunsaturated fat intake, 6–10
    cancers, 7–8
    cardiovascular diseases, 6–7
    chronic kidney disease, 10
    cognition, 8–9
    depression, 9
    diabetes mellitus, 7
    inflammation, 10
    nonalcoholic fatty liver disease (NAFLD), 9–10
    respiratory diseases, 8
    risk factors, 6–7
Dietary supplements, 291
Dietary total fat intake, 3–5
Digestive system, malignant tumor of colorectal cancer (CRC), 91–101
    gastric cancer, 83–87
        anti-inflammatory effects, 85
        apoptosis, 85–86
        cell proliferation, 85–86
        chemotherapeutic agents, 86
        dietary lipids influence, 85–87
        drug-resistant effects, 86–87
        epidemiological evidence, 84
        H. pylori-induced gastric carcinogenesis, 84–85
        PUFAs, 84–86
        synergistic anticancer effect of PUFAs, 86
    liver carcinoma, 87–91
        apoptosis, 88–89
        cancer stem cells, 89–90
        cell proliferation, 88–89
        epidemiological evidence, 87–88
        nonalcoholic steatohepatitis (NASH), 90
        PUFAs, 88–91
    n–3 PUFAs, 91–101
        ameliorate cancer cachexia, 100–101
        ameliorate chemotherapy resistance, 99–100
        BRD4 inhibitor, 98–99
        epidemiological evidence, 91–92
        5-fluorouracil (5-FU), 97–98
        immunomodulatory effects, 93–95
        mitochondrial apoptosis-mediated chemoprevention by fatty acids, 95–97
        paclitaxel, 99
        platinum chemotherapeutic drugs, 98
        radiotherapy and chemotherapy, sensitization to, 97–100
        sensitization to chemotherapy, 97–98
        sensitization to radiotherapy, 100
        sulindac analogues, 99
Direct esterification, 286
Diversity of lipids, 27–29
Docosahexaenoic acid (DHA), 136–138, 141–142
Docosapentaenoic acid, 33

E
Eating disorders (ED), 63–64
Eicosanoids, 34–35
    composition, 244
    metabolism, 246
    pathway, 184
Eicosapentaenoic acid (EPA), 138–140
Endothelial function, 181–183
Endothelin-1 (ET1), 182–183
eNO synthase (eNOS), 181–182
EPA/DHA, 58–59, 64–65
Epanova Program in Crohn's Study (EPIC-1), 234–235
Essential fatty acids (EFAs), 51
Ethanol, 36–37
Exogenous/dietary agents, 36–40
    cholesterol, 37
    ethanol, 36–37
    lipid peroxidation, 37–38
    methyl mercury (MeHg), 39–40
    microparticulate plastic, 39
    plasticizers and microparticulate plastics, 38–39
    reactive oxygen species (ROS), 37–38
    saturated fat-enriched diets, 37
    thyroid hormones (THs), 39
    traumatic brain injury (TBI), 38

F
FA soap complexes, 364
Fasting lipids, 288–289
Fat-soluble nutrients, 358
Fat-to-carbohydrate ratios, 76–78
Fatty acid, 29–30, 136–140, 244, 354–357, 355f, 359–361
    exposure, randomized control trials on, 150–152t
    metabolism, 304–305
Fish oil, antihypertensive effect of, 173
5-fluorouracil (5-FU), 97–98
Folate, 245–246
Free fatty acid (FFA), 135, 293

G
Galactosphingolipids, 29
Gangliosides, 28–29

Gastric cancer, 83–87
　anti-inflammatory effects, 85
　apoptosis, 85–86
　cell proliferation, 85–86
　chemotherapeutic agents, 86
　dietary lipids influence, 85–87
　drug-resistant effects, 86–87
　epidemiological evidence, 84
　H. pylori-induced gastric carcinogenesis, 84–85
　PUFAs, 84–86
　synergistic anticancer effect of PUFAs, 86
G-coupled membrane proteins, 28
Gene-diet interaction, 128
Generally Recognized as Safe (GRAS), 346
Genome-wide association studies (GWASs), 243
Genotype-by-environment interaction (GxE), 128
Gestational diabetes, 131
Glial activation, 235
Glucose metabolism, 289
Glucose transporter-4 (GLUT4), 142–143
Glutamyl transpeptidase (GGT), 136–138
Glycemic control, 130–131
Glycerol, 285
Glycolysis method, 287
Gut-brain axis, 184–185
Gut microbiota, 79–80, 214–216, 364–365
　host lipid metabolism, 215–216
　phylogenetic diversity of, 214–215
　short chain fatty acids, 216

H

1,2,3,4,5,6-hexahydroxycyclohexane, 244–245
High-density lipoprotein (HDL), 129
High-density lipoprotein cholesterol (HDL-C), 3
Higher fat content, 79, 79f
High-performance liquid chromatography (HPLC), 304
Homeostasis model assessment for insulin resistance (HOMA-IR), 5, 130–131

Homocysteine (Hcy)
　cell culture, 277–278
　cystathionine β-synthase (CBS), 273–274
　definition, 273–274
　epidemiological evidence, 274–277
　genetic risk, 276–277
　hyperhomocysteinemia (HHcy), 273–276
　metabolic pathways, 278–279
　methionine synthase (MS), 273–274
　methyltetrahydrofolate reductase (MTHFR), 273–274
　nutritional modulation of, 274
　n-3 PUFAs, 274–275
　　cardiometabolic risk factors, 279–280
　　research, 280–281
　　vitamins, 280
　remethylation, 273–274
H. pylori-induced gastric carcinogenesis, 84–85
Human memory CD8 T cells, 19–21
Hyperhomocysteinemia (HHcy), 273–276
Hypermetabolism, 34–35
Hypertension
　anti-inflammatory response, 183
　blood pressure, dietary supplements of lipids on, 169–173
　cardiometabolic disorder, 173–175
　general/health population, 169–173
　clinical epidemiological traits, 166–167
　cytochrome P450, 182
　Dietary Approaches to Stop Hypertension (DASH), 165
　dietary lipids, longitudinal cohort-based relationship of case-control/cross-sectional studies, 180–181
　high blood pressure, 175–180
　dietary n-3 lipids, antihypertensive effects of, 181–185
　eicosanoid pathway, 184
　endothelial function, 181–183
　endothelin-1 (ET1), 182–183
　eNO synthase (eNOS), 181–182
　evidence based on, 175–181
　fish oil, antihypertensive effect of, 173
　gut-brain axis, 184–185

　lipid medical implications, 168–169
　meta-analytic evidence, 169–175
　metabolites, 167–168
　monounsaturated fatty acids (MUFAs), 165
　n-3polyunsaturated fatty acids (PUFAs), 165
　prevention and management, 168–169
　renin-angiotensin aldosterone system (RAAS), 184
　saturated fatty acids (SFAs), 165
　specialized pro-resolving mediators (SPMs), 183
　systolic BP (SBP), 165
　vascular reactivity, 181–183
　vascular smooth muscle cells (VSMC), 182
Hypertriglyceridemia (HTG), 288

I

Idiopathic pulmonary fibrosis, 148
Immune system, 53–55
Immunity regulation, 159–160
Inflammation, 53
Inflammatory bowel disease (IBD), 233–234, 261–264, 262t
Inflammatory diseases, 225–228
　Alzheimer's disease, 235–237
　inflammatory bowel disease (IBD), 233–235
　nonsteroidal antiinflammatory drugs (NSAIDs), 228
　RCTs, 229–232t
　rheumatoid arthritis (RA), 228–233
Inositol, 244–245
　phospholipids, 29
Insulin, 196
　resistance, 142–143
Interesterification (IE), 201–202

K

Ketogenesis, 212–213
Ketolysis, 213

L

Linoleic acid (LA), 51
Lipid mediators, 29
Lipid medical implications, 168–169
Lipid metabolism
　hepatic triglyceride accumulation, 257–258

plasma/serum lipid metabolism, 255–257, 255–256t
Lipid metabolism disorder (LMD)
 cancer, 217–219
  fatty acid, 217–218
  fatty acid synthase (FASN), 218–219
  4-hydroxynonenal (HNE), 219
  lipid peroxidation metabolites on cancer development, 219
 cardiovascular diseases (CVDs), 211–212, 216–217
  association between ceramides, 216
  association between eicosanoids, 216–217
 gut microbiota, 214–216
  host lipid metabolism, 215–216
  phylogenetic diversity of, 214–215
  short chain fatty acids, 216
 ketogenesis, 212–213
 ketolysis, 213
 lipid peroxidation, 213–214
 lipogenesis, 212
 lipolysis, 212
 neurodegenerative disease, 219–220
 β-oxidation, 212
 total cholesterol (TC), 211–212
Lipid peroxidation, 37–38, 213–214
Lipids synthesized
 fatty acid transport, 35–36
 14C-labeled polyunsaturated fatty acids, 35–36
 uptake from blood, 35
Lipogenesis, 212
Lipokine, 297–301
Lipolysis, 212
Lipoprotein cholesterol (LDL-C), 3
Liver carcinoma, 87–91
 apoptosis, 88–89
 cancer stem cells, 89–90
 cell proliferation, 88–89
 epidemiological evidence, 87–88
 nonalcoholic steatohepatitis (NASH), 90
 PUFAs, 88–91
Long-chain polyunsaturated FAs, 358–359
Low-fat dietary pattern, 112
Low-temperature crystallization, 314–317
Lung cancer, 155–156

M

Maresin 1, 159
Marine n-3 polyunsaturated fatty acids
 inflammatory diseases, 225–228
  Alzheimer's disease, 235–237
  inflammatory bowel disease (IBD), 233–235
  nonsteroidal antiinflammatory drugs (NSAIDs), 228
  RCTs, 229–232t
  rheumatoid arthritis (RA), 228–233
Mass spectrometry techniques, 31–32
Medium-chain and long-chain FAs, 358
Membrane lipids, 29
Mental health
 alpha-linolenic acid (ALA), 51
 brain, lipids metabolism in, 51–53, 52f
 essential fatty acids (EFAs), 51
 immune system, 53–55
 inflammation, 53
 linoleic acid (LA), 51
 microbiota, 53–55
 nervous system, 55–56
 omega-3 fatty acids, 56–65
  addiction, 64
  anxiety disorders, 59–60
  attention-deficit/hyperactivity disorder (ADHD), 60–61
  autism spectrum disorder (ASD), 63
  bipolar disorders (BDs), 62
  dementia, 61–62
  depression, 56–59
  eating disorders (ED), 63–64
  EPA/DHA, 58–59, 64–65
  post-traumatic stress disorder (PTSD), 62
  schizophrenia (SCZ), 63
 oxidative stress, 53
 polyunsaturated fatty acids (PUFAs), 51
 n-3 PUFAs in psychiatry disorders, 65–66t
Meta-analyses, 127t
Metabolic diseases, 295–297, 295f
 cardiovascular diseases, 296–297
 diabetes, 296
 obesity, 295–296
Metabolic health, 365
Methionine synthase (MS), 273–274
Methyl mercury (MeHg), 39–40
Methyltetrahydrofolate reductase (MTHFR), 273–274
Microbial metabolites, 79–80
Microbial oils, 362
Microbiota, 53–55
Microparticulate plastic, 39
Milk fat globules (MFGs), 353–354, 355f
Mitochondrial apoptosis-mediated chemoprevention by fatty acids, 95–97
Monoacylglycerides (MAG), 193–194
4-monomethyl sterols, 330–331
Monounsaturated fatty acid (MUFA), 165, 293
Myelin, 28–29

N

National Birth Defects Prevention Study (NBDPS), 244
Nervous system, 55–56, 365
Neurodegenerative disease, 219–220
Neuroinflammation, 235
Nonalcoholic fatty liver disease (NAFLD), 9–10
 aspartate aminotransferase (AST), 138–140
 biomarkers, 141
 eicosapentaenoic acid (EPA), 138–140
 factors affecting, 141
 fatty acids, 136–140
 polycystic ovary syndrome (PCOS), 138–140
 n-3 PUFA intake, 141–142
 biomarkers, 141–142
 mechanisms, 142–143, 143f
 randomized controlled trials (RCTs), 136–138
 triacylglycerol (TAG), 135
Nonalcoholic steatohepatitis (NASH), 90
Nonpolar lipids, 2
Novel lipid hormone, 294
Nutrigenetics, 128

O

Obesity, 258–260, 258–259t
Olacaceae and Opiliacea family, 317t
Oligodendrocytes, 28
Omega-3 fatty acids, 14, 56–65
 addiction, 64
 anxiety disorders, 59–60

Omega-3 fatty acids (Continued)
  attention-deficit/hyperactivity disorder (ADHD), 60–61
  autism spectrum disorder (ASD), 63
  bipolar disorders (BDs), 62
  dementia, 61–62
  depression, 56–59
  eating disorders (ED), 63–64
  EPA/DHA, 58–59, 64–65
  post-traumatic stress disorder (PTSD), 62
  schizophrenia (SCZ), 63
Omega-3 PUFA deficiency, 34–35
β-oxidation, 212
Oxidative stress, 53

P

Paclitaxel, 99
Palmitoleic acid
  free fatty acids (FFAs), 293
  lipokine, 297–301
  metabolic diseases, 295–297, 295f
    cardiovascular diseases, 296–297
    diabetes, 296
    obesity, 295–296
  monounsaturated fatty acid (MUFA), 293
  novel lipid hormone, 294
  stearoyl-CoA desaturase-1 (SCD-1), 293
Palm oil, 5
Peripheral blood mononuclear cells (PBMCs), 18–19
Peroxisome activation receptor (PPAR), 142–143
Phosphatidylcholine (PC), 28
Phosphatidylserine, 28–29
Phospholipids, 357–358, 358t
Phytosterols
  cardiovascular diseases (CVDs), 329
  cholesterol-lowering effects
    age of subjects, 338
    animal studies, 333–335
    clinical studies, 335–341
    dose response, 335–338
    food matrix type, 339–340
    free versus esterified phytosterols, 341
    intake frequency and occasion, 338–339
    lipid characteristics, 338
    mechanisms, 341–345
    phytostanols, 340
  commercial applications, 345–346
  future perspectives, 346
  4-monomethyl sterols, 330–331
  regulated policy, 345–346
  sources, 329–332
  structure diversity, 329–332
  vegetable oils, 331t
Plant/vegetable seed oil and animal fat, 2
Plasticizers and microparticulate plastics, 38–39
Platinum chemotherapeutic drugs, 98
Pneumonia, 148–153
Polar lipids, 2
Polycystic ovary syndrome (PCOS), 138–140
n-3 polyunsaturated fatty acids (PUFAs), 32
n-3 polyunsaturated fatty acids (PUFAs), 165
Polyunsaturated fatty acids (PUFA), 2, 30–31, 51, 136, 159–160, 200, 353–354
Postprandial dyslipidemia, 196
Postprandial lipemia
  atherogenesis, 196–198
  atherogenic postprandial phenotype, 194–196
  cardiovascular disease (CVD), 193, 204–205
  chylomicron (CM), 197f
  ethnic/genetic influences on, 204
  insulin, 196
  modulators of, 198–203
    dietary fats, 199
    interesterification (IE), 201–202
    polyunsaturated fatty acids, 200
    postprandial triglycerides (ppTG), 202–203
    saturation of fatty acids, 199–200
    triglycerides, fatty acid positioning in, 200–201
  monoacylglycerides (MAG), 193–194
  nonmodifiable factors, 204
  postprandial dyslipidemia, 196
  postprandial lipemia, ethnic/genetic influences on, 204
  postprandial triglycerides, novel mediator of, 203–204
  TG-rich lipoproteins (TRL), 194
  triglycerides (TG), 193
  very low-density lipoprotein (VLDL), 193–194, 197f
Postprandial lipids, 288
Postprandial triglycerides (ppTG), 202–203
  novel mediator of, 203–204
Post-traumatic stress disorder (PTSD), 62
Protein kinase C (PKC), 246–247
n-3 PUFA, 91–101, 114–121
  ameliorate cancer cachexia, 100–101
  ameliorate chemotherapy resistance, 99–100
  BRD4 inhibitor, 98–99
  epidemiological evidence, 91–92, 114–116
  Faecalibacterium, 119–120
  fish fat intake, 117–118t
  5-fluorouracil (5-FU), 97–98
  immunomodulatory effects, 93–95
  long non-coding RNA (lncRNA) regulation, 116–119
  mechanisms, 116–121
  mitochondrial apoptosis-mediated chemoprevention by fatty acids, 95–97
  paclitaxel, 99
  platinum chemotherapeutic drugs, 98
  psychiatry disorders, 65–66t
  radiotherapy and chemotherapy, sensitization to, 97–100
  sensitization to chemotherapy, 97–98
  sensitization to radiotherapy, 100
  sulindac analogues, 99
n-3 PUFA-derived anti-inflammatory lipid mediators, 157–159, 158f
n-6 PUFA-derived pro- and anti-inflammatory lipid mediators, 156–157, 158f
Pulmonary diseases
  asthma, 148–149
  chronic obstructive pulmonary disease (COPD), 147, 153–154
  dietary lipids, 155–156
  influences, 156–160
  fatty acid exposure, randomized control trials on, 150–152t
  idiopathic pulmonary fibrosis, 148
  immunity regulation, 159–160
  lung cancer, 155–156
  Maresin 1, 159
  pneumonia, 148–153
  polyunsaturated fatty acids, 159–160

n-3PUFA-derived anti-inflammatory lipid mediators, 157–159, 158f
n-6PUFA-derived pro- and anti-inflammatory lipid mediators, 156–157, 158f
pulmonary fibrosis, dietary lipids and, 154–155
toll-like receptor 2 (TLR2) activation, 159–160
Pulmonary fibrosis, dietary lipids and, 154–155

R
Randomized controlled trials (RCTs), 5, 18–19, 136–138
Reactive oxygen species (ROS), 37–38
Red blood cells (RBCs), 14–15
Renin-angiotensin aldosterone system (RAAS), 184
Respiratory diseases, 8
Russell-Silver syndrome, 243

S
Santalaceae family, 315–316t
Santalum album, 303
Saturated fat-enriched diets, 37
Saturated fatty acids (SFAs), 32, 165, 199–200
Schizophrenia (SCZ), 63
Selective hydrolysis, 286–287
Single nuclear polymorphisms (SNPs), 243
Sodium valproate (VPA), 245
Specialized lipid mediators (SPMs), 33
Sphingomyelin, 29
Stearoyl-CoA desaturase-1 (SCD-1), 293
Sterol regulatory element-binding protein (SREBP)-1c, 142–143
Sterols, 358
Sulindac analogues, 99
Supercritical fluid extraction (SFE), 318–319
Systolic BP (SBP), 165

T
Telomerase RNA component (TERC), 13
Telomeres
 C-reactive protein, 19–21
 cross-sectional and prospective studies, 14–17
 dietary fatty acid, 14
 human memory CD8 T cells, 19–21
 omega-3 fatty acids, 14
 peripheral blood mononuclear cells (PBMCs), 18–19
 randomized controlled trials (RCTs), 18–19
 red blood cells (RBCs), 14–15
TG-rich lipoproteins (TRL), 194
Thyroid hormones (THs), 39
Toll-like receptor 2 (TLR2) activation, 159–160
Total cholesterol (TC), 3, 211–212
Transintestinal cholesterol excretion (TICE), 345
Traumatic brain injury (TBI), 38
Triacylglycerol (TAG), 135
Triacylglycerol (TG), 2
Triacylglycerols (TAGs), 353, 359–361
Triglycerides, fatty acid positioning in, 200–201
Triximenynin extraction, 319
Type 2 diabetes (T2D), 126–128, 126f
 blood lipids, 128–129
 gestational diabetes, 131
 glycemic control, 130–131
 meta-analyses, 127t
 weight management, 129–130
Type 2 diabetes mellitus (T2DM), 136, 260–261

U
Ulcerative colitis (UC), 233–234
Unsaturated fatty acids, 32

V
Vascular reactivity, 181–183
Vascular smooth muscle cells (VSMC), 182
Vegetable oils, 331t
 animal fat, 361–362
Very-low-density lipoprotein (VLDL), 128–129, 135, 193–194, 197f

W
Weight management, 129–130
Women's Health Initiative Dietary Modification Trial, 112

X
Ximenynic acid
 anticancer activities, 306–307
 antifungal activity of, 309t
 anti-inflammatory activities, 306
 antimicrobial and larvicidal activities, 307–310, 308t
 applications, 304–311
 bioactivities, 304–311, 322f
 biosynthesis, 319–321
 chemical synthesis, 319, 320f
 chromatography, 317–318
 cosmetic industry, 310
 diabetes, 305–306
 distribution of, 314
 fatty acid metabolism, 304–305
 functions, 304–311
 future studies, 321–323
 high-performance liquid chromatography (HPLC), 304
 identification, 312–314
 low-temperature crystallization, 314–317
 natural distribution, 312–314
 NMR spectrum of, 313f
 Olacaceae and Opiliacea family, 317t
 other applications, 310–311
 physical characteristics, 312–314
 safety of, 311–312
 Santalaceae family, 315–316t
 Santalum album, 303
 structure, 312–314
 supercritical fluid extraction (SFE), 318–319
 synthesis of, 319–321
 triximenynin extraction, 319

Printed in the United States
by Baker & Taylor Publisher Services